Normal values

Exact ranges vary between

Haematology see p604			
Hb – Men	13–18g/		
Hb – Women	11.5–16		
MCV	76–96fl	• LØ	1.3–3.5 x 10^9/l (20–45%)
Plts	150–400 x 10^9/l	• EØ	0.04–0.44 x 10^9/l (1–6%)
Ferritin	12–200μg/l	B_{12}	0.13–0.68nmol/l
TIBC	42–80μmol/l	Folate	2–20μg/l

Clotting see p605			
INR	0.8–1.2	D-dimer	<0.3mg/l or <300ng/l
APTTr	0.8–1.2	Fibrinogen	1.5–4.0g/l

U+Es see p606			
Na^+	135–145mmol/l	Ca^{2+}	2.12–2.65mmol/l
K^+	3.5–5mmol/l	PO_4^{3-}	0.8–1.5mmol/l
Urea	2.5–6.7mmol/l	Mg^{2+}	0.75–1.05mmol/l
Creatinine	70–150μmol/l	HCO_3^-	22–30mmol/l
Osmolality	275–295mOsmol/kg	Cl^-	95–105mmol/l

LFTs see p607			
ALP	40–120u/l	Bilirubin	3–17μmol/l
ALT	3–35u/l	Albumin	35–50g/l
γGT	10–55u/l	Total protein	60–80g/l

Other			
Amylase	0–120u/dl	CRP	<10mg/l
Fasting glucose	3.5–5.5mmol/l	ESR	<20mm/h
Immunoglobulins	24–37g/l	CK	25–195u/l
Cholesterol	<6mmol/l	LDH	70–250u/l
Triglycerides	0.5–1.9mmol/l	PSA	0–4ng/ml (p425)

Blood gases see p622			
pH	7.35–7.45	PaO_2	10.6–13.3kPa
Base excess	±2mmol/l	$PaCO_2$	4.7–6.0kPa

OXFORD MEDICAL PUBLICATIONS

Oxford Handbook for the Foundation Programme

Published and forthcoming Oxford Handbooks

Oxford Handbook of Clinical Medicine 7/e (also available for PDAs)
Oxford Handbook of Clinical Specialties 7/e
Oxford Handbook of Acute Medicine 2/e
Oxford Handbook of Anaesthesia 2/e
Oxford Handbook of Applied Dental Sciences
Oxford Handbook of Cardiology
Oxford Handbook of Clinical Dentistry 4/e
Oxford Handbook of Clinical and Laboratory Investigation 2/e
Oxford Handbook of Clinical Diagnosis
Oxford Handbook of Clinical Haematology 2/e
Oxford Handbook of Clinical Immunology and Allergy 2/e
Oxford Handbook of Clinical Pharmacy
Oxford Handbook of Clinical Surgery 3/e
Oxford Handbook of Critical Care 2/e
Oxford Handbook of Dental Patient Care 2/e
Oxford Handbook of Dialysis 2/e
Oxford Handbook of Emergency Medicine 3/e
Oxford Handbook of Endocrinology and Diabetes
Oxford Handbook of ENT and Head and Neck Surgery
Oxford Handbook for the Foundation Programme 2/e
Oxford Handbook of Gastroenterology and Hepatology
Oxford Handbook of General Practice 2/e
Oxford Handbook of Genitourinary Medicine, HIV and AIDS
Oxford Handbook of Geriatric Medicine
Oxford Handbook of Medical Sciences
Oxford Handbook of Nephrology and Hypertension
Oxford Handbook of Nutrition and Dietetics
Oxford Handbook of Neurology
Oxford Handbook of Occupational Health
Oxford Handbook of Obstetrics and Gynaecology
Oxford Handbook of Oncology 2/e
Oxford Handbook of Ophthalmology
Oxford Handbook of Palliative Care
Oxford Handbook of Practical Drug Therapy
Oxford Handbook of Pre-Hospital Care
Oxford Handbook of Psychiatry
Oxford Handbook of Public Health Practice 2/e
Oxford Handbook of Rehabilitation Medicine
Oxford Handbook of Respiratory Medicine
Oxford Handbook of Rheumatology 2/e
Oxford Handbook of Sport and Exercise Medicine
Oxford Handbook of Tropical Medicine 2/e
Oxford Handbook of Urology

Aimée Bartram

Oxford Handbook for the Foundation Programme

Nathalie Hurley

James Dawson

Stephan Sanders

Simon Eccles

OXFORD
UNIVERSITY PRESS

OXFORD
UNIVERSITY PRESS

Great Clarendon Street, Oxford OX2 6DP

Oxford University Press is a department of the University of Oxford.
It furthers the University's objective of excellence in research, scholarship,
and education by publishing worldwide in

Oxford New York

Auckland Cape Town Dar es Salaam Hong Kong Karachi
Kuala Lumpur Madrid Melbourne Mexico City Nairobi
New Delhi Shanghai Taipei Toronto

With offices in

Argentina Austria Brazil Chile Czech Republic France Greece
Guatemala Hungary Italy Japan Poland Portugal Singapore
South Korea Switzerland Thailand Turkey Ukraine Vietnam

Oxford is a registered trade mark of Oxford University Press
in the UK and in certain other countries

Published in the United States
by Oxford University Press Inc., New York

First edition published 2005
Second edition published 2008

British Library Cataloguing in Publication Data
Data available

Library of Congress Cataloguing in Publication Data
Data available

Typeset by Cepha Imaging Private Ltd., Bangalore, India
Printed by L.E.G.O. S.p.A.

ISBN 978–0–19–954773–9

10 9 8 7 6 5 4 3 2 1

Contents

To every doctor who's ever stood there thinking:
'What on earth do I do now?'

Preface

It has been a great pleasure to watch this book become part of daily hospital life over the last three years. Our aim in writing it has always been to help newly qualified doctors and the patients that they treat. It is wonderful to see this in practice and has inspired us to make this edition even better.

Radical changes to junior doctors' training are being implemented and we have revised our guidance on career progression to address this; this new edition has been thoroughly updated with the latest Modernising Medical Careers (MMC) changes, including Specialty Training applications, membership exams and career paths.

Clinical sections of the book have also been thoroughly updated to reflect the most recent practices and to mesh with the expert advice offered in the other Oxford Handbooks. We have also heavily revised the speciality chapters to help foundation doctors gain the most out of their speciality attachments and to allow them to make referrals to other specialities with confidence.

We hope this book encourages those in the Foundation Programme to become more competent and caring doctors.

We are very receptive to suggestions and keen to make this book as useful as possible. Should you have an idea, or spot a mistake, please email us:

ohfp.uk@oup.com

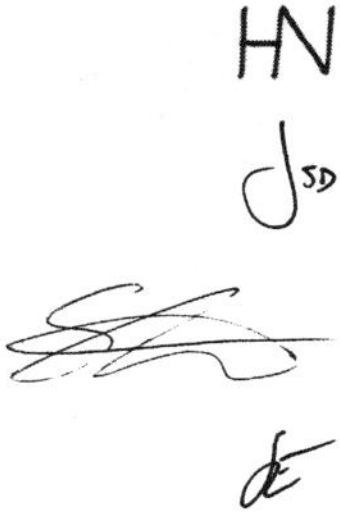

Preface

Acknowledgements

The authors would like to say a huge 'thank you' to the following people for their wisdom, knowledge and support:

- Dr Shreelata Datta for her contribution to the first edition
- Dr Dave Connor, Dr Katie Fletcher, Dr Charlotte Gray, Dr Emmet Griffiths, Dr Ross Hendry, Dr Olly Kemp, Dr Neil Richardson, Dr Naomi Statin and Dr Rebecca Tibbet for field testing the first edition and the many insightful comments that followed
- Mr Naseer Ahmad for his advice on the general surgery chapter
- Dr Mark Benton for his insight into life as a junior doctor and many pearls of wisdom
- Prof Raanan Gillon and Dr Georgia Testa for their advice on medical ethics and Gillick competence
- Dr David Gray for his advice on cardiology
- Dr Imogen Hart for her continued support and being persistently wonderful
- Bev Hurley for major moral support throughout
- Dr Antonia Lile for her advice on the GP chapter in trying conditions
- Paul Wade for his advice on issues relating to Jehovah's Witnesses
- Dr Louise Webster for her advice on the sections on obstetrics and gynaecology
- Dr Phil Webster for his advice on the general medicine sections
- Dr Robert Weinkove for his input into the haematology section
- Dr Joanne Malkin and Dr Vivienne Weston for their advice on microbiology and antibiotics
- Dr Sarah Woodgate for helping to write the psychiatry sections
- Everyone who helped with the first edition; our job was so much easier for all your hard work and we've not forgotten you

We would also like to thank all the staff at Oxford University Press for their help and for making our writing into a book. In particular:

- Anna Winstanley
- Liz Reeve
- Nic Ulyatt
- Kate Wilson
- David Gardner

Acknowledgements

The authors would like to [illegible] thanks to the following people for [illegible] and support:

- Dr [illegible] for [illegible] the [illegible]
- Dr [illegible] Dr [illegible] Gray, Dr [illegible]
- [illegible]
- [illegible]
- [illegible] comments [illegible]
- [illegible] advice on the [illegible]
- [illegible]
- [illegible] versions
- [illegible]
- [illegible] comments [illegible]
- Dr [illegible]
- Dr [illegible] support and [illegible]
- [illegible]
- [illegible] support [illegible]
- Dr [illegible]
- [illegible] issues [illegible]
- Dr [illegible] advice on the section on [illegible]
- [illegible]
- Dr [illegible] advice on the [illegible] sections
- Dr [illegible]
- [illegible]
- [illegible]
- [illegible]
- [illegible]
- [illegible]

We would also like to thank all the [illegible] University Press for their help [illegible] making [illegible] possible:

- [illegible]
- [illegible]
- [illegible]
- [illegible]
- [illegible]

Abbreviations and Symbols

A+E	Accident and emergency (now the emergency department)
AAA	Abdominal aortic aneurysm
ABG	Arterial blood gas
ABPI	Ankle brachial pressure index
ABx	Antibiotics
ACCS	Acute care common stem
ACD	Anaemia of chronic disease
ACEi	Angiotensin-converting enzyme inhibitor
ACF	Academic Clinical Fellowship
ACh	Acetylcholine
ACS	Acute coronary syndrome
ACTH	Adrenocorticotrophic hormone
ADH	Antidiuretic hormone
ADHD	Attention deficit hyperactivity disorder
ADL	Activities of daily living
AED	Automated external defibrillator
AF	Atrial fibrillation
AFB	Acid-fast bacilli
αFP	α-fetoprotein
AFP	α-fetoprotein
AICU	Adult intensive care unit
AIDS	Acquired immunodeficiency syndrome
ALL	Acute lymphoblastic leukaemia
ALP	Alkaline phosphatase
ALS	Advanced Life Support
ALT	Alanine aminotransferase
AMA	Antimitochondrial antibody
AML	Acute myeloid leukaemia
AMPLE	Allergies; Medications; Past medical history; Last meal; Events leading to presentation
AMTS	Abbreviated Mental Test Score
ANA	Antinuclear antibody
ANCA	Antineutrophil cytoplasmic antibody
AO	*Arbeitsgemeinschaft für osteosynthesefragen* (AO screws)
AP	Anteroposterior
APH	Antepartum haemorrhage

APLS	Advanced Paediatric Life Support
APTT	Activated partial thromboplastin time
APTTr	Activated partial thromboplastin time ratio
AR	Aortic regurgitation
ARDS	Acute respiratory distress syndrome
ARF	Acute renal failure
AROM	Artificial rupture of membranes
AS	Aortic stenosis
ASA	American Society of Anesthesiologists
ASAP	As soon as possible
ASD	Atrial septal defect
ASIF	Association for the Study of Internal Fixation
AST	Aspartate transaminase
ATLS	Advanced Trauma Life Support
ATN	Acute tubular necrosis
AV	Atrioventricular
AVPU	Alert, verbal, painful, unresponsive (neurological test)
AVR	Aortic valve replacement
AXR	Abdominal X-ray
B_{12}	Vitamin B_{12}
Ba	Barium
BCG	Bacille Calmette–Guérin (TB vaccination)
bd	*Bis die* (twice daily)
BE	Base excess/Barium enema
BFG	Big friendly giant
β-hCG	β-human chorionic gonadotrophin
BiC	Bicarbonate
BIH	Benign intracranial hypertension
BiPAP	Bilevel/biphasic positive airways pressure
BKA	Below knee amputation
BLS	Basic Life Support
BM	Boehringer–Mannheim meter (capillary blood glucose)/ Bone marrow
BMA	British Medical Association
BMI	Body mass index
BMJ	*British Medical Journal*
BNF	*British National Formulary*
BP	Blood pressure
BPH	Benign prostatic hypertrophy
BSA	Body surface area

BTS	British Thoracic Society
Bx	Biopsy
C+S	Circulation and sensation/culture and sensitivity
C-ANCA	Cytoplasmic ANCA
Ca^{2+}	Calcium
CA	Cancer antigen
ca	Carcinoma
CABG	Coronary artery bypass graft
CAH	Congenital adrenal hyperplasia
CAP	Community acquired pneumonia
CAPD	Continuous ambulatory peritoneal dialysis
CBD	Case-based discussion/Common bile duct
CBT	Cognitive–behavioural therapy
CCF	Congestive cardiac failure
CCST	Certificate of Completion of Specialist Training
CCT	Certificate of Completion of Training
CCU	Coronary care unit
CD	Controlled drugs/cluster of differentiation
CDC	Communicable Disease Control/Centre
CDH	Congenital dislocation of the hip
CDT	*Clostridium difficile* toxin
CEA	Carcinoembryonic antigen
CEPOD	Confidential Enquiry into Perioperative Deaths
CEX	Clinical Evaluation Exercise
CF	Cystic fibrosis
cf	Compare
CHD	Coronary heart disease
CI	Contraindication/Cardiac index
CJD	Creutzfeldt–Jakob disease
CK	Creatine kinase
CK-MB	Creatine kinase MB-isoenzyme (heart-specific)
Cl^-	Chloride
CLL	Chronic lymphocytic leukaemia
CLO	Campylobacter-like organism
cm	Centimetres
CML	Chronic myeloid leukaemia
CMV	Cytomegalovirus
CN	Cranial nerves
CNS	Central nervous system
CO	Carbon monoxide

CO_2	Carbon dioxide
COAD	Chronic obstructive airway disease
COC	Combined oral contraceptive
COCP	Combined oral contraceptive pill
COHb	Carboxyhaemoglobin
COPD	Chronic obstructive pulmonary disease
CPAP	Continuous positive airway pressure
CPK	Creatine phosphokinase
CPN	Community psychiatric nurse
CPP	Calcium pyrophosphate
CPR	Cardiopulmonary resuscitation
CRB	Criminal Record Bureau
CREST	Calcinosis, Raynaud phenomenon, [o]esophageal involvement, sclerodactyly and telangiectasia (syndrome)
CRF	Chronic renal failure
CRP	C-reactive protein
CRT	Capillary-refill time
CSF	Cerebrospinal fluid
CSOM	Chronic suppurative otitis media
CSU	Catheter specimen of urine
CT	Core-training/Computed tomography
CTG	Cardiotocograph
CTPA	CT pulmonary angiogram
CUS	Catheter urine sample
CV	Curriculum vitae
CVA	Cerebrovascular accident
CVP	Central venous pressure
CVS	Cardiovascular system/Chorionic villus sampling
CXR	Chest X-ray
d	Days
D+C	Dilatation and curettage
D+V	Diarrhoea and vomiting
DBP	Diastolic blood pressure
DEXA	Dual-energy X-Ray absorptiometry (DXA)
DH	Drug history
DHS	Dynamic hip screw
DI	Diabetes insipidus
DIB	Difficulty in breathing
DIC	Disseminated intravascular coagulation
DIGAMI	Diabetes Mellitus Insulin–Glucose infusion in Acute Myocardial Infarction Trial

DIPJ	Distal interphalangeal joint
DKA	Diabetic ketoacidosis
dl	Decilitre
DM	Diabetes mellitus
DMARD	Disease-modifying anti-rheumatic drug
DNA	Deoxyribonucleic acid/Did not attend
DNR	Do not resuscitate
DoB	Date of birth
DOH	Department of Health
DOPS	Direct Observation of Procedural Skills
DOTS	Directly observed therapy–short course
DRE	Digital rectal examination
dsDNA	Double-stranded DNA
DSH	Deliberate self-harm
DSM-IV	*The Diagnostic and Statistical Manual of Mental Disorders* 4th revision
DTP	Diphtheria, tetanus and pertussis
DU	Duodenal ulcer
DVLA	Driver and Vehicle Licensing Agency
DVT	Deep vein thrombosis
d/w	Discuss(ed) with
DWP	Department of Work and Pensions
Dx	Diagnosis
DXA	Dual-energy X-Ray absorptiometry (DEXA)
DXT	Deep radiotherapy
EBM	Evidence-based medicine
EBV	Epstein–Barr virus
ECG	Electrocardiogram
Echo	Echocardiogram
ECS	Endocervical swab
ECT	Electroconvulsive therapy
ECV	External cephalic version
ED	Emergency department (formerly A+E)
EDD	Expected due date (pregnancy)
EEA	European Economic Area
EEG	Electroencephalogram
EM	Emergency medicine (formerly A+E medicine)
EMD	Electromechanical dissociation (formerly pulseless electrical activity (PEA))
EMG	Electromyogram
ENA	Extractable nuclear antigen

ENP	Emergency nurse practitioner
ENT	Ear, nose and throat
EØ	Eosinophil
EPO	Erythropoietin
ERCP	Endoscopic retrograde cholangiopancreatography
ERPC	Evacuation of retained products of conception
ESM	Ejection systolic murmur
ESR	Erythrocyte sedimentation rate
ESRF	End-stage renal failure
ET	Endotracheal
ETOH	Ethanol (alcohol)
ETT	Endotracheal tube
EUA	Examination under anaesthetic
EVD	Extra-ventricular drain
EWTD	European Working Time Directive
F1	Foundation year one
F2	Foundation year two
FAST	Focused assessment with sonography in trauma
FB	Foreign body
FBC	Full blood count
FDP	Fibrin degradation product
Fe^{2+}	Iron
FEV_1	Forced expiratory volume in one second
FFP	Fresh frozen plasma
FH	Family history/Fetal heart
FiO_2	Fractional inspired oxygen concentration
fl	Femtolitre
FNA	Fine needle aspiration
FOB	Faecal occult blood
FOOSH	Fall on outstretched hand
FP	Foundation Programme
FRC	Functional residual capacity
FSH	Follicle-stimulating hormone
FTSTA	Fixed-term speciality training appointment
FTU	Fingertip unit
FVC	Forced vital capacity
g	Gram
G+S	Group and save
G6PD	Glucose-6-phosphate dehydrogenase
GA	General anaesthetic

GAD	Generalised anxiety disorder
GB	Gallbladder
GBS	Group B streptococcus/Guillain-Barré syndrome
GCS	Glasgow Coma Score
GFR	Glomerular filtration rate
γGT	γ-glutamyl transpeptidase
GGT	γ-glutamyl transpeptidase
GH	Growth hormone/Gynae history
GI	Gastrointestinal
GMC	General Medical Council
GN	Glomerulonephritis
GnRH	Gonadotrophin-releasing hormone
GORD	Gastro-oesophageal reflux disease
GP	General practitioner
GTN	Glyceryl trinitrate
GTT	Glucose tolerance test
GU(M)	Genitourinary (medicine)
h	Hour
HAART	Highly active antiretroviral therapy
HAI	Hospital-acquired infection
H@N	Hospital at night
HATI	Human anti-tetanus immunoglobulin
HAV	Hepatitis A virus
Hb	Haemoglobin
HbA_{1c}	Glycosylated haemoglobin
HBV	Hepatitis B virus
HCA	Healthcare assistant
HCC	Hepatocellular carcinoma
hCG	Human chorionic gonadotrophin
HCO_3^-	Bicarbonate
HCP	Healthcare professional
Hct	Haematocrit
HCV	Hepatitis C virus
HDL	High-density lipoprotein
HDU	High-dependency unit
HELLP	Haemolysis, elevated liver enzymes, low platelets (syndrome)
Hep B	Hepatitis B
HIT	Heparin-induced thrombocytopenia
HIV	Human immunodeficiency virus
HLA	Human leucocyte antigen

HMMA	4-hydroxy-3-methoxymandelic acid (phaeochromocytoma)
HOCM	Hypertrophic obstructive cardiomyopathy
HONK	Hyperosmolar non-ketosis
HPA	Health Protection Agency
HR	Heart rate
HRT	Hormone replacement therapy
HSP	Henoch–Schönlein purpura
HSV	Herpes simplex virus
HT	Hydroxytryptamine
HTN	Hypertension
HUS	Haemolytic–uraemic syndrome
HVS	High vaginal swab
I+D	Incision and drainage
IBD	Inflammatory bowel disease
IBS	Irritable bowel syndrome
ICD-10	*International Classification of Diseases* 10th revision
ICP	Intracranial pressure
ICU	Intensive care unit
ID	Identification
IDDM	Insulin-dependent diabetes mellitus
IE	Infective endocarditis
Ig	Immunoglobulin
IgA	Immunoglobulin A
IgD	Immunoglobulin D
IgE	Immunoglobulin E
IgG	Immunoglobulin G
IgM	Immunoglobulin M
IGT	Impaired glucose tolerance
IFG	Impaired fasting glucose
IHD	Ischaemic heart disease
ILS	Immediate Life Support
IM/im	Intramuscular
Imp	Impression
IN	Intranasal
INH/inh	By inhalation
INR	International normalised ratio
IPT	Interpersonal therapy
ITP	Idiopathic thrombocytopenic purpura
ITU	Intensive therapy unit
iu	International unit

IUCD	Intrauterine contraceptive device
IUP	Intrauterine pregnancy
IV/iv	Intravenous
IVDU	Intravenous drug user
IVI	Intravenous infusion
IVP	Intravenous pyelogram
IVU	Intravenous urogram
IX	Investigation(s)
JACCOL	Jaundice, anaemia, clubbing, cyanosis, oedema, lymphadenopathy
JDC	Junior Doctors' Committee
JFDI	Just … do it
JIA	Juvenile idiopathic arthritis
JVP	Jugular venous pressure
K^+	Potassium
KCl	Potassium chloride
kg	Kilogram
K-nail	Küntscher nail
kPa	Kilopascal
KUB	Kidneys, ureter, bladder (X-ray)
K-wire	Kirschner wire
l	Litre
LA	Local anaesthetic
LACS	Lacunar circulation stroke
LAD	Left axis deviation/Left anterior descending
LBBB	Left bundle branch block
LCX	Left circumflex artery
LDH	Lactate dehydrogenase
LDL	Low-density lipoprotein
LFT	Liver function test
LH	Luteinising hormone
LHRH	Luteinising hormone-releasing hormone
LIF	Left iliac fossa
LKM	Liver/kidney microsomal (antibody)
LMA	Laryngeal mask airway
LMN	Lower motor neurone
LMP	Last menstrual period
LMWH	Low molecular weight heparin
LN	Lymph node
LOC	Loss of consciousness
LØ	Lymphocyte

LP	Lumbar puncture
LSCS	Lower segment Caesarean section
LTOT	Long-term oxygen therapy
LUQ	Left upper quadrant
LVF	Left ventricular failure
LVH	Left ventricular hypertrophy
MAOI	Monoamine oxidase inhibitor
mane	In the morning
MAP	Mean arterial pressure
M,C+S	Microscopy, culture and sensitivity
MCPJ	Metacarpal phalangeal joint
MCQ	Multiple choice question
MCTD	Mixed connective tissue disease
MCV	Mean cell volume
MDDUS	Medical and Dental Defence Union of Scotland
MDR	Multi-drug resistant
MDU	Medical Defence Union
ME	Myalgic encephalitis
mEq	Milliequivalent
MEWS	Modified Early Warning Score
μg	Microgram
mg	Milligram
Mg^{2+}	Magnesium
MI	Myocardial infarction
min	Minutes
mm	Millimetre
MMA	Methylmalonic acid
MMC	Modernising Medical Careers
mmH_2O	Millimetres of water
mmHg	Millimetres of mercury
μmol	Micromole
mmol	Millimole
MMR	Measles, mumps and rubella
MMSE	Mini-Mental State Examination
MND	Motor neurone disease
mOsmol	MilliOsmole
MPS	Medical Protection Society
MR	Mitral regurgitation
MRCP	Magnetic resonance cholangiopancreatography
MRI	Magnetic resonance imaging

MRSA	Methicillin-resistant *Staph. aureus*
ms	Milliseconds
MS	Multiple sclerosis/Mitral stenosis
MSF	Multisource feedback
MST	Morphine sulphate
MSU	Mid-stream urine
mth	Months
MTPJ	Metatarsal phalangeal joint
MVR	Mitral valve replacement
N+V	Nausea and vomiting
N_2O	Nitrous oxide
NA	Nursing auxillary
Na^+	Sodium
NaCl	Sodium chloride
NAD	Nothing abnormal detected
NAI	Non-accidental injury
NAVY	Nerve, artery, vein, Y-fronts
NBM	Nil by mouth
NCEPOD	National Confidential Enquiry into Perioperative Deaths
NEB	By nebuliser
ng	Nanogram
NG/ng	Nasogastric
NGO	Non-governmental organisation
NGT	Nasogastric tube
NHS	National Health Service
NICE	National Institute of Health and Clinical Excellence
NICU	Neonatal intensive care unit
NIDDM	Non-insulin-dependent diabetes mellitus
NIV	Non-invasive ventilation
NMJ	Neuromuscular junction
nmol	Nanomole
NNH	Number needed to harm
NNT	Number needed to treat
NNTI	Non-nucleotide reverse transcriptase inhibitor
NNU	Neonatal unit
NØ	Neutrophil
nocte	At night
NPA	Nasopharyngeal aspirate
NSAID	Non-steroidal anti-inflammatory drug
NSTEMI	Non-ST elevation myocardial infarction

NTI	Nucleoside reverse-transcriptase inhibitor
NTN	National training number
NVD	Normal vaginal delivery
NYHA	New York Heart Association
O_2	Oxygen
OA	Osteoarthritis
Obs	Observations
OCD	Obsessive-compulsive disorder
OCP	Oral contraceptive pill/Ova, cysts and parasites
od	*Omni die* (once daily)
OD	Overdose
OGD	Oesophagogastroduodenoscopy
OH	Obstetric history
OHA	*Oxford Handbook of Anaesthesia*
OHEM	*Oxford Handbook of Emergency Medicine*
OHAM	*Oxford Handbook of Acute Medicine*
OHCC	*Oxford Handbook of Critical Care*
OHCLI	*Oxford Handbook of Clinical and Laboratory Investigation*
OHCM	*Oxford Handbook of Clinical Medicine*
OHCS	*Oxford Handbook of Clinical Specialties*
OHGP	*Oxford Handbook of General Practice*
OHOG	*Oxford Handbook of Obstetrics and Gynaecology*
OHP	Overhead projector
OHSC	Occupational Health Smart Card
om	*Omni mane* (in the morning)
on	*Omni nocte* (at night)
ORIF	Open reduction and internal fixation
OSCE	Objective structured clinical examination
OT	Occupational therapy
P	Pulse/Plan
P-ANCA	Perinuclear ANCA
PA	Posteroanterior
$PaCO_2$	Partial pressure of arterial carbon dioxide
PACS	Partial anterior circulation stroke/Picture archiving and communication systems
PAD	Peripheral arterial disease
PAN	Polyarteritis nodosa
PaO_2	Partial pressure of arterial oxygen
PAT	Peer Assessment Tool
PBC	Primary biliary cirrhosis

PCA	Patient-controlled analgesia
PCO_2	Partial pressure of carbon dioxide
PCOS	Polycystic ovary syndrome
PCP	Pneumocystis jiroveci pneumonia
PCR	Polymerase chain reaction
PCT	Primary care trust
PCV	Packed cell volume
PDA	Patent ductus arteriosus/Personal digital assistant
PE	Pulmonary embolism
PEA	Pulseless electrical activity
PEEP	Positive end-expiratory pressure
PEFR	Peak expiratory flow rate
PERLA	Pupils equal and reactive to light and accommodation
PET	Positron emission tomography
PI	Protease inhibitor
PICU	Paediatric intensive care unit
PID	Pelvic inflammatory disease
PIH	Pregnancy-induced hypertension
PIP	Peak inspiratory pressure
PIPJ	Proximal interphalangeal joint
Plts	Platelets
PMETB	Postgraduate Medical Education and Training Board
PMH	Past medical history
PMT	Pre-menstrual tension
PND	Paroxysmal nocturnal dyspnoea/postnatal depression
PNS	Peripheral nervous system
PO_4^{3-}	Phosphate
PO/po	*Per os* (by mouth)
pO_2	Partial pressure of oxygen
PoC	Products of conception
POCS	Posterior circulation stroke
PONV	Post-operative nausea and vomiting
POP	Plaster of Paris/Progesterone-only pill
PPH	Postpartum haemorrhage
PPI	Proton pump inhibitor
PR/pr	*Per rectum*
PRHO	Pre-registration house officer
PRN	*Pro re nata* (as required)
PROM	Premature rupture of membranes (pregnancy)
PRV	Polycythaemia rubra vera

PSA	Prostate-specific antigen
PSH	Past surgical history
PT	Prothrombin time
PTH	Parathyroid hormone
PU	Passed urine/Peptic ulcer
PUD	Peptic ulcer disease
PUO	Pyrexia of unknown origin
PUVA	Psoralen–ultraviolet A
PV/pv	Plasma viscosity/Per vagina
PVD	Peripheral vascular disease
qds	*Quater die sumendus* (four times daily)
RA	Rheumatoid arthritis
RAST	Radioallergosorbant test
RAT	Regional action team
RBBB	Right bundle branch block
RBC	Red blood cell
RCA	Right coronary artery
RDW	Red cell distribution width
RF	Rheumatic fever
Rh	Rhesus
RhF	Rheumatoid factor
RIF	Right iliac fossa
RNP	Ribonucleoprotein
ROM	Range of movement
ROS	Review of systems
RR	Respiratory rate
RS	Respiratory system
RSI	Rapid sequence intubation/induction
RTA	Road traffic accident
RUQ	Right upper quadrant
RV	Residual volume (lung)
RVH	Right ventricular hypertrophy
Rx	Prescription
s/sec	Seconds
SAH	Subarachnoid haemorrhage
SALT	Speech and language therapy
Sats	O_2 saturation
SBE	Sub-acute bacterial endocarditis
SBP	Systolic blood pressure/Spontaneous bacterial peritonitis
SC	Subcutaneous

SCBU	Special care baby unit
SCC	Squamous-cell carcinoma
SCD	Sickle-cell disease
SD	Standard deviation
SE	Side-effects
SH	Social history
SHBG	Sex hormone-binding globulin
SHDU	Surgical high-dependency unit
SHO	Senior house officer
SIADH	Syndrome of inappropriate antidiuretic hormone secretion
SIRS	Systemic inflammatory response syndrome
SL/Sl	Sublingual
SLE	Systemic lupus erythematosus
SOA	Swelling of ankles
SOB	Short of breath
SOBAR	Short of breath at rest
SOBOE	Short of breath on exertion
SOL	Space-occupying lesion
SpO_2	Oxygen saturation in peripheral blood
SpR	Specialist registrar (old training system)
SR	Slow release
ssDNA	Single-stranded DNA
SSP	Statutory sick pay
SSRI	Selective serotonin reuptake inhibitor
Stat	*Statim* (immediately)
ST	Specialist Training/Trainee
STD	Sexually transmitted disease
STEMI	ST elevation myocardial infarction
STI	Sexually transmitted infection
STOP	Surgical termination of pregnancy
StR	Speciality Training Registrar
SVC	Superior vena cava
SVR	Systemic vascular resistance
SVT	Supraventricular tachycardia
Sx	Symptoms
SXR	Skull X-ray
T_3	Tri-iodothyronine
T_4	Thyroxine
TAB	Team Assessment of Behaviour
TACS	Total anterior circulation stroke

TB	Tuberculosis
TBG	Thyroxine-binding globulin
TCA	Tricyclic antidepressant
tds	*Ter die sumendus* (three times daily)
TEDS	Thromboembolism deterrent stockings
Temp	Temperature
TENS	Transcutaneous electrical nerve stimulation
TFT	Thyroid function test
THPA	*Treponema pallidum* haemagglutination assay
THR	Total hip replacement
TIA	Transient ischaemic attack
TIBC	Total iron-binding capacity
TIMI	Thrombolysis in myocardial infarction
TIPS	Transjugular intrahepatic portosystemic shunting
TKR	Total knee replacement
TLC	Tender loving care/Total lung capacity
TMJ	Temporomandibular joint
TNF-α	Tumour necrosis factor-alpha
TNM	Tumour, nodes, metastases (cancer staging)
TOE	Transoesophageal echocardiogram
t-Pa	Tissue plasminogen activator
TPN	Total parenteral nutrition
TPR	Total peripheral resistance
TSH	Thyroid-stimulating hormone
$\dot{T}\dot{T}$	Two (two tablets, two puffs etc)
TTA	To take away
TTO	To take out
TTP	Thrombotic thrombocytopenic purpura
TURP	Transurethral resection of prostate
TWOC	Trial without catheter
Tx	Treatment
u/U	Units
U+E	Urea and electrolytes
UA	Unstable angina
UC	Ulcerative colitis
UMN	Upper motor neurone
UO	Urine output
URTI	Upper respiratory tract infection
US(S)	Ultrasound (scan)
USMLE	United States Medical Licensing Exam

UTI	Urinary tract infection
UV	Ultraviolet
V/Q	Ventilation/perfusion scan
VA	Visual acuity
VC	Vital capacity
vCJD	Variant CJD
VDRL	Venereal Disease Research Laboratory (test)
VE	Vaginal examination/Ventricular ectopic
VF	Ventricular fibrillation
VMA	Vanillylmandelic acid
VP shunt	Ventriculoperitoneal shunt
VSD	Ventriculoseptal defect
VT	Ventricular tachycardia
vWF	Von Willebrand's factor
VZV	Varicella zoster virus
WB	Weight-bear
WBC	White blood cell
WCC	White cell count
WHO	World Health Organisation
wk	Weeks
WPW	Wolff–Parkinson–White syndrome
wt	Weight
X-match	Crossmatch
yr	Years
ZIG	Zoster immnue immunoglobulin
ZN	Ziehl–Neelson

Introduction

Welcome to the 2nd edition of the *Oxford Handbook for the Foundation Programme* – the ultimate FP doctor's survival book. It is set out differently from other books; please take 2 minutes to read how it works:

Being a doctor The first six chapters cover the non-clinical side of being a junior doctor; each chapter starts with a contents list:

- ***The job*** (p1) essential kit, efficiency, being organised
- ***Your career*** (p13) the FP, portfolios, MMC, getting ST posts, audits
- ***Communication*** (p51) breaking bad news, translators, languages
- ***Ethics*** (p65) death, confidentiality, consent, religion
- ***When things go wrong*** (p73) errors, incident forms, hating your job
- ***Boring but important stuff*** (p81) NHS structure, money, benefits

Life on the ward (p89) This is the definitive guide to ward jobs; it includes: ward rounds, TTOs, being on-call, night shifts, death certificates, making referrals and writing in the notes.

Prescribing (p143) Covers how to prescribe, best practice, complex patients, interactions and specific groups of drugs eg steroids.

Clinical presentations (p159) These cover common clinical and ward cover problems. They are described by symptoms because you are called to see a breathless patient, not someone with a PE:

- *Emergencies* The inside front cover has a list of emergencies according to symptom (cardiac arrest, chest pain, seizures) with page references. These pages give step-by-step instructions to help you resuscitate and stabilise an acutely ill patient.
- ***Symptoms*** The clinical pages are described by symptom. Each symptom shows the causes, what to ask and look for, relevant investigations and a table showing the distinguishing features of each disease. Relevant diseases are described in the pages following each symptom.
- ***Diseases*** If you know the disease you can look it up in the index to find the symptoms, signs, results and correct management.

Specialities (p443) These will show you how to make the perfect referral, including history, examination and the common questions you will be asked over the phone; common FP placements also have a guide to life as an F1/F2 in that specialty.

Procedures (p551) Each chapter gives instructions on how to perform a specific procedure, the equipment needed and contraindications.

Interpreting results (p603) These pages give a guide to understanding investigations including common patterns, the important features to note and possible causes of abnormalities.

At the back (p635) In front of the index are several pages of useful information including contact numbers, growth charts, unit conversion charts, driving regulations, blank timetables and telephone number lists.

10 tips on being a safe junior doctor

These tips are taken from the National Confidential Enquiry into Patient Outcome and Death (NCEPOD) report *An Acute Problem?*[1] NCEPOD is an independent body which aims to improve the quality and safety of patient care. The report summarises a survey over one month of admissions to UK Intensive Care Units.

(1) More attention should be paid to patients exhibiting **physiological abnormalities.** This is a marker of increased mortality risk (p161).
(2) The importance of **respiratory rate** monitoring should be highlighted. This parameter should be recorded at any point that other observations are being made (p161).
(3) Education and training should be provided for staff that use **pulse oximeters** to allow proper interpretation and understanding of the limitations of this monitor. It should be emphasised that pulse oximetry does not replace respiratory rate monitoring (p161).
(4) It is inappropriate for referral and acceptance to **ICU** to happen at junior doctor (<ST3) level (p452).
(5) Training must be provided for junior doctors in the **recognition of critical illness** and the immediate management of fluid and oxygen therapy in these patients (p162).
(6) Consultants must **supervise** junior doctors more closely and should actively support juniors in the management of patients rather than only reacting to requests for help.
(7) Junior doctors must **seek advice** more readily. This may be from specialised teams eg outreach services or from the supervising consultant.
(8) Each hospital should have a track and trigger system that allows **rapid detection** of the signs of early clinical deterioration and an early and appropriate response (p161).
(9) All entries in the **notes** should be dated and timed and should end with a legible name, status and contact number (bleep or telephone) (p102).
(10) Each entry in the notes should clearly identify the name and grade of the most **senior doctor** involved in the patient episode (p102).

The full report is available on the internet[1] and is well worth reading; there are many learning points for doctors of all grades and specialities.

1 *An Acute Problem?* NCEPOD, 11th May 2005, www.ncepod.org.uk/2005.htm

10 tips on being a happy junior doctor

(1) Book your annual leave Time off is essential. Spend it doing something you really enjoy with people you really like. It can be very difficult to book time off and it is your responsibility to swap on-calls. You usually need to book your leave 6wk in advance and summer is always popular.

(2) Be organised This is important but difficult when you first start as a doctor. Come in early, carry a folder with useful names and numbers, and pick up hints and tips from your predecessor.

(3) Smile You cannot cure most diseases, you cannot make procedures pleasant, you cannot help the fact that you, the ward staff and the patients are in the hospital, but smiling and being friendly can make all the difference.

(4) Never shout at anyone Shouting or being insulting is unprofessional. If you have a problem it should be addressed in private. The job rapidly becomes unpleasant if you get a reputation for being rude and reputations (good and bad) travel quickly.

(5) Phone for senior help Never feel you cannot ask for help, even for something you feel you 'should' know. It is always better to phone someone senior rather than guess, even if it is in the middle of the night.

(6) Check in the *BNF* If you are not familiar with a drug then always check in the *BNF* before you give it. Trust nobody, it will be your name next to the prescription.

(7) Look at the obs Acutely ill patients nearly always have abnormal observations. Always remember to look at the respiratory rate as this is the observation most commonly ignored by junior doctors.

(8) Stay calm It is easy to panic the first time you are called to an acutely ill patient, but staying calm is important to help you think clearly about how to manage the situation. Take a deep breath, work through the 'ABC', perform initial investigations and call someone senior.

(9) Be reliable If you say you are going to do something then do it. If you are unable to do so then let someone know. Nursing staff, in particular, also have many things to remember and constantly reminding doctors of outstanding jobs is frustrating.

(10) Prepare for the future Medicine is competitive, you need to give yourself the best chance. Over the first two years you should:
- plan your career
- create a CV and portfolio
- get good referees and mentors
- undertake an audit
- present interesting cases
- organise speciality taster sessions

The politics of medical careers

Modernising Medical Careers (MMC)

On 1st August 2005, the first stage of the MMC reforms of UK postgraduate training came into effect with the Foundation Programme (FP) replacing the previous PRHO and first year SHO posts. The FP was designed to improve the basic training doctors receive in their first two years, by ensuring the course is more strictly coordinated and supervised with clearer guidance on what is expected of doctors on the programme.

The second stage of reforms was introduced for the 2007 applications with the switch from SHO/SpR jobs to speciality training (ST). The jobs were applied for via MTAS (see box below). The switch over did not go smoothly and the process was changed for 2008 with the introduction of uncoupled training (p26) and Deaneries organised their own recruitment process for most specialties.

> MTAS (Medical Training Application Scheme) this was an on-line system used in 2006/2007 for medical students and junior doctors to apply for FP or ST jobs. A considerable number of problems were encountered, including poorly designed questions, difficulty selecting appropriate trainees, security breaches, website problems and jobs being listed incorrectly. It has now been abandoned.

Tooke Report (www.mmcinquiry.org.uk)

MTAS and the confusion surrounding the new training scheme sparked such an outcry from junior doctors and the medical profession that an independent inquiry was led by Prof Sir John Tooke to investigate what exactly went wrong, why this occurred and how to solve it.

From a junior doctor's perspective the key relevant findings included:
- The process for selection into Specialty Training was rushed in implementation and undervalued clinical experience
- The implementation of Foundation training has been generally successful, but some placements offered to F2s do not provide experience relevant to their desired career

The following recommendations affect junior doctors directly:
- The Foundation Programme should be split in two, with F1 aligned to medical school and F2 as the start of a 3yr core-training programme (similar to the previous system of PRHO and SHO posts)
- There needs to be clearer guidance on the role of doctors at each stage of training and emphasise they are doctors, not just 'trainees'
- The DoH should formally consult with the medical profession and NHS on all significant changes in government policy that affect postgraduate medical education and training
- PMETB and the GMC should merge to become one overall body

It remains to be seen whether all these changes will take place.

> *PMETB* The Postgraduate Medical Education and Training Board was launched in 2005 as an independent regulatory body responsible for junior doctor training. PMETB, working with the royal colleges, amongst others, set the criteria and standards for training.

Chapter 1

Starting as an F1

Before you start

Important organisations

The prices quoted change frequently; they are intended as a guide.

General Medical Council (GMC) To work as a doctor in the UK you need GMC registration; £100 for pre-registration year (F1), £390 each year as F2 or above (full registration).

NHS indemnity insurance This only covers the financial consequences of any mistake you make at work. It automatically covers all doctors in the NHS free of charge; you do not need to subscribe.

Indemnity insurance This is essential; do not work without it. These organisations will support and advise you in any complaints or legal matters that arise from your work. They also insure you against work outside the hospital. There are three main organisations, all offer 24h helplines (p636):

- Medical Protection Society (MPS) – £10 for F1, £40–60 for F2
- Medical Defence Union (MDU) – £14 for F1, £42–60 for F2
- Medical Doctors and Dentist Defence Union of Scotland (MDDUS) – £10 for F1, £40–55 for F2

British Medical Association (BMA) Political voice of doctors; campaigns for better conditions, hours, pay and comments on health issues. Membership includes a weekly subscription to the *BMJ*. Costs £99 as an F1 then £195 as an F2.

Income protection Pays half your basic salary until retirement age if you become too ill to work as a doctor. NHS sickness benefits are poor (only 1mth as an F1 and 4mth the next year):

- Medical Sickness £18/mth as an F1, rises afterwards according to age, pay, illness and risks; many others are available

NHS pension scheme This is the best pension available, do not opt out; a percentage of your pay will be diverted to the pension.

Important documents for your first day

P45/P60 tax form When you leave a job you will receive a P45; if you continue in the same job you will receive a P60 every April. These need to be shown when starting your new job.

Bank details Account number, sort code and address.

Hepatitis B You need proof of hep B immunity and vaccinations. You should be issued with an Occupational Health Smartcard.

GMC registration certificate Proves you are a registered doctor.

Criminal Record Bureau (CRB) certificate Required for most specialities but definitely for paediatrics, obs and gynae and emergency medicine; contact your personnel department to check and give you a form.

Induction pack and contract Sent by the trust before you start; otherwise contact human resources to find out where and when to meet.

Your first day

Leave plenty of time to find the hospital and your room on your first day. Many hospitals organise a session for new doctors to speed up the signing-in process. The following are the essentials:

House If you are living on site this is your top priority. Phone the accommodation office before you start to check their opening hours. It may cost up to £400/month. Avoid leaving your car filled with all your possessions.

Pay roll It can take over a month to adjust pay arrangements so it is vital to give the finance dept your bank details on the first day if you want to be paid that month. Hand in your P45/P60 too.

Parking Check with other staff about the best places to park and 'parking deals'; you will probably need to get several people to sign a form.

ID badge This may also be used to access secure sections of the hospital. If so, insist on getting access to all clinical areas since you will be on the crash team. If the card doesn't give access to all wards return it and get it fixed.

Computer access This allows you to get results, access the internet and your NHS email. Write down all the passwords, usernames etc and keep any documents handed out. Ask for the IT helpdesk phone number in case of difficulty.

Work rota Ideally this should have arrived before the job starts.

Colleagues' mobile numbers This will probably be the last time you are all gathered in one place. Getting numbers makes social activities and rota swaps much easier. Arranging swaps on the first day is also easier.

Important places in the hospital

Try to get hold of a map; many hospitals have evolved rather than been designed. There are often short cuts.

Ward(s) Write down any access codes and find out where you can put your bag. Ask to be shown where things are kept including the crash trolley and blood-taking equipment.

Canteen(s) Establish where the best food options are at various times of day. Note the opening hours – this will be invaluable for breaks on-call.

Cash and food dispensers Hospitals are required to provide hot food 24h a day. This may be from a machine.

Doctors' mess Clearly essential. Write down the access code and establish if there is a freezer. Microwave meals are infinitely preferable to the food from machines.

Radiology Find out which consultants deal with different imaging. You will spend a lot of time chasing investigations so make friends early, including with their secretaries!

Occupational health

Most hospitals have an occupational health department that is responsible for ensuring that the hospital is a safe environment for you and your patients. This includes making sure that doctors work in a safe manner. You can find your local unit at www.nhsplus.nhs.uk.

Common visits

During the Foundation Programme your contact with occupational health is likely to be one of the following:

- ***Initial check*** you will be issued with a smartcard and have a blood test to show you do not have hepatitis C; they will need to see photographic proof of identity eg a passport
- ***Hepatitis B booster*** every 5yr; often your first year as a doctor
- ***Needle-stick/sharps injury/splashes*** see p127
- ***Illness*** that affects your ability to work may require a consultation

Smartcards

When you start work in the NHS you will be issued with an Occupational Health Smart Card (OHSC). This will keep a record of your occupational health details throughout your career. If you need to apply for a card visit www.ohsc-uk.com. If you lose your card you need to contact your postgraduate deanery smartcard office.

Infection control

Patients are commonly infected by pathogens from the hospital and ward staff. The infections are more likely to be resistant to antibiotics and can be fatal. It is important to reduce the risk you pose to your patients:

- If you are ill stay at home, especially if you have gastroenteritis
- Keep your clothes clean including ties and roll up long sleeves
- White coats and sometimes ties and long sleeves are discouraged
- Avoid jewellery (plain metal rings are acceptable) and wrist watches
- Clean your stethoscope with an alcohol swab after each use
- Wash your hands or use alcohol gel after every patient contact, even when wearing gloves; rinsing all the soap off reduces irritation
- Be rigorous in your use of aseptic technique
- Stop unnecessary antibiotics after a full course

Sharps and bodily fluids

As a doctor you will come into contact with bodily fluids daily. It is important to develop good habits so that you are safe on the wards:

- Wear gloves for all procedures that could involve bodily fluids or sharps. Gloves reduce disease transmission when penetrated with a needle – consider wearing two pairs for high-risk patients.
- Dispose of all sharps immediately; take the sharps bin to where you are using the sharps and **always dispose of your own sharps**
- Vacutainers are safer than a needle and syringe
- Mark high-risk bodily fluid samples (eg HIV, hepatitis B+C)
- Consider wearing goggles if bodily fluids might spray
- Cover cuts in your skin
- Avoid wearing open-toed shoes or sandals
- Make sure your hepatitis B boosters are up-to-date

What to carry

Essentials

Pens These are the most essential piece of equipment. Remember you need a biro for writing on blood bottles; all writing must be in black (allows photocopying).

Stethoscope A Littmann® Classic II or equivalent is perfectly adequate, however better models offer clearer sound.

Tourniquet Consider talking to a friendly drug rep, otherwise £4–7. A tied glove can be used if your tourniquet is missing.

Money Out-of-hours, loose change is useful for food dispensers.

ID badge This should be supplied on your first day.

Bleep This will be on the ward, at switchboard or with a colleague.

Optional extras

Clipboard folder see p10

Smartphone/PDA see p6

Pen-torch Useful for looking in mouths and eyes; very small LED torches are available in 'outdoors' shops or over the internet and can fit onto a keyring or attached to stethoscopes to prevent colleagues borrowing and not returning them (although only use these in eyes to certify death as they are too bright for pupillary reactions).

Tendon hammer These are mythical objects, rarely found on wards. Collapsible pocket-sized versions can be bought for £12–15 – try www.medisave.co.uk and search for 'hammer'.

Ward dress

Patients and staff have more respect for well-dressed doctors, however it is important to be yourself; be guided by comments from patients or staff.

Hair Long hair should be tied back.

Piercings Facial metal can be easily removed while at work; while ears are OK, lips and eyebrows ± noses draw comments.

Shoes A pair of smart comfy shoes is essential – you will be on your feet for hours and may need to move fast.

Scrubs Ideal for on-calls, especially in surgery. Generally they should not be worn for everyday work. Check local protocol.

Mobiles Many doctors carry mobile phones in hospital though their use is often banned. If you do carry one keep it on a silent setting and be subtle. Be aware that:

- They may affect some hospital equipment if within 50cm
- You should always turn it off before entering ITU/HDU
- In theory you could be disciplined for breaking trust policy

Smartphones/PDAS

Smartphones are combinations of mobile phones and mini-computers. They can hold entire medical textbooks, medical calculators, word-processing and spreadsheet documents, contact numbers and most other computer files including pictures, videos, games and music. A personal digital assistant (PDA) is essentially a smartphone without the phone.

Basics Smartphones are usually about 11cm by 6cm (smaller than two credit cards) and 1.5–2cm thick. Data can be entered by mini-keyboards, touch-sensitive keyboards or handwriting recognition on a touch-sensitive screen. They can link to a conventional computer to download special programs from the internet or back-up their data.

Different types There are many different types of smartphone and PDA available. Think carefully about which programs you want it to run and look on the internet for reviews. It is also important to see it in a shop to get an idea of its size and usability. Some considerations:

- *Operating system* this is the most important decision as it will affect what programs your phone can use:
  - *Windows Mobile* is the most popular and has many free medical programs available on the internet; can be awkward to use
  - *Palm* used to be the most popular and still has lots of medical software
  - *Symbian* some medical software, a few have touch screens
  - *Blackberry* easy to use, some medical software, no touch screen
  - *iPhone* currently very little medical software, but likely to develop rapidly
- *Battery life* varies widely between devices, check the details of each device and also reviews
- *Memory* make sure there is a memory card slot
- *Software* check what programs each smartphone comes with; most are able to display text or spreadsheet documents without buying any extra software; there are some deals with medical software

Where to buy The internet is the cheapest source; it also provides information and reviews about specific models.

Accessories You may need to buy several extra 'add-ons' before the smartphone is ready to cope with ward life:

- ***Cases*** to prevents broken screens (£15–30)
- ***Screen protectors*** thin plastic sheets to prevent scratches (<£5)
- ***Memory cards*** vital for many programs and textbooks (£15–20)
- ***Software*** see the next page

Phones in hospitals There has been much discussion about using mobile phones near medical equipment. A minority of devices can be affected by a mobile phone <50cm but not at greater distances. It is important to check local hospital policy and follow this otherwise you risk disciplinary action. You should always turn them off before going into ITU or HDU.

Smartphone software

Software is available over the internet from the sites shown in the table below (amongst others); there are literally thousands of programs covering almost every conceivable need. Most programs offer a free trial and some offer the full version free. It is not possible to copy versions you have paid for to share with friends. The following are good, free medical programs:

- *Diagnosaurus* differential diagnosis – www.diagnosaurus.com
- *Medcalc* medical calculator – www.med-ia.ch/medcalc
- *Eponyms* eponymous diseases – www.eponyms.net
- *ePocrates Rx* American version of *BNF* – www.ePocrates.com

Software	Medical software
www.pdatopsoft.com	www.skyscape.com
www.handango.com	www.medspda.com
www.pocketpcsoft.net	www.pdamd.com
www.palmgear.com	www.doctorsgadgets.com
www.mobilefan.net	www.collectivemed.com

Smartphone medical textbooks

There are a wide range of textbooks available for smartphones; the vast majority are not free. It is worth using a free trial if available since the usability of the textbooks varies greatly. You will need a memory card to hold most textbooks, but these are often large enough to store several.

Oxford Handbooks

Several handbooks are available from Skyscape (website above) for about £20 each. They offer the option of searching by index, contents or for specific words. The textbooks link together so if you buy more than one you can quickly jump to the relevant page in another book.

5 Minute Clinical Consult (5MCC)

This is also available from Skyscape; it is a very user-friendly textbook that is easy to navigate on a smartphone. It is written for the US market but is still useful in the UK. Costs about £35.

BNF on PDA

The *BNF* costs about £45 and can work with Windows Mobile, Palm, Blackberry and iPhone operating systems. It is available from Skyscape.

Patient records

There are several programs available for recording your patient's location, diagnoses and investigations (eg Patient Tracker, PatientKeeper). Most hospitals discourage their use (Data Protection Act, confidentiality and security concerns) and in practice it is not efficient since you have to duplicate the patient's details. Bear in mind that only the patient's hospital notes are a legal record of care so these must be kept up-to-date.

How to be an F1

Being an F1 involves teamwork, organisation and communication – qualities that are not easily assessed during finals. As well as settling into a new work environment, you have to integrate with your colleagues and the rest of the hospital team. You are not expected to know everything at the start of your post; you should always ask someone more senior if you are in doubt.

As an F1, your role includes:

- Clerking patients (ED, pre-op clinic, on-call or on the ward)
- Updating patient lists and knowing where patients are (p10)
- Participating in ward rounds to review patient management
- Requesting investigations and chasing their results
- Liaising with other specialities/health-care professionals
- Practical procedures eg taking blood (p554), cannulation (p558)
- Administrative tasks eg theatre lists (p132), TTOs (p106), rewriting drug charts (p145), death certificates (p112)
- Speaking to the patient and relatives about progress/results

Breaks

Missing breaks does not make you appear hard-working – it reduces your efficiency and alertness. Give yourself time to rest and eat (chocolates from the ward do not count); you are entitled to 30min for every 4h worked. Use the time to meet other doctors in the mess; referring is much easier if you know them.

Know your limits

If you are unsure of something, don't feel embarrassed to ask your seniors – particularly if a patient is deteriorating. If you are stuck on simple tasks (eg difficult cannulation) take a break (the patient will welcome this) and try later or ask a colleague to try.

Responsibility

As an F1 you will make many difficult decisions, some with potentially serious consequences. Always consider the worst case scenario and how to avoid it. Ensure you can justify your actions; carefully document events and discussions with relatives.

Expectations

Seniors will expect you to know Mrs Jones' current medication dose, the details of the operation they performed yesterday and the blood results from 5d ago. Initially this seems impossible, but with time your memory for such details will improve.

Your bleep

This quickly becomes the bane of your existence. When the bleep goes off repeatedly, write down the numbers then answer them in turn. Try to deal with queries over the phone; if not make a list of jobs and prioritise them, tell the nurses how long you will be and be realistic. Ask nurses to get an ECG (if appropriate), the obs chart and notes ready for when you arrive. Encourage ward staff to make a list of routine jobs instead of bleeping you repeatedly. The bleep should only be for sick patients and urgent tasks. Learn the number of switchboard since this is likely to be an outside caller waiting on the line. Crash calls are usually announced to all bleepholders via switchboard. If your bleep is unusually quiet, check the batteries. Consider handing over your bleep to a colleague when breaking bad news or speaking to relatives.

- ***Dropping the bleep in the toilet*** This is not uncommon; recover the bleep using non-sterile gloves. Wash thoroughly in running water (the damage has already been done) and inform switchboard that you dropped it into your drink.
- ***Other forms of bleep destruction*** You will usually not have to pay for a damaged bleep; consider asking for a clip-on safety strap.

Learning

You need to be proactive to learn interpretation and management skills as an F1. Formulate a management plan for each patient you see and compare this with your senior's version; ask about the reasons for any significant differences.

Getting organised

Your organisational abilities may be valued above your clinical acumen. While this is not why you chose to become a doctor, being organised will make you more efficient and ensure you get home as early as possible.

Folders and clipboards These are an excellent way to hold patient lists, job lists and spare paperwork along with a portable writing surface. Imaginative improvements can be constructed with bulldog clips, plastic wallets and dividers.

- ***Contents:*** spare paper, drug charts, TTOs, blood forms, radiology forms, phone/bleep numbers, job lists, patient lists, theatre lists, spare pen, computer and ward access codes

Patient lists Juniors are often entrusted with keeping a record of the team's patients (including those on different wards, called 'outliers') along with their background details, investigation results and management plans. With practice most people become good at recalling this information, but writing it down reduces errors.

One means of keeping track is updating a ward-based computer spreadsheet; this also allows every member of the team to carry a copy. It can be invaluable for discussing/referring a patient whilst away from the ward. See p95. **These must be kept confidential and disposed of securely.**

Job lists During the ward round make a note of all the jobs that need doing on a separate piece of paper. At the end of the round these jobs can be allocated amongst the team members.

Serial results Instead of simply writing blood results in the notes try writing them on serial results sheets (with a column for each day's results). This makes patterns easier to spot and saves time.

Timetables Along with ward rounds and clinical jobs there will be numerous extra meetings, teaching sessions and clinics to attend. There are three blank timetables at the end of this book.

Important numbers It can take ages to get through to switchboard so carrying a list of common numbers will save you hours (eventually you will remember them). At the end of this book there are three blank phone number lists for you to fill in. Stickers on the back of ID badges can hold up to 15 numbers.

Ward cover equipment Finding equipment on unfamiliar wards wastes time and is frustrating. You can speed up your visits by keeping a supply of equipment in a box. Try to fill them with equipment from storerooms instead of clinical areas. Alternatively if you are bleeped by a nurse to put in a cannula, you could try asking them nicely to prepare the equipment ready for you for when you arrive (it works occasionally).

Being efficient

Despite the many years spent at medical school preparing for finals and becoming a doctor, being efficient is one of the most important skills you can learn as a house officer.

Working hours When you first start as an F1, you will always work longer hours than those you are paid for, especially towards the beginning of your career. The best way to make your day run as smoothly as possible is to come in early to prepare for the ward round – you will be expected to have the latest bloods, investigation results and any overnight interventions at hand, before your seniors arrive.

Time management You will nearly always seem pressed for time, so it is important to organise your day efficiently. Prioritise tasks in such a way that things such as blood tests can be in progress while you chase other jobs. Requesting radiology investigations early in the day is important as lists get filled quickly, whereas writing blood forms for the next day and prescribing warfarin can wait till later on. TTOs should also be written as soon as the team decides a patient is almost ready for discharge – this will save any unnecessary delays on the day they go home.

On-call It will seem like your bleep never stops going off, especially when you are at your busiest. Always write down every job, otherwise you run the risk of forgetting what you were asked to do. Consider whether there is anyone else you could delegate simple tasks to, such as nurse practitioners and cannulation, whilst you attend to sick patients.

How to be efficient

- Fill in the blood bottle form on p114
- Make a list of common bleeps/extensions, p648
- Establish a timetable of your firm's activities, p649
- Make a folder/clipboard (see p10)
- See organisational tips, p10
- Prioritise your workload rather than working through jobs in order. Try to group jobs into areas of the hospital. If you're unsure of the urgency of a job or why you are requesting an investigation, ask your seniors.
- If you are working with another house officer split the jobs at the end of the ward round so that you share the workload
- Fill out blood forms at the start/end of each day (find out what time the phlebotomists come); if a patient will need bloods for the next 3 days then fill them all out together with clear dates
- Be aware of your limitations eg consent should only be done by the surgeon doing the procedure
- Get a copy of your hospital guidelines/protocols eg pre-op investigations, anticoagulation, DKA, pneumonia etc
- Get a map of the hospital if you haven't got your bearings

Chapter 2

Your career

The Foundation Programme

The concept

The Foundation Programme (FP) is a training programme for all doctors graduating from UK medical schools. It is split into two years:

- F1 (foundation year one)
- F2 (foundation year two)

After successfully completing F1, doctors will gain full registration with the General Medical Council (GMC) and start F2. Once F2 is successfully completed doctors can apply for further training (see p26).

The Foundation Programme was introduced so that all new doctors receive training and assessment in the basic skills of being a doctor (both clinical and non-clinical). Before the FP, junior doctor jobs varied widely in terms of supervision and feedback – hopefully this has improved.

Useful 'foundation terms'

Clinical supervisor	Senior member of staff who supervises your day-to-day learning and training
Educational supervisor	Doctor who will review your progress on a regular basis, check that your assessments are up to date and help you plan your career
Local administrator	A person in each trust or foundation school who keeps a record of all the assessments you complete and organises multi-source feedback
Foundation training programme director (FTPD)	The director of each foundation school who signs you off after each year
Foundation school	The organisation that runs the Foundation Programme locally; it includes medical schools, deaneries, local hospitals (trusts) and PCTs

Other information

You can find more information about the FP and future changes at www.mmc.nhs.uk and www.foundationprogramme.nhs.uk. There are several documents available to download including the Operational Framework (the FP 'rules'), the Curriculum (full list of educational objectives) and Rough Guide to the Foundation Programme; all of these are included in the FP induction pack.

Career structure

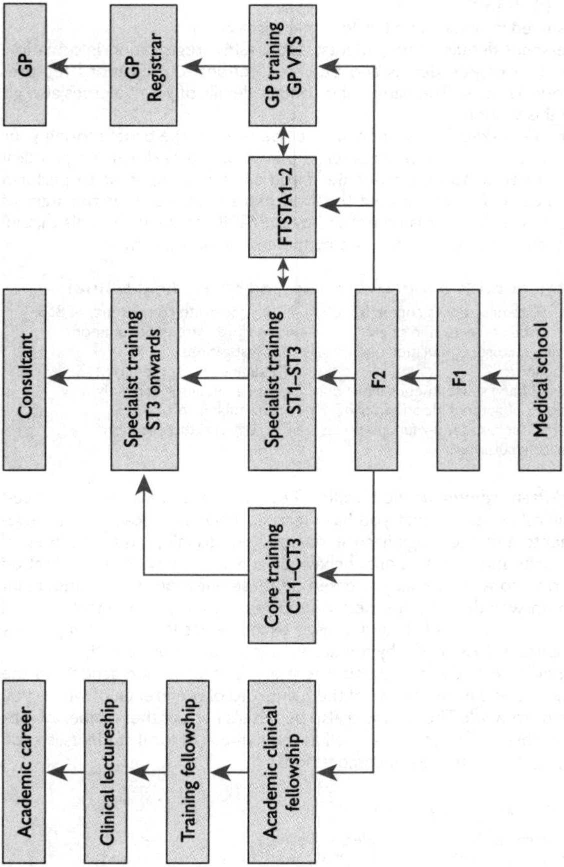

Foundation Programme applications

The application form

This is filled in on-line and has four main areas:

(1) ***Personal details*** Name, address, DoB, GMC registration information, medical degree details and other educational qualifications (eg previous degrees). The names and contact details of your referees also go in this section.

(2) ***Practical skills*** This section will not be seen by the panel scoring your application. You state whether you are able to perform the practical skills below. You must **not lie**; if you are not competent to perform a specific skill you should be given extra supervision at the start of your post. The list is composed by the GMC as the basic skills that all doctors should have attained by the end of medical school.

Practical skills expected by the end of medical school

- Calculate drug doses correctly
- Prescribe correctly and safely
- Venepuncture, cannulation and IV injection
- Give IM and subcutaneous injections
- Carry out arterial blood sampling
- Carry out respiratory function tests
- Perform suturing
- Demonstrate competency in BLS
- Interpret results of common investigations
- Administer O_2 therapy
- Use a nebuliser correctly
- NG tube insertion
- Urethral catheterisation

(3) ***Written communication skills*** These are questions about difficult clinical situations that you have learned from, non-academic achievements and their significance to you/your training and examples of prioritisation, professional behaviour and teamwork. Your application form 'score' will be largely based on these questions so it is important to answer them to the best of your abilities. It is important to read the question carefully and answer exactly what they are asking; many applicants lose marks by not answering the question directly.

(4) ***Ranking Foundation schools*** There are 26 Foundation schools in the UK and you must rank all of them in order of preference of where you want to work. There should also be details here of the number of jobs available in each school as well as the number of local students, so you can get a rough idea of competition.

List of Foundation schools

- Birmingham North
- Birmingham South
- Black Country
- Coventry and Warwick
- East Anglian
- Hereford and Worcestershire
- Leicestershire, Northamptonshire and Rutland
- Mersey Deanery
- North Central Thames
- Trent
- North East Thames
- North Western
- North West Thames
- North Yorkshire and East Coast
- Northern Deanery
- Northern Ireland
- Oxford
- Peninsula
- Scotland
- Severn
- Shropshire and Staffordshire
- South Thames
- South Yorkshire
- Wales
- Wessex
- West Yorkshire

Submission and scoring

Once you have submitted your completed form, it will be scored by a panel from your first choice Foundation school. Each applicant receives an overall score out of 100; up to 45 of these marks are based on your academic performance (this is submitted by your medical school) and the other 55 marks (maximum) come from your application form.

You will receive notification by email of your application results and if you are successful you will also receive details of the school to which you have been allocated. At this point you must decide which hospital/trust you wish to work at within the Foundation school and submit these preferences. Each school will have specific details on how to apply for these, so you should check your school's website for further information on how they match you to a specific programme.

If you are unsuccessful

Do not give up hope. If you feel you have been unfairly marked you may be able to appeal; discuss this with your medical school Dean. Otherwise you will be entered into clearing to be allocated a job from those which are left over. You may not get the exact school you wanted, but you are guaranteed a job.

Choosing your placements

The F1 year usually consists of three placements of 4mth; one of these will be general medicine, one will be general surgery and one will be a speciality (this may be in medicine eg cardiology, surgery eg orthopaedics or a separate speciality eg paediatrics). How these placements are allocated will be decided by the individual Foundation school; details should be shown on their websites. Some will allocate placements alongside the initial application procedure, while others will allocate them at a later date.

What happens in F2?

Most F2 posts will consist of three placements of 4mth; for 80% of F2s one of these will be a GP placement, the other placements will be specialities. You can also arrange week-long 'tasters' in another speciality to help plan your career; to arrange these talk to your educational supervisor and a consultant in the relevant speciality.

Applying for an F2 post

The initial application form is usually for a 2yr Foundation job. However, specific rotations for your F2 year may have not been decided and you will need to apply for them during your F1 year. Once you are on a 2yr Foundation Programme you are guaranteed an F2 post in the same Foundation school, but often in a different hospital. The allocation process will vary between Foundation schools (eg CV, interview, random selection).

FP assessment and portfolios

Throughout the Foundation Programme you will be assessed to prove that you are learning the basic skills of doctoring. You should be given the Foundation Learning Portfolio at the start of the programme which will include examples of the various assessment forms.

Some trusts still use the paper version of the portfolio (available to download and print off from www.foundationprogramme.nhs.uk) but most trusts now use the on-line version (www.nhseportfolios.org). Whichever you are required to use, it is recommended that you also keep a printed version in a folder in case you are required to bring your portfolio (p24) to an assessment where a computer is unavailable.

Whenever you complete one of the assessments below, your assessor should tick the appropriate boxes on the on-line form – when you print out the completed form for your portfolio you should ideally ask the assessor to sign and date the paper version to prove they were the one who marked you. One assessment (either mini-CEX or CbD) per block must be with a consultant. Examples of these forms can be found on the following pages.

Assessments in the Foundation Programme

Direct Observation of Procedural Skills (DOPS)	≥6 in F1, ≥6 in F2
A colleague should watch you perform a procedure (there is a list in the portfolio). The assessor can be anyone who is also able to perform the procedure, but you are not recommended to have medical assessors below you in grade (ie when you are an F2, you should not be assessed by an F1). They then tick boxes about how well you did the various components.	
Initiated by yourself; you choose the time, place and assessor	
Mini-Clinical Evaluation Exercise (Mini-CEX)	≥6 in F1, ≥6 in F2
A colleague should watch you clerk a patient and tick boxes accordingly; they should also give you verbal feedback. The assessor must be a registrar or consultant. You must do at least 2 mini-CEX during each 4-month rotation.	
Initiated by yourself; you choose the time, place and assessor	
Case-based discussion (CbD)	≥6 in F1, ≥6 in F2
You should present a case you have clerked to a doctor (registrar or consultant) and discuss your choice of investigations and management. Once again boxes need ticking and you must do at least 2 CbD per rotation.	
Initiated by yourself; you choose the time, place and assessor	
Multisource/360° feedback (MSF)	1 in F1, 1 in F2
This may be 'Mini-Peer Assessment Tool' (Mini-PAT) or a Team Assessment of Behaviour (TAB). Both essentially involve 10–12 colleagues (consultants, registrars, nurses, physios, GPs, etc) filling in a form about how you are doing. This includes their assessment of your knowledge, practical skills, communication skills, professionalism, approachability, reliability etc.	
Initiated by your local administrator; you choose the assessors	

Direct Observation of Procedural Skills (DOPS)

Please refer to curriculum at www.mmc.nhs.uk for details of expected competencies for F1 and F2

Direct Observation of Procedural Skills (DOPS) - F1 Version

Please complete the questions using a cross: ☒ Please use black ink and CAPITAL LETTERS

Doctor's Surname ☐☐☐☐☐☐☐☐☐☐☐☐☐☐☐☐☐☐☐☐☐☐☐☐☐

Forename ☐☐☐☐☐☐☐☐☐☐☐☐☐☐☐☐☐☐☐☐☐☐☐☐☐

GMC Number: ☐☐☐☐☐☐☐ **GMC NUMBER MUST BE COMPLETED**

Clinical setting: A&E ☐ OPD ☐ In-patient ☐ Acute Admission ☐ GP Surgery ☐

Procedure:

Assessor's position: Consultant ☐ SASG ☐ SpR ☐ GP ☐ Nurse ☐ Other ☐

Number of previous DOPS observed by assessor with <u>any</u> trainee: 0 ☐ 1 ☐ 2 ☐ 3 ☐ 4 ☐ 5-9 ☐ >9 ☐

Number of times procedure performed by trainee: 0 ☐ 1-4 ☐ 5-9 ☐ >10 ☐ Difficulty of procedure: Low ☐ Average ☐ High ☐

Please grade the following areas using the scale below:	Below expectations for F1 completion 1	2	Borderline for F1 completion 3	Meets expectations for F1 completion 4	Above expectations for F1 completion 5	6	U/C*
1 Demonstrates understanding of indications, relevant anatomy, technique of procedure	☐	☐	☐	☐	☐	☐	☐
2 Obtains informed consent	☐	☐	☐	☐	☐	☐	☐
3 Demonstrates appropriate preparation pre-procedure	☐	☐	☐	☐	☐	☐	☐
4 Appropriate analgesia or safe sedation	☐	☐	☐	☐	☐	☐	☐
5 Technical ability	☐	☐	☐	☐	☐	☐	☐
6 Aseptic technique	☐	☐	☐	☐	☐	☐	☐
7 Seeks help where appropriate	☐	☐	☐	☐	☐	☐	☐
8 Post procedure management	☐	☐	☐	☐	☐	☐	☐
9 Communication skills	☐	☐	☐	☐	☐	☐	☐
10 Consideration of patient/professionalism	☐	☐	☐	☐	☐	☐	☐
11 Overall ability to perform procedure	☐	☐	☐	☐	☐	☐	☐

*U/C Please mark this if you have not observed the behaviour and therefore feel unable to comment.

Please use this space to record areas of strength or any suggestions for development.

	Not at all									Highly
Trainee satisfaction with DOPS	1☐	2☐	3☐	4☐	5☐	6☐	7☐	8☐	9☐	10☐
Assessor satisfaction with DOPS	1☐	2☐	3☐	4☐	5☐	6☐	7☐	8☐	9☐	10☐

Have you had training in the use of this assessment tool?: ☐ Face-to-Face ☐ Have Read Guidelines ☐ Web/CD rom

Assessor's Signature: ....

Date: ☐☐ / ☐☐ / ☐☐

Time taken for observation: (in minutes) ☐☐

Time taken for feedback: (in minutes) ☐☐

Assessor's Surname ☐☐☐☐☐☐☐☐☐☐☐☐☐☐☐☐☐☐☐☐☐☐☐☐☐

Assessor's GMC Number: ☐☐☐☐☐☐☐

<u>**Please note:**</u> Failure of return of all completed forms to your administrator is a probity issue 2930518468

Mini-Clinical Evaluation Exercise (Mini-CEX)

Please refer to curriculum at www.mmc.nhs.uk for details of expected competencies for F1 and F2

Mini-Clinical Evaluation Exercise (CEX) - F1 Version

Please complete the questions using a cross: ☒ Please use black ink and CAPITAL LETTERS

Doctor's Surname ☐☐☐☐☐☐☐☐☐☐☐☐☐☐☐☐☐☐☐☐☐☐☐☐☐

Forename ☐☐☐☐☐☐☐☐☐☐☐☐☐☐☐☐☐☐☐☐☐☐☐☐☐

GMC Number: ☐☐☐☐☐☐☐ **GMC NUMBER MUST BE COMPLETED**

Clinical setting: A&E ☐ OPD ☐ In-patient ☐ Acute Admission ☐ GP Surgery ☐

Clinical problem category: Pain ☐ Airway/ Breathing ☐ CVS/ Circulation ☐ Psych/ Behav ☐ Neuro ☐ Gastro ☐ Other ☐

New or FU: New ☐ FU ☐ Focus of clinical encounter: History ☐ Diagnosis ☐ Management ☐ Explanation ☐

Number of times patient seen before by trainee: 0 ☐ 1-4 ☐ 5-9 ☐ >10 ☐

Complexity of case: Low ☐ Average ☐ High ☐ Assessor's position: Consultant ☐ SASG ☐ SpR ☐ GP ☐

Number of previous mini-CEXs observed by assessor with any trainee: 0 ☐ 1 ☐ 2 ☐ 3 ☐ 4 ☐ 5-9 ☐ >9 ☐

Please grade the following areas using the scale below:	Below expectations for F1 completion 1	2	Borderline for F1 completion 3	Meets expectations for F1 completion 4	Above expectations for F1 completion 5	6	U/C*
1 History Taking	☐	☐	☐	☐	☐	☐	☐
2 Physical Examination Skills	☐	☐	☐	☐	☐	☐	☐
3 Communication Skills	☐	☐	☐	☐	☐	☐	☐
4 Clinical judgement	☐	☐	☐	☐	☐	☐	☐
5 Professionalism	☐	☐	☐	☐	☐	☐	☐
6 Organisation/Efficiency	☐	☐	☐	☐	☐	☐	☐
7 Overall clinical care	☐	☐	☐	☐	☐	☐	☐

*U/C Please mark this if you have not observed the behaviour and therefore feel unable to comment.

Anything especially good?	Suggestions for development

Agreed action:

	Not at all 1	2	3	4	5	6	7	8	9	Highly 10
Trainee satisfaction with mini-CEX	☐	☐	☐	☐	☐	☐	☐	☐	☐	☐
Assessor satisfaction with mini-CEX	☐	☐	☐	☐	☐	☐	☐	☐	☐	☐

What training have you had in the use of this assessment tool?: ☐ Face-to-Face ☐ Have Read Guidelines ☐ Web/CD rom

Assessor's Signature: .... Date: ☐☐ / ☐☐ / ☐☐

Time taken for observation: (in minutes) ☐☐

Assessor's Surname: ☐☐☐☐☐☐☐☐☐☐☐☐☐☐☐☐☐☐☐☐☐☐☐☐☐

Time taken for feedback: (in minutes) ☐☐

Assessor's GMC Number: ☐☐☐☐☐☐☐

Acknowledgements: Adapted with permission from American Board of Internal Medicine

Please note:
Failure of return of all completed forms to your administrator is a probity issue

4422256612

Case-based Discussion (CbD)

Please refer to curriculum at www.mmc.nhs.uk for details of expected competencies for F1 and F2

Case-based Discussion (CbD) - F1 Version

Please complete the questions using a cross: ☒ Please use black ink and CAPITAL LETTERS

Doctor's Surname ☐☐☐☐☐☐☐☐☐☐☐☐☐☐☐☐☐☐☐☐☐☐☐☐☐

Forename ☐☐☐☐☐☐☐☐☐☐☐☐☐☐☐☐☐☐☐☐☐☐☐☐☐

GMC Number: ☐☐☐☐☐☐☐ **GMC NUMBER MUST BE COMPLETED**

Clinical setting: A&E ☐ OPD ☐ In-patient ☐ Acute Admission ☐ GP Surgery ☐

Clinical problem category: Pain ☐ Airway/ Breathing ☐ CVS/ Circulation ☐ Psych/ Behav ☐ Neuro ☐ Gastro ☐ Other ☐

Focus of clinical encounter: Medical Record Keeping ☐ Clinical Assessment ☐ Management ☐ Professionalism ☐

Complexity of case: Low ☐ Average ☐ High ☐ Assessor's position: Consultant ☐ SpR ☐ GP ☐

Please grade the following areas using the scale below:	Below expectations for F1 completion 1	2	Borderline for F1 completion 3	Meets expectations for F1 completion 4	Above expectations for F1 completion 5	6	U/C*
1 Medical record keeping	☐	☐	☐	☐	☐	☐	☐
2 Clinical assessment	☐	☐	☐	☐	☐	☐	☐
3 Investigation and referrals	☐	☐	☐	☐	☐	☐	☐
4 Treatment	☐	☐	☐	☐	☐	☐	☐
5 Follow-up and future planning	☐	☐	☐	☐	☐	☐	☐
6 Professionalism	☐	☐	☐	☐	☐	☐	☐
7 Overall clinical judgement	☐	☐	☐	☐	☐	☐	☐

*U/C Please mark this if you have not observed the behaviour and therefore feel unable to comment.

Anything especially good? **Suggestions for development**

Agreed action:

	Not at all 1	2	3	4	5	6	7	8	9	Highly 10
Trainee satisfaction with CbD	☐	☐	☐	☐	☐	☐	☐	☐	☐	☐
Assessor satisfaction with CbD	☐	☐	☐	☐	☐	☐	☐	☐	☐	☐

What training have you had in the use of this assessment tool?: ☐ Have Read Guidelines ☐ Face-to-Face ☐ Web/CD rom

Time taken for discussion: (in minutes) ☐☐

Assessor's Signature: ....

Date: ☐☐ / ☐☐ / ☐☐

Time taken for feedback: (in minutes) ☐☐

Assessor's Surname ☐☐☐☐☐☐☐☐☐☐☐☐☐☐☐☐☐☐☐☐☐☐☐☐☐

Assessor's GMC Number ☐☐☐☐☐☐☐

Please note:
Failure of return of all completed forms to your administrator is a probity issue

8721456665

Multi-source feedback: TAB

Aii) MULTI-SOURCE FEEDBACK: 360° Team Assessment of Behaviour (TAB)

Name of doctor in training		**GMC number**	
Current post		**Date started current post**	

Please use the comments boxes to commend good behaviour and to describe any behaviour which is causing you concern. Give specific examples. This form will be sent to the foundation doctor's educational supervisor, who may ask you privately to enlarge on any concern behaviour you report. At least nine other forms will also be considered. The foundation doctor will receive private feedback, but you will not be identified in person without advance discussion with you.

Attitude and/or behaviour	*No concern*	*You have some concern*	*You have a major concern*	*COMMENTS: Anything especially good? If you cannot give an opinion due to lack of knowledge of the foundation doctor say so here.* ***You must specifically comment on any concern behaviour*** *and this should reflect the trainee's behaviour reflect trainee's behaviour over time – not usually just a single incident.*
Maintaining trust/professional relationship with patients • Listens. • Is polite and caring. • Shows respect for patients' opinions, privacy, dignity, and is unprejudiced.				
Verbal communication skills • Gives understandable information. • Speaks good English, at the appropriate level for the patient.				
Team-working/working with colleagues • Respects others' roles, and works constructively in the team. • Hands over effectively, and communicates well. • Is unprejudiced, supportive and fair.				
Accessibility • Accessible. • Takes proper responsibility. Only delegates appropriately. • Does not shirk duty. • Responds when called. Arranges cover for absence.				

Name of assessor: ____________________ Post/designation: ____________________ Signature: ____________________ Date: ____________

Multi-source feedback: mini-PAT

Please complete the questions using a cross: ☒ Please use black ink and CAPITAL LETTERS

Surname

Forename

User Number:

Please grade the following areas using the scale**:	Below expectations for GLF completion		Borderline for GLF completion	Meets expectations for GLF completion	Above expectations for GLF completion		U/C*
Delivery of Patient Care							
	1	2	3	4	5	6	7
1 Patient consultation	☐	☐	☐	☐	☐	☐	☐
2 Need for drug	☐	☐	☐	☐	☐	☐	☐
3 Selection of drug	☐	☐	☐	☐	☐	☐	☐
4 Drug specific issues	☐	☐	☐	☐	☐	☐	☐
5 Provision of drug product	☐	☐	☐	☐	☐	☐	☐
6 Medicines information and patient education	☐	☐	☐	☐	☐	☐	☐
7 Monitoring drug therapy	☐	☐	☐	☐	☐	☐	☐
Personal Attributes							
8 Organisation	☐	☐	☐	☐	☐	☐	☐
9 Effective Communication Skills	☐	☐	☐	☐	☐	☐	☐
10 Teamwork	☐	☐	☐	☐	☐	☐	☐
11 Professionalism	☐	☐	☐	☐	☐	☐	☐

The Foundation Learning Portfolio

Along with the assessment forms there are several other components to the portfolio that you need to complete. It is important to keep your portfolio up to date and safe; it is essential that you can show evidence that you are competent to move onto the next level of training.

Start of each 4mth placement

- *Self-appraisal-form* complete at the start of each 4mth placement before meeting with your educational supervisor
- *Personal development plan* (PDP) and *Educational agreement* complete at the start of each 4mth placement in the meeting with your educational supervisor
- *Induction meeting* complete at the start of each 4mth placement in the meeting with your clinical supervisor
- *Statement of health and probity* complete at every appraisal

During each 4mth placement

- *Mid-point meeting* this is not compulsory, but it is recommended to have a meeting with your clinical supervisor halfway through each 4mth placement to check how things are going and to discuss which objectives on your PDP you still have to achieve
- *Reflective practice form* and *Self-appraisal of learning* you do not have to complete any of these, but some consultants are very keen on them and they look good in interviews. You can reflect on any event at work that has significance to you; this could be a difficult clinical scenario, an ethical dilemma, problems with colleagues, personal issues when dealing with difficult patients or particularly rewarding or exciting cases.
- *Summary of evidence presented* fill this in as you pass assessments to guide what areas further assessments need to cover

After each 4mth placement

- *End of placement final review* complete at the end of each 4mth placement in a meeting with your clinical supervisor once you have discussed your DOPS/mini-CEX/CbD/MSF forms and gone through your PDP to check you have achieved your objectives
- *Statement of health and probity* complete at every appraisal

End of each year

- *Attainment of competency* this should be completed at the end of your F1 and F2 year to prove you have passed; it can be printed from the on-line portfolio (www.foundationprogramme.nhs.uk)

Data Protection Act

All data collected is covered by the Data Protection Act. This means that you must not keep patient-identifiable data outside the hospital. Using hospital numbers rather than names is considered acceptable.

The paper portfolio

Alongside your on-line portfolio of assessments and appraisals you need to keep a paper portfolio of these documents and other demonstrations of your continued learning and professional development.

Creating a portfolio

Buy a large, smart lever arch file that you will be proud to take to interviews and about 20 dividers. An example of the layout and contents of a portfolio is given below:

Qualifications and CV

- Up-to-date CV
- Proof of qualifications (eg A-Levels, degrees)
- Forms showing completion of placements or years

Assessments and appraisals

- DOPS, mini-CEXs, CbDs, MSFs
- Appraisals
- Reflective learning
- Membership examination results

Clinical work

- Copies of discharge/referral letters (anonymised)
- Copies of clerkings (anonymised)
- Attendance at clinic (date, consultant, learning points)
- Procedures (list of type, when, observing, performing or teaching)
- Details of any complaints made against you and their resolution
- Incident forms you have been involved in (useful for reflective practice and demonstrating that you have learned from your mistakes)
- 'Triumphs' – difficult patients you've diagnosed/treated
- Praise – all thank you letters/cards

Presentations, teaching, audit and research

- Copies of presentations given
- Details of teaching you've done (with feedback if possible)
- Copies of audit or research you've been involved in
- Copies of your publications

Training

- Details of courses you've attended (with certificates of attendance)
- Study leave and associated forms

Important advice

- Start early (when you qualify)
- Keep it up-to-date
- Don't leave assessments till the last minute
- Seize every opportunity to do something you could add to your portfolio to distinguish you from your peers
- Organise it by headings at least every 6mth
- Discuss it yearly with a suitable mentor

Speciality training

After the FP you need to apply for speciality training. You have three main choices:

- *Speciality training* (ST) or *Core-training* (CT), the majority of junior doctors will choose this route
- *Fixed-term speciality training appointment* (FTSTA) single year posts for speciality training for those who cannot commit to, or are unable to secure, a run-through post; there is no equivalent for core-training
- *Academic clinical fellowship* (ACF) for those interested in research see p43 and www.nccrcd.nhs.uk; note that the recruitment process takes place earlier in the year than for other posts (eg November)

Speciality training and run-through

This involves getting a job in a particular speciality (eg paediatrics) and completing a 3–8yr run-through programme in one Deanery (ST1 up to ST8 in some specialities). Assuming you complete all the assessments and membership exams this ends with Certificate of Completion of Training (CCT). This qualifies the doctor for entry to the Specialist or GP Register held by the GMC and entitles them to work as a consultant or GP. This continuous training from ST1 to CCT is called **run-through** training.

FTSTAs are one-year posts that provide an opportunity to gain experience before applying for speciality training at a later date. There is no equivalent in uncoupled specialities, though it may be necessary to develop one in the future.

Core-training and uncoupling

This route offers a two-year core-training programme (three years for psychiatry and emergency medicine) followed by open competition to enter speciality training at ST3 onwards (ST4 for psychiatry and emergency medicine). This split between core-training and speciality training is called **uncoupling**.

For uncoupled specialities, core-training is offered to a large pool of applicants without the option of FTSTAs. Following core-training, the competitive entry into higher speciality training is open to all eligible applicants, including those who have taken alternative routes but have completed appropriate ST1/2 competencies, training and exams.

The job titles for core-training are CT1, CT2 (and CT3 for psychiatry and emergency medicine) depending on the year of training. If you apply to an uncoupled speciality, you will initially train via one of these routes:

- Acute care common stem (ACCS)
- Anaesthetics
- Core medical training
- Psychiatry
- Surgery in general

Speciality training applications

Recruitment process

- *Choose a speciality* (p31) and check the person specification on MMC: www.mmc.nhs.uk → Specialty Training → Person Specifications
- *Check your eligibility* for applying to a training programme eg GMC registration, right to work in the UK, language skills
- *Find suitable jobs* (p30) these can be found on Deanery websites, MMC website or NHS jobs (www.jobs.nhs.uk)
- *Complete the application form* be aware of deadlines as some posts will only be advertised for 72h and you may only have 5d to submit your on-line application form (10d for paper forms)
- *Wait* as applications are reviewed by the Deanery and applicants are shortlisted for interview
- *Interview* (p36) if you are shortlisted; make sure you take your portfolio (p25) and any documentation the Deanery requires
- *Offers* you have a minimum of 48h to accept or decline an offer (not including weekends or bank holidays)
- *Employment checks* and contract signing

National vs. Deanery recruitment

The application process varies between different specialities; some have a nationwide application process (eg GP) whilst others have a separate application process with each deanery (eg medicine). The table on p29 shows which type of application process each of the specialities available to an F2 uses. The table below shows the contact details for the nationwide applications:

Speciality	Contact details
Academic clinical fellowships	National Institute for Health Research Capacity Development Programme www.nccrcd.nhs.uk
General practice	National Recruitment Office for GP Training www.gprecruitment.org.uk
Histopathology	London Deanery www.londondeanery.ac.uk
Neurosurgery	South Yorkshire and South Humber Deanery www.syshdeanery.com
Obstetrics and gynaecology	Royal College of Obstetricians and Gynaecologists www.rcog.org.uk
Paediatrics and child health	Royal College of Paediatrics and Child Health www.rcpch.c.uk/recruitment
Public health	East Midlands Healthcare Workforce Deanery www.eastmidlandsdeanery.nhs.uk

Application forms

These also vary between specialties. Some are on-line applications whilst others require application forms to be posted. They are mostly CV-based.

Speciality training options

There are 25 different training schemes that an F2 can apply to (shown in the table opposite). On top of these there are:

- *Academic clinical fellowships* in most specialities with separate nationwide application procedures (p27)
- *FTSTAs* in the run-through posts, usually applied for with the ST posts. Four of the most common and complex routes are outlined below; for other specialities see the training section in the 'Specialities' (p443)

Acute care common stem (ACCS)

For trainees with an interest in acute specialities ACCS provides experience in acute medicine, anaesthetics, emergency medicine and critical care. ACCS is uncoupled (p26) with application to the local Deanery:

- *Acute medicine* 2yr core-training: CT1 and CT2, then competitive entry to ST3 acute medicine if you have passed the MRCP part 1 (p37). You are also eligible for ST3 in other medical specialities since ACCS acute medicine is equivalent to CT1/CT2 in core medicine.
- *Anaesthetics* 3yr core-training: CT1 and CT2 as for other ACCS specialities then an extra CT2 year of anaesthetics; competitive entry to ST3 anaesthetics if you have passed the Primary FRCA (p37). Anaesthetics can also be applied for directly as a 2yr core-training programme.
- *Emergency medicine* 3yr core-training: CT1 and CT2 as for other ACCS specialities then CT3 year of emergency medicine; competitive entry to ST4 emergency medicine if you have passed MCEM (p37).

Core medical training

This is applied for by deanery and is an uncoupled (p26) training scheme. Two years of core-training (CT1–CT2) in various medical jobs followed by competitive application for ST3 in a specific medical speciality (eg haematology, endocrinology). You need MRCP part 1 to apply for ST3.

General Practice Vocational Training Scheme (GPVTS)

General practice has run-through training (p26) with on-line nationwide application. The application consists of four stages:

- Application form (long-listing)
- Written examinations (short-listing)
- Assessment day and selection
- Job allocation and offer

Successful applicants undertake four 6mth posts in hospital specialities, followed by a year as a GP registrar during which the MRCGP must be completed to join the GP registrar and get a job.

Surgery in general

This is applied for by deanery and is an uncoupled (p26) training scheme. You apply for core-training in a specific surgical speciality (eg general surgery, urology). After two years of core-training (CT1–CT2) there is a competitive application for ST3 in the same surgical speciality (eg general surgery, urology). You need MRCS to apply for ST3. It may be possible to apply for other surgical specialities than the one you did your core-training in if you can demonstrate appropriate competencies.

Training choices available to the F2

Speciality	Application[1]	Type[2]	Competition[3]
Academic clinical fellowship	National	Uncoupled	variable
Acute care common stem (acute medicine)	Deanery	Uncoupled	9.3
Acute care common stem (anaesthetics)	Deanery	Uncoupled	5.5
Acute care common stem (emergency medicine)	Deanery	Uncoupled	8.4
Anaesthetics	Deanery	Uncoupled	4.8
Chemical pathology	Deanery	Run-through	8.8
Clinical radiology	Deanery	Run-through	18.1
Core medical training	Deanery	Uncoupled	5.8
General practice	National	Run-through	6.1
Histopathology	National	Run-through	8.7
Microbiology and virology (microbiology)	Deanery	Run-through	18.0
Microbiology and virology (virology)	Deanery	Run-through	5.3
Neurosurgery	National	Run-through	7.5
Obstetrics and gynaecology	National	Run-through	7.0
Ophthalmology	Deanery	Run-through	8.2
Oral and maxillofacial surgery	Deanery	Uncoupled	8.8
Paediatrics	National	Run-through	4.5
Psychiatry	Deanery	Uncoupled	5.1
Public health	National	Run-through	18.0
Surgery in general (generic)	Deanery	Uncoupled	6.4
Surgery in general (general surgery)	Deanery	Uncoupled	6.8
Surgery in general (otolaryngology)	Deanery	Uncoupled	4.4
Surgery in general (paediatric surgery)	Deanery	Uncoupled	5.2
Surgery in general (plastic surgery)	Deanery	Uncoupled	8.1
Surgery in general (trauma and orthopaedic surgery)	Deanery	Uncoupled	6.8
Surgery in general (urology)	Deanery	Uncoupled	1.9

[1]See p27 for the difference between national and deanery recruitment
[2]See p26 for the difference between run-through and uncoupled
[3]Total number of applicants per post at ST1 level; average of 6.4 applicants per post (source MMC competition ratios, 2007 application)

Choosing a job

Once you have secured a training post you still need to choose which specific jobs to do. There are also jobs outside of speciality training that have a more traditional application process. This page gives ideas about how to find and choose jobs.

Priorities Before looking for a job, write a list of factors that matter to you in making this potentially life-changing decision. Important considerations include:

- *Partner/spouse* can they get a job nearby?
- *Location* could you move? How far would you commute?
- *Family/friends* how far away are you willing to go?
- *Career* is the job in the right speciality/specialities?
- *Duration* can you commit to several years in the same area?
- *Rota/pay* what banding and rota do you want or need?
- *Type of hospital* large teaching hospital vs. district general

If you have no firm career intentions then choose by location and rota since these will affect your life most over the next few months. With this in mind, try the website www.jobscore.co.uk where you can rate previous jobs (confidentially) and see what others thought of yours. Look for suitable jobs on www.jobs.nhs.uk, deanery websites, MMC website or *BMJ Careers*.

Staggering of jobs Jobs come out at different times so it is important to keep checking advertisements. You cannot change your mind after accepting a job (see below); this creates a tricky balance between waiting for the perfect job vs. applying for acceptable ones. In the current competitive climate it is best to err on the side of applying to acceptable jobs.

Competition Medical jobs are competitive; it is important to maximise your chances of getting a job. Apply for several jobs in different regions and/or specialities; check competition ratios (p29, www.mmc.nhs.uk) and person specifications (MMC website); consider a back-up choice eg a less competitive speciality or region. A good CV also helps (p32).

Researching a job Adverts rarely give a true reflection of a job. Phone up hospitals within the Deanery and ask to speak to the person doing the job at the moment. Quiz them on the types of placements available, hours, support, teaching, conditions and what their interview was like. Would they accept the job again?

Contacts With human resource departments and structured interviews, the days of jobs being just a consultant phone call away have gone. There is no doubt that some networking still occurs, with mixed results. Senior contacts are useful for tailored career guidance, CV advice and giving realistic views of where your CV can get you.

Accepting a job Once you have accepted a job it is very bad manners to turn them down at a later date unless you have an extremely good reason (not another job). A doctor has been struck off the GMC register for doing this though there were many other factors involved in this decision.

Specialities in medicine

PMETB currently awards a Certificate of Completion of Training (CCT) in 57 specialities; many of these also have sub-specialities, a selection of which are shown here with bullet points:

Allergy
Anaesthetics
- Paediatric anaesthetics
- Obstetric anaesthetics
- Pain management

Audiological medicine
Cardiology
Cardiothoracic surgery
Chemical pathology (biochemistry)
Child and adolescent psychiatry
Clinical cytogenetics and molecular genetics
Clinical genetics
Clinical neurophysiology
Clinical oncology (radiotherapy)
Clinical pharmacology and therapeutics
Clinical radiology
- Nuclear medicine
- Interventional radiology

Dermatology
Emergency medicine (EM)
Endocrinology and diabetes mellitus
Forensic psychiatry
Gastroenterology
- Hepatology

General (internal) medicine
- Acute medicine

General psychiatry
- Liaison psychiatry
- Substance abuse psychiatry
- Rehabilitation psychiatry
- Forensic psychiatry

General surgery
- Breast surgery
- Colorectal surgery
- Upper GI surgery
- Vascular surgery

Genitourinary medicine
Geriatric medicine
Haematology
Histopathology
- Forensic pathology

Immunology
Infectious diseases
Intensive care medicine
Medical microbiology and virology
Medical oncology
Medical ophthalmology
Neurology
Neurosurgery
Nuclear medicine
Obstetrics and gynaecology
- Family planning
- Reproductive medicine
- Fetal medicine

Occupational medicine
Old age psychiatry
Ophthalmology
Oral and maxillo-facial surgery
Otolaryngology (ENT surgery)
Paediatric cardiology
Paediatric surgery
Paediatrics
- Community paediatrics
- Neonatology

Palliative medicine
Pharmaceutical medicine
Plastic surgery
Psychiatry of learning disability
Psychotherapy
Public health medicine
Rehabilitation medicine
- Stroke medicine

Renal medicine
Respiratory medicine
Rheumatology
Sport and exercise medicine
Trauma and orthopaedic surgery
- Hand surgery
- Spinal surgery

Tropical medicine
Urology

For more details on the career options available to doctors, including all of the above, see *So You Want To Be A Brain Surgeon?* OUP

Your curriculum vitae

What is a CV? This is a Latin phrase which means 'course of life'. In modern days it means a document by which you advertise yourself to a potential employer: a summary of you.

When will I use a CV? You will need a CV for most jobs you apply for after graduating. A few hospital trusts request a CV when final year medical students apply for Foundation jobs.

What is included in a CV? The most important information to include are your contact details, a list of your qualifications (those already acquired and those you are studying for), any outstanding achievements and the details of your referees. Other information can be included, but do not overcrowd your CV.

CV philosophy Your CV should not be a static piece of work, it should evolve with you and reflect your changing skills and attitudes. It is important to keep your CV up-to-date, and from time to time reformat it to freshen it up. Use your CV to demonstrate how you have learnt from your experiences rather than just listing them; a potential employer will be much more impressed if you indicate you learnt about the importance of clear communication whilst working at a holiday resort, than by the actual job itself.

Getting help Human resource departments and educational supervisors can give advice on writing a CV, and often you can find people's CVs or templates on the internet by searching for 'CV'. Try to keep your CV individualised, so do not simply copy someone else's template.

Before writing your CV Ascertain what a potential employer is looking for when sending in your CV; check the essential and desirable criteria and try to echo these. You need to alter the emphasis in your CV to match the position you are applying for eg, highlighting your communication skills or leadership experience.

Layout Your CV should look impressive; for many jobs thousands of CVs are received and yours must stand out. It must be word-processed. It needs to be clearly laid out and easy to follow. The key information and your most important attributes should stand out prominently. Think about the layout before you start writing.

Length Two sides of A4 paper is ideal for a basic CV (and an optional front page); add more as your career progresses.

Remember For most jobs, the candidates applying will have very similar qualifications and so the only way you will stand out to be short-listed for interview is via your CV. Make it as interesting as possible, without it looking ludicrous.

Personal details Name, address which you use for correspondence, contact telephone numbers (home, work, mobile), email address and date of birth are essential. You must state your type of GMC membership (full/provisional) and number. Stating gender, marital status, nationality and other information is optional.

Personal statement This is very much an optional section. Some feel it gives you an opportunity to outline a little about yourself and where you see yourself in 10 years; others feel it is an irritating waste of space.

Education List your qualifications in date order, starting with the most recent or current and progressing backwards in time. Indicate where each was undertaken, the dates you were there and grade. Highlight specific courses or modules of interest. GCSE and A-level results are less important once you have graduated.

Employment and work experience List the placements you have undertaken during the F1 and F2 years starting with the most recent. Include the dates, speciality, your supervising consultant and address of the employer; consider adding key skills that you attained.

Interests An optional section which gives you a chance to outline what you like to do outside of medicine. A well-written paragraph here can show potential employers that you are interesting as well as intelligent.

Publications If you have not yet got your name in print try to get a letter in a medical journal (p38). If you have got publications put the most recent first; ensure they are referenced in a conventional style (see www.pubmed.com for examples).

Referees Your referees should know your academic record as well as your ability to interact with others. State their relationship to you (such as personal tutor) and give contact address, telephone and fax numbers and email address. Ensure they are happy to provide a reference, give them a copy of your CV and tell them when you are applying for jobs.

Headers and footers Having the month and year in either a header or footer shows the reader you keep it up-to-date.

Photographs Some people include a small passport-sized photograph of themselves near the start of their CV; this is optional but not necessarily recommended.

The finished CV Use the spell-checker and get a tutor or friend to read over it to identify mistakes and make constructive criticism; be prepared to make numerous alterations to get it right.

Technical points Use just one clear font throughout. To highlight text of importance use the underline, **bold** or *italic* features. When printing your CV use good quality white paper and a laser printer if possible.

The covering letter Whenever you apply for a job, you must send a covering letter with your CV and application form. This should be short and to the point. Indicate the position you are applying for and briefly say why the job appeals to you.

Post-Foundation Programme CV

Name:	Charles J Flint
Address:	14 Abbeyvale Crescent McBurney's Point McBurney McB1 7RH
Home:	0111 442 985
Mobile:	0968 270 250
Work:	0111 924 9924 bleep 1066
Email:	charles.flint@mcburney.ac.uk
Date of Birth:	12 June 1984 (age 24)
GMC:	0121231 (full)

Personal Statement

I am an outgoing 24-year-old with an enthusiastic yet mature outlook. I have strong communication skills and experience of working independently, both as a team member and leader. I am conscientious, trustworthy, quick to learn and to employ new skills. My long-term aim is to practise an acute speciality within the hospital environment.

Education

2001–2006

University of McBurney, McBurney's Point, McB1 8PQ

MBChB:	2006
BMedSci (Hons):	Upper Second Class, 2004

Employment History

3 Apr 08–date	F2 to Mr Broom, Emergency Medicine McBurney Royal Infirmary
5 Dec 07–2 Apr 08	F2 to Dr Fungi, Microbiology McBurney Royal Infirmary
31 Jul 07–4 Dec 07	F2 to Dr Golfer, General Practice Feelgood Health Centre, Speakertown
3 Apr 07–30 Jul 07	F1 to Mr Grimshaw, General Surgery McBurney City Hospital
5 Dec 06–2 Apr 07	F1 to Dr Mallory, Gastroenterology McBurney City Hospital
31 Jul 06–4 Dec 06	F1 to Dr Haler, Respiratory Medicine McBurney City Hospital

Postgraduate Clinical Experience

During my F1 year I developed my clinical and practical skills and became confident with the day-to-day organisation of emergency and elective admissions in both medicine and surgery.

Since commencing F2 I have built upon these skills and now appreciate the wider role of the doctor in the smooth running of acute admissions and liaison with the community teams prior to, and after, hospital discharge.

Formal skills I have include:

- ALS provider (2008)
- Basic surgical skills, including suturing and fracture management

Research and Audit

- I am currently involved in a research project comparing capillary blood gas analysis with arterial blood gases in acute asthmatics
- I undertook an audit on MRSA screening on surgical wards to investigate which patients were screened and how they were subsequently managed depending on their screening results
- During my SSM I was involved in research investigating the role of caffeine upon platelet aggregation

Interests

I am a keen rock and ice climber and have continued to improve my grade since leaving university. I have organised several climbing trips to Scotland and one to the Alps. I am interested in medical journalism and have spent a week in the editorial office of the *International Journal of Thrombophlebitis*.

Publications

- **Flint CJ**. Letter: Student debt. *Medical Students Journal* 2007; **35**(2): 101
- **Flint CJ** and West DJ. Multiple Sclerosis in social class three. *Journal of Social Medicine* 2006; **12**(9): 118
- Lee S, **Flint CJ** and West DJ. Caffeine as an activator of platelet aggregation. *International Journal of Thrombophlebitis* 2005; **54**(3): 99

References

- Dr Ian Haler, Educational Supervisor, Department of Respiratory Medicine, McBurney's Medical Centre, McBurney's Point, McBurney, McB1 7TS
  Telephone 0111 924 9924 ext 2370. Fax 0111 924 9002.
  Email ian.haler@mcburney.ac.uk
- Mr Ivor Grimshaw, Educational Supervisor, Department of General Surgery, McBurney's Medical Centre, McBurney's Point, McBurney, McB1 7TS
  Telephone 0111 924 9924 ext 4637. Fax 0111 924 9056.
  Email ivor.grimshaw@mcburney.ac.uk

Interviews

Interview preparation Employers must allow you time off to attend the interview itself; try to give them as much notice as possible. For deanery-wide or nationwide interviews look at the competition ratios of the previous round to get an idea of how hard it will be and talk to previous applicants about interview format and questions.

Interview day Arrive at the interview with plenty of time, allow for all sorts of delays on the roads or train, even if this means you have to read the newspaper for an hour. Relax and be yourself with the other candidates before you are called in; most of them will have similar qualifications and experience as yourself and will be just as nervous. Dress smartly in a simple suit and tie for men and suit for women (trouser or skirt). Remember to bring your portfolio (p24).

The interview Relax. The worst that can happen is that you are not offered the job, which is not the end of the world. The format of interviews varies, but there are usually 2–3 interviewers; introduce yourself to all the panel and wait to be offered a seat. Take a few moments to think about the questions before answering and ask for a question to be rephrased if you don't understand it.

Common questions It is impossible to predict the questions you will be asked, but they are likely to include questions about your CV, relevant clinical scenarios and current medical news/issues. Many questions have no correct answer and test your communication skills, common sense and ability to think under pressure:

- What are you most proud of on your CV?
- What is missing from your CV?
- What qualities can you offer our department?
- Why have you chosen a career in…?
- What do you understand by 'clinical governance'?
- Tell us about your audit. Why is audit important?
- If you were the Secretary for Health, where would your priorities lie?
- How would you manage… (specific clinical scenario)?
- Where do you see yourself in 5, 10 years time?
- If you were the ST1 in the hospital alone at night and you were struggling with a clinical problem, what would you do?
- Tell us about your teaching experiences. What makes a good teacher?

Clinical scenarios Interviewers should not ask you specific medical questions (eg what is the dose of…); they can pose scenarios to discuss your management of a situation. These often focus on key issues like communication, prioritisation, calling for senior help when appropriate, multidisciplinary teams, clinical safety.

Results and feedback If you are offered the job and accept it, then you are morally obliged to take up that position and decline all further job offers, even if you think they might be better. If you are unsuccessful, try to obtain some verbal or written feedback about how you could improve your CV or your interview skills. Remember there are always medical jobs so you will find something.

Membership exams

To progress beyond through the ST years you will need to complete the membership exams of your chosen speciality and meet the appropriate level of competency. The exams are difficult (often only ~30% of candidates pass per exam) and expensive. Most membership exams take place 2–3 times a year. You need to apply about 2–4mth before each exam. For the contact details of the various Royal Colleges see p637.

Medicine Regional centres in London, Edinburgh, Glasgow and Dublin, however all centres use the same exams. The MRCP has three sections:

- *Part 1 Written* basic science, £330, ≥18mth after graduation
- *Part 2 Written* clinical, £330, <7yr since Part 1
- *PACES* clinical skills, £520, <2yr and <3 attempts since Part 2

You need to pass Part 1 to apply for the ST3 year. For competitive ST3 posts Part 2 and PACES may be necessary.

Surgery Regional centres in London, Edinburgh, Glasgow and Dublin, however all centres use the same exams. The MRCS has three parts, once you attempt Part A you only have 3yr to complete the MRCS:

- *Part A Written* basic science and clinical, £395, eligible from graduation
- *Part B Interviews (viva)* £395, eligible after part A
- *Part B Clinical and communication* £410, 1mth after Part B interviews

To apply for an ST3 position in surgery you need to have completed the entire MRCS.

General practice You need to be a GP registrar before you can take the nMRCGP exams (this costs about £200 a year and is essential). There are three parts and no time limits though the GP registrar post is a year long:

- *AKT* (written exam) £360
- *CSA* (clinical skills) OSCE stations, £1260
- *WPBA* (portfolio) this is very similar to the FP portfolio and is free

To become a GP you need 2yr GP VTS experience in hospital and 1yr as GP registrar along with having completed the nMRCGP exams.

Other membership exams

Emergency medicine (MCEM) three part exam (two written and one clinical) required to apply for ST4; FCEM exit exam after ST

Anaesthetics (FRCA) Primary exam is required to apply for ST3; the final exam is required prior to progress beyond ST4

Obstetrics and Gynaecology (MRCOG) part 1 (written) eligible after graduation; part 2 (written + OSCE) after further 2yr O+G experience

Pathology MRCP Part 1 required for entry into ST1 except for microbiology and histopathology; MRCPath±MRCP required during ST

Paediatrics (MRCPCH) similar structure to MRCP; part 1 can be taken after graduation; all parts must be completed to progress to ST4

Radiology (FRCR) first part can be taken after graduation (but only allowed three attempts); final part required to complete ST

Psychiatry (MRCPsych) 12mth ST1 psychiatry experience before taking part 1 (three written and one clinical).

Continuing your education

Educational requirements You will be assessed throughout the FP to ensure that you are developing as a doctor and learning new skills. This will be done by Foundation assessments (p18), your portfolio (p24), meetings with your clinical supervisor, informal feedback from ward staff, presentations and attendance at teaching sessions. These assessments should not be difficult but it is essential that you complete them.

Study leave There is no formal provision for study leave for the F1 year; in the F2 year you will be offered the chance to spend taster weeks in specialities of your choice. You may be allowed study leave for specific courses but this will be at the discretion of your clinical supervisor.

Study expenses F2s may get a study leave budget of £300–400 per 6mth though this varies by deanery. Check with your postgraduate centre. You can only use the money for recognised courses and revision courses; never for sitting membership examinations.

Postgraduate courses There are hundreds of these and the costs range from free to >£1000 per day, most are about £100–150 per day. During the FP years Advanced Life Support (ALS) is important and may be compulsory. Check *BMJ* careers adverts section for potential courses and try to speak to other people who have done the course.

Exam planning Once you have decided on a career plan (p31), you will need to consider taking the appropriate membership examination. Membership exams are difficult and expensive but essential for career progression, so start early. See p37 or the relevant Royal College website (p637) for more detail.

Getting published

Having publications on your CV will give you a huge advantage when applying for jobs. There are many ways to get your name in print and you don't have to write a book (which is not great for the social life).

- *Book reviews* Get in touch with a journal and express interest in reviewing books for them; you don't have to be a professor to give an opinion on whether a book reads well or is useful.
- *Case reports* If you have seen something interesting, rare or just very classical then try writing it up. Include images if possible; get a senior co-author and ensure you obtain patient consent.
- *Fillers* Some journals have short stories or funny/moving one-liners submitted by their readers. Write up anything you see which others might be interested in; ensure you obtain patient consent.
- *Letters* If an article is incorrect, fails to mention a key point or has relevance in another field then write to the journal and mention this; it might be worthwhile asking a senior colleague to co-author it with you.
- *Research papers* If you have participated in research make sure you get your name on any resulting publications. If your audit project had particularly interesting results you may be able to publish it.

Audit

Audit is simply comparing practice in your hospital with best practice or clinical guidelines. There are six main stages to the 'audit cycle':

(1) Define standards (eg replace cannulas every 72h)
(2) Collect data (duration of placement for 50 consecutive cannulas)
(3) Compare data to standards (87% of cannulas replaced in <72h)
(4) Change practice (date of placement written on cannula dressings)
(5) Review standards (replace cannulas every 72h unless final dose in <2h)
(6) Since it is a cycle there is no end; once the standards have been reviewed the audit should be repeated to 'close the audit cycle'

Why does audit matter? The aim of audit is to constantly improve the quality of patient care; it allows a unit to applaud areas of strength and improve areas of weakness. Audits will also benefit you as an FP doctor since they are important in job applications and interviews and without at least one it will be hard to get an ST job. Try to do ≥2 during your FP.

Choosing an audit Almost any aspect of hospital/ward life can be audited. Choose something simple that interests you; alternatively look at relevant guidelines and choose one that is simple to measure.

Defining standards Try searching the National Library for Guidelines (accessible via www.library.nhs.uk); alternatively define best practice yourself by asking seniors and supervisors about what is expected.

Collecting data The simpler your audit the quicker and easier this will be. There are many ways of doing this including checking clinical notes, questionnaires and monitoring activities yourself. Try to make your methods objective so that you do the same for every set of notes/subject.

Compare data to standards The method for doing this depends on the type of data you have collected; it is easy to do some simple statistical tests on data, see p44.

Change practice Try to present your audit to relevant clinicians eg an FP teaching session or a ward meeting; use your findings to make feasible changes to practice and discuss these with the audience.

Review standards You may feel that the original standards you defined are still suitable, alternatively the process of auditing may have shown you that these standards need updating.

Close the loop Repeat the data collection to see if the changes to practice have made a difference; it is a good way to stay in touch with old wards and looks fantastic on a CV.

Example audits A few ideas:

- Are ECGs performed within 20min in ED patients with chest pain?
- Are drugs prescribed in accordance with local guidelines?
- Is there soap and alcohol gel in all dispensers?
- Do patients admitted with chest pain have their cholesterol measured?
- How long does it take different doctors to answer their bleep?

Presentations and teaching

The thought of having to give an oral presentation provokes anxiety in most of us. Being able to relay information to an audience is a valuable skill and one which gets easier with time and experience, though it is helped by a logical approach.

Types of presentation There are four main types of presentation: audit/research, journal club (critical appraisal of research), case presentation and a teaching session.

When is the presentation? If you have months to prepare then you can really go to town, whilst if you have only a few hours you need to concentrate on the essentials.

How long should it last? A 5min presentation will still need to be thorough, but less detailed than that lasting an hour. The length of the presentation will also aid you in choosing the topic.

What is the topic? Clarify as early as possible the topic you are to present and any specific aspect of the topic you should be discussing. If you can choose the topic, select something you either know about or are interested in researching.

Audience Are you presenting to your peers, your seniors or juniors? Are they ignorant of the topic or world experts? This information will determine the level of depth you need to go into.

Venue and means of delivery Are you expected to present with acetates on an overhead projector (OHP) or via a computer and projector? If you are using an OHP (now very uncommon) then you should make your slides on computer and print them out.

Sources of information Do you already have books on the subject? Read about the topic on the internet by undertaking a search with an engine such as www.bmj.com. Search *Medline* using keywords; recent review articles are a good place to start.

If there is no information If you cannot find enough information then it is likely you are not searching correctly; ask librarian staff for help. If there really is a lack of information then consider changing the topic, or choose an easier approach to it.

How many slides? This depends on how much detail is present on each slide. On average 20–25 slides will last about 30min.

Slide format Don't get too clever. Slides should be simple; avoid borders and complex animation. PowerPoint has numerous pre-set designs, though remember it is the content of your talk the audience needs to be focused upon.

Presentation format The presentation is in essence an essay which the speaker delivers orally. It should comprise a title page with the topic, speaker's name and an introduction which states the objectives. The bulk of the presentation should then follow and be closed with either a summary or conclusion. Consider ending with a slide acknowledging thanks and a final slide with simply 'questions?' written on it to invite discussion.

Titles Give each slide a title to make the story easy to follow.

Font Should be at least size 24. Ensure the text colour contrasts with the background colour (eg yellow text on blue background). Avoid using lots of effects; stick to one or two colours, **bold**, *italics* or underline features.

Graphics Use graphics to support the presentation; do not simply have graphics adorning the slide to make it look pretty.

How much information Avoid overcrowding slides; it is better to use three short slides than one hectic one. Each slide should deliver one message and this should be in six points or less.

Bullet points Use to highlight key words, not full sentences.

PowerPoint effects Keep slides simple. Never use text flying in from all directions and avoid using sound effects as these distract the audience.

Rehearsing Go through the presentation a few times on your own so you know the sequence and what you are going to say. Then practice it in front of a friend to check timing and flow.

Specific types of presentation

Audit/research Ensure you give a good reason why the audit or research was chosen and what existing research has already been undertaken. State your objectives, your method and its limitations. Use graphs to show numerical data and clearly summarise your findings. Discuss limitations and how your audit/research may have been improved. Draw your conclusions and indicate where further research may be directed. Thank the appropriate parties and invite questions/discussion. See audit/research section, p39/43.

Journal club Begin with a brief explanation of why you have chosen to discuss the particular clinical topic and list the articles which you have appraised. Aim to include why the study was undertaken, the appropriateness of the study, the methods and statistics used, the validity of the study and make comparisons between different studies. Include latest guidelines and invite discussion regarding how the research may affect current clinical practice. Finish with a summary of the studies undertaken, their results and where they were published for future reference.

Case presentation The presentation should tell a story about a patient and let the audience try and work out the diagnosis as though they are clerking the patient for the first time. Name the talk something cryptic, eg 'headache in the traveller'. Present the history and physical examination. Invite audience suggestions for the diagnosis and management. Give the results of investigations and again invite the audience to comment. Give the diagnosis and discuss subsequent management. Summarise with an outline of the topic and management; end with a question/discussion session.

Teaching session It is helpful to base a topic around a patient if this is appropriate. Keep the session interactive; have question slides where the audience can discuss answers. Summarise with learning points; it is helpful to provide a hand-out of your slides for people to take away (see p63).

Giving the presentation

Equipment Ensure that the projector/computer you need will be available well in advance. Ideally check it works and leave enough time to find new equipment if there is a problem.

Timing Arrive early and check your slides project correctly. Leave the title page projected so the correct audience attends.

Speaking You need to talk loudly enough to be heard at the back of the room. This can be daunting, but a good presentation given inaudibly is more disappointing than a poor presentation delivered audibly.

Body language Stand at the front of the audience and avoid walking into the projected image. Direct your talk at the audience, not the screen. This makes you appear more confident and also allows you to gauge if people are confused or bored.

Beginning Introduce yourself and your position, outline the topic you are going to talk about and explain why you chose the topic. This is a good time to interact with the audience; ask if people at the back can hear you.

To use notes or not You should not need notes to prompt you but have them available; points on the slides should be enough.

Style Keep it professional, but show you are human; it is acceptable to be light-hearted and make the audience laugh.

Pacing You probably speak quicker than you think; take your time, pause and allow the audience to read all your points.

Questions Decide in advance if you would like questions to be asked during your presentation or at the end. Anticipate what questions may be asked and prepare for these. Do not be afraid to say you do not know the answer, though offer to find out.

Feedback

Whenever possible ask for constructive criticism from someone who saw your presentation and try to learn from their comments.

Summary of points for a good presentation

- Plan well in advance
- Keep slides simple, avoid unnecessary graphics
- Rehearse your talk
- Try to stay calm and speak clearly
- Look at the audience, not the screen
- Thank the audience for attending

Research and academia

Research Whatever your views on academia it is a fact of medicine that if you want to do well (ie become a consultant/GP) then a spot of research is almost essential. You don't need to cure cancer; it can be a very simple project (eg an audit) so long as it can be published.

Academia Is not turning your back on clinical medicine, but rather adding a new dimension to your clinical experience. Most academic doctors do research alongside clinical work, for example three months on the ward, three months in academia. There are many advantages (interest, world-wide conferences, really understanding your subject, making a difference) but pay is not one of them. MMC includes a training route for academics detailed below. This is not the only way in; if at any stage you want to do research or a PhD there are always opportunities if you look.

Foundation years There are small numbers of two year academic Foundation Programmes. These are often a normal F1 year with a 4mth academic attachment in F2 (eg academic rheumatology); a few have academic components scattered throughout F2±F1.

ST years There are also academic ST positions called Academic Clinical Fellowships available in the same specialities as ST1 posts. They are three years long (equivalent to ST1–3) and are mostly clinical but with 25% of working time set aside for academia. The first year will be almost entirely clinical; the purpose of the second and third years is to give you the opportunity to design a PhD/MD research project and apply for funding. Once you successfully get funding you enter the Training Fellowship.

Training fellowship This is a three year research project designed by yourself with the aim of getting a PhD/MD with small amounts of protected clinical time to maintain your skills.

Clinical lectureship With your PhD/MD under your belt you can now apply for a four year lectureship post. This will give you clinical experience equivalent to ST4/5 and allow you to pursue postdoctoral research interests. You will again need to apply for funding eg a Clinician Scientist Fellowship. Once you have completed this post you will be eligible for consultant or senior lecturer positions.

Finding a project If you get an academic clinical fellowship you may be presented with options for research projects. Outside of fellowships you will need to actively seek out projects (eg *BMJ* careers, approaching professors). Keep three things in mind: (1) do I get on with the supervisor? (2) does the project interest me? (3) where will the project lead? (ie will you be able to apply for the career or subspeciality that you want?).

Funding One of the downsides of academic medicine is that you often need to raise funding to pay for yourself and your research. The process takes a long time (eg 6mth) and involves filling in vast numbers of forms (but form filling is a transferable skill…). If you are on a fellowship your supervisor should help you to search for options.

Medical statistics

Observational studies

Cross-sectional Looks at a sample of the population at one moment in time; used to highlight potential risk factors and determine prevalence.

Case-control (retrospective) Patients with a disease (cases) are asked about their previous exposure to potential risk factors. People without the disease (controls) are asked the same questions and the two groups are compared. Case-control studies are quick, relatively cheap and suitable for rare diseases.

Cohort study (prospective) A defined sample of the population is observed over time to see who develops diseases or complications and what risks they were exposed to. Cohort studies take a long time (years), are expensive and ineffective for rare disease.

Intervention studies/clinical trials

These are trials that compare new treatments against a placebo or the old treatment (as a control). Ideally the trials should be:

- *Randomised* allocating patients to a particular treatment by a random process
- *Blind* the patient is unaware which treatment they were given
- *Double-blind* both the patient and the researcher were unaware which treatment the patient was given

Meta-analysis

This is a powerful technique for answering clinical questions by mathematically combining the results from numerous similar trials into a single paper. The results are dependent on the quality of the trials included.

Level of evidence

Different study designs are ranked according to their 'level of evidence' (below), though a good cohort study may be much better evidence than a bad randomised controlled trial.

The level of evidence

High level ↑	Meta-analysis
	Randomised controlled trial
	Clinical trial
	Cohort study
	Case-control
Low level	Cross-sectional

Evidence-based medicine (EBM)

This is the process of using research results to guide clinical practice so that patients get the best possible care. The aim is to use the highest level of evidence to answer clinical relevant questions. Some useful sources are available via the National Library for Health (www.library.nhs.uk) including *BMJ* clinical evidence and The Cochrane Library.

Population tests (Does one group differ from another?)
These compare the averages of different groups, eg average life expectancy on treatment vs. placebo. Choosing the correct test is based on the type of data (see table below, definitions below and on the next page).

Nominal (categorical) data consists of groups that cannot be arranged in order, eg blood types, eye colour.

Ordinal Data consists of labels (non-numeric eg A-level grades) or subjective numbers (numeric) that can be arranged in order eg rate your pain out of 10.

Metric (interval) data consists of objective numbers. These either have units (eg weight) or count observations (eg number of patients in clinic). The key consideration is that the numbers can be used mathematically: 2 x 35kg = 70kg (metric), but 2 x 2/10 for pain ≠ 4/10 for pain (ordinal).

Type of data	Average	Distribution	Statistical test
Nominal	Mode	Variance	Binomial, Chi-squared, Fisher's
Ordinal non-numeric	Median	Variance	Mann–Whitney, Wilcoxon, Sign test
Ordinal numeric	Median	Range	Mann–Whitney, Wilcoxon, Sign test
Metric non-parametric	Median	Range	Mann–Whitney, Wilcoxon, Sign test
Metric parametric	Mean	Standard deviation	*t*-test, ANOVA

Association tests (Does one variable change with another?)
These are used to investigate whether variables are related, eg survival time vs. size of the tumour. The data should be plotted on a scatter graph to assess the shape. The association could be:

- ***Positive*** the two variables increase together, eg BP and age
- ***Negative*** one variable increases as the other decreases, eg life expectancy and smoking

Correlation is the measure of an association between two variables. It is shown as a coefficient called '*r*' that is between –1.0 (negative association) and +1.0 (positive association). If there is no association the coefficient is 0. The significance of the correlation can be calculated from the coefficient using statistical tables. This table shows the correct test for calculating the correlation coefficient:

Type of data	Statistical test
One or both variables ordinal	Spearman's
Both variables metric	Pearson's

Regression this is the best-fit line on a scatter graph. Make sure the dependent variable is on the X-axis. The equation of the line can be calculated to predict other values.

Statistical definitions

Absolute risk (cf relative) chance of an individual developing a disease in a given time eg 1 in 9 women develop breast cancer during their lives

Average a mid-point of the data, may be a mean, median or mode

Continuous (cf discrete) data with a full range of fractions, eg weight

Dependent (cf independent) a measured variable that is affected by other variables

Discrete (cf continuous) data without fractions, eg number of patients

Distribution how widely the data are spread about the average; may be a standard deviation, range or variance depending on the type of data

Incidence (cf prevalence) number of people developing a disease within a set time; expressed as a number or a proportion of the population

Independent (cf dependent) a variable that is altered by the researcher or one that causes another measured variable to change

Level the number of categories in discrete data, eg gender = 2 levels

Likelihood ratio the increased chance of having a disease based on a test result; calculated from sensitivity and specificity

Matched when a control is chosen because their age/sex/height etc matches those of a case

Non-parametric (cf parametric) metric data that does not follow the 'normal distribution'; if in doubt assume non-parametric

Number needed to harm (NNH) the number of patients receiving a treatment without detectable harm per patient receiving harm

Number needed to treat (NNT) the number of patients who must receive a treatment for one of them to be identified as receiving benefit

Odds ratio the increased chance of contracting a disease following a specific exposure, eg 10:1 for lung cancer from smoking

Paired when two or more observations are made on the same person

Parametric (cf non-parametric) metric data that follows the 'normal distribution'; a graph of frequencies in each group should be bell-shaped

Prevalence (cf incidence) the total number of people with a disease. May be expressed as a number or a proportion of the population.

Relative risk (cf absolute) the change in absolute risk due to a certain action eg if lung cancer is 10 times more common in smokers compared with non-smoking controls the relative risk is '10'

Sensitivity proportion of true-positives correctly identified as positive, irrespective of false-positives; ie a highly sensitive test will always rule-in those with the condition. D-dimer has a high sensitivity for DVT/PE.

Specificity proportion of true-negatives which are correctly identified as negative; ie a highly specific test can be used to safely rule-out those without the condition. D-dimer has a low specificity for DVT/PE.

95% confidence interval the range of values around the mean that represent where the true mean would lie with 95% confidence

Moving and finding a house

Finding a new place to live and moving can be very difficult when there is no gap between your old and new job. It is important to set aside time (often annual leave) to find somewhere suitable as this has a major impact on your future lifestyle.

Hospital accommodation

Most hospitals provide relatively cheap local accommodation. The prices and standards vary widely – view the room before you sign up. Prices usually include utility bills. It should conform to the minimum standards shown on the BMA website (p636). Apply early since rooms may be limited; accommodation departments may have information on other properties too.

Finding a house

Look through local papers which often have weekly property supplements, alternatively visit or phone estate agents and ask them to contact you if a suitable house is available. If you are not living near your new job then the internet is invaluable – make sure you always see the house before signing contracts. The following addresses may help:

- www.rightmove.co.uk — Renting and buying
- www.fish4.co.uk — Renting and buying
- www.findaproperty.com — Renting and buying

Rental accommodation

Most rental contracts are for at least 6mth. You will usually need to pay electricity, water and gas bills and council tax on top of the rent.

Buying a house

Alongside the cost of the house there are many charges that need to be paid up front, often costing thousands of pounds. The largest of these is usually stamp duty which is calculated as a percentage of the house price:

House price	≤£125,000	£125,001–£250,000	£250,001–£500,000	≥£500,001
Stamp duty	0%	1%	3%	4%

Other costs include *solicitor/conveyancing fees* (~£300) and a house survey (~£350) if there is no Home Condition Report in the Home Information Pack (HIP) from the seller.

NHS removal expenses

If you have to move house (bought or rented) to start a new NHS job you may be entitled to receive expenses including a trip to find the property, stamp duty, removal company and all the fees mentioned under 'buying a house' above. Search for 'removal expenses' at www.nhsemployers.org.

Storage units you can store furniture and other possessions securely for about £50–100/mth. Use the internet to find a local company.

Van rental you can rent a decent sized van for about £50–100 a day. You need to have held a driving licence for ≥2yr and be ≥21yr.

Working in the UK (from abroad)

Europe Doctors who are European Economic Area (EEA) or Swiss nationals and trained within the EEA or Switzerland can apply for registration with the GMC without taking further exams.

Outside Europe There are three short cuts to GMC registration:
- *Sponsorship* by a Royal College or approved institute (requires at least 3yr clinical experience), see contacts on www.gmc-uk.org
- Completion of a UK *Membership Exam* eg MRCP, see p37
- Eligibility to enter the UK *specialist or GP register* (see PMETB (www.pmtb.org.uk))

Otherwise doctors must pass three exams:
- *IELTS* (International English Language Testing System) a 3h test of academic English including speaking, reading, writing and listening. It costs about £95 and can be taken around the world. Doctors need to get 7/9 overall with at least 7/9 in speaking and at least 6/9 in all the other sections. See www.ielts.org for more details.
- *PLAB part 1* (Professional and Linguistic Assessment Board) a clinical MCQ that can be taken in test centres around the world for £145
- *PLAB part 2* a 14-station test of clinical skills which must be taken in London and costs £430

The PLAB exams are organised by the GMC and application forms are on their website. Passing these exams entitles the doctor to provisional or full registration with the GMC.

Provisional registration costs £100 for 1yr. It entitles the holder to work in a supervised F1 post in the NHS. Note limited registration no longer exists.

Visa application See www.ukvisas.gov.uk for details by country.

Getting a job this is the hardest part; it is no longer necessary to get a job to obtain registration. Foundation Programme, ST, consultant and GP jobs are very competitive in the UK; Foundation Programme jobs are offered to UK doctors first. There is no longer a deficit in junior doctors so all posts are competitive. It is essential to have a well-presented CV (p32), good references and to apply for appropriate jobs. See p30 for more details. Consider applying through locum agencies (p636).

Job discrimination, including the job application process, is illegal in the UK. Trusts should have an equal opportunities policy that actively prevents such discrimination occurring. If you think that you have been or are being discriminated against then contact the BMA (p636).

Further information look at 'Registration for doctors' and 'International Medical Graduates (IMG)' on the GMC website; see PMETB (www.pmetb.org.uk) for eligibility criteria for specialist or GP register.

Working abroad (from the UK)

When to go The gap between F2 and ST provides an ideal opportunity for jobs abroad and travelling. It also gives more time to consider which career path to follow. There are no set rules and working abroad can be arranged at any stage. The longer you work the more you will be tied down by a training post, finances or family.

Career impact Working abroad is viewed favourably by many employers, but will probably not count towards your training. The key concern is that you are able to justify your trip in an interview. This does not mean that you can't have fun – just make sure there is enough substance to your time out to be able to make it sound good.

Australia and New Zealand These countries are the most popular choice; they are sunny, laid back and provide a reasonable salary for a 38h working week. The health service is similar to the NHS and no special exams are required. Posts may include a stint of working in a rural setting – be sure you know exactly where you will be expected to work.

Europe A British medical degree entitles you to work throughout Europe without extra exams, though obviously language may be a barrier.

USA You must pass the USMLEs which consist of two MCQs (basic sciences and clinical, about $870 each in UK) and a language and clinical skills exam ($1200 in USA only); apply at www.ecfmg.org. With these exams you can apply for a 3yr residency (similar to FP though often in a single speciality) or 4yr fellowship (similar to ST) post via the competitive internet matching scheme (ERAS, www.aamc.org). You will need to attend interviews in the USA. You must do both your residency and fellowship in the USA if you want to work there long term.

Canada The 'evaluating exam' (£510 in UK) and two 'qualifying exams' (£350 and £740 in Canada only) are required for registration.

Finding jobs Talk to your colleagues; many doctors have spent time abroad and may have contacts and ideas. *BMJ Careers* has a short international section. Alternatively the internet is an excellent place to search. Medics Travel (www.medicstravel.co.uk) is also a good starting point. There are numerous companies willing to arrange work for doctors.

Developing world

Medecins Sans Frontieres (www.msf.org) offers placements of 6mth or more in challenging environments. You need at least 2yr post-registration experience, ideally post-membership. Living allowance of about £400 a month.

Voluntary Services Overseas (www.vso.org.uk) placements are of at least 2yr duration; you need at least 2yr post-registration experience. VSO will provide flights, a living allowance and accommodation.

NGOs and mission organisations These can provide diverse jobs all over the world. The Medics Travel website has a selection.

Other If there is a job you want then look for it, it will not look for you.

Working abroad (from the UK)

Chapter 3

Communication

Communication and conduct

Good communication with patients, your team and other health care professionals is an essential part of the job.

All communication

Whenever you are communicating with another health professional you should include the following details:

- Your name and role (eg Dr Charles Flint, F1 on Mercury Ward)
- The patient's name, location and primary problem (eg Eleanor Rigby who has chest pain in bed B4 on Neptune Ward)
- What you wish them to do (eg please give her some paracetamol)
- Urgency (eg as soon as you're free)
- How to contact you if there are any problems (eg I'm on bleep 3366)

Handover

At the start of each day you should receive a handover from the night team regarding any issues that have affected your patients. At the end of your working day you should handover any unwell patients or urgent jobs to the evening/night team. Giving them a piece of paper which clearly details the patient's name, location, medical problems and what you wish them to do makes life much easier.

Ward communication and etiquette

Your team (nurses and seniors)

- Do not hesitate to contact seniors if a patient deteriorates or you are worried; explain why you are worried and what you want them to do
- For non-urgent questions consider writing them down and waiting until you next see a senior
- Make sure that confidential medical information is not overheard
- Try to use the patient's name – this prevents mistakes
- Keep summaries/progress reports brief without missing details
- Never argue with colleagues in front of your patients
- Never make up answers; offer to find them out instead

Your peers (other F1/F2s)

- Keep a jobs list so you both know what is going on
- Have a low threshold for asking for a second opinion
- Help each other and 'share' any difficult tasks/patients
- If you finish your jobs make sure other F1/F2s do not need help before leaving the ward
- If you have serious difficulties working with another F1/F2 you can divide the wards/bays so that you cover different patients

Other health care professionals (HCPs)

- If referring a patient eg SALT/Physio you will need to give the same information as you would if referring to another medical team (p109)
- Listen to any concerns raised and take recommended actions
- Keep them updated about the patient's status, location or care
- See p92 for guidance on the role of different HCPs

Giving information over the telephone

- Establish who the caller is and what they want to know
- If in doubt, take their number and offer to call them back
- For discussions with outside agencies (ie not NHS) see p62
- Make sure you have the patient's permission before disclosing information on their progress to relatives or friends, see p54
- If you are discussing the patient with colleagues (eg a referral), try to use a private office to avoid being overheard

Written communication

Self-discharge If your patient decides to discharge themselves, try to explain why they need hospital management and what might happen if they leave (be blunt but honest). If you think the patient lacks the capacity (p68) to make this decision or requires sectioning (p535) then consult your seniors urgently. If they still want to self-discharge then ask them to wait whilst you contact a senior to discuss their issues. Failing this if they are capable to make the decision then ask them to sign a self-discharge form (saves a lot of paperwork for the nurses). If these are unavailable you can always write your own on a piece of blank paper (below). You, the patient and a second witness (eg nurse) should sign it, recording the time and date and the patient's decision. Keep it in the notes and inform the GP if relevant. Arrange follow-up and TTOs as usual.

16/09/08 *Seabright Ward, McBurney City Hospital*
21:45

I, Iago Trogsplotter state that I am leaving this hospital against medical advice.

Signed:	*Iago Trogsplotter*
Witnessed by:	*CJ Flint (Dr CJ Flint)*
And:	*T Baxter (Senior Nurse T Baxter)*

A self-discharge note

Clinical notes see p102

Referral letters see p110

Sick notes see p108

TTOs see p106

The importance of listening

Listening to your patient helps you gain an insight and appreciation about their worries. Their concerns may be things you can address and reassure them about, eg post-op pain.

Listening to colleagues and peers at work helps you develop your own style and pick up tips. Positive and negative feedback on your performance is important to make you a better doctor, no one starts off perfect.

Professional conduct

As a doctor you are a respected member of the community and a representative of the medical profession. People will expect you to act in a professional manner; this does not mean you cannot be yourself, but you must be aware of expectations:

- Always introduce yourself, especially over the telephone or when answering a bleep; 'Hello' is not acceptable
- Wear your ID badge at all times in hospital
- Never be rude to colleagues/ward staff; you will get a bad reputation
- Never be rude to patients, no matter how they treat you
- Never: shout, swear, scream, hit things or wear socks with sandals
- Avoid inappropriate slang, especially swear words
- Do not gossip about your work colleagues; address any issues you have with a colleague directly and in private
- When you do something wrong, apologise and learn from your mistake; it's a natural part of the learning curve
- If you are going to be late, let the person know in advance especially for handover or ward rounds

In a similar vein, a few simple actions can make life much easier:

- Learn the names of the people you are working with
- For difficult referrals make the effort to speak face to face
- If you think it is not appropriate for you to do a job then run it by the ward staff or your seniors
- Ask for help if you feel overrun with tasks

Patients' relatives

Communication with relatives can be very difficult; they tend to assume the worst and are in a very frustrating position of never knowing what is going on. Added to this they may have a full time job that prevents them simply visiting for the ward round or coming during the day:

- If you are on-call and do not know the patient then be honest about this; explain what times the usual ward staff will be present. If it is a simple request you may be able to help.
- Try to arrange a time when you can discuss the patient's progress at leisure in a quiet room (ask a colleague to hold your bleep)
- To avoid repeating yourself, speak to the family collectively or ask them to appoint a representative
- Check the patient is happy to have their confidential medical details discussed (p67) and encourage them to be present if possible
- Address concerns and answer each question in turn
- Be honest and aware of your limitations; if necessary ask them to arrange a time to meet with a senior
- Keep the meeting professional (see above)
- If things get heated, excuse yourself, take a few moments to calm down (p80) then return. If this doesn't work, speak to your seniors.
- Always document in the notes the date and time, what was discussed and who was present

Patient communication

A patient's perception of your abilities as a doctor depends largely on your communication (and phlebotomy) skills. Remember that patients are in an alien environment and are often worried about their health.

Introductions Always introduce yourself to patients and clearly state who you are. You are more approachable if you use your first name rather than Dr X. Check it is the right patient from their full name and date of birth (this also gives a rough guide to their mental state) and ask what they like to be called. Patients meet many staff members each day so it is important to reintroduce yourself each time you see them:

'Hello, my name is Charles and I'm one of the doctors working on this ward. Are you Doris Green?' 'Yes dear, but I like to be called Vera.' 'OK Vera, what's your date of birth…'

General communication Try to avoid using medical jargon. It is easy to get worse at this as your career progresses and you become more familiar with medical language. Also patients may be unaware of the implications behind conditions; the phrases 'needing help to breathe', 'not reacting to pain' and 'hole in their bowel' could all sound quite innocent.

Honest replies Patients have a right to know what is going on with their body. If a patient asks you a direct question try to give a direct answer; if you are unable to do so then explain why. If you do not know the answer, say so and offer to find out; do not try to guess the answer.

Procedures You should fully explain all procedures and obtain informed verbal or written consent before starting them (p69). Your explanation should include why the procedure is necessary, how much it will hurt (be honest, blood gases can be painful) and what the patient can do to help (keep still, sit up etc).

Results Explain why the investigation was performed, what it shows and what this means. If an X-ray or scan shows a clear image of the problem then show it to the patient. Showing other tests (especially ECGs) can cause more confusion than benefit.

Diagnosis Try to give the everyday name rather than a medical one (heart attack instead of MI). Explain why this has happened and if it is not something the patient has done, then say so. A patient who understands their condition is more likely to comply with medication and seek appropriate help if their symptoms change. Encourage them to learn about the condition and recommend good websites (p636) or support groups.

Prognosis Along with the obvious questions about life expectancy (p57), patients are most interested in how their life will be affected. Pitch your explanation in terms of activities of daily living (ADLs), walking, driving (p646) and working. Bear in mind that patients may want to know about having sex, but are often embarrassed to ask.

Patient-centred care

The traditional medical model made the patient a passive recipient of care. Health care was done *to* people rather than *with* them. Many patients were happy with this, but the patient should be able to be in charge of their own health care should they so wish.

Our task as clinicians is to find out our patients' expectations of their relationship with their doctors and then try to fulfil these. From 'whatever you feel is best doc' to reams of printouts and self-diagnoses from the internet, neither extreme is wrong and our task is to help.

Patient expectations Find out whether your patient wants guidance to be advised what treatment may be best.

Respect their right to make a decision you believe may be wrong. If you feel that they are doing so because they do not fully understand the situation or because of flawed logic, then alert your team to this so that things can be explained again.

Find out their other influences, these can be very powerful. Examples include: religious beliefs, friends, the internet and death/illness of relatives with similar conditions.

Treatment expectations Patients may have clear expectations of their treatment (eg an operation or being given a prescription). These expectations are important sources of discontentment when not fulfilled. Find out what their expectations are and why. Useful questions may include: 'What do you think is wrong with you?' 'What are you worried about?' 'What were you expecting we'd do about this?'

Yourself in their shoes Make time to imagine yourself in your patient's place. Isolation or communication difficulties will heighten fear at an already frightening time. Long waits without explanation are sadly common. Aggression from friends or relatives is often simply a manifestation of anxiety that not enough is being done. Ask yourself 'How would I want my family treated under these circumstances?' then do this for every patient.

Ensuring dignity Hospitals can rob people of their dignity. Wherever and whenever possible help restore this:
- Keep your patients covered in resuscitations
- Ensure the curtains are round the bed on the ward round
- Make sure they have their false teeth in to talk and glasses/wigs on whenever possible
- Help them self-care when possible

Over-examination Patients are often clerked over four times for a single admission. This is frustrating for them and often seen as indicative of a lack of coordination within the hospital. Patients may need to be clerked and examined more than once, but the context of this should be explained carefully – is this to gain more insight about their condition or to allow a training doctor to learn? People rarely mind when they understand the reasons.

Keep examinations which are invasive or cause discomfort to an absolute minimum.

Breaking bad news

Ideally, breaking bad news should always be done by a senior at a predetermined time when relatives and friends± specialist nurses can be present. In reality you are likely to be involved in breaking bad news, often whilst on-call. It can be a positive experience if done well.

Preparation Read the patient's notes carefully and ensure that all results are up-to-date and for the right patient. Be clear in your mind about the sequence of events and the meaning of the results. Consider the further management and likely prognosis – discuss with a senior.

Consent and confidentiality (p69 and p67) A patient has a right to know what is going on or to choose not to know. Ask before the investigations are done and document their response. If a patient does not want their relatives to know about their diagnosis you must respect this. Always ask, do not assume – many families have complex dynamics.

Warning shot Give a suggestion that bad news is imminent so it is not completely out of the blue, eg 'I have the results from . . . would you like anyone else here when I tell you them/shall we go to a quiet room?'

How to do it the SPIKES model is often used:

Setting Ask a colleague to hold your bleep and set aside suitable time (at least 30min); use a quiet room and invite a nurse who has been involved in the patient's care. Arrange the seats so you can make eye contact and remove distractions. Introduce yourself and find out who everyone is.

Perception Find out what the patient already knows by asking them directly; this will give you an idea of how much of a shock this will be and their level of understanding to help you give appropriate information.

Invitation Explain that you have results to give them and ask if they are ready to hear them. It helps to give a very brief summary of events so they understand what results you are talking about.

Knowledge Break the bad news eg 'A doctor has looked at the sample and I'm sorry to say it shows a cancer.' Give the information time to sink in and all present to react (shock, anger, tears, denial). Once the patient is ready, give further information about what this means and the expected management. Give the information in small segments and check understanding repeatedly. Prognosis can be difficult; never give an exact time ('months' rather than '4 months'). Be honest and realistic. Try to offer hope even if it is just symptom improvement or leaving hospital.

Empathy Acknowledge the feelings caused by the news; offer sympathy. This will take place alongside the 'Knowledge' step. Listen to their concerns, fears, worries. This will guide what further information you give and help you to understand their reactions.

Summary Repeat the main points of the discussion and arrange a time for further questions, ideally with a senior and yourself present. Give a clear plan of what will happen over the next 48h.

Remember to document the discussion in the patient's notes (diagnosis, prognosis, expectations) with your name and contact details

Cross-cultural communication

For patients who can't understand or speak the same language as you, the consultation can leave them feeling isolated, frustrated and anxious. You may have to rely on a third party to translate for you.

Family members as interpreters

Address the patient directly and look carefully at the patient's response to gauge their understanding. Record the fact that a family member was used for interpretation in the notes.

Friends and relatives are commonly used as informal interpreters. The main drawbacks are the lack of confidentiality and the bias the relative may have on the patient's decision making – particularly when underlying family issues are present (you may be unaware of these).

Children can interpret for their parents from an early age, but again their views can bias the consultation and its outcome.

Conflict of interests if you think the relative is biasing the conversation or it is an important issue then explain that you are professionally obliged to request a trained interpreter.

Consent relatives cannot consent on behalf of adults, see p69.

Professional interpreters

Professional interpreters can be arranged before the appointment – ask ward staff or phone switchboard:

- Allow extra time for the consultation and check the interpreter is acceptable to the patient
- Address both the patient and the interpreter and look at the patient's non-verbal response to gauge their level of understanding
- Ask simple, direct questions in short sentences to avoid overloading or confusing the interpreter; avoid jargon
- Use pictures or diagrams to explain things wherever possible; provide written/audiovisual material in the patient's own language to take away
- If you cannot organise an interpreter, you may be able to contact a telephone interpreting service who translate for you and the patient directly over the phone (ask nurses or switchboard)
- Document that a trained interpreter has been used with their name and contact details so that the same interpreter can accompany the patient for future appointments
- Never assume you know what the patient wants without asking them

Who can interpret

Family
Friends
Hospital staff (switchboard may have a list)
Hospital interpreters
Local interpreting agencies
Telephone service with which the hospital has a contract

Other means of communication

The NATO phonetic alphabet is often used to prevent mistakes when relaying a list of letters or spelling a word over the telephone; numbers are pronounced differently as well:

Alpha	November	1 WUN
Bravo	Oscar	2 TOO
Charlie	Papa	3 THUREE
Delta	Quebec	4 FOWER
Echo	Romeo	5 FIYIV
Foxtrot	Sierra	6 SIX
Golf	Tango	7 SEVEN
Hotel	Uniform	8 ATE
India	Victor	9 NINER
Juliet	Whisky	
Kilo	X-ray	
Lima	Yankee	
Mike	Zulu	

British sign language (BSL) is used predominantly by the deaf as a means of communication. Below are the hand positions for the English alphabet.

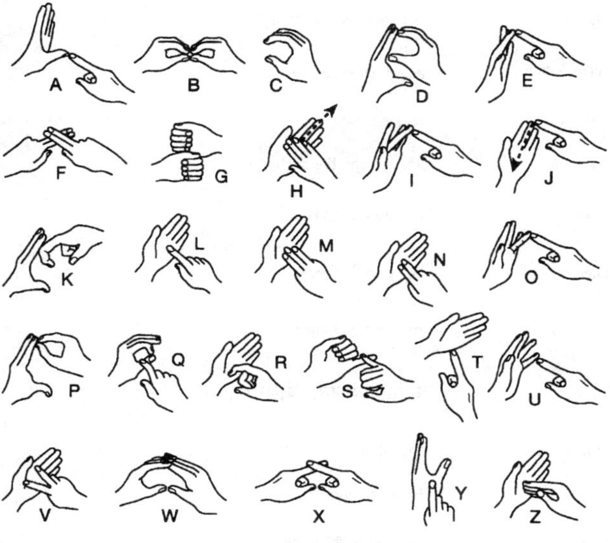

Languages

Ask the patient to point to their language below, which reads: 'I speak (this language)'

Albanian	Flas shqip
Arabic	أتكلم عربى
Bengali	বাংলা বলি
Bosnian	Govorim bosanski
Bulgarian	Говоря български
Cantonese	我 講廣東話
Chinese/Mandarin	我說中國話
Croatian	Govorim hrvatski
Czech	Mluvím česky
Dutch	Ik spreek Nederlands
Farsi/Persian	فارسی حرف میزنم
French	Je parle français
German	Ich spreche Deutsch
Greek	Μιλώ ελληνικά
Gujarati	હું ગુજરાતી બોલું છું
Hebrew	אנימדבר עברית
Hindi	मैं हिंदी बोलता (बोलती) हूं
Indonesian	Saya cakap bahasa Indonesia
Italian	Parlo italiano
Japanese	日本話を語します

Korean	한국말을해요
Latvian	Es runāju latviski
Malay	Saya cakap Melayu
Polish	Mówię po polsku
Portuguese	Falo português
Punjabi	ਮੈਂ ਪੰਜਾਬੀ ਬੋਲਦੀ ਹਾਂ
Romanian	Vorbesc româneşte
Russian	Я говорю по-русски
Serbian	Говорим српски
Slovak	Hovorím slovensky
Somali	Waxaan ku hadlaa luuqada af Soomaliga
Spanish	Hablo español
Swahili	Nisema Kiswahili
Turkish	Türkçe bilirim
Urdu	میں اردو بولتا (بولتی) ہوں

Difficulties with using an interpreter

- The interpreters may misunderstand technical terms or distort your questions
- Your questions and the patient's response may not be translated correctly
- The interpreter may influence the patient's response
- The patient/interpreter may avoid sensitive issues

Outside agencies

Outside agencies who could enquire about your patients include: police, media, solicitors, fire brigade, paramedics, general practitioner, researchers and the patient's employer. Patient confidentiality must be respected.

The rules

- Do you really know who you are talking to?
- Check and arrange to call them back unless certain
- Do they have any right to the information they are seeking?
  - GPs, health care professionals and ambulance staff may well do, police have limited rights (see below), many others do not
- Should you be the one discussing this or should a more senior member of the team?
- Do not talk to the media about a patient/your hospital unless:
  - You have the patient's permission
  - You have permission from your consultant/management (for trust issues)
  - You are accompanied by the trust public relations officer
- Do not 'chat' to a police/prison officer about a patient, no matter what the alleged circumstances; all patients have an equal right to privacy
- Breaching a patient's confidentiality without good cause is treated as misconduct by the General Medical Council.

Confidentiality and the police

Immediate investigation of assaults The police may well ask the clinical condition of an assault victim. 'Is it life-threatening, doctor?' The purpose of this question is to know how thoroughly to investigate the crime scene. It is reasonable to give them an assessment of severity.

In the public interest In situations where someone may be at risk of serious injury, disclosure is permitted by the General Medical Council. This should be a consultant-level decision.

The Road Traffic Act Everyone has a duty to provide the police with information which may lead to the identification of a driver who is alleged to have committed a driving offence. You are obliged to supply the name and address, not clinical details. Discuss with your seniors first.

Being a witness in court

Inform your clinical supervisor; they should accompany you to court. Remember you are a professional witness to the court, you do not represent either side and your evidence should be an impartial statement of the facts. Do not get rattled by the barristers – stick to the facts, do not give opinions, explain the limits of your knowledge/experience. Address your remarks to the judge. Wear your best suit. Ensure you get an expenses form from the witness unit and get this stamped/signed.

Medical research

You may be asked to provide a patient's clinical details for medical research. Ask the researcher to provide you with ID and if they have consent from the patient. It is reasonable to direct researchers towards appropriate patients to get consent.

Teaching medical students

Teaching will benefit you as much as the recipient; it will challenge you to fill any gaps in your knowledge and organise your thinking on the subject. You may not feel that you know enough to teach medical students but you are probably the best teacher on the ward for them, for two reasons:

- You have recently passed the finals exam that they are trying pass, probably at the same medical school
- Finals are meant to test core medical knowledge; this is what you do every day when you clerk and manage a patient

Portfolio keep a record of teaching sessions, ideally with feedback

Teaching principles

Whatever information you are trying to convey it is important to follow a few simple guidelines:

- Be clear about your objectives
- Plan what you are going to teach to give it structure
- Be interactive; this means that the student does some of the work and also they are more likely to remember it
- Try not to use too much medical jargon
- Give relevant examples
- Check the student's understanding and invite questions

Suitable patients

One of the worst parts of being a medical student is finding suitable patients to take a history from or examine. You can use your patient lists (p94) and firsthand experience of the patients to guide medical students to conscious, orientated and friendly folk or those with clinical signs. Better still offer to introduce the student.

Clinical examination

Offer to watch the student examine a patient and give feedback on their technique. You are likely to examine more patients in your first month as a doctor than in all your years as a medical student so your clinical skills will have advanced very quickly.

FP applications

With all the recent changes to medical training many students feel bewildered about what lies ahead. Once again you are in the ideal position to advise since you have already successfully applied for an FP. Simple advice about which are the best jobs, how to fill in the application form or even a copy of your own form can be a great help.

Clinical approach

You can also teach 'how to be a doctor' type skills that are rarely passed on. The trick is to choose a simple subject you know lots about eg:

- Managing chest pain/breathlessness
- Fluid management and volume assessment
- Writing in notes

If you're lacking inspiration try flicking through some of the chapters in this book.

Alternative/complementary medicine

A wide variety of alternative and complementary medicines exist, and many patients access them as either alongside or instead of 'conventional' therapy. Whatever your attitude to complementary medicine it is important that you understand what a patient means when they say they are using a particular type. Some therapies involve 'medications' which may cause reactions; ask about the supplier if this could be relevant.

Evidence supporting the use of these therapies is limited, though it is clear that many people obtain great symptom relief by using them even if the effect is purely placebo (much of your care will be placebo too).

Acupuncture this stems from Chinese medicine. 'Qi' flows around the body in health but in disease is disrupted; insertion of fine needles into certain points on the body helps restore natural flow.

Aromatherapy essential oils are extracted from plants (flowers, leaves, roots, bark etc) and used in massage, inhalation and baths to help restore harmony and balance within the body.

Chiropractice manipulation of the back allows harmony and balance to be restored to the whole body.

'Healing' various forms used, including Reiki (see below), crystal healing, distant healing, sound healing and faith healing.

Herbal medicine extracts of medicinal plants are used to treat illness, in a similar fashion to that of conventional drug therapy.

Homeopathy extracts of plant, animal and mineral are diluted to infinitesimal doses and used to stimulate the immune system.

Hypnotherapy combining elements of counselling and psychotherapy with hypnosis, an altered state of consciousness is induced in the patient to give relaxation and symptomatic relief of certain ailments.

Kinesiology muscle testing is undertaken by tensing, and used in conjunction with massage, touch, nutrition and counselling; used to balance the emotions and promote health, which fights off disease.

Massage stroking, tapping, light friction and kneading of the skin induces relaxation and improves circulation, which together lessen tension and can aid in self-healing and can be used in treating musculoskeletal injuries.

Osteopathy similar to chiropractic but whole musculoskeletal system.

Reflexology stimulation of specific pressure points in the hands and feet improves circulation, balances and relaxes the body and induces a sense of well-being.

Reiki therapist transfers Reiki energy to the recipient by touch or a non-contact method to increase energy levels and stimulate healing.

Shiatsu pressure is applied by the provider's fingers, hands, arms, knees and feet along with stretches and manipulation to stimulate energy flow.

Chapter 4

Ethics

Medical ethics

What is medical ethics?

Ethics are moral values, and in the context of medicine are supported by six main underlying principles:

Autonomy is the right for the individual to make decisions for themselves, and not be overtly pressurised or swayed by others (namely doctors, nurses, relatives etc). Patients should be allowed to contribute when decisions are made about their care. If an individual lacks capacity (p68) then it might not be appropriate to let them make important *autonomous* decisions.

Beneficence is concerned with doing what is right for the patient and what is in their best interests. This does not necessarily mean we should do everything or anything to keep a 90-year-old patient alive who has widespread metastatic disease. There will be times when it is *beneficent* to keep a patient comfortable, and allow them to die naturally.

Non-maleficence ensures care-givers refrain from doing harm to the patient, whether physical or psychological. An example of a breach in *non-maleficence* would be if a patient came to harm as a result of a doctor performing a procedure in which they had inadequate training or supervision.

Justice requires that all individuals are treated equally and that both the benefits and burdens of care are distributed without bias. *Justice* also covers openness within medical practice and the acknowledgement that some activities may have certain consequences – specifically legal action.

Dignity should be retained for both the patient and the people delivering their healthcare.

Honesty is a fundamental quality which doctors (as well as other care-givers) and patients should be expected to exhibit in order to strengthen the doctor–patient relationship.

Ethical conflict

Ethical dilemmas frequently arise in clinical practice and while the principles above do not necessarily provide an immediate answer, they do create a framework on which the various components of the conflict can be teased out and addressed individually, which often allows a harmonious solution to be identified.

Ethics and communication

It is quite common that apparently complex ethical issues arise because of a failure in communication between the patient or their loved ones and healthcare professionals. The solution to most of these conflicts is the establishment of effective and transparent lines of communication.

Patient confidentiality

To breach patient confidentiality is unlawful and unprofessional; several doctors are prosecuted and even struck off the medical register each year for this. You should be careful when talking about patients in public places, including within the hospital environment, and only disclose patient information to recognised healthcare staff as appropriate. Pieces of paper with patient information on must never leave the hospital and should be shredded if they are no longer required. **Do not leave patient lists lying around.** Personal electronic databases of patients should be disguised so individual patients cannot be identified.[1] You should never give any information (names or nature of injuries) to the police, press or other enquirers; ask your seniors to deal with these (see p62).

Publications Most medical journals insist that any article which involves a patient must be accompanied by written consent from the patient for the publication of the material, irrespective of how difficult it would be to track down and identify that patient.

Presentations and images If you are talking about a patient to a group of healthcare workers in your own hospital you do not need to obtain consent. If you are talking to an audience from outside your hospital it is advisable you seek the patient's consent. Equally, if you want to keep copies of radiographs or digital images, ensure these are made anonymous and if this isn't possible obtain the patient's written consent.

Relatives Your duty lies with your patient and if a relative asks you a question about the patient, it is essential you obtain verbal consent from the patient to talk to the relative; alternatively offer to talk to the relative in the presence of the patient. Relatives do not have any rights to know medical information. If the patient lacks capacity then seek senior advice before talking to the relatives. Document all conversations in the notes.

Children As above, if the child has capacity to give consent (see 'Gillick competence'/Fraser guidelines, p68), you must seek verbal consent from the patient to tell the relatives (parents) about their health. If the patient refuses, then offer to talk to the patient about their condition in the presence of their relatives. If you sense the situation will be difficult, seek senior advice/support.

Telephone calls Wards receive many telephone calls asking how patients are and if they have had tests or operations yet. The potential to break patient confidentiality here is great. Often there is a telephone by each bed, so encourage callers to speak to the patient directly. Otherwise, inform the patient who the caller is and relay a message from the patient to the caller. Apologise to the caller for not being able to offer any further information and suggest that you could talk things over with both themselves and the patient when they visit. See 'Outside agencies', p62.

1 Electronic devices on which patient information is stored outside of the hospital should be registered under the Data Protection Act.

Capacity (*OHAM2* p546)

Someone who has capacity can 'comprehend and retain information material [relevant] to the decision, especially as to the consequences of not having the intervention in question, and must be able to use and weight this information in the decision-making process.'[2]

For a patient to have capacity they must:

- Be able to take in and retain the information relevant to making the decision and consequences of refusal
- Believe the information
- Weigh up the information and arrive at a decision

Remember that:

- Patients may have the capacity to make some decisions and not others
- Capacity in the same patient may fluctuate over time

Capacity is most often impaired by chronic neurological pathology such as dementia, learning difficulties and psychiatric illness, but is also impaired by acute states such as delirium, acute severe pain, alcohol and drug intoxication (both recreational and iatrogenic (eg morphine)).

Children and capacity Children under 16yr of age were once regarded as lacking capacity to give consent, but now if the child meets the criteria above then they are regarded as having 'Gillick' competence (Fraser guidelines[3]), and may give consent. It is always advisable, however, to involve the parent or guardian in discussions about the patient's care if the patient allows.

No capacity When the patient does not have capacity and is over 18, family and friends are not able to make a decision on the patient's behalf; their views should, however, be listened to. In this situation, the patient is treated under the 'doctrine of necessity', that is, doing what is in their best interests until they attain capacity to make the decisions themselves.

Gillick competence/Fraser guidelines

Although 16 is the usual age at which young people are allowed to give their own consent, younger people can consent to most treatments or operations if they are capable. This follows a famous case in 1986 when Victoria Gillick went to the courts to get authority to be informed if her daughters sought contraceptive treatments. The law disagreed and decided that if the child was competent they could consent to treatment without their parents' knowledge – this is often referred to as being 'Gillick' competence when it matches the criteria in that case.

2 Department of Health reference guide to consent for examination or treatment.
3 Gillick or Fraser? A plea for consistency over competence in children. *BMJ* 2006;**332**:807.

Consent

Understanding consent and obtaining it satisfactorily can be difficult. If you are ever unsure seek senior help.

Obtaining consent The individual who obtains consent from the patient should be skilled in the procedure to be undertaken, be aware of the risks and benefits and be able to communicate the procedure in a language that the patient will understand. **If you do not regularly perform the procedure yourself then you must not obtain consent for it.**

Informed consent Consent should reflect the fact that the patient is aware of what is going to happen and why. They should be aware of the consequences of not undergoing the procedure, the potential benefits and any alternatives. The common risks and side-effects should be discussed, as should the potentially rare but serious consequences of the procedure. The patient should be provided with information well in advance of the procedure to allow them to think it over and prepare any questions they may wish to ask.

Types of consent There are five main types of consent:

- *Implied* the patient offers you their arm as you approach them with a needle and syringe to take blood.
- *Expressed – verbal* you explain that you are going to site a chest drain to relieve a pneumothorax, by describing the procedure and potential complications and the patient agrees to have it done.
- *Expressed – written* the patient is given an extensive explanation of the procedure and complications and informed of the alternatives. A record of the consultation is made which both patient and doctor sign. This document should be completed within 6mth prior to the planned treatment or procedure.
- *Consultant* if the patient lacks capacity to give consent then two senior doctors can consider the case. If, having considered the opinions of the next of kin, they decide the procedure is in the best interests of the patient, they can jointly give consent for it eg amputating a gangrenous toe which has rendered an elderly patient delirious.
- *Courts* in some rare situations, senior doctors may approach the courts to seek consent to treat a patient.

Difficult situations There are many situations where problems arise with consent issues. If in doubt seek senior advice or consult one of the medical defence unions (p636) which have 24h telephone support.

If a patient has capacity to give or withhold consent, and chooses not to receive treatment even in the face of death, then treating that patient against their will is potentially a criminal offence. This includes patients with psychiatric illness (*OHAM*2 p546).

HIV and consent Consent needs to be obtained from patients to test for their HIV status unless they are unable to give consent (lack capacity or unconscious) and knowing their HIV status would alter their management, or that of others following a needle-stick or other inoculation injury in exceptional circumstances – seek senior consultant advice.

Dealing with death

Fears

It is natural for patients to have a fear of death and dying. It is common to most of us. It should also be noted that many patients, especially the elderly, may be entirely at ease with the prospect of their own death.

If your patient is afraid, it is important to establish exactly what they are afraid of; this may be different from your assumptions:

- loss of dignity and control
- symptoms, eg suffocating/pain
- their relatives seeing them suffering
- the unpleasant death of a relative years ago

Many of these can now be carefully managed or even avoided. When the death is not expected and the deterioration sudden (eg trauma) then your role in talking to the patient and allaying their fear cannot be overstated. This can be emotionally difficult.

Breaking bad news p57

Other sources of help

Even with sudden deteriorations there are many other sources of help:

- Macmillan nurses and the palliative care team (see p122)
- the acute pain team (usually part of anaesthetics)
- the chaplaincy

Do not forget you're working with nursing staff who will know the patient much better than you, so discuss their care with them.

Sorting arrangements

Obviously, marching in and offering a priest and solicitor will be seen as insensitive, but be aware that the hospital will be able to provide legal support or an appropriate religious official if asked. Many patients' strongest wish is to die in comfort, often in their own home. Get the Macmillan and/or palliative care team involved early and this can frequently be arranged.

Do not resuscitate orders

This is a consultant-level decision. It should be clearly written in the notes, on a DNR form, signed and dated. This must be updated as the patient's condition changes. It should be discussed with the patients and/or their relatives. Always inform nursing staff.

Requests for euthanasia

Deliberately quickening a patient's death is illegal. Relieving suffering to the extent that you allow someone to die naturally, with dignity, is not.

- Explain you will always aim to minimise suffering
- Ensure you could justify your actions in court
- Explain to relatives that relieving pain may hasten an inevitable death, before giving opiates (relieving pain removes the adrenergic stimulus which may appropriately lead to a natural death within a few minutes)
- If ever in doubt, involve a senior colleague

Religion

Whatever your personal beliefs it is important to be aware of common religious beliefs as they will influence your patient's views.

Buddhism Started about 2500yr ago with the enlightenment and teachings of Siddhartha Gautama. Buddhists aim to leave the cycle of reincarnation through enlightenment by following the Dharma (teaching); belief in a god(s) varies. ***Features*** no special dress, only monks wear saffron robes; ***region*** Asia and Far East; ***text*** numerous, eg Suttas; ***building*** stupa/temple; ***diet*** vegetarian; ***festivals*** Wesak; ***death*** no special arrangements.

Christianity Began 2000yr ago with Jesus Christ whose life, teachings and resurrection guide followers and allows them to join God in heaven. Includes Catholics, Church of England, Protestants and many other denominations. ***Features*** no special dress; ***region*** predominantly Europe, Africa, Americas and Oceania; ***text*** Bible; ***building*** church; ***diet*** no restraints; ***festivals*** Christmas and Easter; ***death*** no special arrangements.
Jehovah's Witness A Christian denomination who believe that blood products are unacceptable. See p343.

Hindu Originated over 5000yr ago. Though exact beliefs vary widely, many believe in a supreme being (Brahma) who created many gods that perform different functions. Hindus aim to leave the cycle of reincarnation through good karma (consequences of actions) or enlightenment. ***Features*** females may have a bhindi on their forehead; ***region*** predominantly Asia; ***text*** Baghavad Gita and Vedas; ***building*** temple; ***diet*** do not eat beef or pork, may be vegetarian; ***festivals*** Diwali; ***death*** cremation.

Islam (Muslim) Founded 1400yr ago by the prophet Mohammed sent by Allah (God). Followers remain in the grave after death until the Day of Judgement when they may enter paradise. Muslim women may refuse male doctors. ***Features*** many women cover their hair±face; ***region*** predominantly Africa, Middle East and Asia; ***text*** Quran; ***building*** mosque ***diet*** halal meat, no pork; ***festivals*** Eid; the end of Ramadan (month of fasting) ***death*** burial.

Judaism Jews follow the laws of God as written in the Torah about 3300yr ago. Some Jews await a saviour/Messiah. People become Jewish by birth (Jewish mother) or conversion; after death there is an afterlife. ***Features*** males are circumcised and may wear a skullcap; ***region*** predominantly Israel; ***text*** Torah (first five books of the Bible); ***building*** synagogue; ***diet*** kosher food, do not eat pork or shellfish; ***festivals*** Hanukkah, Passover; ***death*** do not leave the body alone; contact a family member.

Sikhism Founded 500yr ago by Shri Guru Nanak due to Muslim and Hindu tensions. Sikhs believe in one god (Waheguru) and in reincarnation after death. ***Features*** men wear a turban (uncut hair), ceremonial knife, underwear, comb and steel bracelet; ***region*** mostly Punjab (India); ***text*** Shri Guru Granth Sahib; ***building*** gurdwara; ***diet*** may be vegetarian; ***festivals*** Vaisakhi; ***death*** do not move the body, cremation is preferred.

Chapter 5

When things go wrong

Medical errors

Every doctor makes mistakes varying from the trivial and correctable to the severe and avoidable.

What to do at once/within an hour

- Stabilise the patient, call for senior help early
- Do not compound the error by trying to cover it up or ignore it
- Correct where possible, apologising to the patient as appropriate
- Don't underestimate the seriousness of the situation; have a low threshold for asking for help to ensure things do not get any worse
- If serious and you have time, start documenting events, including times
- If, some time after an error, you realise you wish to add further details to the notes then do so **but** make it clear when these additions have been written by timing and dating them. This is perfectly acceptable.
- Retrospectively altering notes, so that it appears more had been written at the time than was the case, is serious misconduct

Serious untoward incidents – rare

- An apology is not an admission of guilt, so apologise and explain to the patient early. Apologise that the event has taken place, it is not necessary to 'give confession' at this stage.
- Inform your senior/consultant immediately
- If you believe your error has caused the patient significant harm then you should speak to your defence organization (p636). This is not an immediate priority.

Disciplinary procedures

If you have made a really serious error the hospital may choose to exclude you. That is, to send you home at once and ask you not to return until they have carried out preliminary enquiries. It is not a judgmental act but is designed to allow a calm and quick investigation. You must be informed why you have been excluded. You may be asked not to talk to others involved. If this happens to you, ring your defence organisation at once. You should be given a named person to contact in the hospital. You cannot be excluded for more than 2wk without a review. Go and stay with friends or family, don't be on your own. Let the hospital and others know how to get hold of you.

Less serious errors should be treated as a training issue and dealt with by your consultant initially or the trust clinical tutor/postgraduate dean. A period of close supervision or retraining may be appropriate.

Sources of help

- *Clinical events* your consultant, the clinical tutor, the postgraduate dean, your defence organisation
- *Non-clinical events* your consultant, the postgraduate dean, the BMA

Don't forget friends and family and remember that these events resolve extremely slowly, taking years in the big cases, so don't expect large numbers of answers in the first week.

Complaints

Every doctor has complaints made about them. These can be about your clinical ability, conduct or communication skills. They may be justified or spurious but they are inevitable, therefore do not feel your world has fallen apart when you are told a complaint has been made about you.

How the system handles complaints

There are two types of complaints – formal and informal. If a patient complains to you informally it is in everyone's best interest, and will save many hours of clinical time, if you are able to resolve the situation to the patient's satisfaction there and then. If you are unable to do so, but feel the problem may be solvable by more senior input, then call for help. Don't agree to do something which you are unable to carry out.

How to respond to a complaint

- All formal complaints are collated centrally in the hospital. In the rare event you are sent a complaint personally, do not respond but pass it to the complaints department.
- If a complaint has been made about the care of a patient you saw, you may be asked for a statement. This is an internal document and should be written as a letter, but bear in mind if the case goes to court this document could be requested by the patient's lawyers.
- Simply state the facts as you see them, do not try to apportion blame. You may be able to expand on your notes, particularly the details of conversations which may not have been documented.
- **Do not take it personally**
- If you feel it is clear how any error could be avoided in future then state this as well. Patients are often satisfied by knowing that any mistake they suffered will not be repeated for others.
- All the statements made by the staff involved are then collated and a letter is written on behalf of the chief executive (and usually signed by them) to the patient. This usually ends the matter.
- There are further steps, both with the trust and then regionally, if this is not enough.

Serious errors

- Preventable death of a patient
- Significant harm to a patient, in a predictable way
- Disciplinary offences including:
  - substance abuse
  - being drunk on duty
  - sexual/racial harassment

Incident reporting

Clinical incidents are defined as:

- Anything which harms patients' care or disrupts critical treatment
- An event which could potentially lead to harm if allowed to progress ('near misses'). They range from minor incidents, eg incorrect results, to life-threatening, eg wrong blood group in a blood transfusion.

Non-clinical incidents include:

- Incidents which involve staff, relatives or visitors
- Incidents which involve non-clinical equipment or property

The aim of incident reporting is to highlight any adverse incidents or 'near misses', assess them and to review clinical practice as a result. Ultimately it is designed to reduce clinical risks and improve the overall quality of patient care.

When a clinical incident/near miss occurs

- Make sure the patient is safe
- Complete a trust critical incident reporting form
- Forward the form to the clinical risk coordinator
- Inform staff involved of the outcome

Examples of all too common clinical incidents

- Blood samples from two different patients being confused
- Failure to report or follow up abnormal results
- Equipment failure
- Penicillin prescribed to patients who are allergic to penicillin
- Delay in treatment/management

Completing incident forms

- Fill in an incident form as soon as you can after the event so that you don't forget any relevant information
- Check you are filling in the correct form
- Include the time, date, staff involved as well as the issues being reported
- Check if the named consultant needs to fill in/sign the form
- If you are reporting an incident involving your colleagues, inform them and explain the situation. Learn from their mistakes without judging them.

The critical incident form is copied to clinical risk directors for evaluation at panel meetings, where changes to clinical practice are discussed.

Hints and tips

- If a critical incident form is filed involving yourself, don't assume you're a bad doctor; use it as a learning experience
- Find out the reason and circumstances and clarify the situation with the person filing the report
- Go over the incident and review your actions, asking if there is anything you would change; if it helps, discuss it with a colleague

McBurney City Hospital NHS Trust
Clinical Incident Reporting Form

Serious untoward incident? ~~Yes~~/No *Near miss*

Hospital: *McBurney City Hospital*
Patient's name: *Eleanor Rigby*
Hospital number: *W876470*
Consultant: *Singh*

Name/grade of submitting staff member: *James Smith*
Signature: *J Smith* Bleep: *3296* Date: *16/09/08*

Name of staff involved	Grade and specialty	Agency/locum
C J Flint	*F1, Medicine*	*N/A*

Brief details of incident:
Patient was prescribed co-amoxiclav 625mg/8h PO, despite penicillin allergy (this was stated on drug chart). This was noted by the pharmacist and the patient did not take any co-amoxiclav. The team F1 was contacted and an alternative antibiotic was prescribed.

Severity of outcome: *Nil – action taken beforehand*

Location: *E4 ward*	Date: *16/09/2008*	Time: *16:00*

Immediate action taken: *As above*

Near miss? Yes/~~No~~
Are the file notes attached? *To follow*
Equipment failure? ~~Yes~~/No
FAX/POST THIS FORM TO THE CLINICAL RISK CO-ORDINATOR FOR INVESTIGATION – FAX: 99999 INTERNALLY

Example of a critical incident reporting form.

Colleagues and problems

Most of us have worked with a colleague who worried us professionally – 'I wouldn't want to be treated by Dr X'. When does this become enough to do something? And what do you do?

Clinical incompetence

- The GMC is quite clear that we all have a clinical duty to report colleagues who we believe to be incompetent. This does not equate to pointing out every fault of every other doctor but it does mean that you cannot ignore serious concerns if you believe patients are being put at risk of harm.
- Serious concerns about a trainee should be passed to the relevant consultant. Ask to see them in private. It may be easiest to open the conversation with a question, to ask them to put your mind at rest, for example:

  'I don't know if you are aware that Dr X does not use chaperones? I've always been told we should use them for intimate examinations. I'm here because two women told me that they had felt uncomfortable with Dr X.'
- If the problem is with a consultant then you should either talk to another consultant or, if it is very serious, the medical director.
- If you are unsure whether a problem exists, or how serious it is, then talk to a friendly senior colleague informally (eg your supervisor or a clinical lecturer you got on with at medical school).

Recreational drugs/alcohol

- There is a massive difference between the doctor who drinks too much at weekends or who smokes the occasional joint and one who helps themselves to controlled drugs or has an alcohol problem.
- Likewise, regardless of substance, there is a difference between what someone does that only affects themselves and actions which affect quality of patient care. The badly hungover colleague is better sent to the mess to recover and made to pay the favour back some other time than get drug dosages wrong on the ward.
- Both being drunk on duty and misuse of controlled drugs are serious disciplinary offences and acts of professional misconduct. They are better tackled early whilst solvable than left until they ruin a career.
- It is unlikely that a colleague will change their behaviour simply because you have tackled them over it. Therefore consider discussing the situation with a trusted senior colleague as you may be helping them (in the longer term at least).

Psychological problems

- Every year doctors develop serious psychological illnesses just like the rest of the population and doctors are just as bad at self-diagnosis
- The more common problems include frank depression and hypomania, the rare include psychosis and schizophrenia (p312); the symptoms often come on gradually such that even close colleagues may not notice the transition from mildly eccentric to frankly pathological
- Depression may also mask itself whilst at work
- Talk to your colleague if concerned about their health

Hating your job

Experiencing problems at work is common and is usually transient. If you find that things do not improve try to identify the problem. However difficult things are at work, you should always remain polite, punctual and helpful. If you don't you may be the one perceived to be the problem.

Stress at the workplace

With the responsibility that comes with being a doctor and an intense workload, the demands of your job can leave you physically and mentally exhausted. On top of this there is the pressure of litigation and high expectations from your peers and patients. If you feel things are getting on top of you, take a step back and assess your workload. Speak to colleagues to find out if there are easier ways of doing things. Take some annual leave and upon your return approach your work schedule differently to help regain control over things. Make sure you have plenty of time to relax away from the hospital and keep up your outside interests. If things continue to be stressful, talk to a friend, contact the BMA (p636) for advice or discuss the situation with a trusted senior or mentor.

Bullying at work

Bullying can be from your seniors, peers, other health care professionals, patients or their relatives. If you feel you are being bullied, discuss it with someone, either at work or independently (eg the BMA). Speak to your predecessors to find out if they had similar difficulties and, if so, how they handled the problem. Keep a diary of relevant events, together with witnesses, and approach your consultant. If it is your consultant who is the problem, approach another consultant who you trust or speak to the BMA.

Sexual harassment

This may start very innocently and gradually escalate into intimidating behaviour which may affect your work, social life and confidence. In the first instance make it clear that their advances are not welcome and confide in someone you trust. Find out if other colleagues are also being harassed and report the harassment to your educational supervisor.

Discrimination

All employers must abide by an equal opportunities policy which includes standards on treating all employees. Before deciding to take things further confide in a senior colleague whom you trust. Keep a record of any events that stand out as being discriminatory, documenting dates, times and witnesses. Contact the BMA for advice (p636). You may have to submit a formal letter outlining your concerns, so make sure you are prepared to pursue a formal complaint before committing yourself on paper.

Handing in your resignation

If you can find no other option, you can always leave your job. Find out how much notice you are required to give and who to direct your letter of resignation to. During your last weeks, stay an active member of the team rather than taking a short-timer's attitude. Complete any outstanding work and tidy up loose ends before leaving.

Relaxation

Have a break there are few problems that must be solved immediately. Leave the ward, ask someone to hold your bleep and take 5min to unwind. Try taking deep breaths and concentrating on the feeling of the air rushing in and out of your lungs. Count the breaths and try to clear your mind. Try squeezing the muscles in your feet then feeling them relax; do this with all the muscle groups from your legs to your neck. Think about something you are looking forward to.

Do not let medicine take over your life. It doesn't take much to make life seem massively better; try the following:

- go for a walk
- watch a film
- go shopping
- exercise
- watch a comedy
- take a long bath
- go out for a meal
- talk to friends
- watch sport
- play a game
- have a good cry
- go to the pub
- have a massage
- cook
- plan a holiday
- talk to parents
- have a lie in
- listen to music
- have an early night
- join a class/club
- read a book

Try to avoid the following:
- Smoking
- Excessive alcohol
- Drugs/sleeping tablets
- Excessive caffeine

Causes of stress

Attitude

There is no point worrying about things you have no control over; it is natural to feel concerned about future events but almost everything will turn out well in the end, even if it is not as you have planned it.

The job

See p11 on being efficient. The job gets much easier with time; these skills become second nature and you perform individual tasks quicker.

Yourself

Be honest with yourself; are you tired? Everything is harder, slower and more stressful when you have not had enough sleep.

Think about what makes you stressed and whether this is a problem with your attitude, the way you do the job, other people or the nature of the job. Try to accept, change or avoid these stressors.

Other people

If someone is annoying you then consider telling them so. Plan how you will tell them, do it in private and do not blame them; just explain how it makes you feel. Most people will be apologetic and try to change.

If you feel it is all getting too much and/or nobody cares try speaking to:

BMA counselling (you don't need to be a member)	08459 200 169
Samaritans	08457 90 90 90

Chapter 6

Boring but important stuff

Pay and contracts

The number of hours you are allowed to work in a shift and the total for a given week are determined by two sets of rules:

- *European Working Time Directive* (EWTD), incorporated into UK law
- *'New Deal'* on junior doctors' hours, which is an agreement between the BMA and all the UK Departments of Health

EWTD

- Maximum of 56h of work a week until August 2009
- Maximum of 48h of work a week from August 2009
- 11h of continuous rest each day or compensatory rest must be given
- 24h continuous rest each week or 48h in a fortnight

New deal

- Maximum of 56h of actual work (on your feet) a week
- Maximum of 72h (in total) of duty (including on-calls) a week
- 30min break for every 4h of continuous work
- The New Deal also has detailed requirements about the length of different shifts types. More details on the contract can be found at http://www.dhsspsni.gov.uk/scujuniordoc-2.

Salary

Doctors in training are paid according to a banded contract which comprises:

- *Basic salary* which rises incrementally each year to reflect the trainee's greater experience
- *Banding multiplier* (see opposite) depending on the overall number of hours worked, the intensity of those hours and their antisociability

Monitoring and rebanding

- Monitoring of the actual hours worked by junior doctors is the main method of determining if the actual hours of the job mirror the theoretical hours of the rota. All training posts have to be monitored for at least 2wk by all participants every 6mth. This is a contractual requirement for the employer and employee
- If your post turns out to be monitored as a different band to the one you're paid then your pay can go up but is protected against going down. Your rota cannot be changed in such a way as to affect your salary without the agreement of the majority of the doctors on the rota
- The rules for 're-banding' and for pay protection are complex and are available on the Department of Health website:
    - www.dh.gov.uk/en/Policyandguidance/Humanresourcesandtraining/Modernisingpay/Juniordoctorcontracts/DH_4053873
- If you are a BMA member the *Junior Doctors' Handbook* is a good resource to find out more detail. It is available on-line to members:
    - www.BMA.org.uk/ap.nsf/Content/jdhandbook?OpenDocument&login&Highlight=2,junior,doctors,handbook

The structure of the NHS

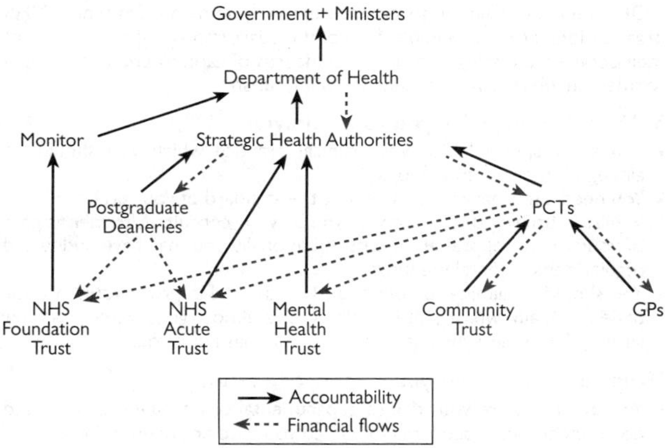

The Banding Contract

- ***Band 1*** total hours of actual work under 48h/wk
- ***Band 2*** total hours of actual work <56h but >48h/wk
- ***Band 3*** total hours of actual work over 56h/wk (now illegal)

Bands 1 and 2 are further subdivided depending on the intensity and antisociability of the out-of-hours component (Bands 2A and 1A the most antisocial, then 2B and 1B, then 1C the least antisocial or intense)

Banding Multiplier

These rates are subject to annual review as part of the doctors' annual pay award

Band 1A	1.5	Band 2A	1.8	Band 3	2.0
Band 1B	1.4	Band 2B	1.5		
Band 1C	1.2				

The latest basic salary rates can be found at:

- www.nhsemployers.org/pay-conditions/pay-conditions-2339.cfm

Clinical governance

DOH definition: 'Clinical governance is the system through which NHS organisations are accountable for continuously improving the quality of their services and safeguarding high standards of care, by creating an environment in which clinical excellence will flourish.'

What this means for you as an individual

- You are responsible for your clinical practice which you should be aiming to improve continuously
- You need a mechanism for assessing the standard of your practice
- Whilst in training this is done for you by your consultant/trainer as part of your regular appraisal process. Additionally you may have audits and regular departmental meetings.
- You should be aiming to continuously learn and improve your care for patients. Again, whilst still in training, this almost goes without saying; revising for endless examinations and diplomas helps too.

What this means for you as part of a team

- You should ensure you stick to departmental or hospital protocols and don't undertake procedures for which you have not been trained
- You will be asked to participate in regular departmental audits, usually of morbidity and mortality. These are used to ensure consistency of practice and to pick up problems early.
- You should attend departmental and hospital-wide audit meetings and grand rounds to keep up to date with changes
- You should answer any responses to complaints promptly

Clinical governance mechanisms

The clinical governance structure in every hospital includes:

- Audit of practice (eg reattendances within 1wk or wound infections)
- Appraisal and revalidation structures
- Regular departmental meetings (eg morbidity and mortality) to allow clinicians to compare their care and highlight common concerns
- Clear routes of accountability for all staff. It can be obvious when these have broken down, leading to problems which everyone can identify but seemingly no one is responsible for fixing.
- A risk management structure to identify practices which jeopardise high-quality patient care (critical incident reporting, p76)
- A complaints department to respond to complaints and ensure lessons are learned from them; may be part of the risk management dept
- A clinical governance committee/structure which oversees and ensures compliance with all of the above

Compliance with clinical governance mechanisms are measured both regionally and nationally.

NHS entitlements

As doctors working and training in the NHS you have certain entitlements, defined under your 'Terms and Conditions of Service'. Those relating to salary are discussed in 'Pay and contracts', p82. The others are listed here.

Accommodation

- Doctors in their first year after graduation are no longer entitled to free accommodation at their employing trust; accommodation should still be available, though there may be a charge for it.
- The standards of accommodation have been agreed between the BMA and the DoH. They are explained on the BMA website (p636) Contact the BMA if you feel your accommodation is unacceptable and the hospital is unwilling to resolve this.
- Substandard accommodation should be free.

Medical staffing/human resources departments

- These are responsible for your employment. They sign you on the payroll and keep track of leave taken. They are the first port of call for employment problems. Your details will be entered on the Electronic Staff Record (the national NHS staff register). Make sure these are correct as they will follow you into every job.

Leave entitlement

- Junior doctors are entitled to 5wk paid annual leave a year plus 2d for the old 'NHS statutory days', a total of 27d/yr or 9d/4mth (13.5d/6mth). You are rarely allowed to carry leave over between jobs/years.
- You will usually need to give 6wk notice for annual leave; your form will need to be signed by your consultant.
- Many posts have 'fixed leave' instead of allowing you to choose when to take it. Swaps are often difficult; ask your consultant or colleagues.
- If you need leave in a forthcoming post (eg getting married) write to let them know. Ask for the rota position which is off for those dates.
- You are allowed leave for bank holidays though not necessarily the days themselves. If you work any part of a bank holiday you are entitled to a day off in lieu.

Maternity/paternity leave

- This is complex. In summary: all women are entitled to 26wk paid maternity leave and must be allowed to return to work after this. If you've been working over 6mth then you can apply for an additional 26wk unpaid leave. Fathers are entitled to up to 2wk paid paternity leave if they have worked for over 6mth. Some trusts try to claim you must have worked the 6mth with them (not just the NHS). This is ill-defined, talk to the BMA if you have a problem.
- More detail is available in the *Junior Doctors' Handbook* from the BMA

Less-than-full-time/flexible training

- Foundation Programme doctors are entitled to train less than full time if they have a valid reason
- A comprehensive list of valid reasons (eg having a baby or ill health) and advice on how to apply is available from your deanery

Money and debt

As the average medical graduate debt now exceeds £20,000, financial management priorities have changed. This section is not comprehensive but aims to give some important pointers and warnings.

Debt clearance

Most graduates have three different types of debt:

(1) ***Short term*** high-interest debts (eg credit cards ±overdraft, if at full charge). Pay these back first and as fast as possible. Don't be tempted to extend them just because you have an income.

(2) ***Medium term*** commercial loans (eg a high street bank graduate studies loan). These should be paid back next, as spare funds allow.

(3) ***Student loans*** at very low rates of interest – pay these back as slowly as you wish provided the APR (Annual Percentage Rate) remains ≤inflation.

Pay close attention to the APR and charges attached to any loan arrangement. Interest-free loans or credit cards can help in the short term but ensure you don't get saddled with a high APR later. Loans are a competitive market so shop around – especially for something like a car loan where the car dealer rarely offers the best rate.

Think 'total cost' not just 'monthly repayments'.

Financial advice

Since you now have a salary increasing every year and virtually guaranteed for life, finance companies will swarm round you like wasps round jam. Beware of some very slick sharks – their aim is only to get you to buy their products. There is no altruism here:

- Truly independent financial advice is hard to obtain – ask how independent they really are
- Check what commission will be received for any product you choose, both to the individual who sold it to you as well as to their company
- Do not buy from the first or most persuasive salesperson, but take your time to consider what you really want and need

Some basic rules for financial planning

- ***Short term*** clear debts with the highest interest as soon as possible. Try to accumulate about one month's salary as 'emergency' savings.
- ***Medium term*** think about trying to save for the deposit on a property (even if just £100/mth). If debt-free consider a medium-term saving scheme (eg ISA) to reduce tax liability.
- ***Long term*** pension and mortgage.

Documents to keep safe for 7 years

P60 – sent every April to all employees
P45 – sent to you every time you change trust
Pay slips – issued every month
Record of additional income – eg locums
Annual interest statements from bank /savings/shares – issued annually

Financial and other products

NHS income support Pays you some income (though less than your basic salary) if you are unable to work for health reasons. Standard NHS benefits are poor especially for the first 2yr of employment.

Critical illness Gives a lump sum if you develop an incapacitating illness. Check if it still pays if you are capable of doing a less demanding job. Check if it pays for all conditions you may get at work.

Life insurance Pays out a lump sum if you die; only really makes sense if you have dependants.

Pension Stay in the NHS pension scheme. Consider a top-up if you can afford one, eg Additional Voluntary Contributions (AVCs); these are often stock-market based but should do well in the long-term. Starting early will cost you far less in the long term.

MDU/MPS Necessary additional protection for problems relating to clinical performance. NHS indemnity doesn't cover everything, eg Good Samaritan acts.

BMA Protection for non-clinical matters eg wrong salary or poor accommodation; the trade union for doctors.

Tax

Now that you are earning a salary you will be paying tax. Most will be collected by PAYE (Pay As You Earn). If you have no other sources of income then you can leave it at that. If you have any other income then you should ask for a tax return and complete it.

Tax codes The box on your first pay-slip will show you your tax code; it illustrates how many tens of pounds you are allowed tax-free (eg 543L = £5435, the basic allowance for 2008-09). You can add unavoidable expenses and subscriptions connected with your job to this, see below. The leaflet '*Understanding Your Tax Code*' is available from the Inland Revenue (IR).

Tax deductible It is possible to claim back the income tax you paid on:

- Job-related expenses (eg stethoscope); make sure you keep receipts
- Professional subscriptions eg GMC, BMA, MDU/MPS, Royal College

Tax returns A tax return is a long form asking for details of all the money you have received which may have tax owing on it. This includes your salary and other income whether earned (eg locum shifts or cremation fees) or unearned (eg lodger/flatmate, bank interest and dividend yields).

- If you are sent one then fill it in
- Return it by the end of September and they will do the maths for you
- Fill it in on-line and the maths is done automatically
- Return it after Jan and they will fine you £100/6mth plus interest
- Claim your deductible allowances but also list your additional income

The IR has been known to ask an undertaker to list all payments to doctors and then cross-check. If your tax is simple then tax returns are not hard to do, otherwise pay a company/accountant to do it for you.

Making more money

There are several ways to make money in addition to your basic income. It is crucial you keep records of all additional income and declare these when you complete your self-assessment to the Inland Revenue at the end of each tax year.[1]

Cremation certificates The cremation form has two parts (p113). The first is completed by a ward doctor (usually the F1) and the second by a senior doctor, often from another department. The first part takes about 10min to complete and the individual is rewarded about £70 for their trouble. The bereavement office usually handles the forms and issues the cheques. Make sure you see the body, checking identity and that there is no pacemaker (p113); they do really explode!

Published articles Several journals and medical newspapers pay authors for articles which appear in print. The amount varies from between £25 to £250 depending on the length and importance. The journals' websites often outline payment and the types of articles they are after.

Research There are usually several research projects being undertaken in most hospitals which require volunteers to have experiments performed on them. These range from a 5min interview to a week-long study and in most circumstances the volunteers are rewarded financially (£5 book token to over £500). These may carry a risk of harm.

Gifts The GMC are quite clear in their message that you should not encourage patients or their families to give, lend or bequeath gifts to yourself, others or to organisations.[2] If you are given a gift then it is acceptable to take it as long as it has negligible financial value. If you are given money then it is sensible to pass this onto the ward sister who can put it in the ward fund account.

Locums Most hospitals employ locum doctors to cover staff sickness or at busy times. Locum doctors often already work for the hospital, but work additional shifts for extra money; alternatively they may be from outside the hospital. It is important to remember that the hours you work as a locum should be added to your basic or regular hours and should not exceed the limits of the New Deal[3] or European Working Time Directive; some contracts may stipulate that you cannot work locum shifts in other hospitals or departments. There are many locum agencies that you can register with (p653), they are often advertised in *BMJ Careers*. Rates of pay vary, but an F1 can expect pre-tax rates of £15–25 per hour, and F2s £20–30. If your own hospital is employing you as a locum, you may be able to negotiate a better rate.

1 http://www.inlandrevenue.gov.uk/sa/
2 http://www.gmc-uk.org/standards/good.htm
3 *Junior Doctors' Handbook* 2007/08. British Medical Association.

Chapter 7

Life on the wards

The medical team

The changes to medical training have caused widespread confusion about the names and roles of different trainees. The medical team or 'firm' usually consists of four grades: (1) consultant-level, (2) registrar-level, (3) SHO-level, (4) F1 (house officer). Many firms have more than one doctor at each level so you may work alongside other F1s under two or more consultants.

Consultant-level These are the most senior doctors on the team; there are several posts at this level:

- ***Academic*** doctors who split their time between research and clinical medicine. They are often called 'honorary consultants' alongside an academic grade (eg senior lecturer, reader, professor).
- ***Consultant*** the most common post at this level reached by completing the CCST which is now called the CCT (p26).
- ***Associate specialist*** a doctor with consultant-level ability and experience who has not got a CCST/CCT. They do not have the accountability or management commitments of consultants.

Consultant role Consultants are responsible for everything that happens on the ward including the actions of junior doctors. They may lead ward rounds, work in clinics, supervise a laboratory or spend time in theatre; their level of involvement in the day-to-day running of the ward varies between specialities and management styles. They will perform your FP appraisals (p24) and are a good source of advice for careers, audits and presentations. If ever you need help and only the consultant is available then do not hesitate to contact them.

Registrar-level If you describe yourself as 'a registrar' most people will assume that you are at this grade. All of these doctors will share an on-call rota that is usually separate from the SHO-level on-call rota. The posts have a natural hierarchy according to experience:

- ***Specialist registrar (SpR)*** doctors training under the old system, this job will slowly be phased out as these doctors complete their training
- ***Staff grade*** a non-training post with equivalent experience to an SpR but not working towards a CCT award
- ***Clinical fellow*** a speciality doctor under the old system who is undertaking research; they may need to secure an ST3/4 post afterwards
- ***Clinical lectureship*** the academic equivalent of ≥ST3/4 they will split their time between clinical and research
- ***Senior speciality training registrar (StR, ≥ST3/4)*** in most specialities this grade starts at ST3, however it is ST4 in emergency medicine, paediatrics and psychiatry. These are the new run-through posts that work towards the CCT award and a consultant post.

Registrar role These doctors supervise the day-to-day running of the ward; they perform similar jobs to consultants (ward rounds, clinics, theatre) but without the management responsibilities. Registrars usually receive referrals from other teams and will spend time reviewing these patients. Their presence on the ward varies between specialities.

SHO-level This is where the training posts get particularly confusing; many senior staff members in the hospital will not be familiar with these new posts. Again there is a hierarchy of experience:

- ***Academic clinical fellow*** the academic equivalent of ST1–2/3 and CT1–2/3 at this level they will perform a similar role except that they have 25% of their time set aside for research
- ***Junior speciality training registrar (StR, ST1–2/3)*** doctors in specialities with run-through training (p26) who will progress to registrar-level specialist training unless they fail to attain competencies or exams. Despite the title it is misleading to call them 'a registrar'.
- ***Core-training (CT1–2/3)*** doctors in specialities with uncoupled training (p26) who can apply for registrar-level specialist training posts if they attain the relevant competencies and exams. The difference between ST and CT posts is the speciality, not experience.
- ***Fixed-term speciality training appointment (FTSTA)*** a post for doctors who were unwilling or unable to secure an ST/CT post. The post lasts one year and will be at ST1, ST2 or ST3 level; at the end of the year they can apply for an ST or FTSTA post at the next level if they have attained the relevant competencies. These posts are only found in run-through specialities (p26).
- ***F2*** doctors in the second year of the Foundation Programme; this will often be their first job in the placement, at the end of the year they will apply for ST/CT/FTSTA posts

SHO role These doctors are your first port of call for help. They can advise on patient management, ward jobs and supervise practical procedures; they often work alongside F1s on the ward though they may have clinic and theatre commitments too. They are an excellent source of advice on careers, applications, exams and training courses.

F1-level These are doctors in their first year with limited registration. They are still often called house officers or PRHOs from the old system.

F1 role F1s manage the day-to-day running of the ward including ward rounds, ward jobs, procedures and reviewing unwell patients; see p93 for more detail.

New career path		Old career path
Consultant		Consultant
ST3 and above		SpR
ST1/ST2	CT1/CT2/CT3	SHO
F2		1st year SHO
F1		PRHO, House Officer

Comparison of common training positions in the new and old system

The multidisciplinary team

Nurses have a 'hands-on' role, ranging from administering medications to attending doctors' rounds. Don't be afraid to ask their advice – their experience means they can often help you out. Most can take blood and perform ECGs, some can cannulate and insert male urinary catheters (all female nurses should be able to insert female catheters).

Bed managers are highly stressed people who are in charge of managing the hospital beds and arranging transfers and admissions. They take the brunt of the 4-hour rule in the ED when patients breach whilst waiting for a bed. They will frequently ask you when patients are likely to be ready for discharge so they can plan ahead for routine admissions.

Discharge coordinators work in conjunction with social workers, physiotherapists and occupational therapists to expedite patients' discharge. They often assist in finding intermediate care placements.

Healthcare assistants (HCAs)/nursing auxiliaries (NAs) perform more basic nursing tasks such as attending to patient hygiene needs and recording observations including finger-prick glucose. They cannot dispense medication or give injections, but many can take blood.

Nurse practitioners are specially trained senior nurses who can assess acutely unwell patients, perform practical procedures (eg cannulation) and assist in theatre. Most cannot prescribe, although there are some who are qualified to using the nurses' formulary.

Nurses specialist include stoma, respiratory, pain, cardiac, diabetes, tissue viability and Macmillan nurses. They are excellent for giving advice and are an important first port of call for the junior doctor.

Occupational therapists work with patients to restore, develop or maintain practical skills such as personal care. Most elderly patients require OT assessment before discharge – nurses usually make the referral.

Pharmacists dispense drugs and advise you on medication. They check the accuracy of every prescription that is written. Most hospitals have a drugs' information-line which you can call for prescribing advice.

Phlebotomists are professional vampires who appear on the wards with the specific aim of taking blood. They often appear at unpredictable times and they may not come at all at weekends. Some can take blood from central lines and perform blood cultures.

Physiotherapists use physical exercises and manipulation to treat injuries and relieve pain. Chest physios are commonly found on respiratory and surgical wards to help improve respiratory function and sputum expectoration by teaching specific breathing exercises. Involve them early in patient management – nurses usually make the referral.

Social workers support patients' needs in the community. They assess patients and help organise care packages (invaluable for elderly patients).

Daily ward duties

First thing
- Handover from night team about any overnight events
- Fill out any missing or extra blood/CXR/ECG requests
- Review new patients, consider writing a brief summary

Ward round
- See p94 for ward round duties, try to keep a jobs' list
- Attempt to do simple jobs (eg TTOs) during ward round

After the ward round
- Spend a few minutes comparing and allocating jobs with the other members of the team; try to group jobs by location and urgency
- Radiology requests (USS, CT, MRI)
- Referrals to other teams eg surgery/cardiology/psychiatry
- Fill out TTOs and other paperwork
- Take blood from patients whom the phlebotomists have been unable to bleed or that have been requested during the ward round

Lunch
- Do you need to do anything for yourself eg book holidays, pay bills?
- You may have teaching/grand round/journal clubs

After lunch
- Review patients you are worried about
- Check and record blood results; serial results sheets help
- Check other results; consider chasing outstanding requests or results from other departments eg radiology/microbiology
- Spend time talking to patients ± relatives
- Fill out blood, X-ray and ECG requests for the next day
- Check the patients' drug cards – do any need rewriting?

Before you go home
- Review results and outstanding jobs with other team members; make a note of anything that needs doing the next day
- Check that all warfarin and insulin doses have been written up
- Prescribe sufficient IV fluids for patients overnight
- Handover patients who are sick or need results chasing to the on-call doctor; write down their ward, name, DoB and hospital number and say exactly what you want the doctor to do

Before weekends
- Only write blood requests for patients who really need them
- Try to prescribe three days of warfarin doses
- Make sure that no drug cards will run out over the next two days, rewrite them if they will (this is infuriating to do as an on-call job)
- Ensure notes contain a brief and easy to find summary of each patient for the on-call team (especially for those who are unwell); include presenting complaint, relevant investigations and plan for the weekend (eg trial of oral fluids, stop IVs if tolerated, home next week)

Ward rounds

A smooth ward round requires preparation of notes, investigations and results. Try to predict requests and start the ward round armed with the appropriate answers.

Before the ward round

- Make an up-to-date patient list with patient details, location, summary of clinical problems/medical history, key investigations/results, referrals made and jobs
- Check notes, drug cards, obs charts, X-rays and blood results are present
- Clearly document all relevant investigation results and reports in the notes with a brief summary on your patient list
- Check all notes have continuation sheets headed with the patient's name, DoB and hospital number/address (can use a hospital sticker)
- Consider writing out the patient's problem list/summary
- If your patients have moved, contact the bed manager to find out where they have been transferred to and phone the receiving ward to ensure their notes, drug card and X-rays have also arrived
- Check or chase the dates/times for outstanding investigations
- Learn your consultant's favourite questions from your predecessor (eg pets, exposure to dyes)
- Consider multidisciplinary issues which may alter further management or delay discharge for the patient
- Think about management dilemmas you want/need answers to

During the ward round

- Ask a nurse to join you on the ward round
- If there are two junior doctors then one can prepare the notes, obs, drug cards and X-rays for the next patient whilst the other presents
- When presenting a patient, always begin in the same logical way eg 'Mrs Smith is a 64-year-old lady who presented with a 4-day history of worsening shortness of breath' then proceed to past medical history, investigation and blood results, then your management plan
- If you have a spare moment start filling in forms or doing the jobs generated on the ward round (eg prescribing fluids)
- If you have any queries about the next step of management or investigation results, ask during the ward round
- Referrals made in the presence of your consultant are often more readily accepted and queries can be discussed directly
- If you have not done something, be honest; never make up results

After the ward round

- Sit down with the rest of the team and go through the jobs generated from the ward round over a cup of tea
- Prioritise the jobs and group by location eg radiology
- Allocate the jobs between your team as appropriate
- If you are unsure of how to approach any of the jobs, ask your seniors
- Clarify any gaps in your understanding of the patients' management

Mr Johnston/Miss Jain's patient list 16–09–08

Patient Details	Problem list	Investigation/Detail	Jobs
Angel Ward			
Eleanor RIGBY *W876470* *26/06/1922*	*Chest pain* *COPD* *Hiatus hernia*	*LBBB on ECG*	*Rpt Cardiac* *TTO*
Seabright Ward			
Annie POPPLE *T589124* *8/9/35*	*Dysphagia* *Haematemesis* *Anaemia*	*3u Bld (11/09/08)* *OGD - Ca stomach*	*Macmillan referral* *Gastro r/v*

Sample patient list

16/09/08 WR: Mr Sutcliff (ST4)
0800 Day 1 post appendicectomy
Patient pain free; slept well overnight
No nausea/vomiting
Good urine output
Obs T 36.5°C, BP 120/78, pulse 66
O/E:

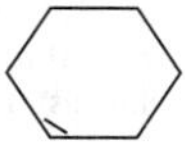

Soft
Non-tender
Bowel sounds present
Wound: clean; no discharge/bleeding

PLAN: 1) FBC/U+E check today
2) Sips, then light diet as able to tolerate
3) Aim for home later today/mane (OP in 6/52)

J Smith
SMITH
F1 6296

Sample of a ward round entry in the patient's notes

Being on-call

Being 'on-call' will occupy a large amount of your time and may involve care of a different group of patients and a greater range of specialities than during the day. Requirements, expectations and priorities are different.

What's important

- Ensure you have a clear handover about which patients are waiting to be seen, how urgently they need seeing and where they are
- Identify the sick and get help early
- Prioritise effectively and stay organised
- Eat and stay well hydrated

How to handle the bleep when tired

- Always try to answer promptly; when you don't it will be the boss or someone really unwell
- Write down who called and the job required
- Learn common extension numbers so you can spot the call from switchboard, the mess or your consultant's office

Being organised on-call

- Document every task, otherwise you **will** forget something – do not use scraps of paper; use a notepad or PDA (p6)
- Have a means of identifying when you've done it (drawing a box to tick when complete helps)
- Visit all the areas you cover in order and tell the wards this is what you'll be doing; ask them to compile a list of non-urgent tasks for when you arrive
- When you order a test on-call, make a note to check the result as it's easy to forget

Prioritising

- Sick patients need seeing first; if you have more than one really sick patient then tell your senior
- If the patient's condition is clearly life-threatening then ask the ward to bleep your senior while you're on your way there
- Check if a task has a deadline (eg before pharmacy closes)
- If you see an abnormal blood result check the patient/notes/previous blood results, see p604–9
- Ask if a task can wait until you're next in that area; tell the staff when this will be and try to stick to it

Taking breaks

You are entitled to a 30min paid break for every 4h work. Whilst you must not ignore a sick patient, there will be a constant supply of work that can usually wait. Breaks are not just about food, they keep you alert and reduce stress and tension headaches. It is in your patients' interests that you recharge. Drink plenty of water. Where possible, arrange to take breaks with the rest of the team on-call – it allows you to catch up and stops you feeling isolated.

Night shifts

Few doctors look forward to their night shifts, especially if they are doing a whole week. That said, on nights you will gain a lot of experience.

Things to take with you

- Food, both a main meal and several quick snacks
- Toothbrush, toothpaste, comb/hairbrush and deodorant
- Stuff for gaps in workload – eg books for private study

Things to check (on the first night)

- What areas and specialities are you responsible for?
- Who are your seniors and what are their bleep numbers?
- When and where is handover?
- What is the policy on short naps?

What is expected of you

- Turn up on time; your colleague will be late home if you don't
- Prioritise work according to urgency – when bleeped to a sick patient ask for obs ±ECG to be done while you get there
- Tour the wards you are covering regularly and delegate simple tasks
- Document all interventions in the notes

Hospital at night (H@N)

This system is now in place in almost half of hospitals in England. It was implemented to improve the efficiency and standard of care provided by the limited number of doctors on duty at night. One of the main areas to affect junior doctors is that all bleeps should go via the Night Sister, who then filters them appropriately eg assessing which jobs can be left for the day team, which jobs could be done by a nurse (eg cannula) and which patients need urgent review by a doctor.

Learning at night

Nights can be a good learning opportunity. Ensure the other doctors on at night know if you have particular skills you wish to learn at that time (eg chest drains). They can then call you to observe or be supervised.

Pitfalls

Many more mistakes are made during night shifts than by day. If you are unsure, check. The following are some of the common problem areas:

- Poor handover; ensure you know who needs review
- Failing to appreciate a sick patient and not calling for help
- Fluid prescriptions (eg failing to note renal/heart failure, DM, electrolyte imbalance)
- Warfarin prescriptions with INRs coming back out of hours

How to cope when not at work

- Go to bed for at least 7h each day, even if you don't sleep you'll rest
- Make your room dark and quiet – eye masks/earplugs help
- Eat enough; have a meal when you get up and before going in
- Travel home safely; if you feel too tired take a 20–30min nap first

Clerking – history

A thorough clerking is an essential skill as a junior doctor and something you will become extremely practised at. See the individual speciality chapters (p443) for unique features in their clerking and p128 for pre-op clerking. The following two pages are a guide to taking and writing a standard clerking.

Taking a history (*OHCM*7 p22)

- Try to be in a setting that offers privacy and has a bed
- Establish the patient's name and check their date of birth
- Introduce yourself and begin with open-ended questions

Heading Your name, position, location, date, time

Dr C J Flint, medical F1, Ward D57
15/9/08, 22:15, Clerking from pt and son

Presenting complaint Why has the patient come to hospital? Write their main problem(s) in their own words along with duration and who referred them; if the referral letter has a different presenting complaint then document this too:

Eleanor Rigby, 83yr old female, with a chest pain for 3 days, GP concerned about new onset of LBBB on ECG

History of presenting complaint(s) Ask questions aimed at differentiating the causes of the presenting complaint and assessing its severity. Try to exclude potentially life-threatening causes first. Ask specifically about previous episodes and investigations/treatments. Use the SOCRATES questions for pain (site, onset, character, radiation, associations, timing, exacerbating/relieving factors, severity). Ask about the effect on their activities of daily living (ADLs). If there are multiple problems ask if they come on together or are related.

Intermittent chest pain for 3/7, comes on suddenly at rest, gradual improvement over ~30min, heavy sensation, 5/10, worst 4hr ago, no change on exertion/breathing/ movement, no radiation, mild SOB, no nausea/sweating, nil previous, no cough/leg pain, mild swelling of ankles
Coping at home, but unable to get to shops 2° SOBOE

Risk factors Document recognised risk factors for important differentials:

Previous IHD x, ↑BP ✓, smoking ✓, FH x, cholesterol ?, DM x

Past medical history Ask about previous medical problems/operations and attempt to gauge the severity of each (eg hospital/ITU admissions, exercise tolerance (ET), treatment); use the drug history to prompt the patient's memory. Consider documenting specifically about asthma, DM, angina, ↑BP, MI, stroke, PE/DVT, epilepsy.

COPD – on inhalers, °home nebs, °LTOT, no recent change
↑BP on treatment °angina/MI/CVA/PE
Hiatus hernia and laparotomy 2° diverticular disease 1992

Drug history Document all drugs along with doses, times taken and any recent changes; always document drug allergies.

Combivent inh ṪṪ/PRN *Lansoprazole 15mg/om*
Beclometasone 100 inh ṪṪ/bd *Lactulose 10ml/PRN*
Bendrofluazide 2.5mg/om
Allergic to penicillin, causes a rash

Family history Ask about relevant illness in the family (eg heart problems, DM, cancer). Are other family members well at the moment?

Sister died of breast cancer aged 67, son alive and well

Social history This is essential: ***home*** ask about who they live with, the kind of house (eg bungalow, residential home), any home help, own ADLs (cooking, dressing, washing); ***mobility*** walking aids (stick/frame), exercise tolerance; ***lifestyle*** occupation, alcohol (units/wk), smoking (cigarettes/d and pack years), recreational drugs:

- *Alcohol*
- *Smoking* – 20 cigarettes/d for 1yr = 1 pack year

Lives alone in a bungalow; exercise tolerence 50m with stick, home help 2/wk for cleaning, ex-smoker for 30yr, 50pack yr

Systems' review Relevant systems' review will often be part of the HPC; a thorough systems' review is only necessary if you are unsure what is relevant or are struggling to explain the symptoms. See *OHCM*7 p24.

CVS	Chest pain, palpitations, SOB, ankle swelling, orthopnoea
Resp	Cough (?blood), sputum, wheeze, SOB
Abdo	Abdo pain, nausea/vomiting, bowel habit (?blood), stool colour and consistency, distension, dysuria, frequency, urgency, haematuria
Neuro	Headache, photophobia, neck stiffness, weakness, change in sensation, balance, fits, falls, speech, changes in vision/ hearing
Systemic	Appetite, weight loss/gain, fever/night sweats, malaise, stiff/ swollen joints, fatigue, rashes/itch, sleep pattern

Summarising Ask if there are any other problems that have not been discussed and repeat back a summary of the history to the patient to check that they agree. It is a good idea to use the ICE questions (**I**deas, **C**oncerns, **E**xpectations) at this point – ask the patient if they have any idea or suspicion of what might be wrong with them, if there's anything in particular that they're worried about (this may prompt them to admit specific concerns eg having cancer) and what they expect will happen to them whilst they are in hospital. Most patients have no idea about tests and investigations and find being admitted to hospital a frightening event, so often value the opportunity to talk about possible options and ask questions.

Always finish your clerking by asking specifically if the patient has any further questions or any other issues they would like to discuss, as frequently they will be too embarrassed/shy/reticent to ask.

Clerking – examination

It is good practice to perform a brief CVS, RS, abdo and neuro exam on all patients but focus your examination according to their history. Check observations (temp, BP, HR, RR, O_2 sats):

- Ask a nurse to chaperone you if necessary
- Get consent before touching the patient, ask where it hurts
- First assess briefly whether the patient looks well or ill

Hands (p504)

- *Look* at the hands for signs of disease
- *Pulse* check the rate and rhythm, ?collapsing pulse

Nails clubbing (IBD, cirrhosis, lung cancer, CF, bronchiectasis, congenital cyanotic heart disease, endocarditis), pitting, koilonychia (concave, ↓iron), Beau's lines, splinter haemorrhages; **hands** palmar erythema, skin turgor, hyperpigmented folds, Dupuytren's disease, muscle wasting, joint swelling, rheumatoid nodules (check elbows), ulnar deviation, Boutonniere's or swan neck deformity, sclerodactyly

Mouth

- Central cyanosis, mucous membranes, stomatitis, beefy tongue (↓iron), candidiasis, ulcers, dental hygiene (risk factor for SBE)

Cardiovascular system (p450)

- *Inspection* JVP (very useful if visible), swollen ankles
- *Palpation* temp of hands, capillary-refill, carotid pulse (volume and character), apex beat, heaves/thrills, hepatomegaly
- *Auscultation* heart sounds, added sounds/murmurs (timing, volume, radiation), carotid bruits, basal crackles

General clubbing, splinter haemorrhages, Janeway lesions, Osler's nodes, Quincke's sign (pulsing nail beds), Corrigan's sign (pulsating carotids), de Musset's sign (head bobbing), Roth's spots (retinal infarcts), xanthelasma, malar flush; **chest** scars, heaves, thrills

Respiratory system (p542)

- *Inspection* asterixis (flap), stridor, JVP, RR and effort (accessory muscles, recession), chest wall movement, peripheral oedema
- *Palpation* trachea, cervical lymphadenopathy, expansion
- *Percuss* right = left, hyperresonant, dull, stoney dull
- *Auscultation* air entry, crackles, wheeze, bronchial BS, rub

General clubbing, nicotine, asterixis (CO_2 flap), muscle wasting, peripheral or central cyanosis, purse-lip breathing, Horner's, (↓pupil, ptosis, ↓sweating), spine or chest wall deformity, cough; **chest** scars, tactile vocal fremitus

Abdomen (p468)

- *Inspection* jaundice, scars, distension, hernias, oedema
- *Palpation* start away from pain and watch patient's face: tenderness, peritonism (guarding, rebound, rigidity, percussion tenderness), masses,

liver, spleen, kidneys and AAA (expansile mass), hernias, ±genitalia, PR (masses, stool, tenderness, prostate, blood/mucus/melaena)
- *Percussion* ascites (shifting dullness, fluid thrill), liver, spleen
- *Auscultation* bowel sounds (absent, reduced, increased, tinkling)

General pallor, leuconychia (white nails, ↓albumin), palmar erythema, asterixis (liver flap), spider naevi, itching, bruising, tattoos, hepatic foetor (pear-drop breath), Virchow's node (left supraclavicular), gynaecomastia, hair distribution; **abdo** visible pulsations/masses, caput medusa, striae, everted umbilicus, liver texture, tenderness, pulsatility, renal bruits, inguinal lymphadenopathy, radio-femoral delay

Peripheral nerves (p510)

See p512 for neuroanatomy.
- *Inspection* posture, movement of limbs
- *Palpation* tone, power (5 normal, 4 weak, 3 against gravity only, 2 not even against gravity, 1 twitch, 0 none), reflexes, plantars, sensation
- *Coordination* finger–nose, slide heel down opposite leg

Extras involuntary movements, muscle wasting, fasciculations, clonus, light touch, pain, vibration, temperature, joint position, dysdiadochokinesis, Romberg's test

Cranial nerves (p509)

- *Inspection* GCS, mental state (p535), speech, posture
- *Eyes* (II, III, IV, VI) acuity, pupil reactivity, fields, movements, fundi
- *Face* (V, VII) sensation and power
- *Mouth* (IX, X, XII) tongue movements, palate position, cough
- *Other* (VIII) hearing, balance, gait (XI), shrug, head movements

Extras (I) familiar smells with each nostril; (II, III, IV, VI) nystagmus, visual inattention, light and accommodation; (V) corneal reflex, mouth muscles; (VII) taste; (VIII) Weber's, Rinne's; (IX, X) gag reflex, swallow

Differential diagnosis

Write a list of differentials in order of likelihood:

Imp *1 Reflux pain 2° hiatus hernia*
2 Musculoskeletal chest pain
3 Need to exclude MI

Management plan

Write the important investigations and treatments the patient requires. Always include symptomatic relief (eg analgesia, antiemetics):

Ⓟ *FBC, U+E, LFT, cardiac markers, ECG, CXR*
O_2, GTN, antacid, paracetamol
Admit overnight for repeat cardiac markers and ECG

Writing in the notes

Most new F1s are unsure about writing in medical notes since this is rarely practised as a medical student. There are a few rules which everyone, irrespective of grade, should conform to:

Notepaper The patient's name, DoB and hospital number or address should identify every sheet (using a hospital sticker is acceptable).

Documentation Each entry should have the date and time. It is useful to have a heading such as 'WR ST2 (Smith)' or 'Discussion with patient and family'. Sign every entry and print your surname and bleep number clearly.

What to write Document the condition of the patient, relevant changes to the history, obs, examination findings, the results of any new investigations and end with a plan. The notes should contain enough information so that in your absence someone else can learn what has happened and what is planned for the patient.

Problem lists It is helpful to write a problem list in the notes either every day if there are frequent changes (eg in ICU/HDU), or once a week for more chronic conditions. This can include both medical and social problems. Having problem lists also makes it much easier for on-call doctors to get up to date with the patient's condition if they are asked to review them, as well as refreshing your memory at the start of a new week of ward rounds.

What not to write Patients can apply to read their medical notes and notes are always used in legal cases. Never write anything that you do not wish the patient to read or that would be frowned upon in court. Documenting facts is accepted (eg obese lady) but not subjective material (eg annoying time-waster). Never doodle in the notes and do not write humorous comments.

How to write Write clearly in black; poorly legible notes result in errors and are indefensible in court. Use only well recognised abbreviations and don't worry about length as long as sufficient information is documented. Always write in the notes at the time of the consultation, even if it means asking the ward round to wait a few moments.

Making changes If you wish to cross something out simply put a single line through the error and initial the mistake. Never cross it out so it cannot be read as this looks suspicious. Previous entries should not be altered, instead make a new entry indicating the change or difference.

Notes and the law It is unlikely that your notes will be used in court. If they are, you want them to show you as a caring and clear-thinking individual; make that clear from how you write. As far as a court is concerned, if it's not documented then it didn't happen.

Hints and tips Bullet points are a useful and clear means of documentation. It is acceptable to write about a patient's mood and it is useful to document if you have cheered them up or discussed some bad news (p57). It is also acceptable to document 'no change' if this is the case.

Example of entries in medical notes

16.09.08	***WR ST4 (Ackerman)***
10:20	*Pt comfortable. No further chest pain.*
	P70 reg, BP 132/81, RR 15, Sats 99% on room air.
	~~CXR shows bilateral pleural effusions~~ (Wrong patient CJF)
	Rpt ECG Ⓝ, no new changes.
	Imp
	• *Atypical chest pain, unlikely to be cardiac.*
	Ⓟ
	• *Await cardiac markers – if Ⓝ, Ⓗ c̄ no f/u.*
	• *Pt wants to discuss risk factors when family arrive.*
	Dr C J Flint F1
	Bleep 3294
16.09.08	***d/w with pt and wife***
11:12	*Pt wanted to talk about cardiac risk factors.*
	Given British Heart Foundation leaflet on risk factors and talked about life-style changes. Cardiac nurse will see pt before discharge.
	Rpt cardiac markers Ⓝ. Pt much relieved.
	Ⓗ later.
	Dr C J Flint F1
	Bleep 3294
16.09.08	***Review; F1 (Flint)***
15:34	*No change. TTO written. Ⓗ.*
	Dr C J Flint F1
	Bleep 3294

Example of a problem list

16/9/08	*Mrs Jones' current problems:*
09:00	*1. Left lower lobe pneumonia - on day 2 IV co-amoxiclav*
	2. Atrial fibrillation (Δ2004) - on digoxin and warfarin
	3. Hypertension - well controlled on ramipril
	4. Previous CVA (1998) with right sided weakness
	5. Previous left knee replacement (1994)
	6. Inability to cope at home – awaiting nursing home

Common symbols in the notes

Ⓗ	Home
Ⓝ	Normal
Ⓟ	Plan
Ⓛ	Left
Ⓡ	Right
Ⓣ	Temperature
dd/DD/$\delta\delta$/$\Delta\Delta$	Differential diagnosis
x/Dx/Δ	Diagnosis
Imp	Impression
Rx	Prescription or drugs
Sx	Symptoms
Tx	Treatment
Ix	Investigations
O/E	On examination
–ve	Negative
+ve	Positive
+/–	Equivocal
+	Presence noted
++	Present significantly
+++	Present in excess
h/o	History of
d/w	Discussed with or discussion with
WR	Ward round
r/v	Review
f/u	Follow up
ATSP	Asked to see patient
IP	Inpatient
OP	Outpatient
c/o	Complains of or complaining of
Pt	Patient
c̄	With
@	At
E+D	Eating and drinking
N+V	Nausea and vomiting
D+V	Diarrhoea and vomiting
BO	Bowels open
PUing	Passing urine
blds	Bloods
°	No/negative (as in °previous MI)
1°	Primary
2°	Secondary
mane	Tomorrow morning

Anatomical terms and planes

The anatomical position	Anatomical planes
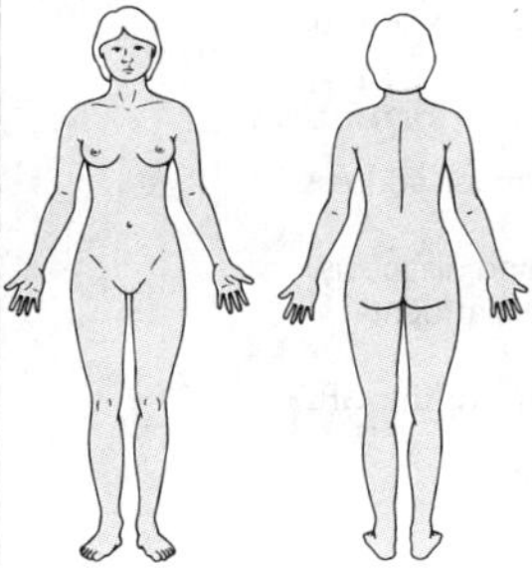	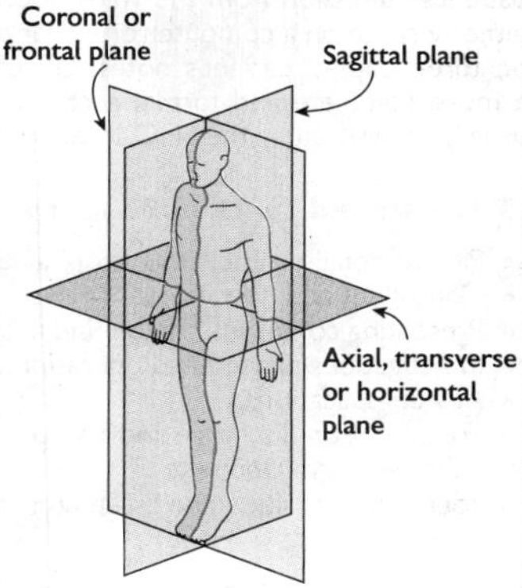

Anterior/ventral	Front of the body
Contralateral	On the opposite side
Coronal/frontal plane	Divides anterior from posterior
Distal	Away from the trunk
Inferior/caudal	Away from the head
Ipsilateral	On the same side
Lateral	Away from the midline
Medial	Towards the midline
Palmar	Pertaining to the palm of the hand
Plantar	Pertaining to the sole of the foot
Posterior/dorsal	Back of the body
Prone	Face down position
Proximal	Close to the trunk
Radial	The lateral (thumb) aspect of the forearm
Sagittal plane	Divides left side from right side
Superior/cephalic	Towards the head
Supine	Face up position
Transverse/horizontal/axial plane	Divides upper and lower sections
Ulnar	The medial (little finger) aspect of the forearm

Commonly used anatomical terms and their meaning

Discharge summaries (TTOs/TTAs)

'TTOs' or 'TTAs' (to take out or away) are written summaries of the patient's admission from the ward doctors to the patient's GP. TTOs are either written on a computer or by hand with carbon copies; there should be three copies: patient's notes, GP, pharmacy. A discharge letter with a more complete and formal account of the patient's hospital stay will usually be written by the SHO-level doctor at a later date.

TTOs should contain the following information

- Patient details: name, DoB, hospital number, address
- Consultant and hospital ward
- Presenting complaint, clinical findings and diagnosis
- Investigations/procedures/operations/treatment
- Any complications
- Treatment on discharge and instructions to the GP
- Follow-up arrangements
- Your name, position and bleep number

When to write TTOs

TTOs should be written as soon as you know the patient will be discharged. This allows the drugs to be dispensed from pharmacy as soon as possible so that the patient's discharge is not delayed.

- Carry TTO forms on ward rounds so that you can write them during any gaps in the ward round; also check any queries with your team
- Check the duration of the medication for discharge (eg ABx) and stop any unnecessary drugs (eg prophylactic enoxaparin)
- Check drug doses and frequencies with the *BNF*, your seniors, a pharmacist or by calling your hospital's drug information-line
- Check who will arrange follow-up appointments (eg the ward clerk or an appointment book)
- Contact the GP (p480) by telephone if the patient needs an early check-up, has a poor social situation or self-discharges
- Hand the TTO and the patient's drug chart to the patient's nurse or inform them that you have completed it to avoid being called later
- If you are unsure whether the TTO has been done check the drug chart; there is often a tick in a box showing if TTOs have been dispensed
- Discuss the diagnosis, results and discharge plan with your patient; if they understand the management plan they are more likely to comply

Controlled drugs for TTOs

These are slightly more complex, but can still be written by F1 doctors. They must be handwritten and include all the information in the table opposite. CD prescriptions are only valid for 28d from the date of signing and only 30d of CDs can be dispensed on a single prescription.

Examples of controlled drugs

Morphine, diamorphine, pethidine, fentanyl, alfentanil, remifentanil, methadone, methylphenidate (ie Ritalin®), cocaine

Controlled drug TTOs must meet the following requirements	
Format rules	• Handwritten
Content rules	• The prescriber's name and work address • Signed and dated by the prescriber • All the information included in a regular TTO
Drug rules	• The drug name, dose, frequency and route • If the drug is a 'preparation' (ie liquid) state the concentration • The total volume (ml) or weight (mg) of the preparation or the total number of tablets/capsules/patches in words and figures

Discharge form McBurney City Hospital

Name: *Eleanor Rigby* — Consultant: *Dr Singh*
DOB: *26/06/1922* — Date of admission: *15/09/2008*
Hospital number: *W876470* — Date of discharge: *16/09/2008*
Ward: *E4*
NHS/~~Private~~ — Inpatient/~~Outpatient/Daycase~~

Presenting complaint: *Chest pain*
Diagnosis: *Musculoskeletal chest pain*
Investigations: *ECG shows LBBB, cardiac markers Ⓝ*

Discharge Plan/Additional notes to GP: *Has had some toothache recently, advised her to see a dentist*

Discharge Medications:

Drug	Dose	Frequency	Route	Duration	GP to continue?
Co-amoxiclav	*625mg*	*tds*	*PO*	*5d*	*No*
Paracetamol	*1g*	*PRN*	*PO*	*7d*	*No*
Oramorph (10mg/5ml)	*5ml*	*bd*	*PO*	*5d*	*No*
	Total = 50ml (fifty millilitres)				

Follow up? *No* — Date: *16-09-2008*
Print name *Flint* — Signature *C J Flint*
Bleep number *3294*

Sample TTO; note oramorph is not usually prescribed in this situation

Morphine oral solution (10mg/5ml); dose: 5ml/12h PO for 5 days
Total= 50ml (fifty millilitres)

Morphine sulphate MR 20mg capsules; dose: 20mg/12h PO for 14 days Total= 560mg (five hundred and sixty milligrams)

Fentanyl 50 patch; dose: one patch every 72 hours for 14 days
Total= 5 (five) patches

Sample TTOs for controlled drugs excluding the patient and prescriber's details.

Sick notes

As the most junior member of the team, the writing of sick notes will usually fall to you. They are commonly required for surgical patients who have been admitted routinely for a procedure as they tend to be younger and require time off work to recover post-operatively. Medical patients may also require them to cover the time they have been in hospital and their recovery time. However, all patients self-certify for the first week of any illness so do not require a sick note if they will be able to return to work within this first week.

You should fill in the note with the patient's name, a brief explanation for their sick leave without mentioning intimate details (eg 'surgical procedure'), your signature and the date. You need to give an appropriate amount of time for the patient to recover from their illness, but some hospitals advise only writing a sick note for 1wk and then request that the patient visits their GP if they require further time off. This guards against patients taking more time than medically necessary off work – check your trust policy or ask your seniors if unsure.

If the patient is claiming state benefits you will need to complete and sign a DWP (Department for Work and Pensions) form – ask the ward clerk if you are unable to find one.

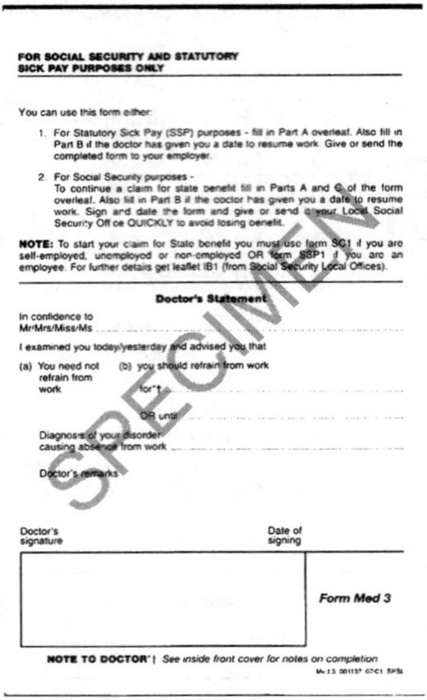

FOR SOCIAL SECURITY AND STATUTORY SICK PAY PURPOSES ONLY

You can use this form either:

1. For Statutory Sick Pay (SSP) purposes - fill in Part A overleaf. Also fill in Part B if the doctor has given you a date to resume work. Give or send the completed form to your employer.
2. For Social Security purposes -
To continue a claim for state benefit fill in Parts A and C of the form overleaf. Also fill in Part B if the doctor has given you a date to resume work. Sign and date the form and give or send it your Local Social Security Office QUICKLY to avoid losing benefit.

NOTE: To start your claim for State benefit you must use form SC1 if you are self-employed, unemployed or non-employed OR form SSP1 if you are an employee. For further details get leaflet IB1 (from Social Security Local Offices).

Doctor's Statement

In confidence to
Mr/Mrs/Miss/Ms ....

I examined you today/yesterday and advised you that

(a) You need not refrain from work

(b) you should refrain from work

for*† ....

OR until ....

Diagnosis of your disorder causing absence from work ....

Doctor's remarks

Doctor's signature

Date of signing

Form Med 3

NOTE TO DOCTOR*† *See inside front cover for notes on completion*

Med 3 001137 07-01 SPSL

Example of sick note (Med 3).

Reproduced with permission from the Department of Work and Pensions. Last accessed 01/02/2008 http://www.dwp.gov.uk/medical/medicalib204/ib204-june04/appendix-h.pdf

Referrals

Referring a patient to another medical team can be one of the most difficult parts of the job. The other doctor is often very busy and will inevitably know more about the patient's condition than you (hence the referral). At times it can feel like they are trying to make you feel stupid. It is important to consider this from the point of view of the other doctor; they are trying to establish:

- How unwell the patient is
- How urgently they need to be seen
- If they are the right person to see them

You will often be asked to refer a patient by a senior, ask them directly:

- Why does the patient need referring?
- What do they want the other team to do (advise over the phone, formal review, take over care, see in clinic, procedure/operation)?
- How urgent is the referral?

Next, think about what information the other doctor will want. You may need to get extra information from history or examination. This varies between different specialities so you will find a separate section on all of the most common ones:

Anaesthetics	p446	GUM	p485	Paediatrics	p528
Breast	p449	Gynaecology	p488	Palliative care	p531
surgery		Haematology	p491	Plastic surgery	p533
Cardiology	p451	Intensive care	p454	Psychiatry	p536
Dermatology	p457	Maxillofacial	p493	Radiology	p539
Endocrine	p467	Microbiology	p495	Renal	p541
ENT	p462	Neurology	p513	Respiratory	p543
Gastro	p469	Obstetrics	p516	Rheumatology	p507
General	p483	Oncology	p519	Urology	p546
surgery		Ophthalmology	p521	Vascular	p549
GP	p480	Orthopaedics	p507	surgery	

Before referring make sure you have the following in front of you:

- Hospital notes with patient's name, DoB, hospital number and ward
- Obs chart (including latest set and trends) and the patient's drug card
- Most recent results or serial results sheet

Phone the relevant specialist, introduce yourself and say, 'My consultant has requested that I refer one of our patients who has [medical condition] with the view to [taking over care, advising on treatment, etc]'.

Offer a brief summary of their condition and management; look up the relevant condition or referral page (above) before calling so that you sound like you know what you are talking about.

Before you put the phone down determine exactly what action the specialist will do and when this will take place. Write the referral and outcome in the notes along with the specialist's name and bleep number.

Referral letters

The basics

Try to make referral letters as professional as possible. Ideally use hospital headed paper and a computer. Like any referral it is essential that it contains the following information:

- Who you are and how to contact you
- Who the patient is (full name, DoB, hospital number, ±address)
- Why you want them to be seen

Diagnoses

List all the patient's active diagnoses and relevant past diagnoses; try to put the ones most relevant to the speciality you are referring to near the top.

Presenting complaint

Start the letter with a statement telling the other doctor what you would like them to do as a result of reading the letter. Give a brief description of the patient's presentation and management during this admission as if you were writing a discharge summary.

Medical information

This will form the bulk of the letter. Think carefully about what information will help the other doctor in deciding when to see the patient and how to manage them, see the relevant referral page (p509). Try to set the letter out like a medical clerking and make sure you include:

- Relevant investigation results
- Latest medications
- Relevant social history (particularly if this will affect how they are seen in clinic eg poor mobility, language difficulties)

Finishing the letter

You should write your name, post and consultant's name. You should also include who the letter is copied to ('cc' stands for carbon copy) which will include the notes and GP. It is recommended practice to send a copy to the patient though this varies between wards and doctors. Some wards send patients a separate letter without medical jargon.

Sending the letter

It depends how much you trust (or have) a ward clerk. It is often easier to print off several copies, sign them and put them in the notes and addressed envelopes yourself. This at least guarantees that it is done.

Faxing a letter

If you need to fax a copy then include a header sheet. This is simply a piece of paper saying who the fax is to, who it is from and the number of pages (and whether this includes the header sheet). You may need to add a number to the fax number to get an outside line eg '9'.

Dr Charles Flint
McBurney City Hospital
McBurney
McB1 4CT

Dr I N Haler
Respiratory Consultant
McBurney City Hospital
McBurney
McB1 4CT

2nd September 2008

Dear Dr Haler,

RE Eleanor Rigby, DoB 26/06/22, Hospital No. W876470

Diagnoses: (1) COPD
(2) Musculoskeletal chest pain
(3) LBBB
(4) Hiatus Hernia

Please review Mrs Rigby in your respiratory clinic to treat her deterioration in respiratory function with COPD.

Mrs Rigby is an 86-year-old lady who presented with chest pain. She was admitted overnight and diagnosed with musculoskeletal chest pain following normal repeat cardiac markers. She was discharged on 1/9/2008. During her admission she was noted to have reduced exercise tolerance (from 200m to 50m). Her current PEFR is 45% of predicted and her latest ABG on air is:

PaO_2	9.3kPa
$PaCO_2$	6kPa

We feel that her COPD is the likely cause of her limited mobility and she has been referred for repeat respiratory function tests.

PMH She was diagnosed with COPD by yourself three years ago following respiratory function tests which showed an FEV1 of 75% predicted. She has not had any acute exacerbations in the last year.

DH She is currently on:

Combivent inhaler	2puffs	qds
Beclometasone 100 inhaler	2puffs	bd
Bendroflumethiazide	5mg	om

SH She lives alone but gets home help for cleaning. She can walk about 50m with a stick. She stopped smoking 30 years ago after 50 pack years.

Yours sincerely,

Dr Charles Flint
F1 to Dr N Stemi
cc GP
Eleanor Rigby
Notes

Example of a referral letter.

Death certificates

Eligibility You can only fill in a death certificate if you have met the patient within the last 14d on their final admission, they are older than 18yr and you understand what occurred. Signing a death certificate means you are confident enough about the cause of death to stand by it in court. Refer to a senior if you are unsure that you meet these criteria.

Coroner Many hospital patients have to be referred to the coroner, see the box below. If you are in doubt, ring the coroner's office (hours vary but often only open during the daytime on weekdays) to discuss the case; they are usually friendly and helpful.

Inform the coroner if: • death <24h since admission • suspicious, accidental or violent deaths (includes RTAs) • suicide • operation, anaesthetic or invasive procedure in the last year (this includes endoscopy, central lines etc) • death from acute effects of alcohol or drugs • death due to industrial disease (coal, asbestos, dyes etc) • unknown cause of death

The coroner is often a lawyer but may have joint degrees in law and medicine; their job is to investigate suspicious deaths. For the majority of deaths you refer to the coroner's office you will be told to issue the death certificate. If you have referred the case to the coroner you need to circle the '4' on the front and the 'a' on the back. If you simply discussed the case then neither of these needs to be circled.

What to write Most of the entries are self-explanatory:

- **Place of death** should be the ward, hospital and city
- Your **residence** should be the hospital address not your home address
- Ring the **digit and letter** above causes of death, often '3' or '4' and 'a' or 'b'
- Tick the box below 'Causes of death' if industrial disease is suspected (there is a table on the back of the certificate)
- **Qualifications**: this is your medical degree eg MBChB
- Remember to fill in the slips to the left and right and the back (you may need to circle 'a' or 'b')

Causes of death	Modes of death
Myocardial infarction, arrhythmia	Cardiac arrest, syncope
Sepsis, hypovolaemia, haemorrhage, anaphylaxis	Hypotension, shock, off-legs
Congestive cardiac failure, pulmonary oedema	Heart failure, cardiac failure, ventricular failure
Bronchopneumonia, pulmonary embolism, asthma, chronic obstructive pulmonary disease	Respiratory failure, respiratory arrest
Cerebrovascular accident	Collapse
Cirrhosis, glomerulonephritis, diabetic nephropathy	Liver failure, renal failure, uraemia
Carcinomatosis, carcinoma of the ...	Cachexia, exhaustion

Cause of death This can be hard. You must avoid using modes of death in preference for causes of death. The table opposite offers common causes – there are many more. You must fill in 'I(a)', but the other three categories may be left blank if there is nothing to put. Do not use abbreviations.

I (a) Direct cause of death eg pulmonary embolism
  (b) Cause of I(a) eg fractured femur
  (c) Cause of I(b) eg steroid-induced osteoporosis

II Other disease or conditions that may have contributed eg rheumatoid arthritis, congestive cardiac failure

Write in the patient's notes that you have completed the death certificate, whether they were referred to the coroner and the responses you gave for the categories 'I(a)', '(b)', '(c)' and 'II' so that the discharge letter can be written to the GP. You **must** see the body to confirm identity.

Post-mortem These used to be carried out regularly, however government legislation means they are now rare. They are usually only carried out if the disease was unusual (with relatives' consent) or if requested by the coroner (do not need relatives' consent).

Cremation forms

If you are asked to fill in a cremation form you **must** see the body to check the patient's identity and whether they have a pacemaker. You also have to sign that they do not have radioactive materials implanted – these are used for palliative treatment of some cancers (eg cervical, bone). You will be paid about £70 for the form (see p88 re tax) – the money comes from the patient's relatives via the funeral director who keeps the money if you refuse. The reason you are paid is because you take responsibility for the fact the body will not be able to be exhumed for evidence if there is any doubt in future as to cause of death.

Checking for pacemakers

You need to check the identity (appearance and wristband) of all patients who you write death certificates for; use the opportunity to check for pacemakers. Look for any scars on the anterior chest wall (usually left side) and palpate the front of the chest for pacemaker boxes. If you are still in doubt, read back through the patient's notes (clinic letters are helpful), check previous ECGs for pacemaker spikes and look at previous CXR. When in the morgue, use the patient's name rather than referring to 'the body', wear gloves and wash your hands afterwards.

Investigation request forms

Whenever you request an investigation the form must contain the following information:

- Full name and at least one other patient identification detail (ie DoB, hospital number or address); G+S/X-match requires at least two more
- Status (inpatient/outpatient) and location (ward or home address)
- Name, position and contact details of doctor ordering the test
- Test requested and reason for request
- Date

Examples of forms that require in-depth clinical details

- **Bloods** blood film, blood cultures, antibodies, hormones (except thyroid), drug levels (doses and timing of doses), genetics
- **Other tissues** CSF, histology, pathology
- **Radiology/procedures** USS, CT, MRI, endoscopy

Clinical information

It is important to include an appropriate level of information on request forms. If in doubt too much is better rather than too little. The clinical information should justify the investigation requested, even if it is a simple blood test.

- *Routine blood tests* It may acceptable to put brief clinical details eg 'chest pain', 'suspected PE'
- *Microbiology* As a bare minimum it must include the sample type (eg urine) and current antibiotics; the more information you include the better the microbiologist will be able to interpret laboratory results
- *Radiology* As radiation is harmful, radiographers will refuse to do tests without clinical information to justify it; an example is shown below

Surname	*Sprinter*	**Date**	*19/08/2008*
Forename	*Ryan*		
Address	*11 Strawberry Fields* *Tarnham* *West Lockington*	**Ward**	*Mary Ward*
		Consultant	*Dr Bentley*
DoB	*21/09/1982*		
Hospital No.	*R445334*		
Examination requested	*CXR please*		
Clinical details	*Previously fit and well young man. Right sided pleuritic chest pain and mild SOB on exertion for 3/7. No cough. P80, RR18, sats 97% on room air. Slightly reduced breath sounds on right, but nil else.* *?pneumothorax, ?pneumonia* *PE unlikely as no risk factors and D-dimer normal*		
Referrer's name/bleep	*Dr J C Flint bleep 3294*	**Signature**	*C J Flint*

Example of a radiology request

How to chase results

As a junior doctor, a large proportion of your time will be spent chasing results. Your consultant will expect scans to be done and reported the same day they request them, and your registrars will expect you to know blood results before you've even had a chance to take the blood. However, with practice and experience, getting things done quickly will become easier. Be careful not to make important decisions on preliminary results – if there is an urgent clinical situation in which you are unsure whether to act on a specific result, ask your seniors.

Radiology

If you are asked to request a certain investigation, ensure you know why it is being requested, how urgent it is and how it will change the patient's management. Request the scan or fill in the form, then go down to the radiology department, find out which consultant is on-call for the day or who has a special interest in your particular investigation, and speak to them directly. Be polite, explain why the test has been requested (and by whom) and ask if there is any way it could be performed today. If this fails and the test is very urgent, ask your registrar to speak to the radiologist directly.

Biochemistry/haematology

Waiting for blood tests to return will be a daily chore and there isn't much you can do to hurry them along apart from take them as early in the day as possible. Often if you send the blood to the lab before the phlebotomists do their rounds, your samples will be processed first.

If you require bloods to be processed urgently, then you can often mark 'urgent' on the blood form and telephone the lab to ask they are done as a priority. At top speed, biochemistry results take approximately 20–30min and haematology results take approximately 30min.

Often results have been processed but are delayed in being uploaded onto the computer system, so it may be worth telephoning the lab for the results of routine bloods after a couple of hours if they're not showing up on the computer screen.

Microbiology

Unfortunately you cannot rush the rate at which bugs grow. The status of cultures at 48h is often stated on the computer system; otherwise consider telephoning the lab at this stage to see if there is any preliminary growth. Most samples are cultured for 5d in total.

Histology

All biopsies which are taken with a provisional diagnosis of malignancy should be processed urgently. The best way to chase results is to telephone the pathology secretaries to ask if it would be possible to fax the histology report to you (on a secure fax machine) instead of waiting for the official printed report to be sent to the ward in the internal mail – this may take 3–7d. Alternatively you could find the secretary's office and pick up a copy of the report by hand.

Difficult patients

Alcoholism Many patients will drink over the daily and weekly recommendations (4 units/d for ♂ and 3 units/d for ♀), though not all of these will be 'alcoholics'. Defining alcoholism is a problem, but if drinking or the effects of drinking repeatedly leads to harm in work or social life, then this is clearly a problem. Answering 'yes' to three out of four of the *CAGE* questions suggests alcoholism: Ever felt you ought to **C**ut down on your drinking? Have people **A**nnoyed you by criticising your drinking? Ever felt bad or **G**uilty about your drinking? Ever had an **E**ye-opener to steady your nerves in the morning?

The medical aspects of alcohol excess and withdrawal are covered on p288. Excessive drinking can be a psychiatric issue in its own right but can also complicate many psychiatric diseases. Modifying drinking behaviour is difficult and only of benefit in patients who want to change.

- ***Abuse*** excessive drinking despite mental or physical harm
- ***Dependence*** alcohol tolerance, withdrawal symptoms if not drinking

Alcoholism management Have a low threshold for commencing benzodiazepine therapy to minimise risk of alcohol withdrawal (see suggested regimen below). In addition, start vitamin B_1 supplementation with either intravenous preparations (Pabrinex® 2 pairs/8h IV for 2d) or oral thiamine 200mg/24h PO and multi-vitamins (1–2 tablets/24h PO).

Chlordiazepoxide doses to prevent alcohol withdrawal

Day 1	20mg/6h PO	Day 5	5mg/6h PO
Day 2	20mg/8h PO	Day 6	5mg/8h PO
Day 3	10mg/6h PO	Day 7	5mg/12h PO
Day 4	10mg/8h PO		

If not treated, thiamine deficiency can lead to Wernicke's encephalopathy (see p303). This is characterised by a triad of nystagmus, ophthalmoplegia and ataxia, but can also present with confusion, altered consciousness, vomiting and headache. This requires urgent treatment with Pabrinex® or oral thiamine, or risks progression to irreversible Korsakoff's syndrome. Korsakoff's is characterised by an inability to acquire new memories associated with a tendency to confabulate to fill in the gaps. Treat as for Wernicke's, but the memory loss is usually permanent.

Other management Alcohol diaries, make a plan for reduced intake or abstinence, individual and group counselling eg Alcoholics Anonymous, pharmacological assistance eg disulfiram, address underlying social and psychiatric problems.

Elderly patients are often taking many medications, so interactions and side-effects are common. As renal function declines, drug excretion falls and lower doses can often be used for renally excreted drugs; equally, elderly patients handle fluid boluses less well and can easily go into heart failure from excessive IV fluids. Other issues to consider: increased susceptibility to infections, higher threshold to pain (can mask fractures or other acute pathology), atypical presentations of disease, poor thermoregulation (become hypothermic easily), malnourishment (if unable to obtain or prepare food), history taking can be difficult if hard of hearing. Elderly patients can suffer with depression and other psychiatric illness (p311) and, like children, social circumstances must always be considered prior to discharge – liaise with OT, physio and social services.

High-risk patient (hepatitis/HIV) (p265/426) Wearing gloves and meticulous handling of sharps (p4) should prevent transmission to yourself and others. Many doctors choose to wear two pairs of gloves (double gloving) when taking blood or using other sharps. All samples of bodily fluids sent for investigation should be labelled with high-risk stickers, as should the forms; they should be transported by porters, not by airtubes. The patient can be nursed on the open ward.

Hypopituitarism Patients with hypopituitarism can have a broad range of symptoms and signs. In the acute situation, these patients tend to present with hypoglycaemia ± coma due to the combined lack of growth hormone, cortisol and thyroxine which all affect insulin function. On the ward, the most important clinical point for junior doctors to be aware of is to ensure the patient is getting their regular steroids (converted to IV if necessary) and to contact an endocrinologist urgently for further management advice.

Immunocompromised patients (p397) Need to be protected from infection. They are reverse barrier nursed in isolation, so that equipment is sterilised before entering the room. Limit contact to essential staff. Before entering, wash hands and wear gloves, apron and mask; remove and dispose of these on leaving the room.

Infectious diseases Contagious infections require isolation and barrier nursing – equipment is sterilised or disposed of on leaving the room. Common reasons include gastroenteritis (especially *C. difficile*), chickenpox, shingles, TB (see below), MRSA (p119), meningitis. You should wear gloves, apron and mask before entering the room and wash hands on leaving.

Intravenous drug users (IVDU) Are commonly admitted with infections (abscesses, cellulitis, endocarditis), DVTs or with pathology unrelated to IV drug abuse. Intravenous cannulation can be difficult and these patients may require temporary central access for prolonged antibiotic therapy. In some circumstances the patient will prefer to take blood samples themselves with a needle and syringe rather than have a junior doctor delving blindly into any potential vein. Treat all bodily fluids as high-risk (see above) unless hepatitis and HIV status has been recently established as negative. IVDU patients should not be allowed off the ward unaccompanied with IV access *in situ*.

Difficult patients (continued)

Substance abuse can cause many psychiatric symptoms (depression, anxiety, psychosis), complicate psychiatric diseases, cause legal issues and result in dependence. It is important to ask whether patients take any illicit drugs as part of the general history.

Street names for commonly misused drugs	
Amphetamines	Speed, uppers
Cannabis	Weed, grass, hash, pot, dope, marijuana, skunk
Cocaine	If snorted: coke, C, Charlie; If smoked: crack
Ecstasy	'E', pills, MDMA
Heroin	Smack, junk, skag
LSD	Acid, trips, tabs
Ketamine	K, special K, ket, vitamin K

Organ transplant Managing patients who have had an organ transplant is a highly specialised area, and one you are unlikely to encounter as an F1. All transplant patients have a lifelong regimen of immunosuppressant drugs which have serious side-effects, increasing the risk of infections and of all types of cancer. The most common drugs used are ciclosporin A, prednisolone and azathioprine. Patients are often very well informed about their medical regime and will have a transplant specialist managing their care, so you should always seek expert advice. Always take fever and illness seriously as immunosuppression masks the 'normal' symptoms. Conversely, a patient may have sepsis without being pyrexial.

Patients on regular steroids (>14d) Are more prone to infections due to relative immunocompromise (p117), but also have suppression of their adrenocortical axis. Sudden withdrawal of (cortico)steroids in such patients can trigger an addisonian-like crisis. Steroid therapy must be maintained or withdrawn slowly. During periods of illness, steroid treatment often has to be increased. If patients are nil by mouth, intravenous steroid preparations are available and equivalent doses can be calculated (p154).

Patient with learning disabilities Have to be individually managed depending on their degree of intellectual function. Some patients are able to give implied consent for simple procedures such as venepuncture, whereas other patients may not have capacity. In this situation, 2 consultants must decide whether a procedure or operation is in the patient's best interest, and sign the appropriate consent form on their behalf. Often patients with learning disabilities can understand their illness if it is explained slowly and in simple terms – some may have relatives or carers with them who are better able to communicate with the patient, but if you are ever unsure, involve a senior colleague. Always ensure you document accurately what is explained to the patient ± their carer or relative.

Patient with MRSA All patients with MRSA should be isolated in a side room if possible, otherwise they should be nursed together in a single bay. Universal precautions such as gloves, gown and hand-washing should be employed during every contact. Don't forget to also clean your stethoscope with an alcohol wipe between patients. Different hospitals have different protocols regarding MRSA eradication, but most trusts use mupirocin (Bactroban®) ointment in the nostrils and any open wounds and antibacterial body wash, both for at least 5d. If you suspect a patient has MRSA bacteraemia, take blood cultures and discuss with a microbiologist regarding antibiotic choice. Most trusts swab MRSA +ve patients weekly.

Patient with tuberculosis (TB) If you suspect TB the patient must be nursed in isolation, ideally a ventilated side room. If TB is suspected or acid-fast bacilli (AFBs) have been seen in their sputum then they and/or their visitor should wear a mask during all contact until three consecutive early morning sputum samples are negative. Children, pregnant women or immunocompromised patients should avoid visiting. Treat sputum samples as high-risk (see above). If the patient has to leave the ward for investigations and procedures the patient should wear a mask.

Pregnant patient (p436) Avoid prescribing medications whenever possible; if a medication is necessary then check Appendix 4 of the *BNF*. X-rays should also be avoided, though the pelvis and lower abdomen can be shielded. Pregnant women have different normal values for some blood results (p438) – discuss with the laboratory or O+G if in doubt.

Psychiatric patient Will often need admission to a medical ward; nurse in a bay in clear view of the nurses' station. Inform a psychiatrist early in complex/serious cases – see p536.

Splenectomy Patients who are undergoing splenectomy require vaccination and lifelong antibiotic prophylaxis in order to minimise their risk of contracting an infection. Ideally they should receive vaccinations at least 2wk prior to splenectomy, (otherwise 2wk afterwards) to maximize their effectiveness. Patients require vaccination against *Haemophilus influenzae* type B and meningococcus groups A+C, with yearly influenza and 5-yearly pneumococcal vaccinations. They should also receive penicillin V 250–500mg/12h PO for life. General measures should include advising the patient to carry a medical card saying they have no spleen and to seek medical advice at the first sign of developing an infection eg fever, productive cough. The patient should also be referred to a haematologist to manage the reactive thrombocytosis post-splenectomy. Some patients may require treatment with low-dose aspirin.

Nutrition

A patient's nutritional state has a huge effect on their well being, mood, compliance with treatment and ability to heal. You should consider alternative nutrition for all patients without a normal oral diet for over 48h. IV fluids are only for hydration, they are not nutrition.

Enteral feeding (via the gut)

Oral Most patients manage to consume sufficient quantities of hospital food to stay healthy. If not, consider simple remedies eg favourite foods, medications for reflux/heartburn (p239) or nausea (p252). If they are still not consuming adequate nutrition then discuss with the dietician who can advise on nutritional supplements and high-energy drinks.

Nasogastric (NG) See p588 for insertion procedure. This is a good short-term measure, however placing the tube is uncomfortable and some people cannot tolerate the sensation of the tube once it is in. Unsurprisingly only liquid foods and medicines can be used; this may require liaison with the pharmacist. Tubes can also be placed naso-duodenally or naso-jejunally if required.

Gastrostomy Often called 'PEGs' (Percutaneous Endoscopic Gastrostomy) these are a good long-term method of feeding in patients who cannot feed orally. They can be sited endoscopically, surgically or radiologically and the procedure is quick. It is also possible to place a jejunostomy if required.

Parenteral feeding (via the blood)

Parentral nutrition (PN) or total parentral nutrition (TPN) requires central access because extravasation of the Ca^{2+} in the feed causes severe burns. Central access can be via a long-line (eg PiCC) or central line (eg Hickman). It is used when the patient cannot tolerate sufficient enteral feeds eg short gut syndrome or when gut rest is required eg severe inflammatory bowel disease.

There is significant risk associated with PN use including line insertion, line infection, embolism/thrombosis and electrolyte abnormalities. It is essential to monitor blood electrolytes regularly including Ca^{2+}, PO_4^{3-}, Mg^{2+}, zinc and trace elements.

Refeeding syndrome

After a prolonged period of malnutrition or parentral nutrition, feeds must be reintroduced slowly (over a few days) to prevent electrolyte imbalance, particularly ↓ PO_4^{3-}. It can be fatal.

Nutritional requirements

Name	Sources	Requirement (per day)	Deficiency
Carbohydrate	Almost all foods	300g	Malnutrition
Protein	Meat, dairy, vegetables, grain	50g	Kwashiorkor
Fat	Nuts, meat, dairy, oily foods	56g	Malnutrition
Calcium	Dairy, leafy vegetables	1g	Osteoporosis
Iodine	Fish, seafood, enriched salt	150μg	Hypothyroid
Iron	Meat, vegetables, grains	15mg	Anaemia
Magnesium	Dairy, leafy vegetables, meat	420mg	Cramps
Potassium	Fruits, vegetables	3.5g	Hypokalaemia
Selenium	Meat, fish, vegetables	55μg	Keshan disease
Sodium	Processed foods, salt	2.4g	Hyponatraemia
Zinc	Cereals, meat	11mg	Hair/skin problems
Vitamin A (retinoid)	Dairy, yellow or green leafy vegetables, liver, fish	900μg	Night blindness
Vitamin B_1 (thiamine)	Bread, cereals	1.2mg	Beri Beri
Vitamin B_2 (riboflavin)	Meat, dairy, bread	1.3mg	Ariboflavinosis
Vitamin B_3 (niacin)	Meat, fish, bread	16mg	Pellagra
Vitamin B_5 (pantothenic acid)	Meat, egg, grains, potato, vegetables	5mg	Neurological problems, paraesthesia
Vitamin B_6 (pyridoxine)	Meat, fortified cereals	1.7mg	Anaemia
Vitamin B_7 (biotin)	Liver, fruit, meat	30μg	Dermatitis
Vitamin B_9 (folate)	Bread, leafy vegetables, cereals	400μg	Anaemia
Vitamin B_{12} (cobalamin)	Meat, fish, fortified cereals	2.4μg	Anaemia
Vitamin C (ascorbic acid)	Citrus fruits, tomato, green vegetables	200mg	Scurvy
Vitamin D	Fish, liver, fortified cereals	5–15μg	Rickets/ osteomalacia
Vitamin E	Vegetables, nuts, fruits, cereals	15mg	None
Vitamin K	Green vegetables, cereals	120μg	↑INR

Palliative care

Palliative care is the non-curative treatment of a disease; originally focused towards terminal cancer, but now covers other disorders. In practice cancer patients are still able to access more services, including the excellent Macmillan nurses who should be involved as early as possible. The aim is to provide the best quality of life for as long as possible – this may include admission to a hospice (usually temporarily).

Pain (p428) This is a common problem in palliative care; opioids are the main treatment. It is important to be creative with treatment, consider:

- Treating the source (urinary retention, bowel spasm, bony mets)
- Non-opioid analgesia (nerve blocks, TENS, neuropathic pain)
- Alternative routes (intranasal, PR, transdermal, SC, IM, IV)

The table below is a guide to converting between opioids, it is not an exact science and changes need to be monitored for over- or under-dosing.

Opioid	Route	Typical dose	24h max	Relative[1]
Codeine	PO	60mg/4h	240mg	0.1
Dihydrocodeine	PO	30mg/4h	240mg	0.1
Tramadol	PO	50mg/4h	600mg	0.2
Oral morphine	PO	10mg/1–4h	N/A	1
Oxycodone	PO	5mg/4h	400mg	2
Morphine	SC/IM/IV	5mg/1–4h	N/A	2
Diamorphine	SC	2.5mg/1–4h	N/A	3
Fentanyl	Topical	25μg/h	2400μg	100–150

[1] Multiply current 24hr dose by this number get equivalent 24h oral morphine dose

Other symptoms Many of the treatments listed below can be used in non-palliative patients. For further information on prescribing in palliative problems see *BNF* and *OHCM*7 p522.

Symptom	Treatments
Breathlessness	O_2, open windows, fans, diamorphine, benzodiazepines, steroids, heliox (helium and oxygen for stridor)
Constipation	See p260, also bisacodyl
Cough	Saline nebs, antihistamines, simple/codeine linctus, morphine
Dry mouth	Chlorhexidine, sucking ice or pineapple chunks, consider Candida (thrush) infection, synthetic saliva
Hiccups	Antacids eg Maalox®, Gaviscon®, chlorpromazine, haloperidol
Itching	Emollients, chlorphenamine, cetirizine, colestyramine (obstructive jaundice), ondansetron
Nausea/vomiting	See p252, also levomepromazine and haloperidol

The dying patient If a patient is very ill and not expected to survive, the decision may be taken by a senior doctor (registrar or consultant) to withdraw active treatment and simply keep the patient comfortable. The patient will often (but not always) be bed-bound with minimal oral intake and reduced GCS.

- Document what the patient and the family have been told and the reasons if they have not been informed (eg unconscious)
- Ask a senior doctor to sign a 'not for resuscitation' form
- Stop unnecessary medications (including anticoagulants, antibiotics, steroids, insulin); anticonvulsants should be converted to a suitable route or a midazolam infusion used instead
- Stop blood tests, IV fluids, O_2 except for symptomatic treatment

Pain Exclude a treatable cause of pain, eg urinary retention, constipation, and prescribe adequate analgesia. If the patient is currently in pain give an immediate diamorphine bolus at the PRN dose:

On opioids Use the table opposite to convert oral opioids to equivalent 24h SC diamorphine dose and prescribe a PRN bolus dose:

- ***Syringe driver*** diamorphine infusion SC at rate calculated
- ***PRN*** diamorphine (dose equivalent to 1/6th of 24h dose) SC max 1hrly

Not on opioids Prescribe a PRN dose

- ***PRN*** diamorphine 2.5–5mg SC max 1hrly

Agitation This may be a sign of pain. Try PRN doses initially; add a syringe driver (with additional PRN dose) if regular doses are required:

- ***PRN*** levomepromazine 6.25mg SC max 4hrly
- ***PRN*** midazolam 5mg SC max 4hrly
- ***Syringe driver*** levomepromazine 12.5mg and midazolam 10mg SC

Nausea + vomiting Continue existing antiemetics in a syringe driver if they are controlling the symptoms; if there is no nausea then prescribe PRN levomepromazine and add a syringe driver if it is needed regularly. If further antiemetics are required use a 5-HT antagonist (eg ondansetron):

- ***PRN*** levomepromazine 6.25mg SC 4hrly
- ***Syringe driver*** levomepromazine 12.5–25mg SC

Secretions The patient's breathing may become rattly due to the build-up of secretions with a poor cough/swallow reflex. Sitting the patient up slightly may help; medication improves the symptoms in about 50%. Start with a PRN dose and add a syringe driver if regular doses are required:

- ***PRN*** hyoscine hydrobromide 400–600μg SC 4–8hrly
- ***Syringe driver*** hyoscine hydrobromide 600–2400μg (0.6–2.4mg) SC

Further care Monitor the patient regularly and include them on your daily ward round. Ask the patient and/or relatives if there are any new symptoms and adjust syringe driver doses accordingly. If you are unable to control symptoms ask for palliative care review.

After death Always remember to inform the GP of the patient's death, especially if it was unexpected. This is both courteous and prevents any unfortunate phone calls from the GP enquiring about the patient's health.

Death

The best medicine in the world can only delay death; it is inevitable for everyone. Patients often die in hospital and the following pages act as a guide for what you will be asked to do.

Declaring death

You will often be bleeped to declare a patient dead. This is not an urgent request, but the patient cannot be transferred to the morgue until it is done. There may be other members of staff who can do this. If you are uncomfortable ask a member of staff to accompany you. Check for:

- Reaction to voice and pain (sternal rub/press on supraorbital nerve)
- Pupil reflexes (pupils will be fixed and dilated, often with a dry appearance)
- Central pulse for 1min (carotid or femoral)
- Heart sounds for 1min
- Respiratory effort and sounds for 1min (may still hear gastro noises)

NB it is helpful to note if there is a pacemaker present (see p113).

In the notes Date and time, contacted to declare the patient dead at (time), summary of your examination, pacemaker present/absent. Remember to sign and print your name and bleep number.

16/09/08 *<u>Asked to verify death.</u>*
03:35

No response to pain
Pupils fixed and dilated
No carotid pulse
No audible heart sounds } *for 60 seconds*
No audible breath sounds

Death declared at 03:35 on 16.09.2008.
No pacemaker palpable.

Dr CJ Flint
FLINT, F1
Bleep 3294

Example of what to write in the notes when a patient dies

What happens to the dead patient

When a patient dies the nurses prepare the body, including: lying them flat with one pillow and their eyes and jaw closed (may be propped closed), washing the body, packing orifices with cotton wool and removing attachments (eg fluids, pumps). Lines and tubes are not removed since these will be inspected if a post-mortem is required. The bed curtains are closed and the patient is completely covered with a sheet.

Once they have been declared dead they are taken to the morgue in a portable coffin. Screens are used to try and hide this from other patients.

Aggression and violence

The majority of patients have respect for NHS staff, however under certain circumstances anyone can become aggressive:

- Pain p428
- Confusion or dementia eg hypoglycaemia p281
- Inadequate communication/fear/frustration p56
- Intoxication (medications, alcohol, recreational drugs)
- Mental illness or personality disorder p303–313

The aggressive patient Ask a nurse to accompany you when assessing aggressive patients. Position yourselves between the exit and the patient and ensure that other staff know where you are. The majority of patients can be calmed simply by talking; try to elicit why they are angry and ask specifically about pain and worry. Be calm but firm and do not shout or make threats. If this does not help, offer an oral sedative or give emergency sedation (see p308) or call security if fit to leave.

The aggressive relative Relatives may be aggressive through fear, frustration and/or intoxication. They usually respond to talking, though make sure you obtain consent from the patient before discussing their medical details. Consider offering to arrange a meeting with a senior doctor. If the relative continues to be aggressive, remember that your duty of care to patients does not extend to their relatives; you do not have to tell them anything or listen to threats/abuse. In extreme cases you can ask security or police to remove the relative from the hospital.

Violence Assault (the attempt or threat of causing harm) and battery (physical contact without consent) by a patient or relative is a criminal offence. If you witness an assault or are assaulted yourself, inform your seniors and fill in an incident form including the name and contact details of any witnesses. If no action is taken on your behalf inform the police yourself.

Abuse Patients of any age can be abused in hospitals or outside. Do not be afraid of asking patients how they received injuries or asking directly if someone caused them. Inform a senior if you believe a patient has been abused physically, sexually or by neglect.

Consent

Obtaining consent satisfactorily is a skill which can be learned from senior colleagues, but you must only take consent for procedures you are competent to perform. It is a good idea to initially shadow your seniors when they are taking consent from a patient to learn how to do it properly. It is also sensible to have a senior colleague supervise you the first few times to ensure you include all the relevant information.

Consent	p69	Capacity	p68

Obtaining informed consent For informed consent to be valid, there are four conditions which must be fulfilled:
- Patient must understand what you are telling them and be able to repeat it back to you in a manner which shows their understanding
- Patient must believe what you are telling them
- Patient must be given information about the intended benefits of the procedure and both the common and serious risks involved. They should also understand what may happen if they refuse the procedure.
- Patient must give consent voluntarily

Common risks to mention (if appropriate) when taking consent:
- Pain
- Bleeding
- Infection
- Failure of procedure
- Risks specific to the procedure eg headache after LP

How to obtain informed consent
- Introduce yourself and check the patient's name and DoB
- Say you would like to explain a procedure which will help in diagnosis and treatment of their condition and/or provide relief from their symptoms
- Check they are happy to discuss the procedure and ask if they would like a relative/friend to be present
- Explain what the procedure entails, the intended benefits and risks involved, approximately how long it will take, when/where it will be done and how long it will take to get results/see benefits
- Explain what other options are available and what happens if the patient chooses not to have the procedure
- Ask the patient to repeat the procedure back to you to check they understand correctly
- Ask if they have any questions and are happy to continue
- Get them to sign a written consent form if appropriate or document in their medical notes that the procedure has been explained (give full details of the conversation) and they have given informed consent

Needle-stick injuries

Many doctors have received needle-stick injuries without serious consequences. However, if you have just been exposed get advice asap.

Immediately

Stop what you are doing. If it is urgent, phone your senior/colleague to do it. Your future health is your top priority.

- *Percutaneous exposure* (needle or sharp) squeeze around the wound so that blood comes out and wash with soap and water; avoid scrubbing or pressing the wound directly
- *Mucocutaneous exposure* (eyes, nose, mouth) rinse with water (or 1l of 0.9% saline through a giving set for eyes/nose)

Within an hour

A colleague should:

- *Talk* to the patient alone, explain what has happened and ask about risk factors:
  - injecting drugs, blood transfusions, tattoos or piercings in foreign countries, unprotected sex (particularly in last 3mth, in a developing country or, if male, with a man), testing for hepatitis B+C or HIV and the results
- *Ask* to take a blood sample for testing for hep B+C and HIV

You should:

- *Phone* occupational health if during office hours or go to the ED and follow their advice exactly
- *Document* the event in the patient's notes and an incident form

Post-exposure prophylaxis

You may be prescribed antiretrovirals (triple therapy, within 1h), 500units of hepatitis B immunoglobulin (within 24h) or hepatitis B booster (within 24h) according to the significance of the exposure. There is currently no post-exposure prophylaxis for hepatitis C.

	Hepatitis B	**Hepatitis C**	**HIV**
UK prevalence	<0.5%	<0.5%	<0.1%
Transmission risk	1 in 3 (without vaccine)	1 in 50	1 in 300
Vaccination	Vaccines at 1, 2 + 12mth	None	None
Post-exposure	Immunoglobulin or booster	None	Triple therapy

Over the next few weeks

The patient's blood tests should take <2d for HIV and hep B+C results. Following high-risk exposure you may be advised to have a blood test in the future (2–6mth); during this time you should practise safe sex (condoms) and not donate blood. **You cannot be forced to have an HIV test.** Discuss with occupational health about involvement in surgery.

Pre-op assessment

Elective patients generally attend pre-admission clinics a few weeks before their operation. This enables you to:

- Assess the patient's problem (ie do they need an operation?)
- Gauge their medical fitness for an anaesthetic and surgery
- Request any pre-op investigations (see NICE guidelines below)
- Check consent (this should only be obtained by the surgeon performing the procedure or a person competent to undertake it, see p126)
- Answer any questions the patient may have

Pre-op investigations[1] (p445)

Investigation	Indication
FBC	To exclude infection or anaemia
Sickle-cell screen	African/Mediterranean patients, +ve family history
U+E	Age >60yr, cardiac/renal disease, patients on steroids, diuretics, ACEi
LFT	Previous or suspected abnormal liver function, biliary surgery
Clotting	Established or suspected abnormal liver function
Urine β-hCG	Women of child-bearing age
CXR	Age >60yr, cardiorespiratory disease, malignancy, major thoracic and upper abdominal surgery, unexplained SOB
ECG	Age >50yr, cardiovascular disease, DM, smokers

[1] NICE guidelines: http://www.nice.org.uk/page.aspx?o=CG003

Requesting blood pre-op

Each hospital will have guidelines on the transfusion requirements for most elective operations; become familiar with these.

Blood for transfusion is in limited supply and should only be cross-matched when necessary. The table below shows commonly accepted blood bank requests for elective surgery.

Summary of operations and blood requirements

Blood request	Operation
No request	Minor day-case surgery (carpal tunnel release, peripheral lipoma excision etc)
Group and save	Laparoscopy, appendicectomy, cholecystectomy, hernia repair, simple hysterectomy, liver biopsy, mastectomy, varicose veins
X-match 2units	Colectomy, hemiarthroplasty, laparotomy, TURP, thyroidectomy, total hip replacement
X-match 4units	Abdominoperineal resection, hepatic/pancreatic surgery
X-match 6units	Aneurysm repair (book ITU bed post-op)

Patients with medical problems

- *DM* see p275, put the patient first on the operating list
- *CVS* inform the anaesthetist if patients have had recent chest pain, an undiagnosed murmur or symptoms of heart failure. The anaesthetist may want you to request an echo or may see the patient personally.
- *Obstructive jaundice* check clotting, FBC, CRP, U+E, LFT
- *Rheumatoid arthritis* inform the anaesthetist as patients with RA may be difficult to intubate and are at risk of atlantoaxial instability – the anaesthetist may request a pre-op C-spine X-ray

Contacting the anaesthetist/ITU

Find out who the anaesthetist is for your list and inform them as soon as possible about any patients who may need further investigations or review prior to surgery. If a patient needs an ITU bed post-op, inform ITU well in advance with the date the bed is required. Phone to confirm that the bed is still available on the day of the operation; if it is not the operation may be cancelled.

Special circumstances

- *Steroids* (p154) patients taking regular steroids must have extra steroid cover during surgery and be converted to IV preparations if NBM. Discuss each patient's needs with your team and the anaesthetist.
- *Warfarin* this should be stopped at least 3d pre-operatively. The INR should be <1.5 for most operations and lower if spinal or epidural anaesthetic techniques are to be employed; warn the anaesthetist. Patients who have prosthetic heart values will need IV heparin whilst warfarin is omitted (p347).
- *Aspirin and clopidogrel* must be stopped 7d prior to surgery
- *Oestrogens and progestogens* HRT can be continued as long as DVT/PE prophylaxis is undertaken. Progestogen-only contraceptives can be continued, but combined oral contraceptives should be stopped 4wk prior to surgery and alternative means of contraception used.
- *Bowel preparation* see next page

Writing the drug chart

Try and do this at pre-admission clinic to save yourself time later. Document any allergies. Things to check include:

- *Prophylactic anticoagulation* usually enoxaparin 40mg/24h SC (all cancer patients, >60y, obese); only use 20mg/24h in young fit patients. Ask haematology for advice on patients with prosthetic heart valves (see p347 for APTT checks)
- *Antibiotics* consider pre-op antibiotics (check local guidelines)
- *Bowel preparation and IV fluid* see below
- *Regular drugs* review these and write up those which should be continued in hospital (stop COCP, aspirin as above etc)
- *TED stockings* prescribe these under regular medications for all patients
- *Analgesia and anti-emetics* (p428 and p252) the anaesthetist will usually write these up during the operation

Pre-op assessment (continued)

Instructions for the patient

- Where and when to go for admission (write this down for them)
- If they are to have bowel prep, they should usually be on clear fluids at least 24h before the operation (see below)
- Tell the patient about any drains, NG tubes or catheters which may be inserted during the operation
- Tell them if they are being admitted to ITU post-op

Bowel preparation

Before endoscopy procedures and many types of GI surgery, patients are given laxatives to clear the bowel. For surgery the aim is to reduce the risk of post-op anastamotic leak and infections. Recent evidence suggests that it does not improve complication rates and may even be harmful.[1] At present it is still common practice, but check your local policy.

Bowel preparation	Procedure
None	OGD, ERCP, closure (reversal) ileostomy
Phosphate enema (on day of surgery)	Anal fissure, haemorrhoidectomy, examination under anaesthetic (sigmoid colon/rectum/perianal area), flexible sigmoidoscopy
Full bowel prep(see below)	Colonoscopy, rectoplexy, right hemi-/left hemi-/sigmoid/pancolectomy, anterior resection, abdominoperineal resection, Hartmann's reversal

Full bowel preparation

- Give 1 sachet Picolax® at 08:00 and 14:00 the day before surgery
- Fleet Phospho-soda® and Klean-Prep® are used in some hospitals
- Patients must drink 2–3l/day of clear fluids whilst taking bowel prep to prevent dehydration
- Elderly patients and those with comorbidities should be admitted for IV fluids from the first dose of bowel prep
- Patients can eat ***low-residue foods*** whilst taking bowel prep eg:
    - ***Breakfast*** 2 slices white bread with thin spread of butter/honey, small amount of cornflakes with milk, tea or coffee with milk
    - ***Lunch*** small quantities of: cream/cottage cheese **or** white meat/fish/prawns with 2 slices white bread (no butter) **or** white pasta/white rice **or** 2 small potatoes (no skin or butter)
    - ***Supper*** clear soup and clear jelly only
- Patients may continue drinking clear fluids until 6h before their operation (02:00 for the morning list, 07:00 for the afternoon list)

1 Guenaga K et al. Mechanical bowel preparation for elective colorectal surgery. *Cochrane Database of Systematic Reviews* 2005, Issue 1. Art. No.: CD001544.

Preparing inpatients for surgery

Checklist

Before your patient goes to theatre, you have a responsibility to check the following have been done:

- The consent form has been signed by the patient and surgeon
- The patient has been seen by the anaesthetist
- The operation site has been marked by the surgeon (imperative if the operation could be bilateral, eg inguinal hernia repair)
- The pre-operative blood results are in the notes
- The pre-operative ECG and/or CXR are available (CXR should be stored on PACS)
- Prophylactic LMWH, TED stockings and antibiotics have been prescribed (do not give enoxaparin <12h pre-op if having spinal/epidural)
- The patient has received bowel preparation if necessary
- The patient has been adequately fasted (see below)
- Blood has been crossmatched and is available if required
- Check if the patient has any last minute questions or concerns and is still happy to proceed with the operation

Oral fluids pre- and post-op

In general, patients should not eat for at least 6h before going to theatre but can have clear fluids until 2h. In emergencies this rule may be overruled, but the risk of aspiration of gastric contents will be increased.

If patients are admitted for an operation which requires bowel preparation, check your hospital guidelines as to what oral intake the patient is allowed whilst taking the laxatives, usually it is either clear fluids only or a low-residue diet (see p130).

Nil by mouth (NBM) Patients cannot have any oral food or significant fluid intake; hydration must be maintained with IV fluids. However, oral medication (eg anti-arrhythmics) may be taken with a sip of water, if not taking them would put the patient at more risk. Non-essential medication such as vitamin supplements may be omitted; check with your seniors.

Clear fluids Include non-carbonated drinks such as black tea, black coffee, water, squash drinks (not milk or fruit juice).

Sips 30ml water/hour orally, usually given for the first day after major abdominal surgery involving bowel anastomoses.

Soft diet This includes food such as soup and jelly. Once patients have been tolerating clear fluids post-operatively for at least 24h, they may be allowed to start a soft diet.

Most patients can safely drink clear fluids up to 2h before surgery. The following increase the risk of aspiration:

- Pregnancy
- Being elderly
- Obesity
- Stomach disorders eg hiatus hernia, reflux
- Pain (+opioids)

Booking theatre lists

Elective lists

Discuss the order of the list with your consultant/registrar (you may need to obtain the operating list from your consultant's secretary or direct from theatre).

The list usually must be submitted by the afternoon before the operating day. You should include:

- Theatre number
- Name of the consultant surgeon
- Name, sex, age, hospital number and location of each patient
- Special patient requirements (eg DM, blood requested, ITU bed booked)
- Operation and side in full (eg open repair left inguinal hernia)
- Sign and leave your bleep number
- If the order of the list needs to be changed, contact theatres and inform them as soon as possible

Booking the order of operations

In general, surgeons tend to prefer a specific order of patients:

- Older patients before younger (except children)
- Patients with comorbidities (eg DM) before healthy
- Clean operations before dirty (eg bowel resection)
- Longer, more complex operations before shorter

Booking emergency operations

- Ensure you discuss the case with the ST1/2 and registrar on-call and that they have agreed to put the patient on the list
- Enter the patient's details as outlined above, noting the time at which the patient last ate
- Inform the on-call anaesthetic ST1/2 and registrar about the patient
- Check the patient has been consented and make sure the results of any relevant investigations are available (including a G+S sample and a pregnancy test in women of child-bearing age)
- You may also need to inform the theatre coordinator

The operating theatre

Theatre design

Operating theatres include an operating area, a scrubbing-up area, a preparation room, a sluice and an anaesthetic room. Most theatres have a whiteboard (to document date, operation and number of swabs used), an X-ray viewing box and an area to write up the operation notes and histopathology forms. Above the operating table, there are usually two mobile lights (satellites).

Theatre staff

Each operating theatre has a team of assistants who clean and maintain the theatre. The 'scrub nurse' scrubs for each operation to select instruments as requested by the surgical team. One other trained nurse and an auxiliary nurse act as 'runners' to fetch equipment for the scrub nurse and to monitor the number of swabs and sutures used (displayed on the whiteboard). An operating departmental assistant (ODA) maintains the anaesthetic equipment and assists the anaesthetist. Each operation is logged, with details of the patient, name of the operating surgeon, patient's consultant and anaesthetist.

Theatre clothing

Fresh scrubs should be worn for each operating list and should be changed between lists, or between cases if they become dirty or potentially infected with MRSA. Theatre shoes are essential for safety purposes and you will not be allowed to enter without them. Theatre scrubs and shoes should not be worn outsides of theatres except in an emergency.

Scrubbing up

Scrubbing up is an art and a key part of minimising infection risk to the patient. If in doubt, a theatre nurse can show you how to do it.

- Prior to scrubbing, remove jewellery and put your mask and a theatre hat on
- Open a gown pack and drop a pair of sterile gloves on top
- When scrubbing up for the first patient, scrub under your nails using a brush with iodine. Wash hands for a further 5min.
- Unravel your gown; ensure that it does not touch the floor
- Touching its inner aspects only, put it on with the end of the sleeves covering your hands
- Put on your gloves. Do not touch the outside of your gloves with your bare hands.
- For high-risk operations (eg Caesarean, HIV +ve) double-glove and protect your eyes with a visor or safety spectacles
- Wait for an assistant to tie your scrub gown from behind
- If your hand becomes non-sterile, change your glove. If your gown becomes non-sterile you need to rescrub; change your gown and gloves.

The operating theatre (continued)

Theatre etiquette

- Check the correct patient is undergoing the correct operation on the correct side (match the consent form to the patient's wristband)
- If you are scrubbed up:
  - ask someone not scrubbed to adjust the lights for you
  - do not pick up instruments which fall to the ground
  - if you are handed an instrument by someone who is not scrubbed, check that you can touch it before accepting it
- In operations involving the abdomen and the perineum, if you are asked to move from the perineum to the abdomen you must rescrub. This is not necessary when swapping from abdomen to perineum.
- If you sustain a needle-stick injury, leave the operation and report to occupational health (p127)
- Always eat/drink and go to the toilet before going to an operating list

Watching an operation

Make sure you can see; get a stool or stand at the patient's head if the anaesthetist allows. Although you are not actively participating in the operation, use the time to learn surgical techniques. If you can't follow what's going on, ask. As the operation finishes, fill in any histology forms or TTOs if appropriate. Check histology samples are labelled accurately.

Some commonly used instruments in theatre

- *Dissecting forceps* used to handle tissue during dissection and suturing. May be toothed or non-toothed, serrated or non-serrated; eg De Bakey forceps
- *Tissue forceps* used to hold static tissue whilst dissecting around it. They are hinged in the middle with a ratchet lock on the handle; eg Allis and Littlewood's forceps
- *Haemostatic (artery) forceps* usually lightweight with spring handles and a delicate tip used to identify and hold bleeding points or vascular pedicles; eg Mosquito, Spencer Wells and Kocher's forceps
- *Abdominal retractors* much loved by junior doctors! eg Langenbeck, Morris and Deaver retractors
- *Operating scissors* may be used to separate and dissect tissue or cut through scar tissue. May be straight/curved with round or bevelled blades; eg McIndoe scissors.
- *Needle-holders* are designed to hold needles securely with a locking mechanism at the handle. They can be straight or curved; eg Mayo and Halsey needle-holders.
- *Needles* may be cutting (triangular in cross-section) for skin or tendon sutures or round-bodied (oval/round in cross-section) for gut and vascular anastomoses. They can be straight or curved.

Surgical tools

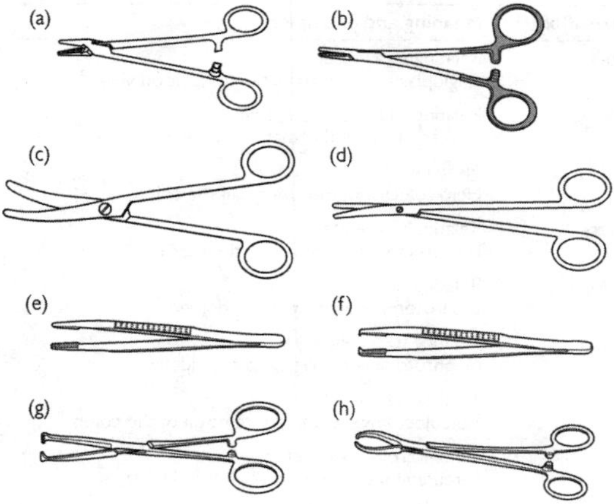

Needle-holders (a) Mayo (b) Halsey
Scissors (c) curved (d) McIndoe
Dissecting forceps (e) non-toothed (f) toothed
Tissue forceps (g) Allis (h) Littlewoods

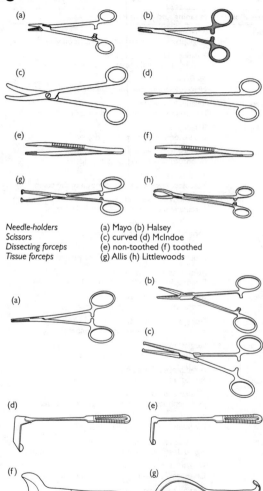

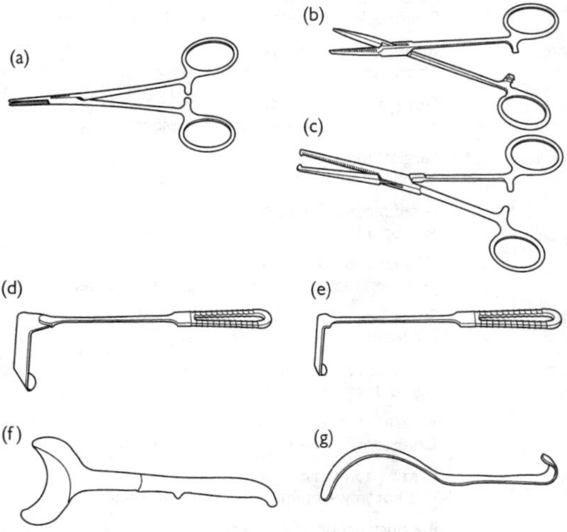

Haemostatic forceps (a) Mosquito Halstead (b) Spencer Wells
(c) Kocher's artery forceps
Retractors (d) Langenbeck (e) Morris (f) Doyen (g) Deaver

Surgical terminology

Prefix/suffix	Meaning and example
Angio-	Relating to a vessel Angioplasty – reconstruction of a blood vessel
Chol-	Relating to the biliary system Cholecystitis – inflammation of the gallbladder
Hemi-	Meaning half of something Hemicolectomy – excising half the colon
Hystero-	Relating to the uterus Hysterectomy – removal of the uterus
Lapar-	Relating to the abdomen Laparotomy – opening the abdomen
Nephr-	Relating to the kidney Nephrotoxic – damaging to the kidney
Pan-	Total/every Pancolectomy – complete removal of the colon
Per-	Going through a structure Percutaneous – going through the skin
Peri-	Near or around a structure Perianal – near the anus/around the anus
Proct-	Relating to the rectum Proctoscopy – examination of the rectum
Pyelo-	Relating to the renal pelvis Pyelonephritis – inflammation of the renal pelvis
Thoraco-	Relating to the thorax Thoracotomy – opening the thorax
Trans-	Going across a structure Transoesophageal – across the oesophagus
-ectomy	Surgical excision Nephrectomy – removal of a kidney
-gram	A radiological image often using contrast medium Angiogram – contrast study of arteries
-itis	Inflammation of an organ Pyelonephritis – inflammation of the renal pelvis
-olith	Stone-like Faecolith – solid, stone-like stool
-oscope	A device for looking inside the body Sigmoidoscope – device for looking into the bowel
-ostomy	An artifical opening between two cavities or to the outside Colostomy – opening of the colon to the skin
-otomy	Cutting something open Craniotomy – opening the cranium (skull)
-plasty	Reconstruction of a structure Myringoplasty – repair of the tympanic membrane

Wound management

Types of wound healing

- *Primary closure* This is most common in surgery, where wound edges are opposed soon after the time of injury and held in place by sutures, steristrips or staples. The aim is to minimise the risk of wound infection with minimal scar tissue formation.
- *Delayed primary closure* This is more commonly used in 'dirty' or traumatic wounds. The wound is cleaned, debrided and then initially left open for 2–5d. Antibiotic cover may be given until the wound is reviewed for closure.
- *Secondary closure* This is much less commonly encountered in surgery. Healing by secondary intention happens when the wound is left open and heals slowly by granulation. This is used in the presence of large areas of excised tissue, infection or significant trauma, where closing the wound would be impossible or would give rise to significant complications.

Abdominal wound breakdown

	Ask about	Examine	Management
Superficial dehiscence	Pink serous discharge, burst sutures	Skin and fat cavity exposed (rectus sheath closed)	Not an emergency but ask for senior review – wound needs packing, may need antibiotics
Deep dehiscence	Pink serous discharge, haematoma, bowel protrusion	Separation of wound edges with bowel exposed	Call for senior help urgently. Cover the bowel with a large sterile swab soaked in 0.9% saline. Check analgesia and fluid replacement, give antibiotics.
Infection	Pyrexia, pain, erythema, white, yellow or bloody exudate from wound site	Tenderness, odorous discharge, swelling	Wound swab, broad-spectrum antibiotics initially

Post-op care

As well as seeing patients pre-operatively, you should review them after the operation, before you go home. This means you can review and discharge day cases with your team, as well as making sure the inpatients are stable after the operation.

Discharging day cases (this may be done by nursing staff)

Before sending day surgery patients home, you should make sure they are alert, have eaten and had fluids without vomiting, have passed urine, are mobilising without fainting and have adequate pain relief. Inspect the operation site and check their observations. Go through the operation procedure, findings and follow-up with the patient.

Organise appropriate follow-up care and clarify if they need dressing changes, suture removal dates and where this can be done (GP surgery, the ED or ward). If the patient develops any post-operative temperatures, pain or bleeding, they should contact their GP or come to the ED.

Common questions about discharge

- Tell the patient if their sutures are dissolvable or if they need to come back to have them taken out (give dates)
- Patients can shower and commence driving again 48h after minor surgery (as long they can perform an emergency stop; see p646)
- Advise patients not to fly for 6wk following major surgery

Inpatient post-op care

Post-op patients are at risk of complications associated with the operation, either directly (eg haemorrhage) or indirectly (eg PE)

When reviewing post-operative patients, document the number of days since the operation and the operation they underwent (eg 2d post left mastectomy)

Ask about pain, ability to eat and drink, nausea/vomiting, urinary output and colour, bowel movements/flatus, mobilisation

Examine wound site, chest, abdomen, legs, drains, stoma bags, IV cannulate, catheter bag, drain entry site, amount drained, colour of any fluid being drained

Look at the observations pyrexia, HR, BP, RR, fluid balance (ie NG tube output, urinary output, drains); document all findings

Review the drug chart for analgesia, antibiotics, fluids

Check post-operative Hb; transfuse if necessary (p340)

Involve other members of the multidisciplinary team if necessary, eg stoma nurse, pain team, physiotherapists, social worker

Post-op problems

Hypotension (p209)

Ask about pre-op BP, fluid input, epidural, drugs

Look for repeat BP, HR, fluid input/urine output, temperature, GCS, orientation, skin temp, cap-refill, signs of hypovolaemia/sepsis, wounds, drain, abdomen, any signs of active bleeding

Management 15min obs, monitor hourly urine output (catheterise bladder). Lie the patient flat, elevate the legs and give oxygen. Get IV access, consider fluid challenge (eg 500ml crystalloid stat, see p210). Send bloods for FBC and crossmatch (blood cultures if you suspect sepsis). Apply pressure to any obvious bleeding points. Call for senior review early.

Pyrexia temp >37.5°C, investigate if this persists/increases after the first 24h post-op; refer to p392

Ask about cough/SOB, wound, dysuria/frequency, abdo pain, diarrhoea

Look for BP, HR, temp, wound, catheter, IV cannulae, chest, abdomen

Management urine M,C+S, FBC, U+E, CRP, blood cultures, CXR, abdominal USS or CT, echo if new onset murmur

Likely causes of post-op pyrexia by day post-surgery

- **Day 1-2** atelectasis; treat with salbutamol/saline nebs and chest physio
- **Day 3-4** pneumonia; treat with antibiotics and chest physio
- **Day 5-6** anastomotic leak; need to take back to theatre
- **Day 7-8** wound infection; treat by opening up wound, antibiotics, may need to return to theatre
- **Day 9-10** DVT/PE; treat with heparin/LMWH then warfarin

Shortness of breath/↓O_2 sats (p219)

Ask about chronic lung/CVS disease, previous PE, chest pain, ankle swelling, new onset cough

Look for BP, HR, temp, pallor, lungs (consolidation, crackles, air entry), signs of fluid overload, leg oedema/calf swelling

Management Sit up and give O_2. FBC, ABG, CXR, ECG. Consider 0.9% saline nebs, antibiotics and regular chest physiotherapy. If you suspect a PE (p225) call for senior help and specialist advice (medical registrar on-call).

Pain	p428
Nausea and vomiting	p252
Low urine output	p317

Common elective operations

Laparoscopic cholecystectomy

Operation to remove the gallbladder

Indications symptomatic gallbladder stones, asymptomatic patients at risk of complications (diabetics, history of pancreatitis, immunosuppressed)

Pre-op no bowel prep required, 6h fasting pre-anaesthetic (see p130)

Procedure involves insufflating the abdomen with CO_2, inserting 4 ports through the anterior abdominal wall to enable laparoscopy and the use of operating instruments to remove the gallbladder

Post-op patients can eat as soon as they recover from the anaesthetic, can usually go home later in the day or the following morning. Not all patients are followed up; some consultants like to review patients in clinic after 6–8wks.

Complications haemorrhage, wound infections, bile leakage, bile duct stricture, retained stones

Colectomy

Operation to remove part or all of the bowel

Indications malignancy, IBD which can no longer be managed medically

Pre-op full bowel prep required, 6h fasting pre-anaesthetic (see p130)

Procedure involves a midline longitudinal laparotomy incision and resection of the diseased bowel. A stoma may or may not be formed.

Post-op sips of fluid orally for 24h post-op, gradually built up to free fluids and then light diet. Hospital stay 7–14 days. All patients followed up in clinic.

Complications haemorrhage, wound infection, wound dehiscence, anastomotic leak

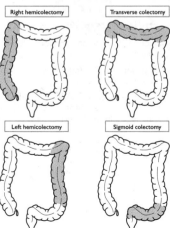

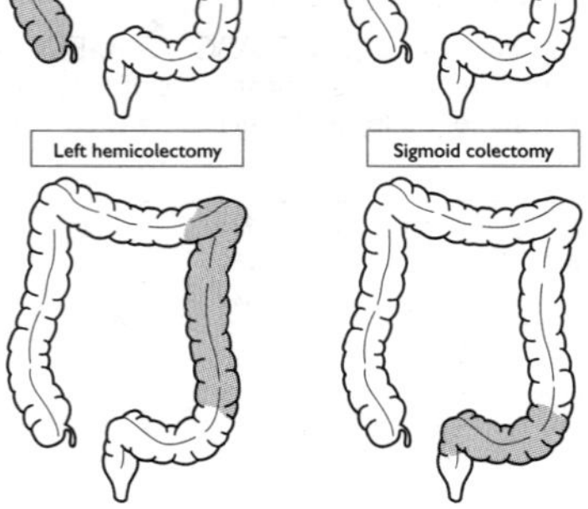

The shaded areas represent the section of colon removed during the operation.

Anterior resection

Operation to resect the rectum with a sufficient margin (usually 5cm) and anastomose the left side of the colon with the rectal stump

Indications rectal carcinoma

Pre-op full bowel prep required, phosphate enema 1h pre-op, 6h fasting pre-anaesthetic (see p130)

Procedure involves a midline longitudinal laparotomy incision and resection of the diseased rectum

Post-op sips of fluid orally for 24h post-op, gradually built up to free fluids and then light diet. Hospital stay 7–14 days. All patients followed up in clinic.

Complications haemorrhage, wound infection, wound dehiscence, anastomotic leak

Anterior resection

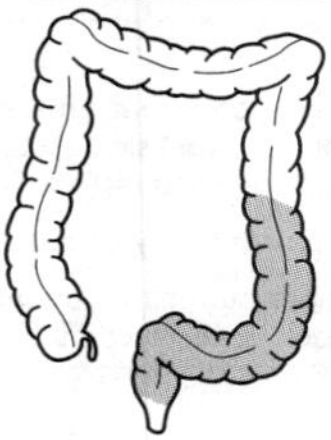

Abdominoperineal resection (AP resection)

Operation to resect the rectum/anus and form a permanent colostomy

Indications low rectal carcinoma where it would be impossible to resect the tumour without removing the anus, can also be performed as part of a panproctocolectomy for ulcerative colitis

Pre-op full bowel prep required, phosphate enema 1h pre-op, 6h fasting pre-anaesthetic (see p130), stoma nurses to be involved

Procedure involves a midline longitudinal laparotomy incision and resection of the diseased rectum and anus

Post-op sips of fluid orally for 24h post-op, gradually built up to free fluids and then light diet. Hospital stay 10–14 days. All patients followed up in clinic.

Complications haemorrhage, wound infection, wound dehiscence, stoma retraction

AP resection

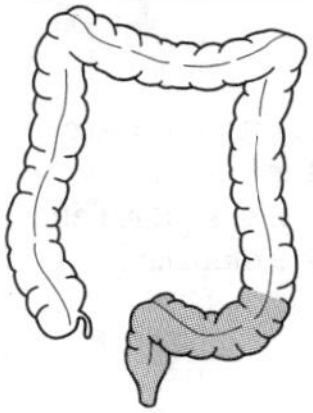

Stomas

Colostomy usually in age >50yr	
Common locations	LIF or right hypochondrium
Features	May be permanent or temporary; mucosa sutured directly to skin
Output	Soft/solid stool; intermittently passed
Indications	Colorectal cancer, diverticular disease, trauma, radiation enteritis, bowel ischaemia, obstruction, Crohn's disease

Ileostomy usually in age 20–50yr	
Common locations	RIF
Features	Usually permanent; bowel mucosa sutured to form a 'spout' to avoid skin contact with bowel contents which are irritating (not flush with skin)
Output	Liquid stool (may be bile-stained); passed continuously
Indications	GI tract cancer, IBD, trauma, radiation enteritis, bowel ischaemia, obstruction

Urostomy usually in age >20yr	
Sometimes referred to as a nephrostomy if originating in renal pelvis	
Common locations	Left or right flank, lower anterior abdominal wall
Features	A ureteric catheter may be protruding from the skin into the stoma
Output	Clear urine passed continuously
Indications	Renal tract cancer, urinary tract obstruction, spinal column disorders, hydronephrosis, urinary fistulae

Common complications

- Electrolyte/fluid imbalance
- Ischaemia/necrosis shortly after formation
- Obstruction/prolapse/parastomal hernia
- Skin erosion/infection
- Psychosocial implications

It is important to refer patients who are likely to need stomas to the stoma care nurse prior to the operation. Patients with stomas also need to alter their diet to avoid excess flatulence or overly watery stool, so should also be referred to the dietician.

Chapter 8

Prescribing

Prescribing – general considerations

Prescribing medicines is rarely taught well in medical school, yet it is one of the first tasks you'll be asked to do on day one. Even the most experienced of doctors will only know the dose and frequency of a maximum of 30-40 drugs, so do not worry if you cannot even remember the dose of paracetamol – for adults it's 1g/4–6h PO max 4g/24h (p428).

Most medical errors in hospital these involve drugs so it is important to consider a few things every time you want to prescribe a drug, rather than just write a prescription as a knee-jerk reaction.

Indication Is there a valid indication for the drug? Is there an alternative method to solve the problem in question (such as move to a quiet area of the ward rather than prescribe night-time sedation).

Contra-indications Are there contra-indications to the drug you are about to prescribe? Does the patient have asthma or suffer with Raynaud's syndrome, in which case β-blockers may create more problems than they solve.

Route of administration If a patient is nil by mouth, then it is pointless prescribing oral medications on the whole; use the *BNF* or ask the pharmacist to help you use alternative routes of administration. Remember IM and SC injections are painful, so avoid these if possible.

Drug interactions Some drugs are incompatible when mixed together (eg morphine and cyclizine), and other drug combinations should ring alarm bells (ACEi with K^+-sparing diuretics). Look through the patient's drug chart to spot obvious drug interactions (p147).

Adverse effects All drugs have side-effects. Ensure the benefits of treatment outweigh the risk of side-effects and remember some patients are more prone to some side-effects than others (eg Reye's syndrome in children with aspirin or occulogyric crises in the young with metoclopramide).

Administering drugs Sometimes it's necessary for doctors to prescribe and administer a drug to the patient. Always double check the drug prescription and the drug with another member of staff (qualified nurse, doctor or pharmacist). This is not a sign of uncertainty, this is a sign that you are meticulous and will greatly limit the chance of a drug error occurring, which would make you look careless.

If in doubt Never prescribe or administer a drug you are unsure about. Even if it is a dire emergency seek senior help or consult the *BNF* or a pharmacist.

How to prescribe – best practice

Knowing how drugs work and their common side-effects is very useful, but you must also be able to safely prescribe them to the patient. There are a few basic rules about prescribing; and if you are even slightly unsure ask the ward or hospital pharmacist or *BNF* – it's not a sign of failure.

The basics There are usually at least four drug sections on the drug card; once-only, regular medications, PRN medications and infusions (fluids) (p146). Other sections might include O_2, anticoagulants, insulin, medications prior to admission and nurse prescriptions.

Labelling the drug card As with the patient's notes, the drug card should have at least three identifying features: name, DoB, hospital number or address. There are usually spaces to document the ward, consultant, date of admission and number of drug cards in use (1 of 2, 2 of 2 etc).

The allergy box Ask the patient about allergies and check old drug cards if available. Document any allergies in this box and the reaction which was precipitated; eg penicillin → rash. If there are no known drug allergies, then record this too. Nurses are unable to give any drugs unless this box is complete.

Writing a prescription Use black pen and write clearly, ideally in capitals. Use the generic drug name (diclofenac, not Voltarol®) and clearly indicate the dose, route, frequency of administration, date started and circle the times the drug should be given. Record any specific instructions (such as 'with food') and sign the entry, writing your name and bleep number clearly on the first prescription.

Common abbreviations

- IV – intravenous
- PO – by mouth
- IM – intramuscular
- SC – subcutaneous
- PR – by rectum
- INH – inhaled
- NEB – nebulised
- stat – immediately
- g – gram
- microgram - avoid mcg or μg
- unit - never write 'U' or 'IU'
- †,†† one tablet, two tablets
- od – once a day/24h
- om – every morning
- on – every night
- bd – twice a day/12h
- tds – three times a day/8h
- qds – four times a day/6h
- international units – avoid 'IU'
- PRN – as required
- mg – milligram
- ml – millilitre

Controlled drugs See page 149.

Changes to prescriptions If a prescription is to change do not amend the original; cross it out clearly and write a new prescription (see page 146). Initial and date any cancelled prescriptions and record a reason if appropriate (eg β-blocker stopped in wheezy asthmatic patient).

Rewriting drug cards When rewriting drug cards ensure the correct drugs, doses and original start dates are carried over and that the old drug card(s) are crossed through and filed in the notes.

Drug			Date/Time	-/--	--/--/--
PARACETAMOL			0600		
Route	Dose	Start	0800		
PO / PR	1g	18.09.08	1000		
Additional instructions			1200		CJF
			1400		
Signature		Pharmacy	1800		
Dr C J Flint			2200		
			0000		

Example of cancelled drug prescription for a regular medication

Drug			Date	18.09.08	
IBUPROFEN					
Route	Dose	Start	Time	12:35	
PO	400mg	16.09.08			
Max frequency		Max dose/24 hr	Dose	400mg	
8 hourly		2.4g			
Indications for use			Route	PO	
Analgesia / fever					
Signature		Pharmacy	Given by	SN Jones	
Dr C J Flint					

Example of drug prescription for a prn medication

Date	Drug	Dose	Route	Time	Prescribed	Given by	Time
16.09.08	ASPIRIN	300mg	PO	STAT	C J Flint	SN Jones	15:35

Example of a once-only (stat) medication

Verbal prescriptions

You may prescribe common drugs over the telephone, but you must say the prescription to two nurses and sign for it as soon as possible. Try to avoid verbal prescribing, but it is occasionally necessary. Check your hospital policy first.

Self-prescribing

F1s can only prescribe on inpatient drug cards and TTOs. The GMC has recommended that doctors should not self-prescribe and seek to consult with their own GP instead.

Drug interactions

A list of specific drug interactions are shown in Appendix 1 of the *BNF*

Pharmacokinetic interactions occur when one drugs alters the *absorption, distribution, metabolism* or *excretion* of another drug which alters the fraction of active drug, causing an aberrant response to a standardised dose. See the examples below:

- **Absorption** metal ions (Ca^{2+}, Fe^{2+}, Mg^{2+}) form complexes with tetracyclines and decrease their absorption
- **Distribution** warfarin is highly bound to albumin, so drugs such as the sulphonamides which compete for binding sites cause displacement of warfarin, increasing both its free fraction and anticoagulant effect
- **Metabolism** rifampicin is a potent enzyme inducer (p150) and increased metabolism of the OCP reduces its clinical effectiveness; other forms of contraception should be used in such circumstances
- **Excretion** some of the NSAIDs compete with methotrexate for active sites in the kidney, and as a consequence methotrexate toxicity can be precipitated

Pharmacodynamic interactions occur when two or more agents have affinity for the same site of drug action, such as:

- Salbutamol and propranolol (a non-specific β-blocker) have opposing effects at the β-adrenergic receptor; clinical effect is determined by the relative concentrations of the two agents and their receptor affinity

Drugs which commonly have interactions include digoxin, warfarin, anti-epileptics, many antibiotics, antidepressants, antipsychotics, theophylline and amiodarone. **If in doubt, look in the *BNF*.**

Reporting adverse drug reactions

The Yellow Card Scheme has been running for over 40 years, and is coordinated by the Medicines and Healthcare products Regulatory Agency (MHRA). Yellow tear-out slips in the back of the *BNF* are completed and sent off and used to monitor adverse drug reactions. The forms can be completed by any healthcare worker and even patients.

Common drug reactions such as constipation from opiates, indigestion from NSAIDs and dry mouth with anticholinergics are well recognised and considered minor effects and do not need reporting

Sinister drug effects such as anaphylaxis, haemorrhage, severe skin reactions etc must be reported via the Yellow Card Scheme, irrespective of how well documented they already are. Any suspected reaction from a new drug (drugs marked with an inverted triangle (▼) in the *BNF*) must also be reported by this scheme.

24 hour contact can be made with the MHRA via telephone (0800 731 6789) or the internet (www.yellowcard.gov.uk), though this service is not designed to offer clinical advice on adverse events, it is merely a drug monitoring facility

Special considerations

Every prescription should be carefully considered with specific consideration of the patient in question. If in doubt, consult the *BNF* or speak to the pharmacist or a senior. There are some groups of patients for whom prescriptions must be even more carefully considered.

Patients with liver disease see Appendix 2 of the *BNF*. The liver has tremendous capacity and reserve so liver disease is often severe by the time the activity of most drugs is altered. The liver clears some drugs directly into bile (such as rifampicin) so these should be used cautiously if at all. The liver also manufactures plasma proteins (namely albumin) and hypoproteinaemia can result in increased free fractions of some agents (phenytoin, warfarin, prednisolone) and result in exaggerated pharmacodynamic responses. Hepatic encephalopathy can be made worse by sedative drugs (night sedation, opiates etc), and fluid overload by NSAIDs and corticosteroids is well documented in liver failure. Hepatotoxic drugs (such as methotrexate and isotretinoin) should only be used by experts as they may precipitate fulminant hepatic failure and death. Patients with established liver failure have an increased bleeding tendency so avoid IM injections.

Patients with renal disease see Appendix 3 of the *BNF*. Patients with *impaired* renal function should only be given nephrotoxic drugs with extreme caution as these may precipitate fulminant renal failure; these include NSAIDs, gentamicin, lithium, ACEi and IV contrast. Any patient with renal disease (impairment or end-stage renal failure) will have altered drug handling (metabolism, clearance, volume of distribution etc) and specialist advice must always be sought when prescribing for these patients (*BNF*, pharmacist or senior); the amount, dosing frequency, and choice of drug needs careful thought. Remember that a creatinine in the 'normal' range does not mean normal renal function, see p321.

Pregnant patients see Appendix 4 of the *BNF*. Many drugs can cross the placenta and have effects upon the fetus. In the first trimester (weeks 1–12) this usually results in congenital malformations, and in the second (weeks 13–26) and third (weeks 27–42) trimesters usually results in growth retardation or has direct toxic effects upon fetal tissues. There are no totally 'safe' drugs to use in pregnancy, but there are drugs known to be particularly troublesome. The minimum dose and the shortest duration possible should be used when prescribing in pregnancy and all drugs avoided if possible in the first trimester.

- ***Drugs considered acceptable*** penicillins, cephalosporins, heparin, ranitidine, paracetamol, codeine
- ***Drugs to avoid*** tetracyclines, streptomycin, quinolones, warfarin, thiazides, ACEi, lithium, NSAIDs, alcohol, retinoids, barbiturates, opioids, cytotoxic drugs and phenytoin

Breast-feeding patient see Appendix 5 of the *BNF*. As with pregnant patients, drugs given to the mother can get into breast milk and into the feeding baby. Some drugs become more concentrated in breast milk than maternal plasma (such as iodides) and can be toxic to the child. Other drugs can stunt the child's suckling reflex (eg barbiturates), or act to stop breast milk production altogether (eg bromocriptine). Check Appendix 5 of the *BNF* or speak to a pharmacist before prescribing any drug to a mother who is feeding a child breast milk.

Children see the *British National Formulary for Children*. Neonates are unpredictable in terms of pharmacokinetics and pharmacodynamics; prescriptions for this age group should be undertaken by experienced paediatric staff and drugs double-checked prior to administration. After the first month or two the gut, renal system and metabolic pathways are more predictable. Almost all drug doses still need to be calculated by weight (eg mg/kg) or by body-surface area (BSA). There are a few drugs which should never be prescribed in children by a non-specialist, including tetracycline (causes irreversible staining of bones and teeth), aspirin (predisposes to Reye's syndrome); others should be used with caution such as prochlorperazine and isotretinoin. **Always consult the *BNF for children* when prescribing for paediatric patients.**

Controlled drugs

Controlled drugs (CDs) are those drugs which are addictive and most often abused or stolen, and are subject to the prescription and storage requirements of the Misuse of Drugs Regulations 2001; they include the strong opiates (morphine, diamorphine, pethidine, fentanyl, alfentanil, remifentanil, methadone), amphetamine-like agents (methylphenidate (Ritalin®)) and cocaine (a local anaesthetic). These agents are stored in a locked cabinet and a record of their use on a named patient basis is required to be kept by law. Some other drugs may be kept in the CD cupboard such as KCl, ketamine, benzodiazepines and anabolic steroids, but this is not a legal requirement and will depend upon local policy. The weaker opiates (codeine, tramadol) are not treated as controlled drugs though they are still often misused.

Prescribing controlled drugs for inpatients is just like prescribing any other drug and the benefits should be balanced against potential side-effects for each individual patient. Morphine, diamorphine and pethidine are the most commonly prescribed CDs on the ward. As with all prescriptions, write the details clearly and make sure a maximum dose and a minimal interval between doses is documented (see p428 for management of pain).

Controlled drugs for TTOs see p106.

Enzyme inducers and inhibitors

The term *enzyme inducers* is used to describe agents (usually drugs, but not always) which alter the activity of hepatic enzymes, namely the cytochrome P450 enzymes which are involved in phase 1 metabolism. Agents which *induce* cytochrome P450 activity result in increased metabolism and reduced activity of other drugs; *inhibitors* of cytochrome P450 have the reverse effect and result in exaggerated drug responses. Common inducers and inhibitors are listed below.

Inducers

The following table shows drugs that induce enzymes. Each of the drugs on the left can induce the enzymes so that all of the drugs on the right (and any of the other drugs on the left) will have reduced plasma levels:

Enzyme inducers		Plasma levels reduced
Phenobarbitone/barbiturates		Warfarin
Rifampicin		Oral contraceptives
Phenytoin	→	Corticosteroids
Ethanol (chronic use)		Ciclosporin
Carbamazepine		(all drugs on left)

Inhibitors

The following table shows drugs that inhibit enzymes. Specific drugs on the left can inhibit the enzymes so that specific drugs (only the ones on the same line) on the right will have increased plasma levels:

Enzyme inhibitors		Plasma levels increased
Disulfiram	→	Warfarin
Chloramphenicol	→	Phenytoin
Corticosteroids	→	Tricyclic antidepressants
Cimetidine	→	Amiodarone, phenytoin, pethidine
MAO inhibitors	→	Pethidine
Erythromycin	→	Theophylline
Ciprofloxacin	→	Theophylline

Therapeutic drug monitoring

Monitoring of therapeutic drug levels is routine for some drugs and is useful in cases where under-dosing or over-dosing is suspected.

Taking blood for many drugs it is necessary to have a 'trough' level taken just before a dose (lowest plasma level) and a 'peak' level (timing of which varies for different drugs). Most drugs are assayed from a clotted sample (p557); as a rule antibiotic drug levels are sent to microbiology while all others to clinical chemistry – check with your laboratories.

Interpreting results of therapeutic drug monitoring can be very difficult. Potentially toxic drug levels should be telephoned to the ward and usually advice given on dose changes. Otherwise dose changes should be made by someone who is familiar with the kinetics of the drug and aware of potential interactions with other agents; this is likely to be your senior. As a general rule: high peak, reduce dose; high trough, reduce frequency.

Drugs commonly monitored advice on when to take blood and expected ranges are listed below with toxic levels associated and clinical features, where appropriate. Individual hospitals may have different therapeutic ranges depending on the type of assay used – check locally.

Amikacin	*peak 1h post IV dose* 20–30mg/l; *trough* <10mg/l
Carbamazepine	*random sample* 20–50µmol/l (4–12mg/l); *toxic* >50µmol/l (>12mg/l)
Ciclosporin	*trough* 50–200µg/l; *toxic* >200µg/l
Digoxin	optimum sampling time *6–12h post oral dose* 1–2.6nmol/l (0.8–2µg/l); *toxic* >2.6nmol/l (>2µg/l). Toxicity can occur at levels <1.3nmol/l if patient has ↓K^+; *signs of toxicity* arrhythmia (heart block, bradycardia), confusion, insomnia, agitation, yellow vision (xanthopsia), delirium, nausea and vomiting (*OHAM*2 p808)
Gentamicin	usually after 3rd dose *peak 1h post IV dose* 9–18µmol/l (5–10mg/l); *trough* <4.2µmol/l (<2mg/l); *toxic* >12mg/l (22µmol/l); *signs of toxicity* tinnitus, deafness, nystagmus, vertigo, renal failure (*OHCM*7 p739). Will vary with once-daily regimen, check locally.
Lithium	optimum sampling time *12h post dose* 0.4–0.8mmol/l; *early signs of toxicity* (Li^+ >1.5mmol/l) tremor, agitation, twitching, thirst, polyuria, N+V; *late signs of toxicity* (Li^+ >2mmol/l) spasms, coma, fits, arrhythmias, renal failure (*OHAM*2 p820)
Phenobarbital	*trough* 60–180µmol/l (15–40mg/l); *toxic* >180µmol/l (>40mg/l)
Phenytoin	*trough* 40–80µmol/l (10–20mg/l); *toxic* >80µmol/l (>20mg/l); *signs of toxicity* ataxia, nystagmus, dysarthria, diplopia
Sodium valproate	*trough* 200–700µmol/l (50–120µg/ml); *toxic* >200µg/ml (>1400µmol/l)
Theophylline	stop infusion 15min prior to sampling, take sample *4–6h after commencing an infusion* 10–20mg/l (55–110µmol/l); *toxic* >20mg/l (>110µmol/l); *signs of toxicity* arrhythmia, anxiety, tremor, convulsions (*OHAM*2 p836)
Vancomycin	usually after 3rd dose (check locally) *peak 1h post IV dose* 20–40mg/l; *trough* 5–15mg/l; *toxicity* can occur within therapeutic range

Endocarditis prophylaxis

Who requires prophylaxis for bacterial endocarditis remains unclear as there is little evidence which supports or refutes the prophylactic use of antibiotics. Patients are classified as special high-risk if they have a prosthetic heart valve (metal or tissue) or have had endocarditis previously. Standard high-risk patients are those with any intra-cardiac shunt, acquired valve disease, or mitral prolapse with regurgitation. Patients with mitral prolapse without regurgitation and those with innocent murmurs do not need prophylaxis and are not considered at risk at all.

Procedures which warrant antibiotic prophylaxis is equally lacking in an evidence base. Generally any breach or potential breach of a mucosal surface is considered high-risk, including all dental work (other than a simple examination or plain radiological investigation). The *BNF* (Section 5.1, Table 2), the British Heart Foundation (www.bhf.org.uk) and the British Society for Antimicrobial Chemotherapy (www.bsac.org.uk) have guidelines which should be consulted if in doubt.

Antibiotic regimens for those under 16yr consult the *BNF for Children*. For adults:

Dental procedures under local anaesthesia

- *Standard high-risk* amoxicillin 3g PO 1h before procedure. If penicillin allergic or >1 prophylactic dose of a penicillin in the last 28d, oral clindamycin 600mg PO 1hr before procedure
- *Special high-risk* amoxicillin 1g IV and gentamicin 120g IV at start of procedure, then amoxicillin 500mg PO 6h later

Dental procedures under general anaesthesia

- *Standard high-risk* either amoxicillin 1g IV at induction, then amoxicillin 500mg PO 6h later **or** amoxicillin 3g PO 4h before induction, then amoxicillin 3g PO as soon as possible after the procedure.
- *Special high-risk* amoxicillin 1g IV and gentamicin 120g IV at induction, then amoxicillin 500mg PO 6h later
- *If penicillin allergic* (irrespective of special risk or not): vancomycin 1g IV over 100min and gentamicin 120mg IV at induction **or** teicoplanin 400mg IV and gentamicin 120mg IV at induction **or** clindamycin 300mg IV over 10min then clindamycin 150mg IV/PO 6h later

Upper respiratory tract procedures

- As for dental procedures; post-operative dose may be given IV if swallowing is painful

Genitourinary procedures

- As for special risk patients undergoing dental procedures except that clindamycin is avoided in penicillin-allergic patients given its limited spectrum of activity covering genitourinary flora

Obstetric, gynaecological and gastrointestinal procedures

- Only required in patients with prosthetic valves or previous endocarditis, as for genitourinary procedures

Night sedation

Patients develop tolerance and dependence to hypnotics (sedating drugs) if they are prescribed long term. They are only licensed for short-term use and should be avoided if possible.

Causes of insomnia anxiety, stress, depression, mania, alcohol, pain, coughing, nocturia (diuretics, urge incontinence), restless leg syndrome, steroids, aminophylline, SSRIs, benzodiazepine withdrawal, sleep apnoea, poor sleep hygiene, levothyroxine

Try to dose regular medications so that stimulants (steroids, SSRIs, aminophylline) are given early in the day, whilst sedatives (tricyclics, antihistamines) are at night. Encourage sleep hygiene (below), ear plugs, eye shades and treat any causes of insomnia.

Sleep hygiene *avoid* caffeine in evening (tea, coffee, chocolate), alcohol, nicotine, daytime naps, cerebral activity before sleep; *encourage* exercise, light snack 1–2h before bed, comfortable + quiet location (ear plugs and eye shades), routine

If the patient is still unable to sleep and there is a temporary cause (eg post-op pain, noisy ward) then it is appropriate to prescribe a one-off or short course (≤5d) of hypnotics. Some patients may be on long-term hypnotics; these are usually continued in hospital. If long-term hypnotics are stopped the dose should be weaned to minimise withdrawal.

Common oral hypnotics

Diazepam	5–10mg/24h	Significant hangover effect, useful for anxious patients
Temazepam	10–20mg/24h	Shorter action than diazepam, less hangover
Zopiclone	3.75–7.5mg/24h	Less dependence and risk of withdrawal than diazepam and less hangover effect

Contra-indications respiratory failure and sleep apnoea.

Side-effects Include hangover (morning drowsiness), confusion, ataxia, falls, aggression and a withdrawal syndrome similar to alcohol withdrawal if long-term hypnotics are stopped suddenly.

Discharge if a patient is not on hypnotics when they enter hospital they should not be on hypnotics when they leave. GPs get irritated if patients are discharged with supplies of addictive and unnecessary medications.

Violent/aggressive patients See p308 for emergency sedation.

Pre-op sedation Diazepam and temazepam can be used for sedation before a procedure or anaesthetic; this is usually prescribed by the anaesthetist 1–2h beforehand. **Midazolam** is a rapidly acting IV sedative; it should only be used by experienced doctors under monitored conditions (sats, RR, BP and cardiac monitor) with a crash trolley present. Give 1–2mg boluses then wait 5min for the full response before repeating; >5mg is rarely needed.

Steroid therapy

Steroids given for >14d should never be abruptly discontinued as this can precipitate an addisonian crisis (p421). Patients can need >60mg prednisolone per day for severe disease and this must be converted to an appropriate intravenous corticosteroid dose if they are NBM, eg surgery. Long-term steroid use should raise concerns about osteoporosis and prophylactic steps considered.

Conversion of oral prednisolone to IV hydrocortisone

Prednisolone/24h PO	Hydrocortisone/6–8h IV
60mg	240mg
50mg	200mg
40mg	160mg
30mg	120mg
20mg	80mg
10mg	40mg

Steroid conversion (See *BNF* 6.3.2)

These are equivalent corticosteroid doses compared to 5mg prednisolone, but do not take into account dosing frequencies or mineralocorticoid effects

- Hydrocortisone 20mg – usually given IV 6–8h
- Methylprednisolone 4mg – usually given once daily
- Dexamethasone 750µg – usually given once daily

Steroid side-effects and treatment options

GI ulceration	Consider PPI or H_2-receptor antagonist
Infections and reactivation of TB	Low threshold for culturing samples or CXR
Skin thinning/poor wound healing	Pressure care and wound care
Na^+ and fluid retention	Twice-daily BPs
Hyperglycaemia	Twice-daily BMs if taking high-dose steroids
Osteoporosis (p475)	Bone protection (Ca^{2+} + bisphosphonate)
Hypertension	Twice-daily BPs

Withdrawing steroid therapy It is an art and must be performed gradually if steroids have been used for >14d. Large doses (>20mg prednisolone or equivalent) can be reduced by 5–10mg/wk until dose is 10mg prednisolone/d. Thereafter the doses must be reduced more slowly, by 2.5mg/wk until the dose is 5mg/d. Thereafter reduce the dose by 1mg/wk down to zero. See p118. Consider using alternative day doses.

Topical corticosteroids

Topical steroids are used in the treatment of many inflammatory skin diseases. As with corticosteroids given orally or intravenously the mechanism of action is complex. Corticosteroids offer symptomatic relief but are seldom curative. The least potent preparation (see table below) should be used to control symptoms. Withdrawal of topical steroids often causes a rebound worsening of symptoms and the patient should be warned about this. The amount of steroid needed to cover various body parts is shown in the table below. Always wash hands after applying topical steroids.

Side-effects of topical steroids are predominantly related to skin atrophy (especially on face and flexures) although excessive or prolonged use can result in systemic effects (cushingoid features, p204).

Topical corticosteroid potencies

Potency	Example
Mild	Hydrocortisone 1% eg hydrocortisone
Moderately potent	Clobetasone butyrate 0.05% eg *Eumovate*®
Potent	Betamethasone 0.1%, hydrocortisone butyrate 0.1% eg *Betnovate*®
Very potent	Clobetasol propionate 0.05% eg *Dermovate*®

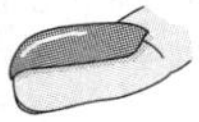

ONE adult fingertip unit (FTU)*

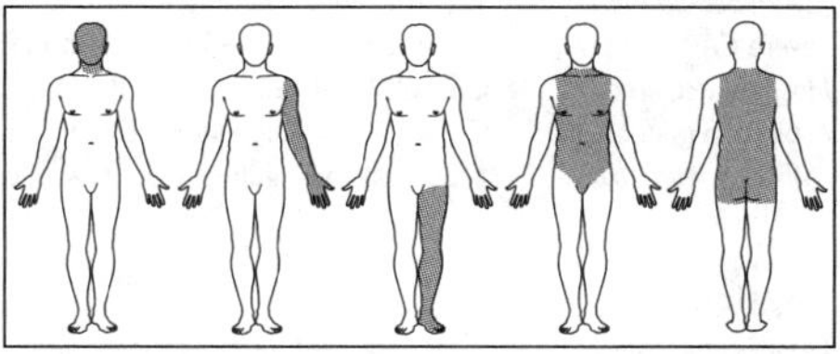

Age	Number of fingertip units (FTUs)				
	Face & neck	Arm & hand	Leg & foot	Trunk (front)	Trunk (back) inc. buttocks
Adult	2½	4	8	7	7
Children:					
3–6 months	1	1	1½	1	1½
1–2 years	1½	1½	2	2	3
3–5 years	1½	2	3	3	3½
6–10 years	2	2½	4½	3½	5

*One adult fingertip unit (FTU) is the amount of ointment or cream expressed from a tube with a standard 5mm diameter nozzle, applied from the distal crease ot the tip of the index finger

Reproduced with permission from Long, C.C. and Finlay, A.Y. (1991) Clinical and Experimental Dermatology, 16: 444–7. Blackwell Publishing.

Empirical antibiotic treatment

Choice of suitable antibiotic will depend upon many factors, including likely pathogen and their usual antimicrobial sensitivity profile, patient factors such as age and coexisting disease, drug availability and local guidelines. Always think of the drug's potential side-effects (see *C. difficile* opposite). Below are some common infections and a suggested antibiotic regimen (suitable for an otherwise healthy 70kg adult).

Local antibiotic guidelines should be available in every hospital as organism sensitivity varies throughout the country as does drug availability. Do not hesitate to contact the on-call microbiologist if in doubt.

Taking cultures prior to commencing antibiotic therapy is very useful as it will allow subsequent therapy to be more specifically tailored. However, cultures should not delay treatment in the unwell patient.

Urinary tract	Trimethoprim 200mg/12h PO/nitrofurantoin 50mg/6h PO
Cellulitis	Flucloxacillin 1g/6h IV
Wound infection	Await wound swab, otherwise as for cellulitis
Meningitis	Ceftriaxone 2g/12h IV
Encephalitis	As for meningitis + aciclovir 10mg/kg per 8h IV
Endocarditis (empirical therapy)	Benzylpenicillin 1.2 g/6h IV + gentamicin (p151) (take 3 sets of blood cultures first; d/w microbiology)
Septic arthritis	Flucloxacillin 2g/6h IV

Pneumonia

Community-acquired (CAP), non-severe	Amoxicillin 500mg/8h PO + erythromycin 500mg/6h PO
Severe CAP	Co-amoxiclav 1.2g/8h IV + clarithromycin 500mg/12h IV
Hospital-acquired	Consult local guidelines – d/w microbiologist
Aspiration pneumonia	Consult local guidelines – d/w microbiologist
?MRSA pneumonia	Consult local guidelines – d/w microbiologist

Septicaemia

Urinary tract sepsis	Cefuroxime 1.5g/8h IV, ±gentamicin (p151)
Intra-abdominal sepsis	Cefuroxime 1.5g/8h IV + metronidazole 500mg/8h IV
Meningococcal sepsis	Ceftriaxone 2g/12h IV
Neutropenic sepsis	Tazocin®[1] 4.5g/8h IV ±gentamicin (p151); see p396
Skin/bone source	Flucloxacillin 2g/6h IV – d/w microbiologist
Unknown source	d/w microbiologist

[1] Tazocin® 4.5g = piperacillin 4g + tazobactam 500mg.

Clostridium difficile (C. diff)

Bacteriology C. difficile is a Gram-positive anaerobe which consists of spore-forming rods (bacilli). It colonises the intestines of some individuals (often those in long-term care), and the use of antibiotics (particularly the cephalosporins, quinolones and clindamycin) alters the balance of the gut flora, and in some cases allows the overgrowth of *C. difficile*.

Transmission via the faecal–oral route. The spores which are released are heat-resistant and can lay dormant in the environment for long periods tautology. The spores are resistant to stomach acid and begin to multiply once in the colon.

Symptoms diarrhoea and abdominal pains are the commonest features of *C. difficile* overgrowth, and result from pseduomembranous colitis. In the elderly and frail this can result in dehydration and even death.

Treatment is with metronidazole 400mg/8h PO or vancomycin 125mg/6h PO, barrier nursing and thorough hand hygiene.

Surveillance as *C. difficile* is now one of the largest causes of hospital-acquired infections (HAI), most local infection control teams should be made aware if a case is identified or even suspected; they will often advise ward and medical staff on how the patient should be managed.

Antibiotics and Clostridium difficile

Due to the increasing awareness of the role of certain antibiotics in the establishment of *Clostridium difficile* diarrhoea, many trusts are limiting the use of cephalosporins, quinolones and clindamycin. Therefore check local antibiotic guidelines before prescribing these agents.

Chapter 9
Clinical presentations

Early warning scores

Early detection of the 'unwell' patient has repeatedly been shown to improve outcome. Identification of such patients allows suitable changes in management, including early involvement of critical care teams or transfer to critical care areas (HDU/ITU) where necessary.

Identification of the 'at risk' patient relies on measurement of simple physiological parameters, which generally deteriorate as the patient becomes more unwell; these include RR, HR, BP, O_2 saturation, level of consciousness, urine output and temp. Remember that the sick patient might not look that unwell from the bottom of the bed.

Scoring of these parameters can be carried out in many ways and is usually undertaken by nursing staff. One common example, the Modified Early Warning Score (MEWS), is shown opposite. Normal observations are awarded a score of 0, whilst abnormal observations attract higher scores. The values for each physiological parameter are added together. If this total score reaches a 'threshold' value (eg ≥ 4 on the example opposite), the nursing staff should alert either a senior nurse or a doctor to review the patient, depending on local policy/guidelines.

Trends in physiological parameters are often more useful than one-off observations. Some patients may have abnormal scores even when they seem relatively 'well' because of compensatory mechanisms. These patients may be given higher thresholds, but are also likely to deteriorate much more quickly.

Patients who should be monitored by such scores include:
- Emergency admissions
- Unstable patients
- Elderly patients
- Patients with pre-existing disease (cardiovascular, respiratory, DM)
- Patients who are failing to respond to treatment
- Patients who have returned from ITU/HDU
- Postoperative patients

Early warning scores are not used in all hospitals, though their principles can be used by anyone to help prioritise clinical need when faced with several referrals over the telephone or in an admissions unit.

ALERT™

Acute Life-threatening Events – Recognition and Treatment

This is an evolving course that aims to guide people in early recognition of the unwell patient and in their immediate resuscitation. This course complements the Immediate Life Support (ILS) and Advanced Life Support (ALS) courses (p164). Further information can be found at www.alert-course.com

Adult Modified Early Warning System Observation Score (MEWS)

If score ≥4 notify junior doctor immediately. If any individual measure = 3 notify junior doctor immediately.

Score	3	2	1	0	1	2	3
RR		≤8	9–10	11–20	21–25	26–30	≥31
HR		≤40	41–50	51–100	101–110	111–130	≥131
Systolic BP (mmHg)	≤84	85–89	90–100	101–199		≥200	
SpO_2	≤87	88–91	92–94	95–100			
GCS or AVPU	≤8	9–13	14 New agitation or confusion	15 A	V	P	U
Temp °C		≤35.0	35.1–35.9	36.0–37.4	37.5–38.4	≥38.5	
Urine	≤10ml/h for 2h	≤30ml/h for 2h					

Peri-arrest

Airway	Check airway is patent; consider manoeuvres/adjuncts with C-spine control in trauma
Breathing	If no respiratory effort – **CALL ARREST TEAM**
Circulation	If no palpable pulse – **CALL ARREST TEAM**
Disability	If GCS ≤8 – **CALL ANAESTHETIST**

Airway – if irreversibly obstructed CALL ARREST TEAM
- **Look** inside the mouth, remove obvious objects/dentures
- Wide-bore **suction** under direct vision if secretions present
- **Listen** airway impaired if stridor, snoring, gurgling or no air entry
- **Jaw thrust**/head tilt/chin lift with cervical spine control in trauma
- **Oropharyngeal** or **nasopharyngeal** airway as tolerated
- If still impaired ***CALL ARREST TEAM***

Breathing – if poor or absent respiratory effort CALL ARREST TEAM
- **Look** for chest expansion (does R = L?), fogging of mask
- **Listen** to chest for air entry (does R = L?)
- **Feel** for expansion and percussion (does R = L?)
- **Non-rebreathe** (trauma) mask and 15l/min O_2 in all patients
- **Bag and mask** if poor or absent breathing effort
- **Monitor** O_2 sats and RR
- **Think** tension pneumothorax

Circulation – if no pulse CALL ARREST TEAM
- **Look** for pallor, cyanosis, distended neck veins
- **Feel** for a central pulse (carotid/femoral) – rate and rhythm
- **Monitor** defibrillator ECG leads and BP
- **Venous access**, send bloods if time allows
- **12-lead ECG**
- Call for **senior help** early if patient deteriorating

Disability – if GCS ≤8 or falling CALL ANAESTHETIST
- Assess **GCS** (p280) and check glucose
- **Look** for pupil reflexes and unusual posture
- **Feel** for tone in all four limbs and plantar reflexes

Exposure
- **Remove** all clothing, check **temp**
- **Look** all over body including perineum and back for rash or injuries
- **Cover** patient with a blanket

Common causes

Arrhythmia	p186	Hypoxia	p219
Myocardial infarction	p177	Pulmonary oedema	p226
Hypovolaemia	p212	Pulmonary embolism	p225
Sepsis (UTI/pneumonia)	p214	Metabolic (↑↓K^+)	p326
Hypoglycaemia	p271	(Tension) pneumothorax	p227

In-hospital resuscitation

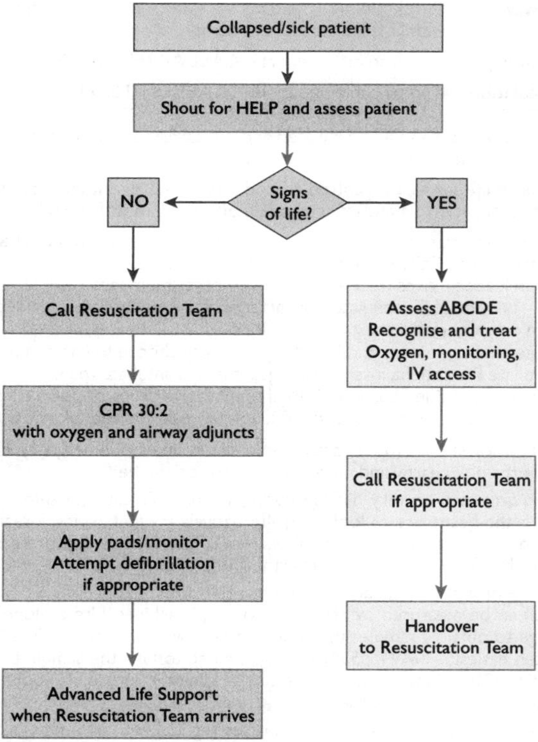

In-hospital resuscitation algorithm, 2005 guidelines
Reproduced by kind permission of the Resuscitation Council (UK).

Signs of life

Good respiratory effort
Palpable pulse
Moving limbs
Making noises

Advanced life support (ALS)

Airway	Check airway is patent; consider manoeuvres/adjuncts with C-spine control in trauma
Breathing	If no respiratory effort – **CALL ARREST TEAM**
Circulation	If no palpable pulse – **CALL ARREST TEAM**

Basic life support should be initiated and the cardiac arrest team called as soon as cardiac or respiratory arrest is identified.

Advanced life support is centred around a 'universal algorithm' (opposite) which is taught on a standardised course offered by most hospitals.

The cardiac arrest team usually consists of a team leader (medical StR), F1, anaesthetist, CCU nurse and senior hospital nurse:

- Team leader – gives clear instructions to other members
- F1 – provide BLS, cannulate, take arterial blood, defibrillate if trained, give drugs, perform chest compressions
- Anaesthetist – airway and breathing, they may choose to bag-and-mask ventilate the patient, insert a laryngeal mask or intubate (p582)
- Nurses – provide BLS, defibrillate if trained, give drugs, perform chest compressions, record observations, note time points and take ECGs

Needle-stick injuries (p127) are commonest in times of emergency. Have the sharps box nearby and never leave sharps on the bed.

Cannulation can be very difficult during a cardiac arrest. The antecubital fossa is the best place to look first; alternatively try feet, hands, forearms, or consider external jugular if all else fails. Take bloods if you are successful, but don't allow this to delay the giving of drugs.

Blood tests are occasionally useful in cardiac arrests, especially K^+ which can often be measured by arterial blood gas machines. Use a blood gas syringe to obtain a sample (the femoral artery with a green needle (21G) is often easiest – NAVY, p556) and ask a nurse to take the sample to the machine. Other blood tests depend on the clinical scenario, if in doubt fill all the common blood bottles.

Defibrillation is taught on specific courses (eg ILS, ALS) and must not be undertaken unless trained. The use of automated external defibrillators or AEDs (p573) are becoming more common.

Cardiac arrest drugs are now prepared in pre-filled syringes: adrenaline (epinephrine) 1mg in 10ml (1:10,000), atropine 3mg in 10ml, amiodarone 300mg in 10ml. Always give a large flush (20ml saline) after each dose to encourage it into the central circulation. See inside back cover for further emergency drug doses.

Cardiac arrest trolleys are found in most areas of the hospital. Know where they are for your wards. Ask the ward sister if you can open the trolley and have a good look at the equipment within it as they differ between hospitals. They are often arranged so the top drawer contains **A**irway equipment, the second contains **B**reathing equipment, the third contains **C**irculation equipment and the lower drawer contains the drugs and fluids. You'll seldom need anything that isn't on the trolley.

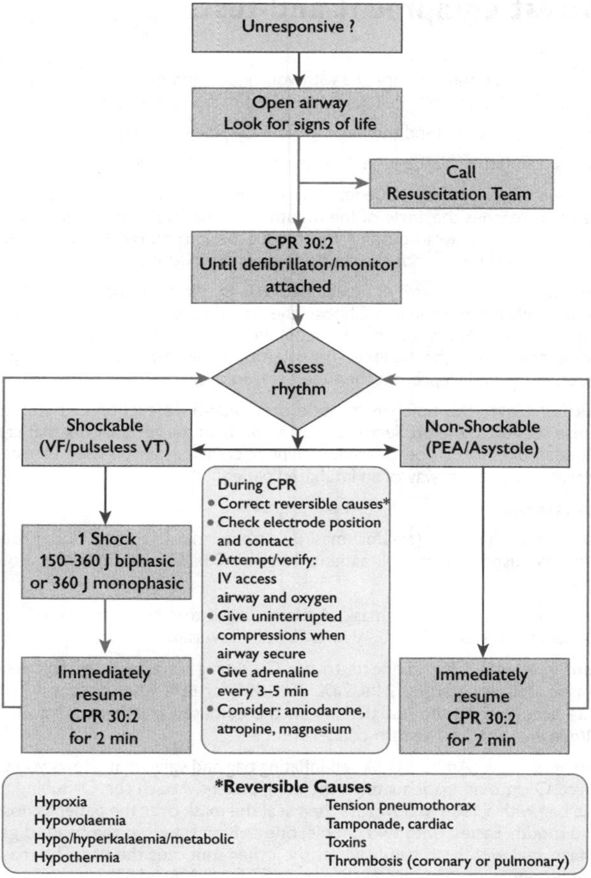

Adult Advanced Life Support algorithm, 2005 guidelines
Reproduced by kind permission of the Resuscitation Council (UK).

Arrest equipment and tests

Airway

Jaw thrust Pull the jaw forward with your index and middle fingers at the angle of each mandible. Pull hard enough to make your fingers ache.

Head tilt Gently extend the neck, avoid if C-spine injury risk.

Chin lift Pull the chin up with two fingers, avoid if C-spine injury risk.

Oropharyngeal airway (Guedel) A rigid, curved plastic tube; choose the size that reaches the angle of the mouth from the tragus of the ear. Insert upside down to avoid pushing the tongue back, then rotate 180° when inside the mouth (do not insert upside down in children).

Nasopharyngeal airway A flexible, curved plastic tube, not to be used with significant head injury. Choose the size that will easily pass through the nose (size 6–7mm in most adults); insert by lubricating and pushing horizontally into the patient's nostril (not upwards). Use a safety pin through the end to prevent the tube being lost.

Suction Cover the hole on the side of a wide-bore suction catheter to cause suction at the tip. Secretions in the parts of the oropharynx that can be seen directly can be cleared. A thinner catheter can be used to clear secretions in the airway of an intubated patient.

Breathing

Non-rebreath mask (trauma mask) A plastic mask with a floppy bag attached; used in acutely ill patients to give ~80% O_2 with a 15l/min flow rate

Standard mask (Hudson mask) A plastic mask that connects directly to O_2 tubing; delivers ~50% O_2 with a 15l/min flow rate

Venturi A mask that connects to the O_2 tubing via a piece of coloured plastic, delivering either 24%, 28%, 35%, 40% or 60% O_2. Adjust the flow rate according to the instructions on the coloured plastic connector, eg 4l/min with the 28% Venturi connection.

Bag and mask (Ambu bag) A self-inflating bag and valve that allows you to force O_2 into an inadequately ventilating patient. Attach the O_2 tubing to the bag with a 15l/min flow rate then seal the mask over the patient's nose and mouth. Easiest with two people; one person stands at the head to get a firm seal with both hands whilst the other squeezes the bag. The mask can be removed to attach the bag to an ETT or LMA (p582).

Pulse oximeter Plastic clip with a red light that measures blood O_2 saturations. Clip onto the patient's index finger. Do not rely on the reading unless there is an even trace on the monitor and the patient has a pulse; use on the different arm from the BP cuff.

Nebuliser This is a 3cm-high cylinder that attaches beneath a mask. The cylinder is made of two halves that can be untwisted so that the nebulised fluid can be inserted. The nebuliser can be connected to a pump or directly to an O_2 or medical air supply.

Circulation

Defibrillator ECG leads Red to right shoulder, yellow to left shoulder and green to apex; turn the defibrillator onto 'monitor' (p568).

Defibrillator paddles You can get a rhythm trace by holding the paddles in position (right paddle to right upper sternal edge, left paddle to apex (p573)) or via the adhesive hands-free electrodes (p573) and turning the defibrillator onto 'monitor'.

Defibrillation (p573) Only defibrillate if you have been trained:

- Check the gel pads are on the chest before you pick up the paddles
- Never hold the two paddles in the same hand
- Charge the paddles by pressing the charge button
- Tell staff to stand clear and stand clear yourself
- Check the O_2, staff and you are clear (O_2, top, middle, bottom, self)
- Check the rhythm is still shockable then press the buttons on both paddles to deliver the charge

Blood pressure Attach the cuff to the patient's left arm so it is out of the way and leave in place. If it does not work or is not believable (eg tachyarrhythmia) then obtain a manual reading.

Venous access Ideally two brown/grey venflons in the antecubital fossae; however, get the best available (biggest and most central). Remember to take bloods (20ml syringe) but don't let this delay giving drugs.

Disability

Glucose Use a spot of blood from the venous sample or a skin prick to get a capillary sample; clean skin first with water to avoid false readings

Examination GCS, pupil size and reactivity to light, posture, tone of all four limbs, plantar reflexes

Exposure

Get all the patient's clothes off; have a low threshold for cutting them off. Inspect the patient's entire body for clues as to the cause of the arrest, eg rashes, injuries. Measure temp. Remember to cover the patient with a blanket to prevent hypothermia and for dignity.

Other investigations

Arterial blood gas Attach a green (21G) needle to a blood gas syringe, feel for the femoral pulse (½ to ⅔ between superior iliac spine and pubic symphysis) and insert the needle vertically until you get blood. Press hard after removal. Even if the sample is venous it can still offer useful information.

Femoral stab (p556) If no blood has been taken you can insert a green needle into the femoral vein which is medial to the artery (NAVY, p556). Feel for the artery then aim about 1cm medially. If you hit the artery take 20ml of blood anyway and send for arterial blood gas and normal blood tests, but press hard after removal.

ECG Attach the leads as shown on p568

CXR Alert the radiographer early so that they can bring the X-ray machine for a portable CXR

Advanced trauma life support (ATLS)

ATLS is designed to quickly and safely stabilise the injured patient. The purpose of ATLS is not to provide definitive care of all injuries, but to recognise the immediate threats to life and to address these. As with ALS, in ATLS the patient's care is delivered by a team which will consist of a leader and various members. Details of how to undertake an ATLS course are given at the bottom of this page.

The primary survey allows a rapid assessment and relevant management to be undertaken. If a life-threatening issue is found this must be treated before moving on to the next step of the primary survey. The primary survey is as follows: Airway with cervical spine protection; Breathing: ventilation and oxygenation; Circulation with haemorrhage control; Disability: brief neurological examination; Exposure/Environment; Adjuncts to primary survey; Reassess patient's ABCDE and consider need for patient transfer.

The secondary survey follows once all life-threatening issues have been identified and dealt with; the secondary survey is a top-to-toe examination looking for secondary injuries which are unlikely to be immediately life-threatening. The secondary survey is as follows: AMPLE history (p465) and mechanism of injury; Head and maxillofacial; Cervical spine and neck; Chest; Abdomen; Perineum/rectum/vagina; Musculoskeletal; Neurologic; Adjuncts to the secondary survey.

ATLS and the F1 doctor it is highly unlikely the F1 doctor will be the first person to attend to a major trauma patient, though ATLS can be applied in principle to any patient who has sustained an injury. Having a logical, step-wise approach to injured patients minimises the risk of missing life-threatening complications or injuries which subsequently may become debilitating if left unrecognised and untreated.

ATLS course

In the UK, ATLS courses are coordinated by the Royal College of Surgeons. The course is currently three days long, and details of where and when courses are run can be obtained from the College (see p636 for contact details). There is usually a long waiting list for places as this is a popular course; the cost for the three-day course is nearly £600.

Paediatric basic life support

Airway	Check airway is patent; consider manoeuvres/adjuncts
Breathing	If poor respiratory effort – **CALL ARREST TEAM**
Circulation	If HR <60bpm – **CALL ARREST TEAM**
Disability	If unresponsive to voice – **CALL ARREST TEAM**

Call the **arrest team** if severely unwell; call **senior help** early

Airway – if irreversibly obstructed CALL ARREST TEAM
- Airway manoeuvres: (**head tilt**), **chin lift, jaw thrust** (see table opposite)
- **Oropharyngeal** or **nasopharyngeal** airway if responding only to pain
- If still impaired ***CALL ARREST TEAM***

If you suspect **epiglottitis** (stridor, drooling, septic) do not look in the mouth, but give O_2 call your senior help urgently and an anaesthetist and ENT surgeon

Breathing – if poor or absent respiratory effort CALL ARREST TEAM
- **Bag and mask** with 15l/min O_2 if poor or absent breathing effort
- **Non-rebreath mask** and 15l/min O_2 in all other patients
- **Monitor** pulse oximeter
- **Effort** stridor, wheeze, RR, recession, grunting, accessory muscle use (head bobbing in infants), nasal flaring
- **Efficacy** chest expansion, air entry (does R=L?), O_2 sats
- **Effects** HR, pallor, cyanosis (late sign), agitation, drowsiness

Circulation – if HR <60 or absent CALL ARREST TEAM
- Start **CPR** if HR absent or <60bpm
- **Monitor** defibrillator ECG leads
- **Status** HR + rhythm, pulse volume, cap refill (≤2s normal), BP
- **Effects** RR, mottled/pale/cold skin, urine output, agitation, drowsiness
- **Venous access** (consider intraosseous) check glucose and send blds
- Consider **fluid bolus** (20ml/kg IV 0.9% saline stat) if shocked
- **Exclude heart failure** ↑JVP, gallop rhythm, crepitations, large liver

Disability – if unresponsive to voice CALL ARREST TEAM
- Assess **AVPU** (**A**lert, responds to **V**oice, responds to **P**ain, **U**nresponsive); check **glucose** if not already done
- **Look** for pupil size and reflexes; assess posture and tone
- See p286 for **seizures**

Exposure
- **Look** all over body for rashes, check **temp**, **cover** with a blanket

Life-threatening conditions

Croup (exclude epiglottitis)	Dehydration (DKA)
Inhaled foreign body	Sepsis, meningitis, pneumonia
Bronchiolitis	Anaphylaxis
Asthma	Heart failure (especially infants)

Advanced Paediatric basic life support

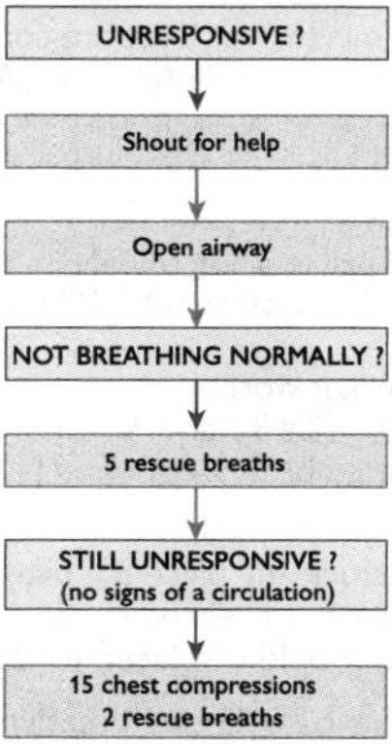

After 1 minute call resuscitation team then continue CPR

Resuscitation Guideline 2005, reproduced with the kind permission of the Resuscitation Council (UK).

Main age-related differences in paediatric life support

Feature	Infant <1yr	Child >1yr	Post-puberty
Airway position	Neutral	Slightly extended	Slightly extended
Breaths	Mouth and nose	Mouth, ±nose	Mouth only
Pulse	Brachial	Carotid	Carotid
CPR position	1 finger above xiphisternum	1 finger above xiphisternum	2 fingers above xiphisternum
For CPR use	1 finger	1 or 2 hands	2 hands
Compressions:breaths	15:2	15:2	15:2

Common emergency drug doses:

- **Fluid bolus** 20ml/kg 0.9% saline IV
- **Glucose** 5ml/kg 10% glucose IV
- **Adrenaline (arrest)** 0.1ml/kg 1:10,000 IV
- **Adrenaline (anaphylaxis)** 0.01ml/kg 1:1,000 IM
- **Diazepam** 0.5mg/kg PR
- **Lorazepam** 0.1mg/kg IV
- **Ceftriaxone** 80mg/kg IV

Normal range for observations by age

Age	RR (/min)	HR (/min)	Systolic BP (mmHg)
<1yr	30–40	110–160	70–90
2–5yr	20–30	95–140	80–100
6–12yr	12–20	80–120	90–110
>12yr	12–16	60–100	100–120

Neonatal Life Support (NLS)

If no improvement after 2min (earlier if you are concerned) of resuscitation then fast bleep a senior or CALL THE NEONATAL ARREST TEAM

Preparation
- Put non-sterile gloves on
- Turn on the heater and place warm towels on the resuscitaire
- Turn on O_2/air and check pressure, set PIP/PEEP to 30/10cmH_2O for term babies
- Turn on suction and check it works
- Get the laryngoscope and size 3.5 and 4.0 (term babies) airways ready
- Check gestation, estimated birth weight and history

Drying
- Post-delivery **start the clock** and place the baby on the resuscitaire
- **Dry** vigorously with a warm towel and cover
- Babies <30/40 gestation should be placed directly in a plastic bag

Meconium delivery if the baby is not breathing suck out meconium from the mouth and beneath the vocal cords under direct vision with a laryngoscope before drying; if the baby breathes then stop and resuscitate as usual

Airway and breathing
- **Assess** RR and HR, if either impaired and not improving:
  - Place the baby's head in the **neutral position**
  - Place **Neopuff** over nose and mouth, jaw thrust; give **5 inflation breaths**:
  - Cover the Neopuff hole for 2–3s then uncover for 2–3s
  - Look for **chest movement**, improved HR, colour
- If unsuccessful reposition head and give a further **5 inflation breaths**
- If unsuccessful ***CALL ARREST TEAM*** and consider intubation
- **Look for** oropharynx obstruction and consider a Guedel airway
- **Continue** Neopuff breaths at lower pressures (eg 20/5, 1s on 1s off)

Circulation – if HR <100 after breaths CALL ARREST TEAM
- **Assess** the HR by gripping the umbilicus or listening to the heart
- Start **CPR** if HR <60/absent despite inflation breaths
  - grip round the chest and use both thumbs over lower sternum
  - aim for a rate of 120 (twice a second)
  - ratio of 3:1 compressions to breaths
- Attempt to get **IV access** eg umbilical venous catheter, check glucose

Drugs – if needed CALL ARREST TEAM
- **Adrenaline** 0.1–0.3ml/kg of 1:10,000 IV if HR not improving
- **Na^+ bicarbonate** 4.2% 2–4ml/kg IV if acidotic and not improving
- **Dextrose** 10% 2.5ml/kg IV if hypoglycaemic
- **0.9% saline** 10ml/kg IV if large blood loss suspected

Life-threatening conditions

- Prematurity
- Hypoxia
- Meconium aspiration
- Congenital abnormality

Neonatal life support algorithm

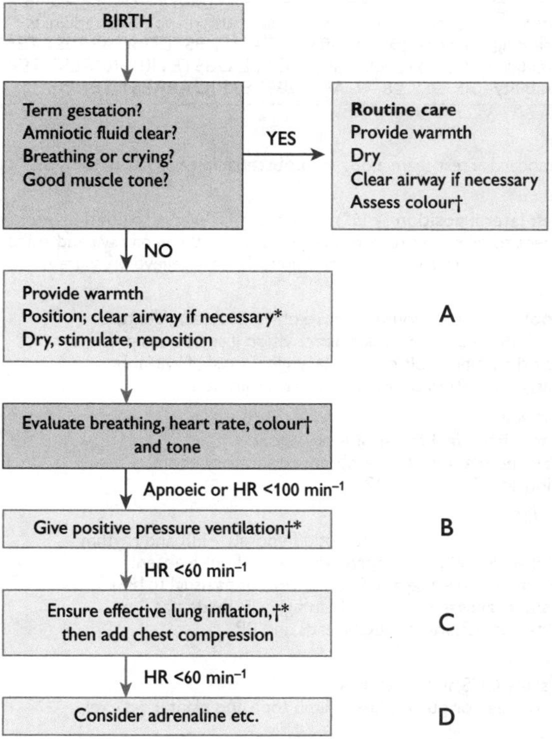

* Tracheal intubation may be considered at several steps
† Consider supplemental oxygen at any stage if cyanosis persists

Resuscitation Guideline 2005. Reproduced with the kind permission of the Resuscitation Council (UK).

Apgar scores (scored out of 10 at 1min, 5min and 10min)

	0	1	2
Colour	Blue all over	Pink body, blue extremities	Pink
HR	Absent	<100	>100
Stimulation	No response	Grimace or feeble cry	Good cry, sneeze, cough, pulls away
Tone	None	Reduced	Normal
Breathing	Absent	Irregular	Strong and regular

Obstetric arrest

Airway	Check airway is patent; consider manoeuvres/adjuncts
Breathing	If no respiratory effort – **CALL OBSTETRIC ARREST TEAM**
Circulation	If no palpable pulse – **CALL OBSTETRIC ARREST TEAM**
Disability	IF GCS ≤8 – **CALL OBSTETRIC ARREST TEAM**

Staff

- Standard arrest team along with **obstetrician** and **neonatologist**

Position

- **Left lateral position** (>15°) using a Cardiff Wedge, pillows or your knees to take the pressure of the uterus off the vena cava and aorta
- **Push the uterus** to the left and up to further relieve pressure

Airway

- **Look** inside the mouth, remove obvious objects/dentures
- Wide-bore **suction** under direct vision if secretions present
- **Jaw thrust**/head tilt/chin lift; **laryngeal mask** if available
- **Early intubation** to prevent gastric aspiration

Breathing

- **Look/listen/feel** for respiratory effort
- **Bag and mask** if poor or absent respiratory effort
- **Monitor** O_2 sats and RR

Circulation

- **Feel** for a central pulse (carotid/femoral) – HR and rhythm
- Mid-sternal **chest compression** (30:2) if pulse absent
- **Arrhythmias** – use a defibrillator/drugs as usual (p186)
- **Venous access**, send bloods and give IV fluids stat
- **Monitor** defibrillator ECG leads and BP

Disability

- **Assess** GCS and check **glucose**
- **Look/feel** for pupil reflexes, limb tone and plantar reflexes

Surgery

- **Emergency Caesarean** if resuscitation is not successful by 5min
  - improves maternal chest compliance and venous return
- The **mother's needs** take priority in all decisions

Obstetric causes, see also p162

Haemorrhage/hypovolaemia	p212	Pre-eclampsia/eclampsia	p438
Excess magnesium sulphate		Pulmonary embolism	p225
Acute coronary syndrome	p177	Amniotic fluid embolism	
Aortic dissection	p183	Stroke	p290

Chest pain emergency

Airway	Check airway is patent; consider manoeuvres/adjuncts
Breathing	If no respiratory effort – **CALL ARREST TEAM**
Circulation	If no palpable pulse – **CALL ARREST TEAM**

Call for **senior help** early if patient deteriorating

- **Sit patient up**
- **15l/min O_2** in all patients
- **Monitor** pulse oximeter, BP, defibrillator ECG leads if unwell
- Obtain a full set of **observations** including BP in both arms and **ECG**
- Take brief **history** if possible/check **notes**/ask ward staff
- **Examine patient**: condensed CVS, RS, abdo exam
- Establish **likely causes** and rule out **serious causes:**
  - consider **thrombolysis** (p576)
  - consider giving **aspirin** 300mg PO stat
  - consider **needle decompression** (p227)
- **Initiate further treatment**, including analgesia, see following pages
- **Venous access**, take bloods:
  - FBC, U+E, LFT, CRP, glucose, cardiac markers, D-dimer
- Request urgent **CXR**, portable if too unwell
- Call for **senior help** if no improvement or worsening
- Repeat **ECG** after 20min if no improvement
- **Reassess**, starting with A, B, C …

Life-threatening causes

- Myocardial infarction
- (Tension) pneumothorax
- Acute coronary syndrome
- Pericardial effusion/cardiac tamponade
- Aortic dissection
- Pulmonary embolism
- Sickle-cell crisis

Chest pain

> Worrying features ↑↓HR, ↓BP, ↑RR, ↓GCS, sudden onset, sweating, nausea, vomiting, radiating to back or left arm, ECG changes

Think about ***common*** myocardial infarction, acute coronary syndromes, angina, pulmonary embolism, musculoskeletal, pneumonia, pneumothorax (tension or simple), pericarditis, reflux and peptic ulcer disease; ***uncommon*** aortic dissection, cardiac tamponade, sickle-cell crisis

Ask about site (site of onset and radiation), quality (heavy, aching, sharp), intensity (scale of 1–10), timing (onset), associated symptoms (sweating, nausea, palpitations, breathlessness), exacerbating/relieving factors (breathing, position, exertion, eating), recent trauma/exertion, similarity to previous episodes; ***PMH*** cardiac or respiratory problems, DM, acid indigestion; ***DH*** cardiac and respiratory medications, antacids; ***SH*** smoking, exercise tolerance

Risk factors:
- ***IHD*** ↑BP, ↑cholesterol, FH, smoking, obesity, DM, previous IHD
- ***PE/DVT*** previous PE/DVT, immobility, ↑oestrogens, recent surgery, FH, pregnancy, hypercoagulable states, smoking, long distance travel
- ***GI*** acid indigestion, known peptic ulcer, alcohol binge

Obs HR, BP (both arms), RR, sats, temp.

Look for pulse rate/rhythm/volume, sweating, pallor, dyspnoea, cyanosis, ↑JVP, asymmetric chest expansion/percussion/breath sounds, chest wall tenderness, mediastinal shift, tracheal tug, swollen ankles, calf pain/swelling/erythema.

Investigations ***ECG*** (p568/610 for procedure/interpretation); ***blds*** FBC, U+E, LFT, D-dimer (if PE suspected), cardiac markers; ***ABGs*** taken on O_2 if patient acutely unwell (see p562/622 for procedure/interpretation); ***CXR*** if you suspect a tension pneumothorax clinically perform immediate needle decompression (p227), otherwise request a portable CXR if the patient is severely ill (poorer image quality) or standard CXR, see p620 for interpretation; ***urgent echo*/CT** if large proximal PE or aortic root dissection suspected (discuss with cardiologist on-call).

Treatment 15l/min O_2 in everyone initially. Consider intravenous opiates (and an antiemetic) if pain is severe.

Diagnoses to exclude Even if you cannot confirm a diagnosis immediately, use the following criteria to rule out life-threatening causes:
- ***Cardiac ischaemia*:** normal ECG, normal cardiac markers (p179)[1]
- ***PE*:** normal ECG, ABG, D-dimer, echo, low clinical risk for DVT/PE
- ***Pneumothorax*:** clinically and radiologically no pneumothorax
- ***Aortic dissection*:** no evidence of shock, left and right systolic BP differ by <15mmHg, no mediastinal widening on CXR, normal echo

Contact cardiology registrar on-call for advice if necessary.

1 The various cardiac markers rise at different times, so check locally which you should assay for and at what time-point post onset of chest pain (p179).

	History	Examination	Investigations
STEMI	Sudden onset pain, radiating to left arm/jaw, >20min, breathlessness, sweating, nausea	Dyspnoea, ±arrhythmia, sweating, non-tender	ST elevation or new LBBB, ↑cardiac markers. Cardiac markers are not needed to make the diagnosis of STEMI
NSTEMI	Sudden onset pain, radiating to left arm/jaw, >20min, breathlessness, sweating, nausea	Dyspnoea, ±arrhythmia, sweating, non-tender	ST depression or T wave inversion, ↑troponin
Unstable angina	Anginal pain at rest or with ↑frequency, severity or duration	Dyspnoea, ±arrhythmia, sweating, non-tender	ST depression, T wave inversion, troponin not elevated
Stable angina	Exertional pain, radiating to left arm/jaw, <20min, breathlessness, ↓by rest/GTN	Dyspnoea, tachycardia, non-tender, may be normal after pain resolves	Transient ECG changes, normal cardiac markers, +ve stress ECG + coronary angiography
Pericarditis	History of viral-like illness, pleuritic pain, ↑on lying, ↓sitting forwards	Pericardial rub, otherwise normal CVS and RS examinations	Saddle-shaped ST segments on most ECG leads, ↑CRP/ESR
Aortic dissection	Sudden onset severe interscapular pain, tearing in nature, breathlessness	Tachycardia, ↓BP, difference in brachial pulses and pressures, ↑RR	±Widened mediastinum on CXR, aortic dilatation on echo/CT, aortic leak on angiogram
Pulmonary embolism	Breathlessness, PE risk factors, may have pleuritic chest pain and haemoptysis	Often normal, may have evidence of DVT (swollen red leg), tachycardia, dyspnoea, ↓BP	ABG: PO_2↔/↓, CO_2↓, clear CXR, ↑D-dimer, sinus tachycardia, $S_1Q_3T_3$ (rare), thrombus on echo
Pneumothorax	Sudden onset pleuritic pain, ±trauma, tall and thin, COPD	Mediastinal shift, unequal air entry and expansion, hyperresonance	Pleura separated from ribs on CXR, other investigations often normal
Pneumonia	Cough, productive with coloured sputum, pleuritic pain, feels unwell	Febrile, asymmetrical air entry, coarse creps (often unilateral), dull to percussion	↑WCC/↑NØ/↑CRP, consolidation on CXR (p620)
Musculoskeletal chest pain	Lifting, impact injury, may be pleuritic, worse on palpation or movement	Tender (presence does not exclude other causes), respiratory examination normal	ECG to exclude cardiac cause, normal CXR
GORD	Previous indigestion/reflux, known hiatus hernia, ↓by antacids	May have upper abdo tenderness, normal CVS and RS examinations	ECG to exclude cardiac cause, normal CXR, trial of antacids

Acute coronary syndromes (ACS) (*OHCM7* p104)

Nomenclature The definition of ACS has been changed to allow a prospective diagnosis to be made rather than a retrospective diagnosis which was the traditional style; the aim of this is to improve both acute management and subsequent patient outcome.

Acute coronary syndrome (ACS) classification in patients with typical cardiac-sounding chest pain lasting >20min

ECG findings	Troponin (12h post-pain)	Diagnosis
ST elevation or new LBBB	Not needed to make a dianosis, but will be ↑	STEMI (p180)
Ischaemia (other than ST elevation), though may be normal	Trop T ≥0.1ng/ml or Trop I ≥1ng/ml	NSTEMI (p181)
	Trop T <0.1ng/ml or Trop I <1ng/ml	Unstable angina (p182)

Serum cardiac markers in suspected acute IHD

The term 'cardiac enzymes' is incorrect when referring to the troponins as these are structural/regulatory proteins and have no enzymic activity.

Troponins (I or T)	Identification of these in the blood is highly suggestive of myocardial injury, though they can be raised in PE, renal failure, septicaemia and following tachyarrhythmias (but CK is seldom concurrently raised in these conditions). Detection is usually possible 6h after myocardial injury and levels remain elevated for up to 14d. Troponins are also used as a prognostic indicator in NSTEM/UA (p181/182).
Creatine kinase (CK)	Enzyme found in all muscle and released in muscle cell lysis; not specific for cardiac muscle. Peaks within 24h post-MI and usually returns to normal within 48–72h.
CK-MB	Cardiac isomer of CK enzyme, so more specific than total CK. Rises and falls in similar fashion to total CK.
AST LDH	These were once used to retrospectively aid in the diagnosis of acute MI but have been superseded in recent years.

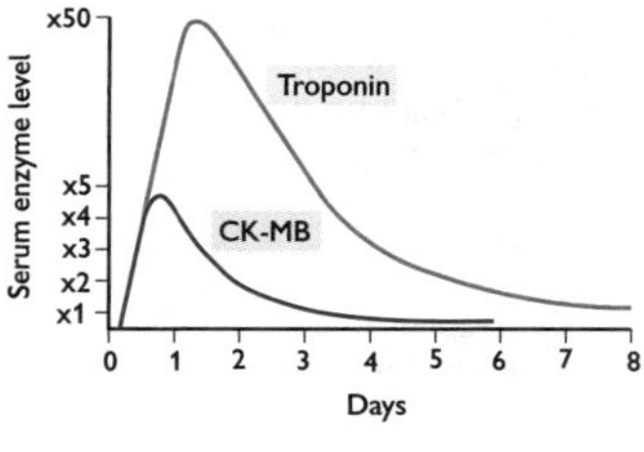

Changes in cardiac markers following an acute myocardial infarction.

STEMI (ST Elevation MI) (*OHCM7* p106)

Worrying signs features of LV failure, cardiac dysrhythmia

Symptoms central, crushing, heavy chest pain (>20min), ±radiating to left arm/jaw, shortness of breath, nausea, sweating, palpitations, anxiety

Risk factors smoking, obesity, DM, ↑BP, ↑cholesterol, FH, previous IHD

Signs tachycardia, cool and sweaty ('clammy'), ±LV failure or hypotension

Investigations ***ECG*** ST elevation, peaked T waves, new LBBB; subsequent Q waves (commonly), ±T wave inversion; ***CXR*** cardiomegaly, signs of LV failure; ***cardiac markers*** will be raised but diagnosis and treatment should not be withheld to wait for these results as ECG findings and history alone are sufficient for the diagnosis to be made

Acute treatment O_2, aspirin (300mg), clopidogrel (300mg), diamorphine (2.5–5mg IV), antiemetic (p252), GTN (two puffs sublingually), thrombolysis if meets criteria (p576) – seek senior help to perform thrombolysis; alternatively consider for percutaneous transluminal coronary angioplasty if available (PTCA, see *OHAM*2 p24). Consider β-blocker, eplerenone and tight glycaemic control (insulin-sliding scale, p275 (continuous DIGAMI regime)). LMWH. Needs CCU.

Secondary prophylaxis ↓modifiable risk factors (smoking, obesity, DM, ↑BP, ↑cholesterol), β-blockade, statin, anti-platelets, eplerenone, ACEi, symptom management (nitrates, Ca^{2+} channel antagonists)

Complications arrhythmias (heart block, bradycardia, VF/VT), LVF, valve prolapse, ventricular septal rupture, ventricular aneurysm formation, pericarditis (Dressler's syndrome, *OHAM*2 p182)

Sequential ECG changes following an acute STEMI

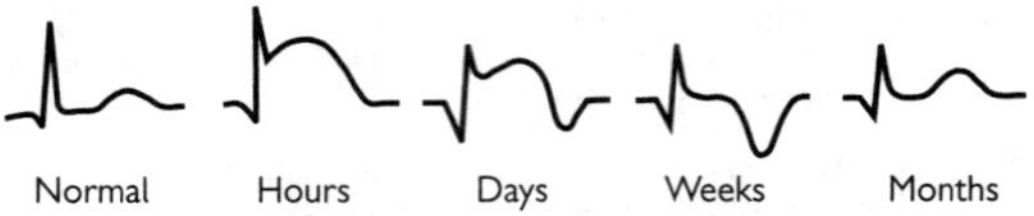

Post-myocardial infarction care (*OHCM7* p106)

Bed rest for 48h with continuous ECG monitoring
Daily 12-lead ECG and thorough clinical examination of CVS/RS
Thromboembolism prophylaxis (p346)
β-blockade unless contraindicated
ACEi/angiotensin II receptor antagonist
Statin
Address modifiable risk factors
Exercise ECG (p570)
Consider coronary angiography
Review in outpatients at 5wk and 3mth for symptoms and to check lipids, BP

NSTEMI (Non-ST Elevation MI) (*OHAM2* p44)

Worrying signs features of LV failure, cardiac dysrhythmia
Symptoms central, crushing, heavy chest pain (>20min), ±radiating to left arm/jaw, shortness of breath, nausea, sweating, palpitations, anxiety
Risk factors smoking, obesity, DM, ↑BP, ↑cholesterol, FH, previous IHD
Signs tachycardia, cool and sweaty ('clammy'), ±LV failure or hypotension
Investigations ***ECG*** ST depression, inverted T waves; subsequently ±Q waves, ±T wave inversion; ***CXR*** cardiomegaly, signs of LV failure; ***cardiac markers*** elevated troponin (trop T ≥0.1ng/ml or trop I ≥1ng/ml)
Acute treatment O_2, aspirin (300mg), clopidogrel (300mg), diamorphine (2.5–5mg IV), antiemetic (p252), GTN (two puffs sublingually). Consider treating pain with IV nitrate infusion (0.05% Isoket® starting at 4ml/h increased to 10ml/h by increments of 2ml/h every 10min according to BP; keep systolic >90mmHg). Anticoagulation with LMWH (p347). Continue O_2 and opiates as required. Glycoprotein IIb/IIIa inhibitors may be indicated under local guidelines (see also *BNF*) and consideration of percutaneous coronary angiography should be made by a cardiologist for high-risk patients (TIMI risk stratification below). Needs CCU.
Secondary prophylaxis ↓modifiable risk factors (smoking, obesity, DM, ↑BP, ↑cholesterol), β-blockade, statin, anti-platelets, eplerenone, ACEi, symptom management (nitrates, Ca^{2+} channel antagonists)
Complications arrhythmias (heart block, bradycardia, VF/VT), LVF, valve prolapse, ventricular septal rupture, ventricular aneurysm formation, pericarditis (Dressler's syndrome, *OHAM2* p182)

Thrombolysis in myocardial infarction (TIMI) risk scoring in NSTEMI/UA[1]

Risk factor	Yes	No
Age >65y	1	0
>3 risk factors for IHD (FH, ↑BP, ↑cholesterol, DM, smoker)	1	0
Known coronary artery disease with >50% stenosis	1	0
Aspirin use within the previous 7d	1	0
Severe angina (≥2 episodes within last 24h)	1	0
ST segment changes of >0.5mm	1	0
Elevated troponin	1	0
Risk score	/7	

Risk score	Risk	Risk of second event within 14d
0 or 1	Low	5%
2	Low	8%
3	Moderate	13%
4	Moderate	20%
5	High	26%
6 or 7	High	41%

[1] Antman *et al.* 2000. Journal of the American Medical Association **284:** 835–42.

Unstable angina (*OHAM2* p46)

Worrying signs features of LV failure, cardiac dysrhythmia

Symptoms central, heavy chest pain radiating to left arm and jaw at rest or precipitated by minimal exertion and poorly relieved by rest or GTN, shortness of breath, nausea, sweating, palpitations; episodes lasting longer (>20min), more frequently and more severe than typical angina

Risk factors smoking, obesity, DM, ↑BP, ↑cholesterol, FH, previous IHD

Signs tachycardia, cool and sweaty ('clammy'), anxiety, pallor. Often no acute signs after episode has settled

*Investigations **ECG*** ST depression, flat or inverted T waves, signs of previous MI; ***cardiac markers*** trop T <0.1ng/ml or trop I <1ng/ml. If resting ECG normal and no rise in troponin, consider exercise ECG (p570), thallium scan or coronary angiography.

Acute treatment O_2, aspirin (300mg), clopidogrel (300mg), diamorphine (2.5–5mg IV), antiemetic (p252), GTN (two puffs sublingually). Consider treating pain with IV nitrate infusion (0.05% Isoket® starting at 4ml/h increased to 10ml/h by increments of 2ml/h every 10min according to BP – keep systolic >90mmHg). Anticoagulation with LMWH (p347). Continue O_2 and opiates as required. Glycoprotein IIb/IIIa inhibitors may be indicated under local guidelines (see also *BNF*) and consideration of percutaneous coronary angiography should be made by a cardiologist for high-risk patients (see p451). Needs CCU.

Secondary prophylaxis ↓modifiable risk factors (smoking, obesity, DM, ↑BP, ↑cholesterol), β-blockade, statin, anti-platelets, ACEi, symptom management (nitrates, Ca^{2+} channel antagonists)

Complications MI, arrhythmias (heart block, bradycardia, VF/VT)

Stable angina (*OHCM7* p102)

Worrying signs features of LV failure, cardiac dysrhythmia

Symptoms central, heavy chest pain (lasting <20min) radiating to left arm and jaw, precipitated by exertion and relieved by rest or rapidly by GTN (<5min), shortness of breath, nausea, sweating, palpitations

Risk factors smoking, obesity, DM, ↑BP, ↑cholesterol, FH, previous IHD

Signs tachycardia, cool and sweaty ('clammy'), anxiety, pallor. Often no acute signs after episode has settled.

*Investigations **ECG*** transient ST depression, flat or inverted T waves, signs of previous MI; ***cardiac markers*** not detectable (trop T <0.01ng/ml or trop I <0.1ng/ml). If resting ECG normal and no enzyme rise, consider exercise ECG (p570), thallium scan or coronary angiography.

Acute treatment as for unstable angina until pain settles. If pain lasting >20min, investigate and treat as for NSTEMI/UA.

Primary prophylaxis assessment and reduction of modifiable risk factors (smoking, obesity, DM, BP, cholesterol), β-blockade, statin, anti-platelets, ACEi, symptom management (nitrates, Ca^{2+} channel antagonists)

Aortic dissection (*OHCM7* p586 or *OHAM2* p170)

Symptoms sudden onset severe chest pain, anterior or interscapular, tearing in nature, dizziness, breathlessness, sweating, neurological deficits

Risk factors smoking, obesity, DM, ↑BP, ↑cholesterol, FH, previous IHD

Signs unequal radial pulses, tachycardia, hypotension/hypertension, difference in brachial pressures of >15mmHg, aortic regurgitation, pleural effusion (L>R), neurological deficits from carotid artery dissection

Investigations ***ECG*** may be normal or show LV strain/ischaemia (p610); ***CXR*** classically widened mediastinum >8cm (rarely seen), enlargement of aortic knuckle and small left pleural effusion can develop from blood tracking down; ***echo*** may show aortic root leak, aortic valve regurgitation or pericardial effusion. Also consider MRI/CT/conventional angiography

Acute treatment if **hypotensive**, treat as shock (p210). O_2, two large-bore cannulas, crossmatch 10 units, analgesia (IV opiates), seek immediate cardiology/senior assessment. If **hypertensive** aim to keep systolic BP <100mmHg (p201)

Chronic treatment surgery or medical management (*OHAM*2 p174)

Musculoskeletal chest pain

Symptoms localised chest wall pain, worse on movement and/or breathing, recent trauma or exertion (eg lifting)

Signs focal tenderness, erythema, absence of other signs in CVS or RS

Investigations only investigate if you cannot satisfy yourself of the diagnosis on clinical grounds; ***ECG*** normal (no ischaemia/MI); ***CXR*** normal (no pneumothorax); ***D-dimer*** normal

Acute treatment reassurance and simple analgesia (p428)

Chronic treatment should settle within 2wk, prevention from further injury (no more heavy lifting for a few weeks), adequate regular analgesia to allow activities of daily living to be carried out and to allow deep inspiration and coughing (to prevent chest infection), stop smoking

Pericarditis (*OHAM*2 p178)

Symptoms pleuritic chest pain, worse on lying flat and deep inspiration, relieved by sitting forwards, recent viral illnesses

Signs may be no abnormalities, ±pericardial rub

Investigations ***ECG*** saddle-shaped ST segments on most leads (concave upwards); ***blds*** ↑WCC and inflammatory markers, ±↑viral titres; ***echo*** ±pericardial effusion

Acute treatment reassurance and analgesia; paracetamol, NSAIDs, weak opiates

Chronic treatment should settle within 2–4wk; recurrence common

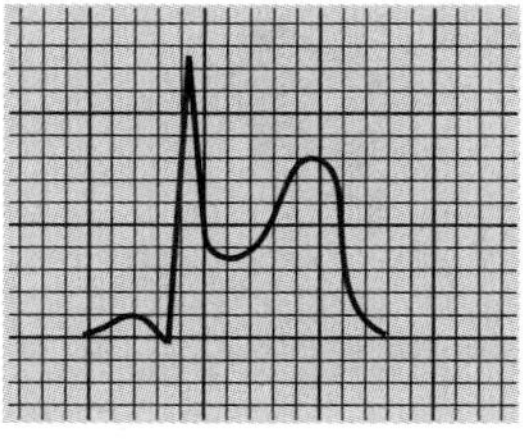

Typical saddle-shaped ST segment seen in pericarditis.

Tachyarrhythmia emergency

Airway	Check airway is patent; consider manoeuvres/adjuncts
Breathing	If no respiratory effort – **CALL ARREST TEAM**
Circulation	If no palpable pulse – **CALL ARREST TEAM**

Call for **senior help** early if patient 'unstable':

Signs of an unstable patient include:

- Reduced conscious level
- Systolic BP <90mmHg
- Chest pain
- Heart failure

- **Sit patient** up unless hypotensive, then lay flat with legs elevated
- **15l/min** O_2 in all patients
- **Monitor** pulse oximeter, BP, defibrillator ECG leads if unwell
- Request full set of **observations** and **ECG**
- Take brief **history** if possible/check notes/ask ward staff
- **Examine patient**: condensed CVS, RS, ±abdo exam
- Establish **likely causes** and rule out **serious causes**
- **Initiate further treatment**, see following pages
- **Venous access**, take bloods:
  - FBC, U+E, D-dimer, cardiac markers, TFT
- Consider requesting urgent **CXR**, portable if too unwell
- Call for **senior help**
- **Reassess**, starting with A, B, C…

Life-threatening causes

- Ventricular tachycardia (VT) or ventricular fibrillation (VF)
- Torsade de pointes
- Supraventricular tachycardia with haemodynamic compromise
- Fast atrial fibrillation/flutter with haemodynamic compromise
- Sinus tachycardia
  - secondary to shock, including PE
  - iatrogenic (drugs)

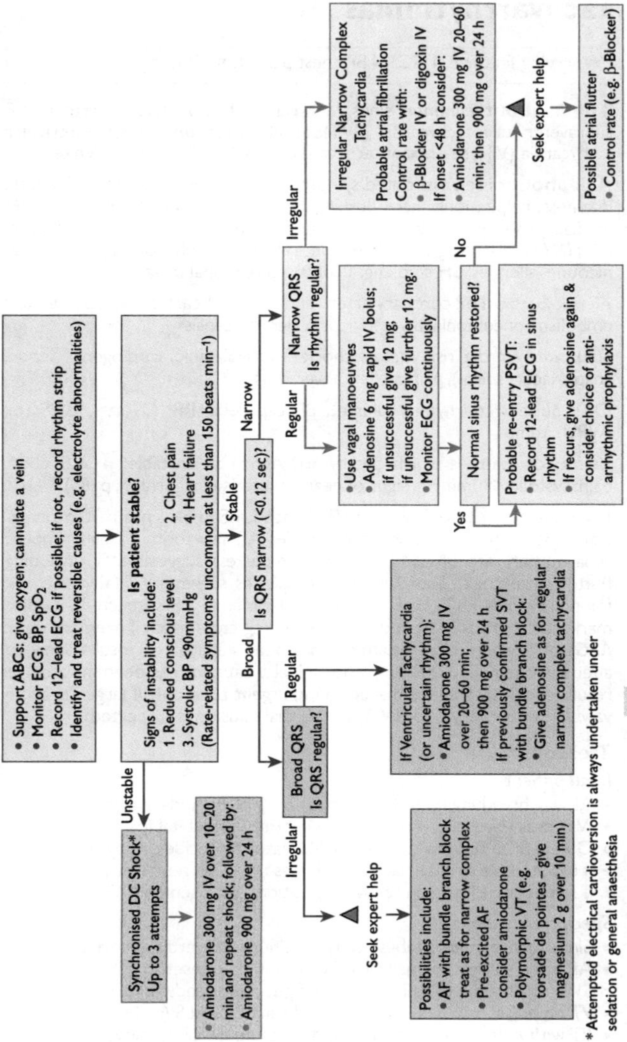

Tachycardia algorithm (with a pulse), 2005 guidelines.
Reproduced by kind permission of the Resuscitation Council (UK).

Tachyarrhythmias

Worrying features ↓GCS, ↓BP, chest pain, heart failure

Think about ***common*** sinus tachycardia, fast ventricular rate in AF, supraventricular tachycardia (SVT), atrial flutter; ***uncommon*** ventricular tachycardia (VT), re-entrant tachycardia (eg Wolff–Parkinson–White)

Ask about onset, associated symptoms (chest pain, shortness of breath, dizziness, palpitations, facial flushing, headache), previous episodes; ***PMH*** cardiac problems (IHD, valvular lesions, hypertension), thyroid disease, DM; ***DH*** cardiac drugs, levothyroxine, salbutamol, anticholinergics, caffeine, nicotine, allergies; ***SH*** smoking, alcohol, recreational drug use

AF risk factors ↑BP, coronary artery and valvular heart disease, pulmonary embolism, pneumonia, thyrotoxicosis, alcohol, sepsis

Sinus tachycardia risk factors shock (hypovolaemic, cardiogenic, septic, anaphylactic, spinal), pain/anxiety, fever, drugs

Obs pulse (rate/rhythm/volume), BP, cap refill, RR, O_2 sats, GCS (or AVPU), temp

Look for features which classify arrhythmia as 'unstable': ↓GCS, chest pain, systolic <90mmHg, signs of heart failure (see algorithm, p185)

Investigations *ECG* P waves before each QRS imply sinus rhythm, irregular QRS without clear P waves implies AF, saw-tooth baseline implies atrial flutter, rate of ≥140 (narrow complexes) suggests SVT (including flutter with block), broad regular complexes suggests VT (always check for pulse); ***blds*** FBC, U+E, TFT, CRP, D-dimer (if PE suspected), cardiac markers, others as indicated by suspicion (eg crossmatch if haemorrhage); ***ABGs*** only when initial treatment has been initiated or results likely to alter management; ***CXR*** only once initial treatment has been initiated or results are likely to alter management; ***urgent echo*** only if large PE, acute valvular lesion, very poor LV or pericardial effusion is suspected

Treatment

In all patients

- Airway, breathing (with O_2), circulation (HR, BP and capillary refill)
- IV access (two large-bore cannula in both antecubital fossa)
- Obtain ECG or view trace on defibrillator to decide on rhythm
- If hypotensive or dizzy lay flat with legs up – Call senior help
- If semi-conscious lay in recovery position – Call senior/ARREST TEAM

Specific arrhythmias

- ***Sinus tachycardia:*** establish cause of sinus tachycardia, ?shock (p210)
- **AF** is the patient normally in AF or is this new onset? (p188)
- ***SVT*** usually time to call for help and get drugs ready (p189)
- ***VT no pulse:*** call ARREST TEAM and start BLS/ALS (p164)
- ***VT with pulse:*** call senior help and anaesthetist for cardioversion (p572). May respond to amiodarone (p189).

ECG features of tachyarrhythmias

	Rate	Regular	P waves	Broad/narrow
Sinus tachycardia	>100	✓	✓	Narrow (unless BBB)
Fast AF	>100	✗	✗	Narrow (unless BBB)
SVT	≥140	✓	✓	Narrow (unless BBB)
VT (with pulse)	≥150	✓	✗	Broad
VT (pulseless)	As for 'VT with pulse'; always perform a pulse-check (carotid)			
VF	Chaotic irregular electrical activity; never has a pulse			

Typical appearance of various tachyarrhythmias

	ECG, lead II view (rhythm strip)
Sinus tachycardia	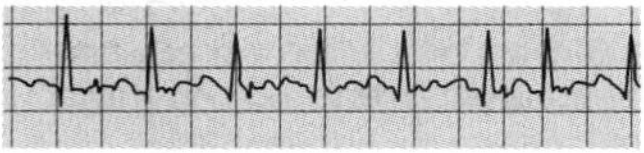
Fast AF	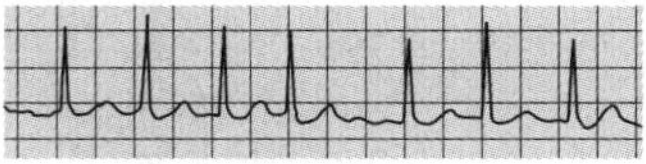
SVT	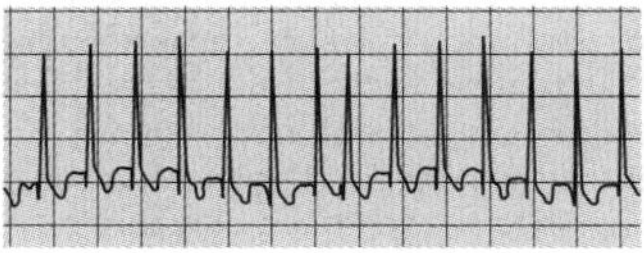
VT with or without a pulse	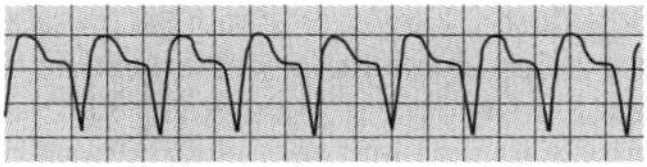
VF	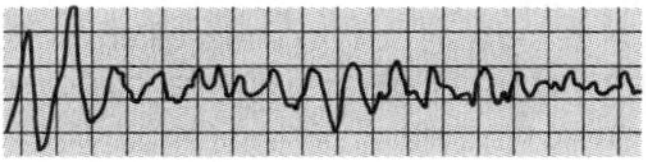
Torsade de pointes	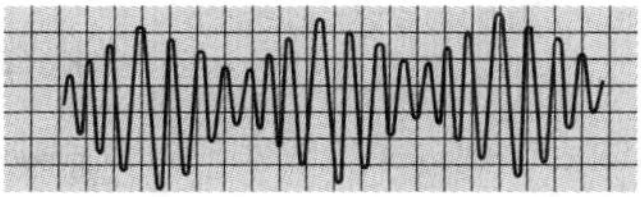

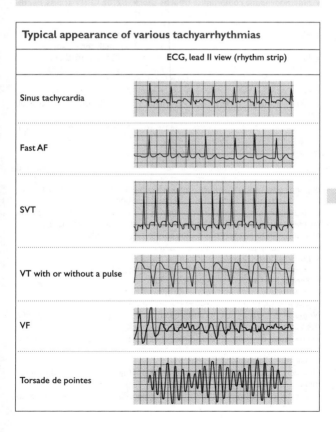

Fast atrial fibrillation (AF)/flutter (*OHAM*2 p84)

Worrying signs heart failure, hypotension, ↓GCS or chest pain

Symptoms palpitations, shortness of breath, dizziness, ±chest pains

Risk factors previous AF, ↑BP, IHD, valvular heart disease, PE, pneumonia, thyrotoxicosis, alcohol (acute excess, chronic use or withdrawal), dilated cardiomyopathy, ↑age, acute illness

Signs irregularly irregular pulse, hypotension if cardiovascular compromise, signs of concurrent/precipitant disease (pneumonia, thyrotoxicosis)

Investigations ***ECG*** absent P waves, irregularly irregular QRS complexes in AF; saw-tooth appearance of baseline in atrial flutter; ***blds*** FBC (↑WCC), U+E, TFT, alcohol, ±D-dimer (PE); ***CXR*** heart size, pulmonary oedema, pneumonia; ***echo*** LV dilatation/impairment, valvular lesion

Acute treatment

- ***Haemodynamic compromise*** treat as shock (p210); O_2, IV access, needs rapid rate-control or restoration of sinus rhythm (DC cardioversion, see below). Seek immediate senior help.
- ***Haemodynamically stable*** and AF present for >2d, load with digoxin (below) and anticoagulate with LMWH (p347). Seek senior advice.
- ***Haemodynamically stable*** and AF present for <2d, aim to chemically cardiovert with flecainide or amiodarone and anticoagulate with LMWH (p347). Seek senior advice for dosing regimen.

Chronic management identify precipitant of AF (echo, stress ECG, TFT, CXR), anticoagulate, revert to sinus rhythm chemically or, if unsuccessful, consider elective DC cardioversion

Complications thromboembolic disease (eg ischaemic stroke commonly). Drug side-effects (amiodarone, warfarin, β-blockers, digoxin etc)

Starting digoxin therapy (*OHAM*2 p88)

Control of the ventricular rate in fast AF can be achieved with several drugs, as well as with DC cardioversion. The maintenance dose of digoxin depends upon ventricular rate (may need higher dose if rate poorly controlled) and patient factors (such as renal function)

Digoxin does not restore sinus rhythm, it merely slows conduction at the atrioventricular node, limiting the number of impulses passing from the atria through to the ventricles thus controlling ventricular rate

Urgent loading as follows (also see *BNF*)

- Loading dose 500μg/over 30min IVI (in saline or glucose)
  - use 250μg if patient very elderly, small or frail
- Repeat loading dose of 500μg/over 30min IVI 8h later
  - use 250μg if patient very elderly, small or frail
- Commence maintenance dose (62.5-500μg/24h PO) 8h later

Non-urgent loading can be undertaken orally; 1mg divided over 24h PO, then commence the likely maintenance dose (eg 62.5μg/24h PO)

Therapeutic monitoring should be undertaken if toxicity is considered (usually presents with N+V) or if compliance is questioned. Sample should be taken 6–12h post-oral dose (p151)

Digoxin toxicity (p197) is increased in ↓K^+, ↓Mg^{2+} or ↑Ca^{2+} and in renal impairment, therefore use a reduced dose

If rate not controlled after loading with digoxin, discuss with senior or cardiologist (p451)

Supraventricular tachycardia (SVT) (*OHAM*2 p78)

Worrying signs heart failure, hypotension, ↓GCS or chest pain
Symptoms palpitations, shortness of breath, dizziness, ±chest pains
Risk factors previous SVT, structural cardiac anomaly, alcohol, ↑T_4
Signs tachycardia, anxiety, hypotension if haemodynamic compromise
Investigations ***ECG*** narrow complex tachycardia (unless concurrent BBB) with P waves (which may merge into QRS), regular QRS complexes, rate usually ≥140; **further investigations** only required if diagnosis in question, otherwise initiate treatment as below
Acute treatment O_2, large-bore IV access (antecubital fossa). Monitor rhythm on defibrillator

- ***Vagal manoeuvres*** see pXXX
- ***Chemical*** see pXXX

Chronic treatment if recurrent, seek cardiology advice as may require electrophysiological testing of cardiac conduction pathways
Complications hypotension, heart failure in individuals with existing cardiac disease, deterioration into more sinister arrhythmia

Wolfe–Parkinson–White syndrome (WPW) (*OHAM*7 p112)

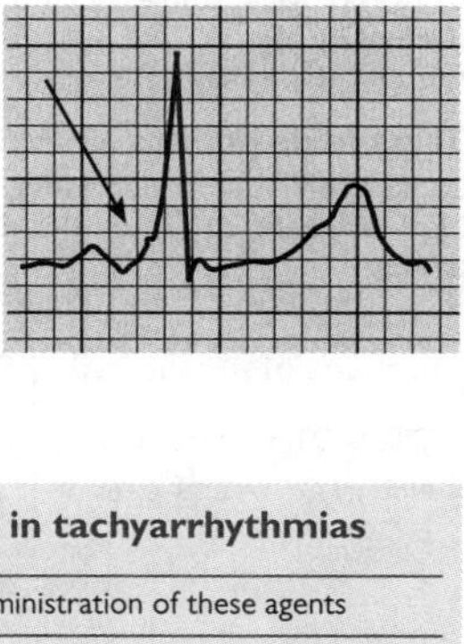

Aetiology This is a re-entrant tachycardia which results from an accessory conduction pathway between the atria and the ventricles (bundle of Kent). It classically appears as a short PR interval and a δ/delta wave (shown by arrow in the illustration).

Treatment Avoid digoxin and verapamil. Refer to a cardiologist for consideration of electrophysiology and ablation of accessory pathway.

Anti-arrhythmics commonly used in tachyarrhythmias

Patient must be in a monitored bed during administration of these agents

Amiodarone (should be given via a central vein, but can be given peripherally in an emergency)	**Loading dose** 300mg/over 60min IVI via central line followed by 900mg/over 23h IVI via central line OR 200mg/8h PO for 1wk then 200mg/12h PO for 1wk **Maintenance dose** 200–400mg/24h PO
Verapamil (avoid if pt on β-blockers)	5mg/over 2min IV repeated every 5min to maximum 20mg OR 40–120mg/8h PO
Flecainide (avoid if pt has IHD)	2mg/kg/over 10min IV (maximum 150mg) OR 100–200mg/12h PO

Ventricular tachycardia (VT) (*OHAM*2 p98)

Worrying signs heart failure, hypotension, ↓GCS, chest pain or absent pulse (pulseless VT)
Symptoms palpitations, dizziness, shortness of breath, ±chest pain, arrest
Risk factors IHD, trauma, hypoxia, acidosis, long QT
Signs tachycardia, anxiety, pallor, hypotension, ↓GCS, shock
Investigations ECG broad complex tachycardia, absence of P waves, rate usually >150; ***blds*** check urgent U+E (especially K^+) and Mg^{2+}; ***other investigations*** should be directed by clinical situation though cardioversion is main priority at this stage

Acute treatment

- *Pulseless VT:* Call ARREST TEAM, commence BLS/ALS (p164) after precordial thump (if witnessed and monitored arrest)
- ***VT with a pulse:*** O_2, two large-bore IV cannula in antecubital fossa, call senior help. Restoration of sinus rhythm with either drugs (eg sotalol, amiodarone, Mg^{2+}) or DC cardioversion. Seek senior advice.
- ***Possible SVT with bundle branch block or VT:*** treat as VT

Chronic treatment may need drug therapy to maintain sinus rhythm, electrophysiological studies/ablation or implantable cardioverter/defibrillator (*OHAM*2 p74)
Complications may deteriorate into VF or other dysrhythmia

Torsade de pointes (*OHAM*2 p72)

Looks like VF but has a rotating axis (p187). Caused by ↑QT interval. Give Mg^{2+} sulphate 2g (8mmol) over 15min (4ml 50% solution) ±overdrive pacing.

Causes of prolonged QT interval

QTc = QT/√(RR interval)

Normal QTc = 0.38–0.46s (9–11 small squares)

Congenital	Romano-Ward syndrome (AD) Jervell, Lange-Neilsen syndrome (AR, associated with deafness)
Drugs	Anti-arrhythmics (amiodarone, sotalol, quinidine) Antipsychotics (thioridazine, pimozide) Antihistamines (terfenadine, astemizole) Antimalarials (halofantrine)
Electrolyte disturbance	↑/↓K^+, ↓Mg^{2+}, ↓Ca^{2+}
Severe bradycardia	Complete heart block, sinus bradycardia
IHD	Ischaemia, myocarditis
Intracranial bleed	Subarachnoid haemorrhage

Bradyarrhythmia emergency

Airway	Check airway is patent; consider manoeuvres/adjuncts
Breathing	If no respiratory effort – **CALL ARREST TEAM**
Circulation	If no palpable pulse – **CALL ARREST TEAM**

Call for **senior help** early if patient has 'adverse signs':

Adverse signs include:

- Systolic BP <90mmHg
- HR <40bpm
- Ventricular arrhythmia
- Heart failure

- **Sit patient up** unless hypotensive/dizzy, then lay flat with legs elevated
- **15l/min O_2** in all patients
- **Monitor** pulse oximeter, BP, defibrillator's ECG leads if very unwell
- Request full set of **observations** and **ECG** with long **rhythm strip**
- Take brief **history** if possible/check **notes**/ask ward staff
- **Examine patient**: condensed CVS, RS, ±abdo exam
- Establish **likely causes** and rule out **serious causes**
- Consider **IV atropine**, 500µg, repeat at 2–3min intervals (max 3mg)
- **Initiate further treatment**, see following pages
- **Venous access**, take bloods
    - FBC, U+E, LFT, cardiac markers, TFT
- Consider requesting urgent **CXR**, portable if too unwell
- Call for **senior help**
- **Reassess**, starting with A, B, C…

Life-threatening causes

- Complete (3rd degree) heart block (±following MI)
- Möbitz type II
- Pauses >3s on ECG
- Hypoxia in children

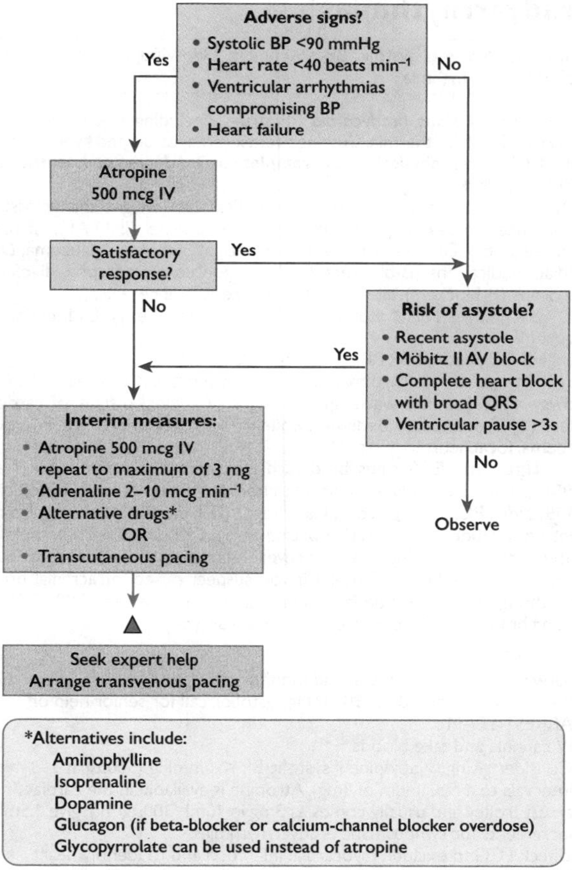

Bradycardia algorithm, 2005 guidelines.
Reproduced by kind permission of the Resuscitation Council (UK).

Bradyarrhythmias

> Worrying features systolic BP <90mmHg, HR <40bpm, heart failure, ventricular arrhythmia

Think about ***sinus bradycardia*** MI, drugs (including digoxin toxicity), vasovagal, ↓T_4, hypothermia, Cushing's reflex (bradycardia and hypertension 2° to ↑ICP), sleep, physical fitness; ***complete or 3rd degree atrioventricular (AV) heart block***

Ask about dizziness, postural dizziness, fits/faints, weight change, visual disturbance, nausea, vomiting; ***PMH*** cardiac disease (IHD/AF), thyroid disease/surgery, DM, head injury or intracranial pathology, glaucoma; ***DH*** cardiac medications (β-blockers, Ca^{2+} antagonists, amiodarone, digoxin), eye drops (β-blockers), allergies; ***SH*** exercise tolerance

IHD risk factors ↑BP, ↑cholesterol, FH, smoking, obesity, DM, previous angina/MI

Obs HR, BP, postural BP, RR, sats, temp, GCS

Look for pulse rate/rhythm/volume, pallor, shortness of breath, ↓GCS, drowsy, ↑JVP (cannon waves in 3rd degree AV block), signs of cardiac failure (↑JVP, pulmonary oedema, swollen ankles), features of ↑ICP (papilloedema, focal neurology – p300)

Investigations ***ECG*** sinus bradycardia or complete heart block (see p195), evidence of ischaemia or infarction (p610) or of digoxin toxicity (p195); ***blds*** FBC, U+E, glucose, Ca^{2+}, Mg^{2+}, TFT, cardiac markers, digoxin level, coagulation (if considering pacing-wire); ***CXR*** unlikely to be helpful in the immediate setting, but may reveal heart size and evidence of pulmonary oedema; ***head CT*** useful if you suspect raised intracranial pressure, though patient will be *in extremis* (about to cone, see p280) if ↑ICP causing bradycardia (speak to on-call neurosurgeon)

Treatment

- Airway, breathing (with O_2) and monitor circulation
- If either ↓GCS or ↓BP (<90mmHg systolic), call for senior help or ARREST TEAM
- IV cannula and take bloods
- Consider giving IV atropine if systolic BP <90mmHg (500μg at 2–3 min intervals to a maximum of 3mg). Atropine is available in the cardiac arrest trolley and usually comes as 3mg in 10ml (300μg/ml); give 1.5ml increments for symptomatic bradyarrhythmias.
- Check ECG to exclude myocardial infarction and to identify heart block or extreme sinus bradycardia or very slow atrial fibrillation

ECG features of bradyarrhythmias and types of heart block

Sinus bradycardia	P waves precede each QRS, rate <60
1st degree AV block	P–R interval >5 small squares (>0.2s)
Möbitz I (Wenkebach)	P–R interval lengthens until failure of AV conduction
Möbitz II	Intermittent P waves fail to conduct to ventricles, but P–R interval does not lengthen, unlike Möbitz type I
High-grade AV block	Only 3rd or 4th P wave conducts to the ventricle (3:1, 4:1 etc)
3rd degree AV block	Complete dissociation between P waves and QRS
Digoxin effect/toxicity	Down-sloping ST segment (reversed tick), inverted T waves
Rate controlled AF	No P waves; irregularly irregular rhythm

Typical appearance of various bradyarrhythmias and types of heart block

	ECG, lead II (rhythm strip) view; arrows indicate P wave
Sinus bradycardia	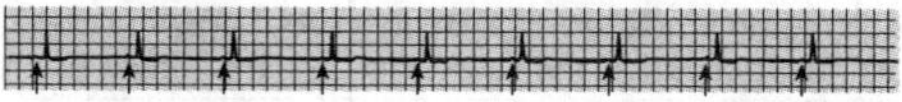
1st degree AV block	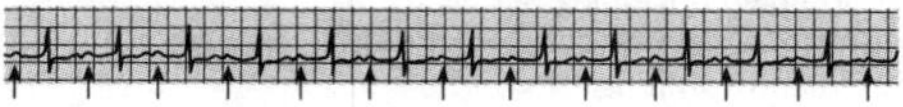
Möbitz type I	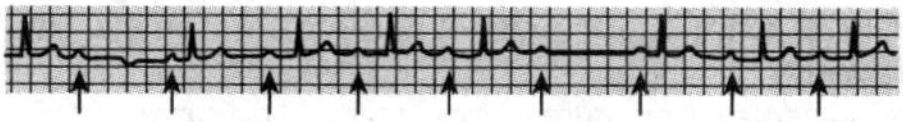
3:1 AV block	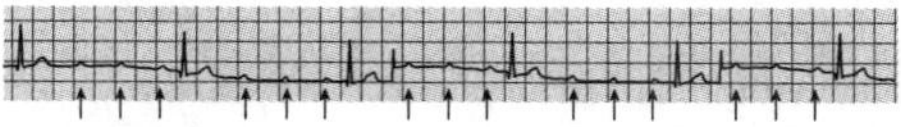
3rd degree (complete) AV block	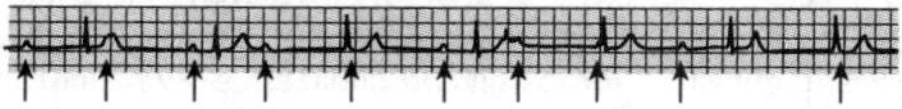
Digoxin effect/ toxicity	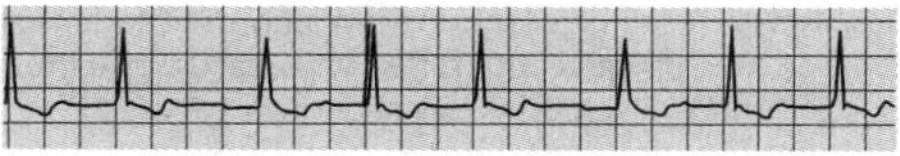

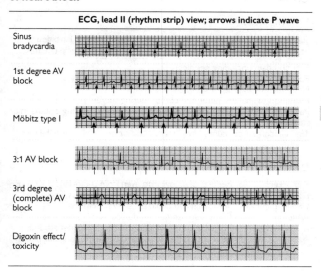

Sinus bradycardia (*OHAM*2 p102)

Worrying signs features of heart failure, hypotension, ↓GCS
Symptoms asymptomatic, dizziness (±on standing), palpitations, shortness of breath, symptoms of either ↑ICP, hypothermia or $\downarrow T_4$
Signs orthostatic ↓BP, hypothermia, evidence of ↑ICP (p300) or $\downarrow T_4$ (p473)
Investigations *ECG* QRS complex will be preceded by a P wave, rate <60, QRS will be narrow unless BBB; exclude ischaemia/infarction; ***blds*** FBC, U+E, Ca^{2+}, Mg^{2+}, TFT, cardiac markers, coagulation (if considering pacing-wire); ***CXR*** unlikely to be helpful in immediate resuscitation phase
Acute treatment if symptomatic (dizzy or GCS <15) or systolic <90mmHg, monitor heart rate on defibrillator, lay flat with legs elevated (as long as ↑ICP not suspected). O_2, secure IV access and take bloods. Call senior help/ ARREST TEAM. Titrate 500μg atropine IV every 2–3min (to a maximum of 3mg) followed by a large flush, until HR improves. Identify and correct precipitant. Consider external pacing/pacing-wire via central line (p574) though obtain senior advice; a rhythmical precordial thump can be used in extremis when an external pacing machine is not immediately available.
Chronic treatment may need permanent pacemaker (*OHCM*7 p118)
Complications severe bradycardia and high vagal tone can deteriorate into asystole so prompt treatment is required. Remember to regularly check for a pulse since pulseless electrical activity (PEA) is common and the ECG trace will not change.

Vasovagal attacks

Sudden reflex bradycardia from unopposed parasympathetic inhibition upon heart rate is common and several factors are known to precipitate this.

Fear and pain (including needles)
Post-micturition (especially in men)
Nausea and vomiting
Dilatation of anal sphincter and cervix (during surgery)
Pulling of extra-ocular muscles and pressure on eye (during ophthalmic surgery)
↑Intra-abdominal pressure (during laparoscopic surgery, straining on the toilet)

Drugs which can precipitate bradycardia

β-blockers	Reports of bradycardia even from β-blocking eye drops
Digoxin	Rhythm likely to be AF, but may be sinus if reverted
Ca^{2+} antagonists	Verapamil and diltiazem slow heart rate
Amiodarone	Can cause conduction defects and bradycardia
α-agonists	Phenylephrine is mainly used by anaesthetists and can cause reflex bradycardia by increasing peripheral vascular resistance

Sick sinus syndrome

Dysfunction of the sinoatrial node often precipitated by ischaemia/fibrosis. Results in bradycardia (±arrest), sinoatrial block or SVT with alternating bradycardia/asystole (tachy-brady syndrome). Needs pacing if symptomatic.

Complete (3rd degree) heart block (*OHAM*2 p106)

Worrying signs features of heart failure, hypotension, ↓GCS

Symptoms asymptomatic, dizziness (±on standing), palpitations, shortness of breath, ±chest pain

Causes congenital, fibrosis, ischaemic, post-cardiac surgery, drug-induced (amiodarone, β-blockers, Ca^{2+}channel blockers), infective, neuromuscular

Signs ↓BP (and potentially ↓GCS), cannon waves in ↑JVP (due to asynchronous contraction of the right atria against a closed tricuspid valve), signs of heart failure, features of underlying disease

Investigations ***ECG*** complete dissociation of P waves from QRS complexes; narrow QRS implies proximal lesion (may respond to atropine), broad QRS implies distal lesion (unlikely to respond to atropine); look for evidence of myocardial infarction; ***blds*** FBC, U+E, cardiac markers, coagulation (if considering pacing-wire); ***CXR*** unlikely to be helpful in immediate resuscitation phase

Acute treatment if symptomatic (dizzy or GCS <15) or systolic <90mmHg, monitor heart rate on defibrillator, lay flat with legs elevated. O_2 supplementation, secure IV access and take bloods. Call senior help/ARREST TEAM. Titrate 500μg atropine IV every 2–3min (to a maximum of 3mg), followed by a large flush, until HR improves. Identify and correct precipitant. Consider external pacing/pacing-wire via central line (p574) though obtain senior advice; a rhythmical precordial thump can be used in extremis when an external pacing machine is not immediately available.

Chronic treatment likely to need permanent pacemaker (*OHCM*7 p118) and/or correction of precipitant

Complications severe bradycardia and high vagal tone can deteriorate into asystole so prompt treatment is required. Remember to regularly check for a pulse since pulseless electrical activity (PEA) is common and the ECG trace will not change.

Other types of heart block (*OHAM*2 p106)

1st degree AV block and Möbitz I do not require treatment unless the patient is symptomatic or there is a reversible cause (usually drugs)

Möbitz II and high-grade AV block may deteriorate into complete heart block and may require temporary/permanent pacing, especially when associated with an ACS or general anaesthesia – seek cardiology advice

Digoxin toxicity (*OHAM*2 p808)

Symptoms	Nausea, vomiting, confusion, diarrhoea, yellow and blurred vision
Bloods	Toxicity precipitated by renal failure, ↓K^+, ↓Mg^{2+} and ↓T_4 Check digoxin level (p151); toxic if >2.6nmol/l (>2μg/l).
ECG (p195)	Tachy- and bradyarrhythmias. ST depression/T wave inversion
Complications	↑K^+, cardiac dysrhythmias (tachy- and bradyarrhythmias)
Management	Airway, breathing, and circulation Continuous ECG monitoring Treat tachy- and bradyarrhythmias as described Consider *digoxin-binding antibody fragments* if cardiovascular compromise, resistant ventricular tachyarrhythmias or ↑K^+

Hypertension emergency

Airway	Check airway is patent; consider manoeuvres/adjuncts
Breathing	If no respiratory effort – **CALL ARREST TEAM**
Circulation	If no palpable pulse – **CALL ARREST TEAM**
Disability	If GCS <8 – **CALL ANAESTHETIST**

Call for **senior help** early if patient deteriorating
If **systolic >200** or **diastolic >120** (BP this high is often seen in clinic):

- **Sit patient up**
- **15l/min O_2** in all patients
- **Monitor** pulse oximeter, BP, defibrillator ECG leads if unwell
- Request full set of **observations** and **ECG**
- Take brief **history** if possible/check notes/ask ward staff
- **Examine patient**: condensed RS, CVS, abdo and eye examination
- Rule out **serious causes** and establish **likely causes**
- **Do not** give stat dose of antihypertensive without senior review
- **Initiate further treatment**, see following pages
- **Venous access**, take bloods:
  - FBC, U+E, cardiac markers, TFT, fasting glucose, cortisol
- Consider requesting urgent **CXR**, portable if too unwell
- Urinalysis and β-hCG
- Call for **senior help** for advice
- Re-assess, starting with A, B, C…

Life-threatening causes

- Pre-eclampsia/eclampsia
- Malignant hypertension >200/120
- Hypertensive encephalopathy
- Phaeochromocytoma
- Thyrotoxic storm
- Cushing's reflex (raised ICP)

Hypertension (systolic >160 or diastolic >100)

Worrying features ↓HR, ↓GCS, chest pain, retinal haemorrhages, systolic >200, diastolic >120, renal failure, seizures

Think about ***life-threatening*** malignant hypertension (BP>200/120), pre-eclampsia; ***other*** anxiety, pain, primary (essential) or secondary hyper–tension (including thyroid storm and phaeochromocytoma)
Ask about visual symptoms, headache, chest/back pains, new motor weakness, facial flushing, diarrhoea, weight gain/loss, pregnancy (pre- or post-partum), change in hat size/change in facial features, haematuria; majority asymptomatic; ***PMH*** previous hypertension, Cushing's syndrome, acromegaly, Conn's syndrome, phaeochromocytoma, coarctation, thyroid disease, DM, renal artery stenosis; ***DH*** cardiac and antihypertensive medications, steroids, contraceptive pill, levothyroxine/carbimazole, MAOI, antipsychotics, recreational drugs (cocaine, amphetamines); ***FH*** hypertension, endocrine disease, polycystic kidney disease; ***SH*** exercise tolerance, smoking
Obs HR, BP (both arms and postural), sats, temp, GCS, repeat BP after a period of relaxing (both arms and postural)
Look for *signs of underlying disease* radiofemoral delay, striae, buffalo hump, central obesity, large hands/feet/face, tremor, exophthalmos, thyroid mass/bruit, proximal myopathy, gravid uterus, renal bruits/polycystic kidneys; ***signs of end-organ damage*** left ventricular hypertrophy (LVH – displaced apex beat), retinopathy (see table p201), Cushing's reflex (raised ICP) and proteinuria/haematuria
Investigations ***serial BP*** repeat BP manually to confirm diagnosis; ***ECG*** features of LVH (see table p611); ***blds*** FBC, U+E, glucose, cholesterol, TFT; ***urine*** blood, protein, β-hCG (<20wk); ***CXR*** unlikely to be helpful in the immediate setting, but may reveal heart size and aortic contours; ***renal USS/arteriography*** small kidneys/stenotic renal arteries; ***24h urine*** VMA (p629), cortisol (p609); ***24h ambulatory BP*** may reveal 'white-coat hypertension' which settles at home or during sleep

Treatment

- Airway, breathing (with O_2 if sats <95%) and monitor circulation
- If ↓GCS call for senior help, p280
- IV cannula and take bloods
- Check ECG to exclude myocardial infarction
- A sudden drop in BP can cause a stroke, aim to lower the BP gradually, see p201, unless benefits outweigh the risks (eg pregnancy, MI, aortic dissection or hypertensive encephalopathy)

Indications for admission

Diastolic persistently >120mmHg
Retinal haemorrhages
Newly diagnosed/recognised renal impairment

Malignant hypertension (*OHAM*2 p166)

Hypertensive emergency with acute retinopathy (see opposite).
Symptoms headache, visual loss, confusion and drowsiness

Signs BP usually >200/120, retinopathy (see p201), ↓GCS

Investigations as for hypertension in general (p199) to exclude a secondary cause and as a baseline investigation of renal function and size. Needs formal (ophthalmic) assessment for retinal disease.

Diagnosis relies on retinopathy being present, ±vasculitis, ±papilloedema, together with the symptoms and signs above. Additional features: renal failure, heart failure, microangiopathic haemolytic anaemia and DIC in severe cases.

Acute treatment needs admission to monitored area (HDU/ITU), with close monitoring of BP, ECG, neurological state and fluid balance (consider arterial line, central line, catheterisation). Aim to reduce diastolic BP to <100mmHg over first 24h (see opposite for treatment options). Patients with early features may be commenced on oral therapy, though late features need treating with IV agents. If no evidence of LVF use labetalol, though if LVF present commence furosemide (40–80mg IV) with either nitroprusside or hydralazine. Consider ACE inhibitor to counteract high circulating levels of renin.

Chronic treatment BP needs checking regularly once discharged from hospital. Ensure GP knows what investigations have been undertaken, their results and what the therapeutic plan/target BP is.

Hypertensive encephalopathy (*OHAM*2 p168)

Medical emergency. Cerebral oedema secondary to loss of autoregulation of cerebral blood flow. Rare in patients with chronic hypertension.

Symptoms headache, nausea, vomiting, confusion, visual changes/loss

Signs hypertension (BP rise only needs to be moderate), retinopathy (see opposite), confusion or ↓GCS, seizures, coma

Investigations as for hypertension in general (p199) to exclude a secondary cause and as a baseline investigation of renal function and size. Needs formal (ophthalmic) assessment for retinal disease and CT/MRI head to exclude other intracranial pathology.

Diagnosis of exclusion (stroke, encephalitis, tumour, bleeding, hypoglycaemia, vasculitis)

Acute treatment needs admission to monitored area (HDU/ITU), with close monitoring of BP, ECG, neurological state and fluid balance (consider arterial line, central line, catheterisation). Aim to reduce diastolic BP to <100mmHg over first 1–2h (see opposite for treatment options). Correct electrolyte abnormalities and give furosemide 40–80mg IV. Nitroprusside as first-line agent, labetalol and Ca^{2+} channel blockers as second-line agents. Avoid clonidine or methyldopa as these are sedating. Consider ACE inhibitor to counteract high circulating levels of renin.

Chronic treatment BP needs checking regularly once discharged from hospital. Ensure GP knows what investigations have been undertaken and their results and what the therapeutic plan/target BP is.

Emergency treatment of hypertension

Most cases of hypertension do not need emergency treatment and oral therapy is usually sufficient to control BP. Never use stat doses of sub-lingual nifedipine. If BP needs to be rapidly reduced use an intravenous agent in a high-dependency/critical care area.

Before commencing therapy confirm diagnosis by repeating BP and ensuring that the BP cuff is sited correctly and an appropriate size (width of the cuff should be at least 40% of the arm circumference and bladder of the cuff should be centred over brachial artery). Check baseline bloods and initiate investigations to exclude secondary causes.

IV antihypertensives for acute management of hypertension[1] (*OHAM*2 p164)

Patient must be in HDU/ITU, ideally with invasive BP monitoring. Intravenous therapy results in rapid falls in BP so drugs must be titrated cautiously.

Drug	Dose	Comment
Isoket® 0.05%[2] (0.5mg/ml)	2–10ml/h IVI (1–5mg/h)	Venodilates. Useful in LVF/angina. Easy for nurses to set up infusion. Drug of choice.
GTN	1–10mg/h IVI	Venodilates. Useful in LVF and angina.
Hydralazine	5–10mg/20min IVI	Vasodilates, can cause compensatory rise in heart rate; use with a β-blocker.
Labetalol	20–80mg/10min	Drug of choice in phaeochromocytoma or aortic dissection. Avoid in LVF.
Nitroprusside	0.25–8μg/kg/min	Rapid onset. Useful in LVF or hypertensive encephalopathy. Rarely used now.

Oral antihypertensives for acute management of hypertension[1] (*OHAM*2 p165)

Drug	Dose	Comment
Atenolol	50–100mg/24h PO	Many β-blockers available. Contraindicated in asthma, peripheral vascular disease, DM.
Hydralazine	25–50mg/8h PO	Vasodilator. Safe in pregnancy.
Nifedipine	10–20mg/8h PO	Avoid sublingual as rapidly drops BP. OK to use in conjunction with β-blocker (avoid verapamil or diltiazem with β-blockers).

Hypertensive retinopathy

Grade 1 Tortuous retinal arteries, silver wiring
Grade 2 Grade 1 + AV nipping
Grade 3 Grade 2 + flame-shaped haemorrhages and cotton wool spots
Grade 4 Grade 3 + papilloedema

1 Aim to reduce BP by 25% in 1–4h, then more slowly to a diastolic of <100mmHg.

2 Available as 50ml 0.05% solution (25mg in 50ml).

Essential (primary) hypertension (*OHCM*7 p124)

Accounts for 95% of cases of hypertension.
Worrying signs BP>200/120, signs of retinopathy or encephalopathy (p200)
Symptoms most often asymptomatic, may present with end-organ damage (IHD, retinopathy, nephropathy, neuropathy)
Signs BP>160/90, ±end-organ dysfunction
Investigations as for hypertension in general (p199) to exclude a secondary cause and as a baseline investigation of renal function and size. Needs formal (ophthalmic) assessment for retinal disease.
When to treat BP>140/90
Acute treatment if BP<200/120 but >160/100 and no clear cause identified, commence oral antihypertensive therapy unless there are other indications to reduce BP more rapidly (eclampsia, MI, aortic dissection). If BP>200/120 consider commencing IV anti-hypertensive therapy (p201) in a monitored environment (HDU/ITU); discuss with senior/cardiologist.
Chronic treatment BP needs checking regularly once discharged from hospital. Ensure GP knows what investigations have been undertaken, their results and what the therapeutic plan is. Inform patient about need to comply with medication regime and identify lifestyle changes and modifiable risk factors (opposite).
Antihypertensive drugs include: ACE inhibitors, β-blockers, Ca^{2+} channel blockers and diuretics
Complications end-organ damage, malignant hypertension

Secondary causes of hypertension

Renal (p321)	Intrinsic renal disease (glomerulonephritis, polycystic kidneys) Renovascular disease (renal artery stenosis, AAA)
Endocrine (p204)	Cushing's syndrome, Conn's syndrome, phaeochromocytoma, acromegaly, hyperparathyroidism, thyrotoxicosis
Drugs	Steroids, MAOI, oral contraceptive pill
Others	Coarctation, gestational, pre-eclampsia/eclampsia

Lifestyle changes and modifiable risk factors

Lifestyle	Stop smoking Reduce salt and alcohol consumption Reduce stress Take regular exercise
Modifiable risk factors (to limit risk of IHD)	Diagnose and aggressively treat DM Diagnose and treat dyslipidaemia

Management of hypertension in adults in primary care

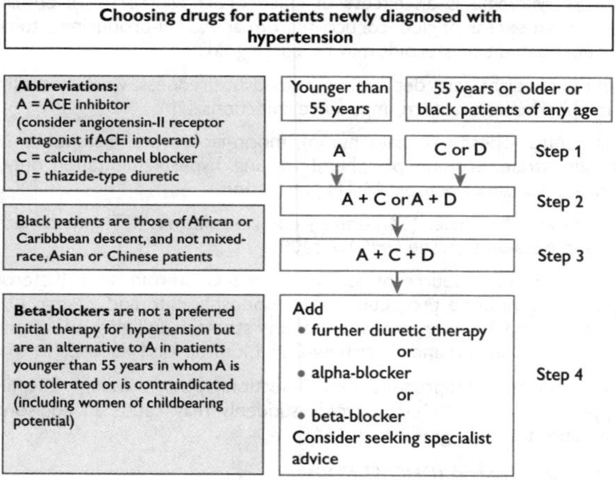

NICE clinical guideline 34, 2006. Reproduced with permission of NICE.
www.nice.org.uk/nicemedia/pdf/CG034NICEguideline.pdf

Starting an ACE inhibitor

Can be undertaken as inpatient, outpatient or by GP

Contraindications	Renal artery stenosis, aortic stenosis, hyperkalaemia, known allergy to ACEi, pregnancy/lactation
Side-effects	Dry cough, postural hypotension, renal impairment and hyperkalaemia, taste disturbance, urticaria and angioneurotic oedema. If cough is problematic for the patient, consider ATII receptor antagonist, or other anti-hypertensive agent.
Before starting	Check U+E, document starting BP
First dose	Start with lowest dose and give at bedtime to limit any problems with first-dose hypotension
Day 4–7	Recheck U+E, ask about postural symptoms and check lying and standing BP
Day 10–14	Recheck U+E, ask about postural symptoms and check lying and standing BP
Week 3	Increase dose if tolerating and no new renal impairment
Week 4	Recheck U+E, ask about postural symptoms and check lying and standing BP
Week 5	Increase dose if tolerating and no new renal impairment. Continue weekly until target/maximal dose achieved

Cushing's syndrome (*OHCM*7 p208)

Cushing's syndrome is an excess of glucocorticoids (cortisol); *Cushing's disease* is an excess of glucocorticoids from an ACTH-producing pituitary tumour. A patient on steroids may be 'cushingoid'.

Symptoms weight gain, depression, psychosis, tiredness, weakness, oligo- or amenorrhoea, hirsutism, impotence, infections, DM

Signs central obesity (buffalo hump), moon-face, water retention, ↑BP, thin skin, striae, bruising, peripheral wasting, hyperpigmentation only in Cushing's disease or ectopic ACTH production

Investigations ↑glucose, ↑24h urinary cortisol, plasma ACTH, dexamethasone suppression test; see *OHCM*7 p209

Treatment remove source of cortisol or reduce steroid dose. If steroid-dependent give bone protection with bisphosphonate and vitamin D, eg alendronic acid 70mg once a week (empty stomach, full glass of water, sit up for at least 30min) and Calcichew-D_3®. Monitor for ↑glucose.

Complications osteoporosis, DM, infection, poor healing, infertility. Stopping long-term (>14d) steroids suddenly may cause an addisonian crisis; taper the dose gradually (p154).

Conn's syndrome (*OHCM*7 p212)

Excess of aldosterone, usually from an adrenal cortex tumour.

Symptoms thirst, polyuria, weakness, muscle spasms, headaches

Signs hypertension

Investigations ↓K^+, normal or ↑Na^+, metabolic alkalosis, measure plasma renin and aldosterone together, consider CT abdo

Treatment spironolactone 200–300mg/24h PO for 4wk followed by surgical removal of adrenal lesion

Secondary hyperaldosteronism diuretics, heart failure, liver failure and renal artery stenosis cause ↑renin and aldosterone, producing the features of Conn's. Spironolactone and ACEi combat this effect.

Phaeochromocytoma (*OHCM*7 p212)

Excess of catecholamines (eg adrenaline) from adrenal medulla tumour or ectopic source.

Symptoms episodic anxiety, chest tightness, breathlessness, tremor, palpitations, headaches, sweating, abdo pain, vomiting

Signs episodic hypertension

Investigations glycosuria during attack, 24h urine for VMA/HMMA

Treatment phenoxybenzamine (α-blocker), followed by propranolol (β-blocker), followed by surgery

Anaphylaxis in adults

Airway	Check airway is patent; consider manoeuvres/adjuncts
Breathing	If no respiratory effort – **CALL ARREST TEAM**
Circulation	If no palpable pulse – **CALL ARREST TEAM**

Call for **senior help** early if anaphylaxis suspected

- **Sit patient up** unless hypotensive, then lay flat with legs elevated
- **15l/min O_2** in all patients
- **Monitor** pulse oximeter, BP, defibrillator ECG leads if unwell
- Request full set of **observations**
- Take brief **history** if possible/check **drug chart**/ask ward staff
- **Examine patient:** look for early signs of anaphylaxis (see below)
- Establish **likely cause** and stop further exposure (eg IV antibiotics)
- **Adrenaline**, 1:1000 solution, 0.5ml **intramuscular**
  - repeat every 5 minutes if no improvement
- Large-bore **venous access**, take bloods if time permits:
  - FBC, U+E, mast cell tryptase (see p207)
- Intravenous infusion of **1l 0.9% saline**, stat
- Consider nebulised beta-agonist for **bronchospasm**
  - salbutamol 5mg, or
  - adrenaline 1:1000 solution, 5ml (5mg)
- Re-assess
- Consider **adjuncts** to treatment
  - antihistamine, chlorphenamine, 10mg slow IV
  - hydrocortisone 200mg slow IV
- Ensure **senior help** has been requested

Intramuscular adrenaline is relatively safe and should be given if the diagnosis of anaphylaxis is likely

Early signs of anaphylaxis

- Urticaria
- Flushing
- Bronchospasm/stridor
- Abdominal pain
- Vomiting and/or diarrhoea
- Sense of impending doom

Anaphylaxis (*OHCM*7 p780)

Commoner precipitants

Drugs	Penicillins, anaesthetic drugs, contrast medium, blood products
Environmental	Latex, stings, eggs, fish, strawberries, nuts

Worrying signs BP <90mmHg systolic, ↓O_2 sats, chest tightness, stridor
Symptoms chest tightness, wheeze, breathlessness, itching, swelling
Signs hypotension, tachycardia, tongue/periorbital swelling, wheeze, urticaria, erythema, cyanosis
Investigations if you suspect anaphylactic shock commence treatment; seconds count. Subsequently check for serum mast cell tryptase to confirm global mast cell degranulation; three samples of clotted blood, one during the reaction once adrenaline has been given, one about 1h post-reaction, and one between 6h and 24h post-reaction.
When to treat all patients with physical signs
Acute treatment call senior help; early involvement of ITU/anaesthetist

- 15l/min O_2
- Secure airway if compromised
- Remove precipitant (eg stop antibiotic IVI etc)
- Lay flat or with legs elevated if patient dizzy
- **Give 0.5mg adrenaline (epinephrine) IM (0.5ml of 1:1000)**
  - every 5min until improvement in BP and respiratory symptoms
- Secure IV access, give 1l 0.9% saline stat
- Chlorphenamine 10mg IV and hydrocortisone 200mg IV
- Nebulised salbutamol 5mg or adrenaline 5ml of 1:1000 solution (5mg)
- Ensure senior help available

Chronic treatment follow-up by immunologist; may need EpiPen

Adrenaline (epinephrine) preparations

1:1000	Preparation – 1ml ampoule. Give 0.5ml (0.5mg) IM 1mg in 1ml
1:10,000	Preparation – 10ml syringe in cardiac arrest drugs, or 10ml ampoule 1mg in 10ml

Intramuscular adrenaline is relatively safe and should be given if the diagnosis of anaphylaxis is likely

Hypotension emergency

Airway	Check airway is patent; consider manoeuvres/adjuncts
Breathing	If no respiratory effort – **CALL ARREST TEAM**
Circulation	If no palpable pulse – **CALL ARREST TEAM**

Call for **senior help** early if patient deteriorating
Systolic <100:
- Lay patient flat and **elevate the legs** if dizzy
- **15l/min O_2** in all patients
- **Monitor** pulse oximeter, BP, defibrillator ECG leads if unwell
- Request full set of **observations** and **ECG**
- Take brief **history** if possible/check **notes**/ask ward staff
- **Examine patient:** condensed RS, CVS, abdo and neuro exam
- Establish **likely cause of shock**
- Large-bore **venous access**, take bloods:
  - FBC, U+E, CRP, D-dimer, cardiac markers, blood cultures
- Intravenous infusion of **1l 0.9% saline** stat
- **Initiate further treatment**, see following pages
- **Arterial blood gas**, but don't leave the patient alone
- Consider requesting urgent **CXR**, portable if too unwell
- Call for **senior help**
- **Reassess**, starting with A, B, C…

Life-threatening causes

- Hypovolaemic/haemorrhagic shock (p212)
- Septic shock (p214)
- Cardiogenic shock (tamponade/tension pneumothorax/heart failure) (p216)
- Anaphylactic shock (p206)
- Neurogenic shock (spinal shock) (p217)

Hypotension (systolic<100)

Worrying features ↓GCS, ↑↓HR, stridor, ↓O_2 sats, bleeding, chest pain, dizziness, ↓urine output, renal failure, severe back pain, non-blanching rash

Think about *life-threatening* shock (hypovolaemic/haemorrhagic, septic, cardiogenic, anaphylactic, neurogenic), dysrhythmia (brady- or tachyarrhythmia); ***other*** postural hypotension, vasovagal episode, Addison's disease/adrenal insufficiency, iatrogenic (β-blockers, ACE inhibitors, Ca^{2+} channel blockers, diuretics, nitrates)
Ask about palpitations, chest pain, shortness of breath, feeling faint/dizzy on standing, blood loss (haematemesis, melaena, PV bleeding), trauma, abdominal/back/loin pain, diarrhoea, vomiting, indigestion, polyuria, fever, sweats, cough, urinary symptoms, itch/urticaria, chest tightness, spinal trauma or anaesthetic, weight loss, skin darkening; ***PMH*** AAA, gastroduodenal ulcers, pregnancy, diabetes insipidus and DM, infections (urinary, chest, cardiac, blood), immunocompromise, angina, MI, previous DVT/PE, Addison's disease, postural hypotension; ***DH*** blood transfusions, antibiotics, cardiac medications (β-blockers, ACE inhibitors, Ca^{2+} channel blockers, diuretics, nitrates) heparin/warfarin, recent anaesthetics, steroids (?withdrawal); ***FH*** PE/DVT, Addison's/autoimmune disease; ***SH*** smoking, alcohol, recreational drug abuse
Obs HR, BP, postural BP, RR, sats, temp, GCS, fluid balance
Look for volume status (p319), pulse rate/rhythm/volume, evidence of diarrhoea or vomiting, source of bleeding (limbs, chest, abdomen, back, mouth, anus, vagina and head), palpable abdominal aortic aneurysm, abdominal guarding or tenderness, warm peripheries or fever, flushed appearance, sweating, urticaria, dyspnoea, focal signs in the chest (consolidation, pneumothorax (tension) or pulmonary oedema), calf swelling or tenderness, wasting of small muscles of the hands or ↑skin pigmentation (signs of Addison's disease)
Investigations ***serial BP*** repeat BP manually to confirm diagnosis and check bilateral BP; ***ECG*** arrhythmia, evidence of LVH/strain/MI; ***blds*** FBC, U+E, glucose, G+S (crossmatch if haemorrhage), CRP, D-dimer, cardiac markers, clotting, blood cultures, mast cell tryptase if anaphylaxis suspected; ***CXR*** do not request if you suspect tension pneumothorax – perform immediate needle decompression (p227); consolidation, mediastinal width; ***urine*** catheterise, dipstix and C+S; ***urgent echo*** LV function, aortic root dilation/dissection, pericardial fluid (tamponade effect), massive PE, aortic/mitral valve prolapse; ***other*** pelvic X-ray in trauma, CT chest may be necessary if aortic dissection suspected, central venous pressure monitoring may be needed via a central line, continuous arterial pressure can be monitored via an arterial line

Treatment

- Airway, breathing (with 15l/min O_2) and monitor BP; elevate legs
- IV access, 14G (orange/brown) cannulae in both antecubital fossa
- If bleeding give IV colloid and consider blood
- Otherwise give 1l 0.9% saline stat
- Establish and treat likely cause
- Call for senior help early

Shock

Classification of shock

Shock has many definitions, but is essentially a problem at the cellular level and results from inadequate tissue perfusion. There are several causes of this, and the key to treating shock successfully is establishing what is the precipitating factor(s). Cutaneous signs and a very brief history often allows the cause of shock to be quickly identified (see opposite).

Hypovolaemic or haemorrhagic shock (p212) is caused by a reduced circulating volume. The patient is usually pale, cool to touch, has moist skin and is tachycardic.

Septic shock (p214) is mediated by a loss in vascular tone, usually by pathogenic toxins and endogenous inflammatory mediators. The circulatory volume is likely to be normal, but loss of peripheral vascular resistance results in ↓BP and inadequate tissue perfusion. The patient is usually warm, flushed, vasodilated and tachycardic.

Cardiogenic shock (p216) results from pump failure (heart failure) or inadequate filling of the pump (massive pulmonary embolism). This can occur as part of a chronic picture or acutely following a massive MI. The patient is pale and clammy, feels cool to touch and usually tachycardic, though a profound bradycardia may itself result in cardiogenic shock. ↑JVP and peripheral oedema if right ventricular failure, basal lung crepitations if left ventricular failure – both if biventricular failure.

Anaphylactic shock (p206), like septic shock, results from loss of vascular tone, mediated by histamine release, amongst other endogenous factors. Like septic shock, the patient is often flushed and peripherally warm, with a rapid weak pulse; wheeze, stridor, urticaria and oedema are also well recognised features.

Spinal shock (p217) also results from loss of vascular tone, but mediated by either trauma to the cord or following spinal anaesthesia. Loss of sympathetic innervation of the vascular beds or the heart can produce a drop in BP and a reduced cardiac output (rate and force of contraction). Patients have mixed cutaneous clinical signs, but neurological deficit will be the most striking feature.

Fluid challenges

A bolus of fluid is helpful in treating most types of shock, and is also useful in determining the cause of shock. The purpose of a fluid challenge is to assess if the patient responds to this fluid bolus. Note the patient's baseline observations (HR, BP, RR, sats, cap refill, urine output), then give 500ml of 0.9% saline over 5min, and repeat the observations. A slowing of the HR or a rise in BP (usually diastolic) suggests the patient has responded well to the fluid challenge, and another 500ml should be considered. Failure to respond to a fluid challenge either means the patient is grossly fluid depleted, or adequately filled and this is not the cause of shock. You are highly unlikely to push any adult patient into heart failure by giving 500ml of 0.9% saline. If in doubt, call for senior help.

Clinical markers in shock – how to differentiate between the types of shock

	Hypovolaemia/ haemorrhage	Sepsis	Cardiogenic	Anaphylaxis	Spinal
HR	↑	↑	↑	↑	↓
BP	↔/↓	↓	↓	↔/↓	↓
JVP	↓	↓	↑	↓	↓
Peripheries	Cool	Warm	Cool	Cool/warm	Warm

Main causes of shock

Haemorrhagic/ hypovolaemic	• External blood loss (eg scalp laceration)
	• Internal blood loss (eg ruptured AAA/pelvic fracture)
	• Severe dehydration
	  • inadequate fluid intake (eg starvation)
	  • excessive fluid loss (eg diarrhoea, polyuria)
	  • 3rd space loss (eg pancreatitis)

Septic	• Septicaemia • blood-borne infection, ?source

Cardiogenic	• Pump failure/ineffective pump
	  • severe LV dysfunction
	  • outflow tract obstruction (eg aortic dissection)
	  • dysrhythmia (tachy- or bradyarrhythmia)
	• Inadequate pump filling
	  • pulmonary embolism
	  • cardiac tamponade
	  • tension pneumothorax (or large simple)

Anaphylactic	• Systemic inflammatory response/dilatation

Spinal	• Loss of sympathetic (vascular) tone ± ↓cardiac output
	  • dilatation of arterioles/venous pooling
	  • loss of sympathetic drive of the heart (T1–T4)

Estimated blood loss – classification of haemorrhagic shock

Based on a 70kg adult man

	Class I	Class II	Class III	Class IV
Blood loss (ml)	<750	750–1500	1500–2000	>2000
Blood loss (% blood volume)	<15%	15–30%	30–40%	>40%
HR	↔/↑	↑	↑↑	↑↑
BP	↔*	↔	↓	↓↓

* A postural drop in BP is often the first sign of shock.

Hypovolaemic/haemorrhagic shock (*OHAM*2 p263)

Common causes

Haemorrhage	Trauma (external/internal bleeding), ruptured AAA, GI bleed
Salt + water loss	Diarrhoea, vomiting, burns, polyuria (DI and DM)
'3rd space' loss	Acute pancreatitis, ascites

Worrying signs BP<90mmHg, ↓GCS/restlessness, oliguria, mottled skin, unresponsive to fluid challenge, ongoing bleeding – call senior help
Symptoms dizziness on standing (±lying), SOB, ±chest pain
Symptoms of underlying disease trauma to limb/chest/abdomen/pelvis, back/loin pain, melaena/haematemesis, diarrhoea, urinary frequency, epigastric pain radiating to back, abdominal swelling/bloating
Signs BP <100mmHg systolic, tachycardia, weak/thready pulse, postural hypotension, cool peripheries/cap-refill >2s, ↓JVP, ↓GCS/restlessness, oliguria, mottled skin in severe hypotension
Signs of underlying disease obvious source of external (wound/GI bleed) or internal (haemothorax, ascites/tense abdomen, pelvic instability, swollen thighs) bleeding, burns, palpable AAA, tender epigastrium, Grey-Turner's sign/Cullen's sign, melaena on pr examination
Investigations ***blds*** FBC (↓Hb, though may be normal in acute blood loss), U+E (↑urea in GI bleed, ↓K^+ in diarrhoea/vomiting), LFT, amylase, clotting, osmolality, crossmatch (in severe bleeding: 4 units O-ve + 4 units type-specific + 4 units full match); ***ABG*** acidosis in haemorrhage, DKA and pancreatitis, alkalosis in vomiting; ***ECG*** ischaemia; ***CXR*** haemothorax; ***pelvic X-ray*** pelvic fracture; ***abdo USS*** (FAST scan) AAA (though if ruptured AAA likely to need theatre before USS) or free intra-abdominal fluid; ***urine*** Na^+ and osmolality in diabetes insipidus ***stool*** M,C+S (ova, cysts and parasites, *C. diff.* toxin)
When to treat all hypotensive patients, especially if HR >100. A BP of 100mmHg systolic may be critically low if the patient is normally hypertensive (eg elderly), use HR and other clinical markers as a guide.
Acute treatment of severe haemorrhage O_2, 1l 0.9% saline stat, call senior help, lay flat and elevate legs if patient dizzy, attempt to stop bleeding by compression if appropriate, further 1l 0.9% saline stat if no improvement in BP or slowing of HR, identify likely cause of haemorrhage and commence appropriate management (see opposite). Early involvement of ITU. 'Permissive hypotension' is employed in the early phase of resuscitation in haemorrhagic shock so do not push systolic BP >100mmHg.
Acute treatment of non-haemorrhage hypovolaemia O_2, 1l 0.9% saline stat, call senior help, lay flat and elevate legs if patient dizzy, further 1l 0.9% saline stat if no improvement in BP or slowing of HR, identify likely cause of hypovolaemia and commence appropriate treatment; pancreatitis (see opposite), severe diarrhoea (p256), vomiting (p252), burns (p416), fever and sweating (p392), ascites (p590). Early involvement of ITU.
Chronic treatment once appropriate management initiated, recheck observations, including glucose, repeat U+E and FBC (±ABG); catheterise and monitor urine output; continually reassess starting with A, B, C
Complications hypotension results in underperfusion of vital organs and subsequent disruption in their physiology (brain – ↓GCS/coma, kidneys – renal failure, heart – myocardial ischaemia)

Severe GI bleeding (p244)

Haematemesis	Melaena/fresh PR bleeding
A, B, C – CALL ARREST TEAM if compromised **Call for senior help** Give 15l/min O_2; lay flat with legs elevated if BP <100mmHg systolic Secure 14G cannulae in both antecubital fossae, take blood for 6 unit crossmatch 1l 0.9% saline stat, followed by 1l 0.9% saline stat if no improvement	
Needs urgent upper GI endoscopy ?Sengstaken tube if varices Check U+E/LFT/clotting	Needs urgent upper GI endoscopy ± lower GI endoscopy Check U+E/LFT/clotting

Probable ruptured AAA (p240)

A, B, C – CALL ARREST TEAM if compromised
Call for senior help, vascular surgeon and anaesthetist
Give 15l/min O_2; lay flat with legs elevated if BP <100mmHg systolic
Secure 14G cannulae in both antecubital fossae, take blood for 8 unit crossmatch
1l 0.9% saline stat, aim to keep BP 90–100mmHg systolic
NEEDS THEATRE STAT

Severe external bleeding (p168)

A, B, C – CALL ARREST TEAM if compromised
Call for senior help
Give 15l/min O_2; lay flat with legs elevated if BP <100mmHg systolic
Apply pressure to bleeding source
Elevate bleeding source
Secure 14G cannulae in both antecubital fossae, take blood for 4 unit crossmatch
1l 0.9% saline stat, followed by 1l 0.9% saline stat if no improvement
NEEDS THEATRE STAT

Pancreatitis (p241)

A, B, C – CALL ARREST TEAM if compromised
Call for senior help
Give 15l/min O_2
Secure intravenous access, take bloods, glucose and ABG
1l 0.9% saline stat, followed by 1l 0.9% saline over 30min
Analgese with IV morphine as required
Catheterise; hourly urine measurement
Needs surgical input/surgical HDU bed

Septic shock (*OHAM*2 p266)

Common sources of infection resulting in septicaemia

Chest Pneumonia
Skin/soft tissues Cellulitis/gangrene
Heart Endocarditis
Intra-abdominal Perforation/biliary tract
Urinary tract UTI/pyelonephritis
Post-op Wound infection, bowel leak

Worrying signs BP <90mmHg, ↓GCS, oliguria (renal failure), DIC, mottled skin, petechial rash, unresponsive to fluid challenge; call senior help
Symptoms dizziness on standing (±lying), SOB, ±chest pain
Symptoms of underlying disease hot and cold, sweats, shivers, nausea and vomiting, breathlessness, cough, dysuria, urinary frequency, abdominal pain, wound/skin pain, headache, confusion
Signs fever, BP <100mmHg systolic, tachycardia, ±bounding pulse, warm peripheries, ↓JVP, ±↓GCS/restlessness, oliguria, mottled skin in severe hypotension, non-blanching petechial rash in meningococcal septicaemia. Signs of underlying disease such as cellulitis, consolidation in pneumonia or abdominal/loin/suprapubic tenderness in intra-abdominal infections
Investigations ***blds*** FBC (↑WCC, ±↓Hb), U+E, LFT, ↑CRP/ESR, glucose, clotting/fibrinogen; ***bld cultures*** take 2–3 sets from different sites; ***ABG*** acidosis, ↓BE, ↑lactate; ***ECG*** ischaemia; ***urine dipstix*** blood, protein, nitrites, leucocytes, C+S; ***Erect CXR*** consolidation, free air under diaphragm sputum C+S; ***skin/wound swabs*** C+S; ***echo*** valvular lesion/vegetation (transoesophageal more sensitive than transthoracic); ***other imaging*** as appropriate
When to treat all hypotensive patients, especially if HR >100. A BP of 100mmHg systolic may be critically low if the patient is normally hypertensive (eg elderly), use HR and other clinical markers as a guide.
Acute treatment O_2, 1l 0.9% saline stat, call senior help, lay flat and elevate legs if patient dizzy, give IV antibiotics appropriate to likely source of infection (see over and p156), repeat 1l 0.9% saline bolus stat if no improvement in BP or slowing of HR. Consider central line to monitor CVP and arterial line for serial ABGs and invasive BP monitoring. Early involvement of ITU as may need inotropic/ventilatory support. **Goal-directed therapy** in sepsis aims to restore tissue perfusion and O_2 delivery and ensure early administration of antibiotics; this has been shown to greatly improve outcome in sepsis.
Chronic treatment continue broad-spectrum antibiotic therapy until advised of alternative, more targeted therapy by microbiologist. Aggressive fluid therapy to ensure adequate tissue perfusion.
Complications hypotension results in underperfusion of vital organs and subsequent disruption in their physiology (brain – ↓GCS/coma, kidneys – renal failure, heart – myocardial ischaemia) and in multi-organ failure. Sepsis can precipitate DIC which can result in necrosis and gangrene, as well as profound bleeding (p345).
Toxic shock is a specific form of septic shock, caused by the production of a toxin by Gram-positive bacteria. It is commonest amongst females (in association with the use of tampons) but can occur in anyone. Treatment is the same: fluid resuscitation, broad-spectrum antibiotics initially, **remove source of infection/pus**, support impaired organ function.

Sepsis definitions

SIRS (**S**ystemic **I**nflammatory **R**esponse **S**yndrome) present if ≥2 of:
- HR>90
- Temp <36 or >38°C
- RR >20 or $PaCO_2$ <4.3 kPa
- WCC <4 or >12x10^9/l

Sepsis if 'SIRS' + proven or highly suspicious source of infection
Severe sepsis if 'sepsis' + signs of hypoperfusion or organ failures including ↓urine output, elevated urea or creatinine, abnormal LFTs, coagulation disturbance, hypoxia or ARDS, or a raised lactate 2mmol/l
Septic shock where hypotension persists despite adequate fluid challenge, or requires use of vasopressors or inotropes

Empirical antibiotic treatment in sepsis

For dosing regimens see p156

Pneumonia	
Community-acquired	Co-amoxiclav + clarithromycin
Hospital-acquired	Consult local guideline and discuss with microbiologist
Intra-abdominal	Cefuroxime + metronidazole
Biliary tract	Tazocin®[1] ±gentamicin (p151)
Meningitis	Ceftriaxone; discuss with microbiologist
Skin	
Cellulitis	Flucloxacillin; discuss with microbiologist p495
Necrotising fasciitis	
Urinary tract	
Community-acquired	Cefuroxime IV ±gentamicin (p151)
Hospital-acquired	Consult local guideline and discuss with microbiologist
Unsure of origin	Consult local guideline and discuss with microbiologist

Causes of lactic acidosis – metabolic acidosis with ↑lactate

Tissue hypoxaemia
- Inadequate perfusion
- Severe anaemia
- Severe hypoxia
- Catecholamine excess (↑SVR)
- Severe exercise

Non-hypoxaemic tissues
- Sepsis
- Renal and hepatic failure
- Uncontrolled DM
- Acute pancreatitis
- Paracetamol overdose

Drug-induced
- Metformin
- Methanol
- Ethanol
- Aspirin (salicylates)
- Cyanide

Rare hereditary causes
- Glucose-6-phosphatase deficiency
- Fructose-1,6-diphosphatase deficiency

1 Tazocin® 4.5g = piperacillin 4g and tazobactam 500 mg.

Cardiogenic shock (*OHCM*7 p788)

Common causes

Pump failure	LV dysfunction (post-MI/ACS), aortic dissection, dysrhythmia
Inadequate filling	Pulmonary embolism, pneumothorax, cardiac tamponade

Worrying signs BP <90mmHg, ↓GCS/restlessness, oliguria (renal failure), mottled skin, chest pain, hypoxaemia; call senior help
Symptoms dizziness on standing (±lying), SOB, ±chest pain
Symptoms of underlying disease chest pain, ±pleuritic, ±radiating to back/left arm/jaw, breathlessness, palpitations
Signs BP <100mmHg systolic (check both arms), tachycardia or bradycardia, weak/thready pulse, cool peripheries, ↑JVP, ±↓GCS, oliguria, mottled skin in severe hypotension
Signs of underlying disease stigmata of hyperlipidaemia, ↓O_2 sats, signs of pneumothorax (↓expansion, ↑percussion note, ↓breath sounds on affected side, tracheal deviation), pulmonary oedema, Beck's triad in cardiac tamponade (shock, ↑JVP, muffled heart sounds), pitting oedema
Investigations if you suspect cardiogenic shock identify most likely cause and treat prior to undertaking investigations; seconds count. Most useful investigation will be immediate ***echocardiogram*** (bleep cardiologist on-call) for dissection, PE, cardiac tamponade, LVF; ***ECG*** ischaemia, small complexes; ***CXR*** pneumothorax, cardiomegaly; ***ABG*** hypoxaemia; ***blds*** FBC, U+E, glucose, clotting, crossmatch; ***other imaging*** as appropriate
When to treat all hypotensive patients, especially if HR >100. A BP of 100mmHg systolic may be critically low for some normally hypertensive patients, so use HR and other clinical markers as a guide
Acute treatment 15l/min O_2. Further management depends on pathology:

Bradyarrhythmia	p194	Aortic dissection	p183
Tachyarrhythmia	p186	Pulmonary embolism	p225
Heart failure	p226	Pneumothorax	p227

Cardiac tamponade (*OHCM*2 p184)

Collection of fluid (usually blood) in pericardium resulting in external compression upon ventricles and inability for heart to fill/pump.
Causes trauma, pericarditis, post-MI, dissecting aortic aneurysm
Signs tachycardia, hypotension, Beck's triad (see above)
Investigations ***echo*** pericardial fluid, poor stroke volume; ***CXR*** cardiomegaly, pulmonary oedema; ***ECG*** small complexes, tachycardia, ischaemia
Acute treatment 15l/min O_2, IV access, needle pericardiocentesis

Emergency needle pericardiocentesis (*OHAM*2 p890) get senior help

- Monitor heart rhythm on ECG monitor, have drip running and defibrillator close
- Clean skin on chest/upper abdomen with antiseptic
- Long 18G cannula to 20ml syringe via a 3-way tap
- Advance needle to the left of xiphisternum, aiming for tip of left scapula
- Withdraw syringe as advancing, watching for ectopics on ECG
- Ectopics imply needle in myocardium, withdraw a little into the pericardial space
- Aspirating 20–40ml can improve BP, but fluid likely to reaccumulate
- Patient needs definitive cardiothoracic input urgently

Anaphylaxis (*OHCM*7 p780), see also p206

Spinal (neurogenic) shock

Common causes

Trauma	Traumatic transection of spinal cord at any level
Iatrogenic	Spinal anaesthesia

Symptoms usually has motor/sensory dysfunction below level of lesion, bowel and bladder dysfunction

Signs hypotension, warm peripheries, may not be able to mount tachycardia if lesion above T1–T4 (origin of sympathetic supply to the heart), focal neurology, up-going plantar relaxes, loss of anal tone

Investigations imaging of spinal cord as appropriate

When to treat BP <100mmHg systolic, symptomatic of ↓BP, organ failure

Acute treatment O_2, 1l 0.9% saline stat, call senior help, lay flat with legs elevated if patient dizzy and spinal injury not suspected. Catheterise. If trauma involve spinal/orthopaedic surgeons. If iatrogenic, (eg epidural) consult anaesthetist. Early involvement of ITU.

Postural (orthostatic) hypotension

Common causes

Volume depletion	Dehydration, anaemia, vasovagal
Iatrogenic	Antihypertensives, diuretics, nitrates, antidepressants
Autonomic neuropathy	DM, Guillain–Barré, syphilis, Parkinson's disease, ageing

Drop in the systolic BP of >20mmHg upon standing from sitting or lying position; can occur when sitting from a lying position in severe disease.

Symptoms dizziness, ±loss of consciousness (LOC) when standing

Signs fall in systolic BP of >20mmHg upon standing

Investigations lying/standing BP usually diagnostic. Other investigations as appropriate to investigate cause of syncope/collapse (p350).

When to treat all symptomatic patients

Acute treatment review medications and identify likely precipitants; can these be stopped or changed for a drug without this side-effect? Optimise control of DM. Identify and treat other precipitating disease (see above). Ensure patient is going to be safe in immediate period.

Chronic treatment advise simple lifestyle changes such as getting out of chairs slowly or holding onto something as one stands. Graduated stockings for lower legs may help if poor venous circulation. Steroids/mineralocorticoids may be useful in some situations, though benefit needs to outweigh risks.

Complications falls and subsequent bone and soft tissue injuries including intracranial bleeding and fractured neck of femur

Breathlessness and low sats emergency

Airway	Check airway is patent; consider manoeuvres/adjuncts
Breathing	If no respiratory effort – **CALL ARREST TEAM**
Circulation	If no palpable pulse – **CALL ARREST TEAM**

Call for **senior help** early if patient deteriorating

- **Sit patient up**
- **15l/min O_2** in all patients if acutely unwell
- **Monitor** pulse oximeter, BP, defibrillator's ECG leads if unwell
- Obtain a full set of **observations** including temp
- Take brief **history** if possible/check **notes**/ask ward staff
- **Examine patient**: condensed RS, CVS, ±abdo exam
- Establish likely causes and rule out serious causes
- Initiate **further treatment**, see following pages
- **Venous access**, take bloods:
  - FBC, U+E, LFT, CRP, bld cultures, D-dimer, cardiac markers
- **Arterial blood gas**, but don't leave the patient alone
- **ECG** to exclude arrhythmias and acute MI
- Request urgent **CXR**, portable if too unwell
- Call for **senior help**
- Reassess, starting with A, B, C…

Life-threatening causes

- Asthma/COPD
- Pulmonary oedema (LVF)
- (Tension) pneumothorax
- MI/arrhythmia
- Pneumonia
- Pulmonary embolism (PE)
- Pleural effusion
- Anaphylaxis/airway obstruction

Breathlessness and low sats

Worrying features RR >30, sats <92%, systolic <100mmHg, chest pain, confusion, inability to complete sentences, exhaustion, tachy/bradycardia

Think about *life-threatening* see box on previous page; ***most likely*** COPD/asthma, pneumonia, pulmonary oedema (LVF), pulmonary embolism (PE), myocardial infarction (MI); ***other*** pneumothorax, pleural effusion, arrhythmia, acute respiratory distress syndrome (ARDS), sepsis, metabolic acidosis, anaemia, pain, panic, foreign body/aspiration; ***chronic*** COPD, lung cancer, bronchiectasis, fibrosing alveolitis, TB

Ask about speed of onset, cough, sputum (quantity, colour and blood), chest pain (pleuritic (worse on deep inspiration or coughing), related to movement or tender), palpitations, dizziness, difficulty lying flat, recent travel, weight loss; ***PMH*** cardiac or respiratory problems, malignancy, TB; ***DH*** inhalers, home nebulisers, home O_2, cardiac medication, allergies; ***SH*** smoking, pets, exercise tolerance, previous and current occupation

- ***PE risk factors*** recent surgery/immobility/fracture/travel, oestrogen (pregnancy, HRT, the pill), malignancy, previous PE/DVT, thrombophilia, varicose veins, obesity, central line

Obs temp, RR (11–20 is normal), BP, HR, sats (should be >92%[1]), O_2 requirements (improving or worsening?)

Look for confusion, cyanosis, CO_2 tremor, clubbing, rashes, itching, swollen lips/eyes, raised JVP, tracheal shift and tug, use of accessory muscles, abnormal percussion, unequal air entry, crackles, stridor, wheeze, bronchial breathing, swollen/red/hot/tender legs, swelling of ankles, cold peripheries

Investigations *PEFR* if asthma or COPD suspected (may be too ill); ***blds*** FBC, U+E, LFT, CRP, D-dimer (if PE suspected), cardiac markers, blood cultures; ***sputum*** may need physio help, inspect and send for M,C+S; AFBs if TB risk; ***ABGs*** see p622, keep on O_2 if acutely SOB; ***ECG*** see p610; ***CXR*** see p620; portable if unwell, though image quality may be poor; ***Spirometry*** this should be done once the patient has been stabilised to help confirm the diagnosis, see p624

Treatment Sit all patients up and give 15l/min O_2 – this saves lives. This can be reduced later and CO_2 retention in COPD takes a while to develop. Check sats and ECG in all patients:

- ***Stridor*** – call an anaesthetist, p230
- ***Wheeze*** – give nebuliser, p221/223
- ***Unilateral resonance with reduced air entry and shock*** – treat urgently as tension pneumothorax (p227)
- ***Asymmetrical crackles and air entry*** – consider pneumonia, p226
- ***Symmetrical crackles and air entry with raised JVP*** – consider LVF, p226
- ***Normal examination*** – consider PE, cardiac and systemic causes

1 Patients with chronic lung disease may normally have sats <92%.

	History	Examination	Investigations
COPD	Known respiratory problems, smoker, productive cough worse than usual	±wheeze/crackles, ±cyanosed/purse-lip breathing, look for infection and pneumothorax	$\downarrow$PEFR; CXR hyperexpanded, exclude pneumonia and pneumothorax, flat diaphragms common in COPD
Asthma	Known asthma, recent cold or exposure to allergens	Wheeze ±crackles, look for signs of infection or pneumothorax	
Pneumonia	Productive cough, dark sputum, feels unwell, ±pleuritic chest pain	Febrile, asymmetrical air entry, crackles and percussion	$\uparrow$WCC/NØ/CRP, consolidation or blunted angles on CXR (p620)
Pulmonary embolism	PE risk factors, leg pain, ±pleuritic chest pain and haemoptysis	$\uparrow$JVP, $\uparrow$HR, may have swollen red legs, can be severely shocked	$\downarrow pCO_2$, ±hypoxia on ABGs, $\uparrow$D-dimer, CXR often normal
Pulmonary oedema	Known cardiac problems, orthopnoea, swollen legs	$\uparrow$JVP, symmetrical fine crackles, pink frothy sputum, oedema, cold peripheries	Big heart + signs of oedema on CXR (p620), ECG may show evidence of previous MIs
Pneumothorax	Sudden onset pleuritic chest pain, trauma, previous episodes, tall and thin	Unequal air entry and expansion, hyperresonant, displaced trachea (late)	Treat tension pneumothorax first, CXR shows pleura separated from ribs
Pleural effusion	Gradual onset breathlessness, ±pleuritic chest pain	Reduced expansion, stony dull base	Effusion on CXR
ARDS	Concurrent severe illness	Hypoxic	Bilateral infiltrates on CXR
Anaemia/MI/ arrhythmias	Chest pain, palpitations, dizziness, tiredness	Irregular or fast pulse, shocked, pale	Abnormal ECG (p610), $\downarrow$Hb, $\uparrow$cardiac markers
Anaphylaxis	Sudden onset, itching, swelling, urticarial rash, new drugs/food	Stridor, ±wheeze, shock, swollen lips and eyes, blanching rash	Treat with IM adrenaline (epinephrine) (p206)

COPD/emphysema (*OHAM2* p218)

Worrying signs ↓GCS, rising CO_2
Symptoms breathlessness, cough, ↑sputum, tight chest, confusion, ↓exercise tolerance, (ex-)smoker

Signs wheeze, cyanosis, barrel-chested, poor expansion, tachypnoea

Investigations ***↓PEFR, ABGs*** are often deranged in COPD, compare with previous samples and check the O_2 concentration. Repeat at 30min in seriously ill patients; ***CXR*** hyperexpanded, flat diaphragm (look for evidence of infection, pneumothorax or bullae); ***spirometry*** ↓FEV_1, ↓FEV_1:FVC ratio (<70%), see p624

Acute exacerbation sit the patient up and give the minimum amount of O_2 to maintain sats ≥90% (aim for PaO_2 ~8kPa) but avoid profound hypoxaemia (sats <90%). Give salbutamol 5mg NEB ±ipratropium (Atrovent®) 500μg NEB and prednisolone 30mg PO (hydrocortisone 200mg IV if unable to take tablets). Sputum for M,C+S. Get an ABG and CXR (portable if unwell). Use ABG results and clinical observations to guide further management:
- ***Normal* ABG** (for them) continue current O_2 and give regular nebs
- ***Worsening hypoxaemia*** ↑O_2, repeat ABGs <30min, watch for confusion which should prompt a repeat ABG sooner
- ***↑CO_2 retention or ↓GCS*** request senior help **urgently**; consider:
  - **ITU** input/assessment
  - **aminophylline** 5mg/kg IV bolus over 20min unless the patient is on oral aminophylline or theophylline
  - **Mg^{2+} sulphate** 2g (8mmol) IV over 20min (no evidence base)
  - **NIV**, see below

Antibiotics consider prescribing antibiotics (doxycycline 100mg/12h PO for 1d then 100mg/24h PO or amoxicillin 500mg/8h PO) if the patient has increased SOB, worsening cough or purulent sputum

Chronic treatment See p472 or *OHCM*7 p168. Stop smoking, exercise, inhalers (p222 for colours and types), home nebulisers, long-term O_2 therapy (if PaO_2 ≤8kPa), long-term oral steroids, antibiotics. Avoid giving O_2 >28% unless acutely SOB; this can reduce respiratory drive in some patients causing CO_2 retention and confusion

Complications exacerbations, infection, cor pulmonale, pneumothorax, respiratory failure, lung cancer

Non-invasive ventilation (NIV)

These are machines that help ventilate patients through a tightly fitting mask instead of intubation. They are commonly used in COPD patients with a pH ≤7.35 and CO_2 ≥6.0kPa to get them through acute illness. BiPAP is the most common. CPAP is not a type of NIV since it does not help with the mechanics of ventilation (see p226), but is sometimes used in acute respiratory failure (commonly pulmonary oedema). Patients who need NIV are usually allocated specialist beds on the respiratory ward or on HDU/ITU.

Common inhalers for asthma and COPD

Type of drug	Colour	Medication	Trade
Short-acting β-agonist	Blue	Salbutamol	Ventolin®
	Blue	Terbutaline	Bricanyl®
Inhaled steroids	Brown	Beclometasone	Qvar®
	Brown	Budesonide	Pulmicort®
	Orange	Fluticasone	Flixotide®
Short-acting anticholinergic	White + green	Ipratropium	Atrovent®
Short-acting β-agonist and anticholinergic	White + orange	Salbutamol and ipratropium	Combivent®
Inhaled steroids with long-acting β-agonist	Red Purple	Budesonide and formoterol Fluticasone and salmeterol	Symbicort® Seretide®
Long-acting β-agonist	Green	Salmeterol	Serevent®
Long-acting anticholinergic	Grey	Tiotropium	Spiriva®

Pulmonary rehabilitation

There is good evidence that patients with chronic lung disease who take part in a pulmonary rehabilitation programme see increased exercise tolerance and improved well-being. These programmes do not reverse the pathological process or improve spirometry measurements.

Most hospitals and general practices have access to such programmes, and patients generally take part in a structured programme for 8–12wk. Exercise is encouraged which becomes progressively more strenuous. Diet and other lifestyle advice is also usually covered.

Once discharged from the programme, patients are encouraged to continue the exercises they have learnt, either as part of their daily lives at home or at leisure centres.

The British Lung Foundation can be contacted to find local programmes; 08458 50 50 20.

Online respiratory resources

British Thoracic Society	www.brit-thoracic.org.uk
British Lung Foundation	www.lunguk.org
SIGN	www.sign.ac.uk
NICE	www.nice.org.uk

Asthma[1] (*OHAM2* p210)

Severe	Incomplete sentences, PEFR <50% of best, HR >100, RR >25
Life-threatening	As for severe plus any of: PEFR <33% of best, silent chest, HR <60, systolic <100mmHg, confusion, sats <92%, PaO_2 <8kPa, poor respiratory effort, normal $PaCO_2$ (exhaustion), cyanosis
Near-fatal	Any CO_2 retention – call ITU

Symptoms breathless, tight chest and wheezy episodes (exercise, allergens, cold), night and morning cough, excess sputum, previous wheeze, hayfever, eczema, relatives with asthma, previous admissions/ITU

Signs wheeze, prolonged expiration, tachypnoea, hyperinflation

Investigations ***PEFR*** reduced compared with their best; ***ABG*s** normal to mild hypoxia with a $\downarrow CO_2$ due to hyperventilation; ***CXR*** hyperexpanded, exclude pneumonia and pneumothorax; ***spirometry*** $\downarrow FEV_1$, $\downarrow FEV_1$:FVC ratio

Acute exacerbation sit up and give 15l/min O_2. Salbutamol 5mg nebs, ±ipratropium (Atrovent®) nebs 500μg and prednisolone 40mg PO (or hydrocortisone 200mg IV). Connect the nebuliser mask to the O_2 supply, do not use air. Repeat salbutamol 5mg nebs every 15–30min and monitor with 15–30min PEFRs and sats.

- ***No improvement*** Call for **senior help**. Consider:
  - **ITU** input/assessment
  - **Aminophylline** 5mg/kg IV bolus over 20min unless the patient is on oral aminophylline or theophylline
  - **Mg^{2+} sulphate** 2g (8mmol) IV over 20min
- ***Improving*** gradually reduce the % of O_2 and frequency of salbutamol as tolerated – this can be done over several days

Chronic treatment See p472 or *OHCM7* p166. Avoid smoking and allergens, monitor PEFR, check inhaler technique, inhalers (see p222 for colours and types), oral steroids for exacerbations.

Complications exacerbations, infection, pneumothorax, death

Simplified stepwise management of asthma[1]

	Step 1	Step 2	Step 3*	Step 3*	Step 4	Step 5
Oral steroids						✓
High-dose steroid inhaler				✓	✓	✓
Long-acting β-agonist			✓		✓	✓
Low-dose steroid inhaler		✓	✓			
Salbutamol/terbutaline	✓	✓	✓	✓	✓	✓

* Either low-dose steroid inhaler and long-acting β-agonist or high-dose steroid inhaler

1 See BTS Asthma guidelines.

Pneumonia (*OHAM*2 p194)

Worrying signs CURB-65 score ≥3 (see below)
Symptoms cough, increased sputum (green), pleuritic chest pain, breathless, haemoptysis, fever, unwell, confusion, anorexia

Signs ↑temp, ↑RR, ↑HR, ↓sats, unequal air entry, bronchial breathing, dull percussion, reduced expansion

Investigations ***blds*** ↑WCC and NØ ↑CRP; ***ABGs*** hypoxic if severe with a ↓CO_2 due to hyperventilation; ***CXR*** focal consolidation

Severity can be assessed using the CURB-65 criteria, see BTS algorithm below, which helps decide on whether to admit and antibiotic use

Treatment sit up and give 15l/min O_2. Give antibiotics according to local policy or see p156 empirical treatment. If admitting to hospital consider giving IV fluids if dehydrated. If symptoms are not resolving within 3d consider repeating the CRP and CXR to exclude pleural effusion/empyema.

Complications empyema (pleural effusion of pus), respiratory failure, sepsis, confusion

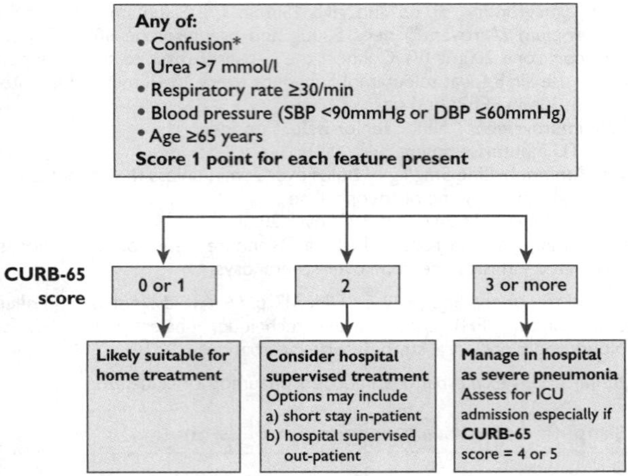

***Defined as a Mental Test Score of 8 or less, or new disorientation in person, place or time.**

CURB-65, from BTS pneumonia guidelines 2004. Reproduced with permission of BMJ Publishing Group Ltd.

Pulmonary embolism (*OHAM*2 p146)

Symptoms often none except breathlessness, may have pleuritic chest pain, haemoptysis, dizziness, leg pain; see risk factors below

Signs ↑JVP, ↑RR, ↑HR, RV heave, hypotension, pleural rub, ±pyrexia. Often a tachycardia is the only clinical sign.

Investigations ***D-dimer*** these are raised by most inflammatory conditions, however a normal D-dimer makes a PE very unlikely; ***ECG*** ↑HR, RBBB, inverted T waves V1–V4 or $S_1Q_3T_3$; ***ABG***s ↓CO_2, ± ↓O_2; ***V/Q scan***

Acute treatment sit up and give 15l/min O_2. If life-threatening get an urgent CT or echo followed by thrombolysis. Otherwise LMWH (p347), eg enoxaparin 1.5mg/kg/24h SC and pain relief; IV fluids if hypotensive.

Chronic treatment warfarin (INR 2–3) for 6mth or for life if second episode or thrombophilia. See p348

Clinically assessing risk of pulmonary embolism[1]

Major risk factor	Minor risk factor
Recent major surgery	Indwelling central line
Late pregnancy	Oral oestrogens (OCP/HRT)
Fracture or varicose veins	Long distance travel
Malignancy	Obesity
Previous proven DVT/PE	Thrombotic disorder

(1) The patient must have:
- breathlessness and/or tachypnoea (±pleuritic chest pain, ±haemoptysis)

(2) If so, does the patient have:
- A) absence of another reasonable explanation for these symptoms?
- B) the presence of a major risk factor?

If the answer to A and B is 'yes' then there is HIGH probability of PE
If the answer to A or B is 'yes' then there is INTERMEDIATE probability of PE
If the answer to A and B is 'no' then there is LOW probability of PE

Management

HIGH probability; no D-dimer test required
- Start LMWH and request radiological imaging (CT-PA/VQ scan)

INTERMEDIATE or LOW probability; check D-dimer:
- If positive start LMWH and request radiological imaging (CT-PA/VQ scan)
- If negative no imaging required, identify alternative diagnosis

[1] Adapted from British Thoracic Society guidelines for the management of suspected acute pulmonary embolism. *Thorax* 2003; **58**:470–84.

Pulmonary oedema (*OHAM*2 p108)

Symptoms breathless, frothy sputum, worse laying flat, usually sleeps with >2 pillows (orthopnoea), swollen legs, previous heart problems

Signs ↑JVP, tachypnoea, fine inspiratory basal crackles, wheeze, pitting oedema ankles and/or sacrum, cold hands and feet

Investigations ***blds*** FBC, U+E, CRP, cardiac markers, look specifically for anaemia, infection and MI; ***ABGs*** may show hypoxia with ↑↓$PaCO_2$; *ECG* exclude arrhythmias and acute STEMI, may show old infarcts, LV hypertrophy or strain (p610); ***CXR*** cardiomegaly (not on portable), signs of pulmonary oedema (p620); ***echo*** poor LV function/ejection fraction

Acute treatment sit up and give 15l/min O_2. If the attack is life-threatening call an anaesthetist early as CPAP and ITU may be required. Otherwise monitor HR, BP, RR and O_2 sats whilst giving furosemide 40–120mg IV and diamorphine 1mg boluses IV (repeat up to 5mg, watch RR).

- ***Systolic >100*** Give 2 sprays of sublingual GTN followed by an IV infusion of GTN (p181) starting at 4mg/h and increasing by 2mg/h every 10min, aiming to keep systolic >100; usual range 4–10mg/h
- ***Systolic <100*** The patient is in shock, probably cardiogenic. Get senior help as inotropes are often required. Do not give nitrates.
- ***Wheezing*** Treat as for COPD alongside above treatment.
- ***No improvement*** Give furosemide up to 120mg total (more if chronic renal failure) and consider CPAP (see below). Insert a urinary catheter to monitor urine output, ±CVP monitoring. Request senior help. Consider HDU/ITU.

Once stabilised, the patient will need daily weights, ±fluid restriction; spironolactone can be prescribed in patients already on high dose of furosemide (always monitor U+E). An echo should be performed to assess LV function and cardiac markers at >12h to exclude MI as a precipitant. ACE inhibitors and β-blockers improve long-term life expectancy in heart failure.

Continuous positive airway pressure (CPAP)

Application of positive airway pressure throughout all phases of the respiratory cycle limits alveolar and small airway collapse, though the patient must still initiate a breath and have sufficient muscular power to inhale and exhale. Purse-lip breathing has a similar effect, and is often observed in patients with chronic lung disease. CPAP is often used in the acute treatment of pulmonary oedema or the chronic treatment of sleep apnoea (may use nasal CPAP).

Simple pneumothorax (*OHAM2* p236)

Risk factors ***primary*** tall, thin, male; ***secondary*** COPD, asthma, infection, trauma, recent central line or pleural aspiration, mechanical ventilation
Symptoms breathlessness, ±chest pain
Signs hyperresonant and reduced air entry on affected side, tachypnoea, may have tracheal deviation or fractured ribs
Investigations **CXR** lung markings not extending to the peripheries, line of pleura away from the periphery
Treatment sit up and give 15l/min O_2. Chest drain/aspiration as directed by BTS guidelines (p228). Primary pneumothoraces arise in otherwise healthy individuals, whereas secondary pneumothoraces arise in patients with underlying lung disease. For aspirating a pneumothorax, or inserting a chest drain see p578 and p580.

Tension pneumothorax (*OHAM2* p242)

Symptoms breathlessness, ±chest pain
Signs hypotensive, tachycardia, tachypnoea, unilateral hyperresonance with ipsilateral reduced air entry, ↑JVP, may have tracheal deviation
Acute treatment sit up and give 15l/min O_2. This is an emergency, it will rapidly worsen if not treated. Treat prior to CXR. Insert a large cannula (brown/grey) into the 2nd intercostal space, midclavicular line directly above the 3rd rib. Listen for a hiss and leave it in situ, open; insert a chest drain on the same side. If there is no hiss, consider alternative diagnoses; leave the cannula in situ and a chest drain is usually still required to prevent a tension pneumothorax accumulating.

Pleural effusion (*OHAM2* p248)

Causes ***transudates*** (protein <30g/l) pulmonary oedema, cirrhosis, nephrotic syndrome; ***exudates*** (protein >30g/l) malignancy, infection, vasculitidies, rheumatoid, haemothorax; ***empyema*** (pH is <7.2) infection
Symptoms may be breathless with pleuritic chest pain
Signs stony dull to percussion with reduced air entry, tachypnoea
Investigations CXR loss of costophrenic angle with a meniscus, p620
Treatment sit up and give 15l/min O_2. Investigate the cause; if the effusion is large, pleural aspiration may relieve symptoms and aid diagnosis, see p578 (draining >1.5l/24h may cause pulmonary oedema).

Acute respiratory distress syndrome (ARDS) (*OHAM2* p230)

Acute onset respiratory failure following a pulmonary insult (eg pneumonia, gastric aspiration) or systemic insult (shock, pancreatitis, sepsis).
Symptoms breathless, often multi-organ failure
Signs hypoxic, signs of respiratory distress and underlying condition
Investigations bilateral infiltrates on CXR
Treatment sit up and give 15l/min O_2. Refer to HDU/ITU and treat underlying cause. Often requires ventilation.

Algorithm for the treatment of primary pneumothorax[1]

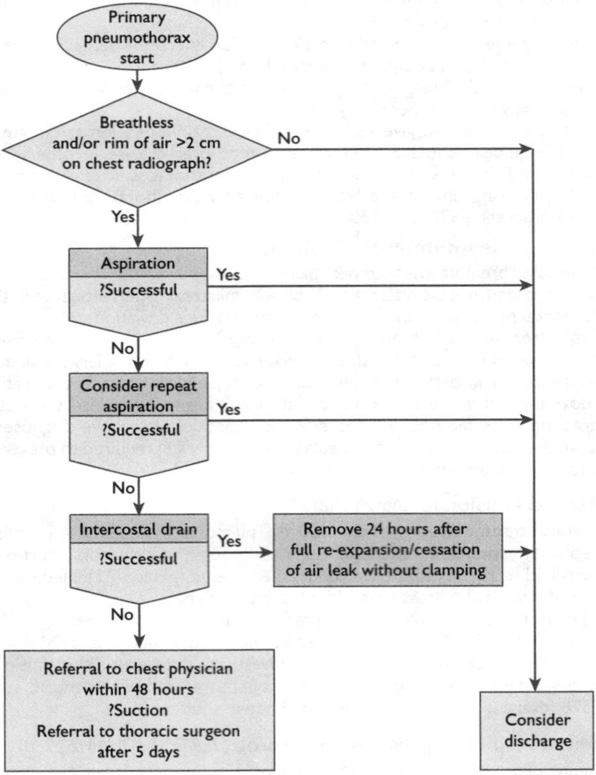

1 Adapted from BTS guidelines for the management of spontaneous pneumothorax. Thorax 2003; 58(Suppl II):ii39-52

Algorithm for the treatment of secondary pneumothorax[1]

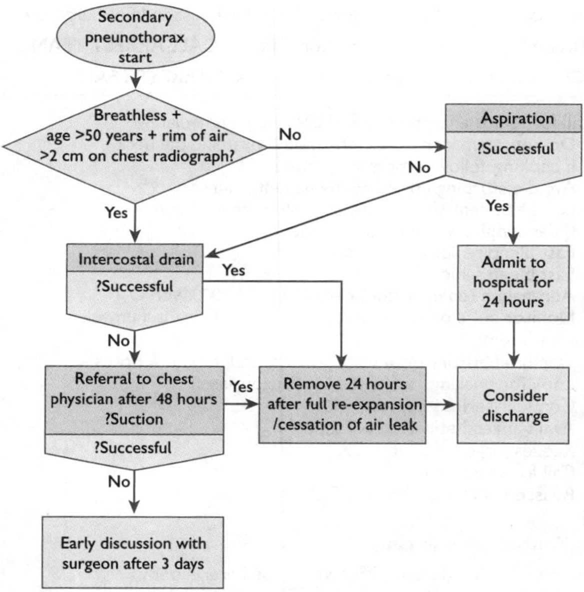

1 Adapted from BTS guidelines for the management of spontaneous pneumothorax. Thorax 2003; 58(Suppl II):ii39-52

Stridor in a conscious adult patient

Airway	Acute stridor: bleep anaesthetist and ENT urgently
Breathing	If poor respiratory effort – **CALL ARREST TEAM**
Circulation	If no palpable pulse – **CALL ARREST TEAM**

Call for **senior anaesthetics** and **ENT help** immediately

- **Do not** attempt to look in the mouth/examine the neck
- If **choking**, follow algorithm opposite
- Avoid **disturbing/upsetting** the patient in any way
- Let the **patient sit** in whatever position they choose
- Offer **supplemental O_2** to all patients
- **Fast bleep** senior anaesthetist
- **Fast bleep** senior ENT
- **Adrenaline (epinephrine) nebs** (5ml of 1:1000 with O_2)
- **Monitor** pulse oximeter, ±defibrillator's ECG leads if unwell
- Check **temp**
- Take brief **history** from relatives/ward staff or check **notes**
- **Look for** swelling, rashes, itching (?anaphylaxis)
- Consider **serious causes** (below)
- Await **anaesthetic** and **ENT** input
- Request urgent portable **CXR**
- Call for **senior help**
- **Reassess**, starting with A, B, C…

Life-threatening causes

- Infection (epiglottitis, abscess)
- Tumour
- Trauma
- Foreign body
- Post-op
- Anaphylaxis

SVC obstruction (*OHAM7* p514)

Symptoms breathless, orthopnoea, facial/arm swelling, headache

Signs facial plethora (redness), facial oedema, engorged veins, stridor

Pemberton's test elevating the arms over the head for 1min results in increased facial plethora and ↑JVP

Investigations *CXR/CT* mediastinal mass, tracheal deviation; ***venogram*** venous congestion distal to lesion; ***other*** sputum cytology for atypical cells

Treatment sit up and give 15l/min O_2. Dexamethasone 4mg/6h PO/IV. Consider nebulised β-agonist (salbutamol 5mg/PRN neb) if stridor prominent. Otherwise symptomatic treatment. Seek senior input as tissue diagnosis needed.

Adult choking algorithm

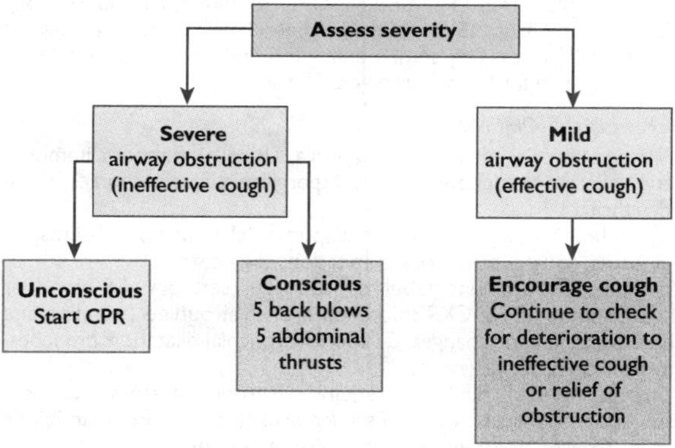

Adult choking algorithm, 2005 guidelines
Reproduced by kind permission of the Resuscitation Council (UK).

Cough

Causes of coughs	
Acute	URTI, post-viral, post-nasal drip (allergy), pneumonia, LVF, PE
Chronic	asthma, COPD, bronchitis, bronchiectasis, smoking, post-nasal drip, oesophageal reflux, pneumonia, TB, parasites, interstitial lung disease, heart failure, ACE inhibitors, lung cancer, sarcoid, sinusitis, cystic fibrosis, habitual
Bloody	***massive*** bronchiectasis, lung cancer, infection (including TB and aspergilloma), trauma, AV malformations; ***other*** bronchitis, PE, pulmonary oedema, mitral stenosis, aortic aneurysm, vasculitidies, parasites

Haemoptysis coughing up blood, ≥400ml is considered 'massive'.
Management FBC, U+E, LFT, clotting, G+S, sputum C+S and cytology, ABG, ECG, CXR. Sit up, 15l/min O_2. Codeine 60mg PO (may ↓cough) **if massive:** good IV access (≥green), monitor HR and BP, immediate referral to respiratory team for bronchoscopy ±CT thorax

Bronchiectasis (*OHCM7* p158)
Causes cystic fibrosis, infection (pneumonia, TB, HIV), tumours, immunodeficiency, allergic bronchopulmonary aspergillosis, foreign bodies, rheumatoid arthritis
Symptoms chronic cough with purulent sputum, ±haemoptysis, halitosis
Signs clubbing, course inspiratory crepitations, ±wheeze
Investigations FBC, immunoglobulins, aspergillus serology; ***CF*** blood or sweat test; ***sputum*** C+S; ***CXR*** thickened bronchial outline (tramline and ring shadows), ±fibrotic changes; ***CT thorax*** bronchial dilatation; ***bronchoscopy*** to exclude other diagnoses
Acute treatment O_2 ±BiPAP as required, ±bronchodilators ±corticosteroids. Infections likely to be *Pseudomonas* (consult local antibiotic guidelines). Chest physiotherapy to mobilise secretions.
Chronic treatment postural drainage (chest physio), inhaled/nebulised bronchodilators/corticosteroids, surgery may be considered, consider prophylactic antibiotics (rotating choice of agent ~every 3mth)
Complications recurrent pneumonia, pseudomonal infection, massive haemoptysis, cor pulmonale

Abdominal pain emergency

Airway	Check airway is patent; consider manoeuvres/adjuncts
Breathing	If no respiratory effort – **CALL ARREST TEAM**
Circulation	If no palpable pulse – **CALL ARREST TEAM**

Call for **senior help** early if patient deteriorating

- **15l/min O_2** in all patients
- **Monitor** BP, pulse oximeter, defibrillator's ECG leads if unwell
- Obtain a full set of **observations**, are they haemodynamically stable?
- Take brief **history** if possible/check **notes**/ask ward staff
- **Examine patient**: condensed RS, CVS, abdo, ±wound exam
- Consider **serious causes** (below) and treat if present
- Initiate **further treatment**, see following pages
- **Venous access**, take bloods:
  - FBC, U+E, LFT, amylase, CRP, clotting, X-match 4 units, bld cultures
- Give IV **fluids** if hypovolaemic or shocked (p212)
- **Analgesia** as appropriate
- **Arterial blood gas**, but don't leave the patient alone
- **Erect** CXR (portable if unwell) and **plain** AXR (cannot be portable)
- **ECG**
- **Urine dipstick** and β-**hCG** (all pre-menopausal women), ±catheter
- Keep patient **NBM** if likely to need theatre
- Call for **senior help**
- **Reassess**, starting with A, B, C …

Life-threatening causes and emergencies

- Perforation
- Bowel infarction/ischaemia
- Bowel obstruction
- Acute pancreatitis
- Acute cholangitis
- Appendicitis
- Leaking abdominal aortic aneurysm (AAA)
- Strangulated hernia
- Testicular or ovarian torsion
- Ruptured ectopic pregnancy
- Referred pain (MI, aortic dissection)

Abdominal pain

> **Worrying features** sudden onset, ↑HR, ↓BP, ↓GCS, distension, peritonism, expansile mass, recurrent vomiting, haematemesis, frank PR bleeding

Think about *life-threatening*, see box on previous page; ***common*** gastroenteritis, gastroduodenal ulcer, gastro-oesophageal reflux disease (GORD), constipation, IBD, irritable bowel syndrome (IBS), diverticular disease, adhesions, mesenteric adenitis, renal colic, UTI, urinary retention, biliary colic, pancreatitis; ***obs/gynae*** ectopic pregnancy, ovarian cyst, ovarian torsion, PID, endometriosis, labour; ***other*** MI, pneumonia, sickle-cell crises, DKA, renal disease, psoas abscess, trauma

Ask about nature of pain (constant, colicky, changes with eating/vomiting/bowels), duration, onset, frequency, severity, radiation to the back, dysphagia, dyspepsia, abdominal swelling, nausea and vomiting, stool colour, change in bowel habit, urinary symptoms, weight loss, breathlessness, rashes, lumps, chest pain, recent surgery, last period; ***PMH*** DM, IBD, IHD, jaundice, pancreatitis; ***DH*** NSAIDs; ***SH*** alcohol

Obs temp, HR, BP, RR, sats, finger-prick glucose, urine output.

Look for jaundice, sweating, pale, pulse volume, lung air entry, clubbing, leuconychia (white nails), lymphadenopathy (Virchow's node), abdominal scars, distension, ascites, visible peristalsis, tenderness, peritonitis (tenderness with guarding, rebound or rigidity), loin tenderness, hepatomegaly, splenomegaly, masses (?expansile/pulsatile), check hernial orifices, examine external genitalia (if male examine for testicular vs. epididymal tenderness), femoral pulses, bowel sounds; ***PR*** perianal skin tags, fissures, warts; tenderness, masses, prostate hypertrophy, stool, check glove for blood, mucus, melaena and stool colour.

Investigations ***urine*** dipstick, **β-hCG** in all pre-menopausal women of reproductive age, MSU; ***blds*** FBC, U+E, LFT, amylase, Ca^{2+}, glucose, ±cardiac markers, clotting, bld cultures; ***ABGs*** if the patient is unwell; ***ECG*** to exclude MI; ***erect CXR*** to exclude perforation; ***plain AXR*** to exclude bowel obstruction; ***KUB or IVU*** for renal colic; ***USS*** especially if hepatobiliary cause suspected; ***CT abdo*** discuss with senior.

Treatment Give all patients O_2, analgesia and anti-emetics; insert a urinary catheter if unwell. Keep NBM until urgent surgery is ruled out:

- ***Shocked*** IV fluids, urgent senior review
- ***Peritonitic*** with IV fluids, IV antibiotics, urgent senior review
- ***>50yr in severe pain*** ?AAA, IV fluids, urgent senior review
- ***Abdo pain and vomiting*** consider obstruction, IV fluids, NG tube, AXR, p238, urgent senior review
- ***GI bleed*** resuscitate with IV fluids, see p244, urgent senior review

	History	Examination	Investigations
Perforation	Short onset, severe abdominal pain	Peritonitis, no bowel sounds	Gas under diaphragm, acidotic
Bowel obstruction	Pain, distension, nausea, vomiting, constipation	Distension, tenderness, tinkling bowel sounds	Dilated loops of bowel on AXR
Bowel ischaemia/ infarction	Sudden onset, severe pain, previous arterial disease	Shock, generalised tenderness	↑WCC, acidotic, ± AF or previous MI on ECG
Appendicitis	RIF pain, anorexia, nausea, vomiting	Slight temp, RIF tenderness, ±peritonitic	↑WCC, ↑CRP
Strangulated hernia	Sudden onset pain, previous hernia	Shocked, tender hernial mass	Needs urgent surgery
GORD/ gastroduodenal ulcer	Dyspepsia, heartburn, anorexia, NSAIDs	Epigastric tenderness	Seen on OGD, +ve CLO test
Gastro-enteritis	Rapid onset, vomiting, diarrhoea	↑temp, epigastric tenderness, no peritonitis	↑WCC, ↑CRP
Inflammatory bowel disease	Weight loss, mouth ulcers, PR bleeding, vomiting, diarrhoea	Distended, tender, ±peritonitis	↑WCC, ↑CRP, dilated bowel on AXR, lesions on colonoscopy
Diverticular disease	Pain, diarrhoea, constipation, PR bleeding	Tenderness, ±peritonitis	↑WCC, ↑CRP, diverticulae on colonoscopy
Acute pancreatitis	Constant epigastric pain radiating to back, vomiting, anorexia, ↑alcohol or gallstones	Shock, epigastric tenderness, ↓bowel sounds	↑↑↑amylase, ↑WCC, ↑CRP, ↑glucose, ↓Ca^{2+}
Abdominal aortic aneurysm (AAA)	Abdominal and back pain, collapse, prev heart disease/↑BP, age >50yr	Expansile mass, unwell, often ↓BP, ↓leg pulses	Straight to theatre if leaking, may be seen on portable USS
Renal colic	Sudden severe colicky flank pain, radiates to groin, nausea/vomiting	Sweating, restless, loin tenderness	90% of stones visible on KUB, lesion on IVU/CT
Hepatobiliary disease	Constant or colicky RUQ pain, gallstone	RUQ tenderness, ±jaundice	Deranged LFT
Obs/gynae disease	Lower abdo pain, PV bleeding, irregular/ absent periods	Lower abdo tenderness, PV exam abnormal	β-hCG +ve, lesions seen on USS
Testicular torsion	Sudden onset severe unilateral groin pain	Tender testicle, ±swelling	Urgent surgery

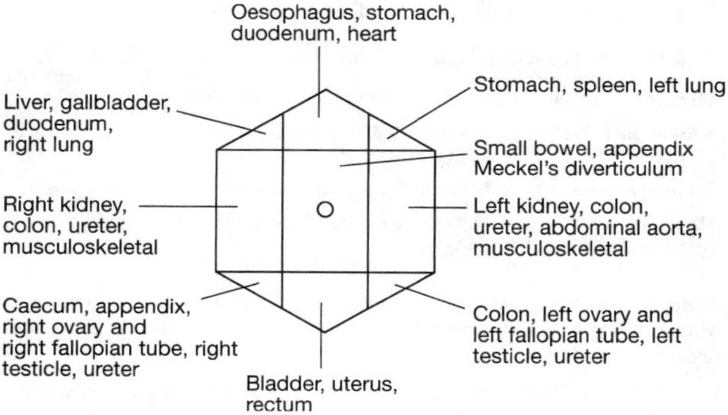

Abdominal regions and structures in each

GI bleed	p244	Testicular torsion	p242
Inflammatory bowel disease	p259	Hernias	p377
Irritable bowel syndrome	p258	Renal disease	p240
Gastroduodenal ulcer	p247	Obs and gynae	p242
Hepatobiliary disease	p242	Gastroenteritis	p257

Perforation (*OHCM*7 p580)

Causes gastroduodenal ulcer, appendicitis, diverticulitis, inflammatory bowel disease, bowel obstruction, GI cancer, gallbladder

Symptoms acute abdominal pain worse on coughing or moving; ***PMH*** gastroduodenal ulcer, cancer, IBD; ***DH*** NSAIDs; ***SH*** alcohol

Signs ↑HR, ±↓BP, ↑RR, peritonism (abdo tenderness, guarding, rebound, rigidity), reduced or absent bowel sounds

Investigations ↑WCC, ↓Hb, ↑amylase, erect CXR shows air under the diaphragm, ±obstruction on AXR, acidosis on ABGs

Management resuscitate with IV fluids, 15l/min O_2, good IV access (large ×2), analgesia (eg morphine 5–10mg IV with cyclizine 50mg/8h IV), NBM and urgent X-match 2–4units: IV antibiotics (cefuroxime 1.5mg/8h, metronidazole 500mg/8h) insert NG tube and urinary catheter, prepare for emergency laparotomy (see p131)

Bowel obstruction (*OHCM*7 p598)

Causes of intestinal obstruction

Outside the bowel	Adhesions, hernias, masses, volvulus
Within the bowel wall	Tumours, IBD, diverticular disease, infarction, congenital atresia, Hirschsprung's disease
Inside the bowel	Impacted faeces, FB, intussusception, strictures, polyps
Paralytic ileus (pseudo-obstruction)	Post-op, electrolyte imbalance, uraemia, DM, anticholinergic drugs

Symptoms vomiting (may be faeculant), colicky abdo pain, pain improves with vomiting, constipation (±absolute – no flatus or stool), bloating, anorexia, recent surgery

Signs ↑HR, ±↓BP, ↑RR, swollen abdomen, absent or tinkling bowel sounds, peritonitis, scars from previous surgery, hernias

Investigations mild ↑WCC and ↑amylase, ±acidosis, look for dilated bowel (?small or large) or volvulus on supine AXR (p626), erect CXR to exclude perforation

Management may need fluid resuscitation and analgesia, treat according to the type and location of the obstruction:

- ***Strangulated*** Constant severe pain in an ill patient with peritonitis (acute abdomen); can be small or large bowel. This will require urgent surgery especially if caused by a hernia.
- ***Small bowel*** Early vomiting with late constipation, usually caused by hernias, adhesions or Crohn's. Treated conservatively with NBM, an NG tube and IV fluids (0.9% saline 1l/4–6h) – often referred to as drip and suck – until the obstruction resolves, or by surgery if patient unwell. K^+ is often lost into the bowel and needs to be replaced in fluids (eg 20mmol/l).
- ***Large bowel*** Early absolute constipation with late vomiting, usually caused by volvulus (sigmoid or caecal), tumours, faeces or diverticulitis. IV fluids, NBM and refer to a senior surgeon. Urgent surgery may be required if the caecum is >8cm across on AXR otherwise a colonoscopy or water-soluble contrast enema may be ordered to investigate the cause. Surgery is usually required except for:
  - sigmoid volvulus – sigmoidoscopy and flatus tube insertion
  - faecal obstruction – laxative enemas, see p260
- ***Paralytic ileus*** Loss of bowel motility can mimic the signs and symptoms of a mechanical blockage. It is a response of the bowel to inflammation locally (eg surgery) or adjacently (eg pancreatitis). The main distinguishing feature is the relative lack of abdo pain, however the pathology responsible for the ileus may cause abdo pain itself. A USS abdo, contrast enema or CT may be required to exclude mechanical obstruction. Treat conservatively with NBM, NG tube, IV fluids (0.9% saline 1l/4–6h) until the underlying pathology improves. K^+ is often lost into the bowel and needs to be replaced in fluids.

Complications strangulation, bowel infarction, bowel perforation, ↓K^+, hypovolaemia

Adhesions

Causes previous surgery, abdominal sepsis, IBD, cancer, endometriosis
Symptoms and signs chronic intermittent abdominal pain and tenderness, may develop bowel obstruction (distension, vomiting, constipation)
Management analgesia and stool softeners; may need division of adhesions, but this may lead to new adhesions forming

Bowel ischaemia/infarction (*OHCM7* p594)

Symptoms unwell, sudden onset severe constant abdominal pain; ***PMH*** AF, MI, polycythaemia
Signs ↑HR (?irregular), ±↓BP, ↑RR, ↑temp, cold extremities, generalised tenderness but few specific signs
Investigations ↑WCC, ↑amylase, acidotic (metabolic), ±AF on ECG
Management NBM, resuscitate with IV fluids; analgesia, IV ABx (cefuroxime 1.5g/8h, metronidazole 500mg/8h), anticoagulate with IV heparin (p347) and treat AF if present (digoxin, p188), consider ITU care, laparotomy is usually necessary. Very poor prognosis.

Appendicitis (*OHCM7* p582)

Differential UTI, diverticulitis, gastroenteritis, mesenteric adenitis, perforated ulcer, IBD, diverticulitis; ***gynae*** ectopic pregnancy, ovarian torsion, ruptured ovarian cyst, salpingitis
Symptoms central, abdominal colicky pain worsening over 1–2d then developing into constant RIF pain, worse on moving, anorexia, nausea, vomiting, may have constipation, diarrhoea, dysuria, oliguria
Signs ↑temp, ↑HR, ±↓BP, RIF tenderness ±guarding/rebound/rigidity, RIF pain on palpating LIF (Rovsing's sign), PR tender on right
Investigations ↑WCC, ↑ESR, ↑CRP, bld cultures (if pyrexial), G+S
Management surgery – NBM, IV fluids, analgesia, IV ABx (cefuroxime 750mg–1.5g/8h and metronidazole 500mg/8h). If peritonitic send for immediate surgery, otherwise reassess regularly whilst awaiting surgery.

Gastro-oesophageal reflux disease – GORD (*OHCM7* p236)

Common risk factors smoking, alcohol, obesity, pregnancy, hiatus hernia
Symptoms burning retrosternal or epigastric pain, worse on bending and lying, waterbrash (excess saliva), acid reflux, nausea, vomiting, nocturnal cough, symptoms improved by antacids
Signs epigastric tenderness (no peritonitis)
Investigations *H. pylori* testing (see p247), endoscopy if symptoms persistent, difficulty swallowing or weight loss; 24h ambulatory pH monitoring
Management ***conservative*** weight loss, avoid foods/drugs which exacerbate symptoms; ***medical*** Gaviscon®, ranitidine, regular PPI (eg lansoprazole); ***surgery*** fundoplication (rarely) if severe

Diverticular disease (*OHCM7* p594)

- ***Diverticulosis*** diverticulae (out pouchings) in the large bowel
- ***Diverticulitis*** inflammation of diverticulae; acutely symptomatic

Symptoms abdominal pain/cramps (usually left sided, improves with bowel opening), irregular bowel habit, flatus, bloating, PR bleeding
Signs ↑temp, ↑HR, ±↓BP, LIF tenderness, ±peritonitis, distension
Investigations ***blds*** ↑WCC, ↑CRP, diverticulae may be seen on barium enema (may lead to perforation in diverticulitis) or colonoscopy
Management ***diverticulosis*** high-fibre diet, antispasmodics (eg mebeverine), laxatives (eg senna, p260); ***diverticulitis*** NBM, analgesia, fluids and ABx (cefuroxime 1.5g/8h IV, metronidazole 500mg/8h IV)
Complications obstruction, perforation, abscess, adhesions, strictures, fistula, PR bleeding (usually painless)

Abdominal aortic aneurysm (AAA) (*OHCM7* p586)

If you suspect a ruptured/leaking AAA:

- Fast-bleep for senior help and vascular surgeon immediately
- Order urgent O-ve blood and urgent X-match 8 units

Symptoms severe constant or colicky abdominal pain radiating to the back, collapse or feeling faint
Risk factors ↑age, male, ↑BP, smoking, IHD, ↑cholesterol
Signs expansile abdominal mass (pushes hands apart, not just pulsing) – examination will not cause rupture, ↑HR, ±↓BP, ↑RR, pale, sweating, cool extremities, distension, tenderness, ↓peripheral pulses
Investigations none if the patient is unstable; seniors may order an urgent USS/CT abdo if diagnosis is doubted
Management emergency give O_2, resuscitate, IV access for bloods and stat infusion of colloid/blood (keep systolic BP 90–100mmHg, important not to raise too much as ↑risk of leak from AAA); once senior help arrives get the patient to theatre; ***if the patient is stable/not leaking*** keep NBM, prep for theatre, with observations every 15min

Renal colic (*OHCM7* p284)

Exclude a AAA (if the patient is >50yr) and other causes of abdominal pain especially if no previous renal stone disease.
Symptoms acute onset severe unilateral colicky loin pain, nausea and vomiting, sweating, haematuria, dysuria, strangury (frequency as the stones pass); iliac fossa or suprapubic pain suggests another pathology
Signs ↑HR, sweating, patient restless and in severe pain, usually no tenderness on palpation unless superimposed infection
Investigations blood/Hb on urine dipstick (~90% of cases), imaging (KUB, IVU, CT according to policy), FBC and U+E, pregnancy test in ♀
Management analgesia (NSAID first, then opiates), if <5mm should pass spontaneously. If evidence of infection give IV ABx (check local policy). If evidence of infection and hydronephrosis refer urgently to urologist for nephrostomy or stent depending upon local expertise
Complications pyelonephrosis, renal dysfunction

Acute pancreatitis (*OHCM*7 p584)

Varies from a mild self-limiting illness to severe and life-threatening.
Causes 'GETSMASHED': gallstones (50%), ethanol (25%), trauma, steroids, mumps, autoimmune, scorpion bites (rare), hyperlipidaemia, hypercalcaemia, ERCP, drugs (eg thiazide diuretics), idiopathic
Symptoms constant severe epigastric pain radiating to the back, improved with sitting forward, nausea, vomiting, anorexia
Signs ↑HR, ±↓BP, ↑temp, cold extremities, epigastric tenderness with peritonitis, abdominal distension, ↓bowel sounds, mild jaundice, Cullen's (bruised umbilicus) or Grey–Turner's (bruised flanks) sign
Results ↓Hb, ↑WCC, ↑↑↑amylase, ↑glucose, ↓Ca^{2+}, deranged clotting (±DIC), deranged LFT; ***USS*** gallstones; ***CT*** pancreatic necrosis
Management resuscitate with IV fluids and O_2, analgesia, NG tube, urinary catheter, monitor fluid balance, NBM, if the patient has a high Ranson score, is unwell or shocked call for senior review ±ITU/HDU. Monitor obs, glucose and daily U+E, FBC, CRP; prophylactic LMWH (p346).
Complications DIC, renal failure, respiratory failure, haemorrhage, thrombosis, sepsis, pseudocyst, abscess, thrombosis, chronic pancreatitis

Ranson criteria for acute pancreatitis severity – score one for each criteria

Timing	Measure	Criteria
On admission	Age WCC Glucose AST LDH	>55yr >16 x 10^9/l >11mmol/l >250u/l >350u/l
Over next 48h (can be fulfilled at any time during this period)	Fall in haematocrit Urea increase Ca^{2+} PaO_2 Base deficit Estimated fluid sequestration	>10% >1.8mmol/l <2mmol/l <8kPa >4MEQ/l (eg–5) >6l
Add up all the criteria that have been fulfilled to get a total score		
Score 0–2	Mild pancreatitis	2% mortality
Score 2–5	Moderate pancreatitis	10–20% mortality
Score >5	Severe pancreatitis	>50% mortality

Chronic pancreatitis (*OHCM*7 p272)

Causes usually alcohol, but can be due to gallstones (which may also cause recurrent pancreatitis), familial, cystic fibrosis, hyperparathyroidism
Symptoms general malaise, anorexia, weight loss, recurrent epigastric pain radiating to back, steatorrhoea, bloating, DM
Signs cachexia, epigastric tenderness
Investigations glucose (?DM, p277), USS (±endoscopic), ERCP, CT
Management analgesia, advise to stop drinking alcohol; ***diet*** refer to dietician: low fat, high calorie, high protein with fat-soluble vitamin supplements; ***pancreatic enzymes*** eg Creon® before eating; ***surgery*** coeliac-plexus block, stenting of the pancreatic duct, pancreatectomy

Biliary colic

Contraction of the gallbladder or cystic duct around gallstones.
Symptoms recurrent colicky or constant RUQ/epigastric pain, especially on eating fatty foods, nausea, vomiting, bloating
Signs RUQ tenderness, non-peritonitic, not jaundiced
Results bloods normal, USS shows gallstones
Management analgesia and elective cholecystectomy
Complications gallstone rarely passes into common bile duct where it may cause cholestatic jaundice, cholangitis or acute pancreatitis

Acute cholecystitis

Gallstone impacted in the neck of the gallbladder with inflammation.
Symptoms continuous RUQ/epigastric pain, unwell, vomiting
Signs ↑temp, RUQ tenderness and peritonitis, Murphy's sign (pain on inspiration if two fingers placed on RUQ, not present on LUQ)
Results ↑WCC, ↑CRP, uss shows gallstones
Management NBM, analgesia, cefuroxime 1.5g/8h IV and metronidazole 500mg/8h IV; consider urgent cholecystectomy

Testicular torsion (see p377)

This is an emergency – if you suspect torsion, get a senior review immediately as testicular tissue can become completely necrosed in only 4h.
Symptoms lower abdominal pain, swollen/painful testis, nausea, vomiting
Signs ↑HR, high riding, horizontal-lying testis, thickened spermatic cord (early sign), –ve Prehn's sign (elevating testis does not relieve pain), absent cremasteric reflex
Differential diagnosis epididymo-orchitis, hydrocele, femoral hernia, indirect inguinal hernia, saphena varix, lymphadenopathy, aneurysm, ectopic testis, skin lumps, psoas abscess, testicular tumour
Management NBM, analgesia, IV access to take blood and for fluids, inform seniors immediately as emergency surgical exploration is required; call theatres and put the patient on the emergency list
Complications testicular necrosis, contralateral torsion if not fixed

Pelvic inflammatory disease (PID)

Infection of the upper genital tract commonly with *Chlamydia trachomatis* or *Neisseria gonorrhoeae*.
Symptoms pyrexia, vaginal discharge (may be foul-smelling), intermenstrual/postcoital bleeding, dysuria, dyspareunia, lower abdominal pain, nausea, vomiting, infertility, general malaise
Signs abdomen tenderness; ***PV*** adnexal tenderness, cervical excitation
Risk factors young age at first intercourse, multiple sexual partners, no barrier contraception, smoking
Differential diagnosis appendicitis, endometriosis, ovarian cysts, ectopic pregnancy, other STIs, HIV, urinary tract infection
Investigations MSU; ***triple swab*** for M,C+S (p484); ***blds*** FBC, CRP, cultures, USS (to exclude ovarian cyst)
Management IV access for fluids, analgesia, broad-spectrum antibiotics eg metronidazole and doxycycline, refer to gum for contact tracing
Complications tubo-ovarian abscess, septicaemia, recurrence, secondary infertility, ectopic pregnancy, chronic pelvic pain

Ovarian cyst/torsion

Torsion most commonly occurs with fibromas and dermoid cysts.
Symptoms severe, sudden onset lower abdominal pain, iliac fossa pain radiating to the flank, nausea, vomiting, fever
Signs ***abdomen*** tenderness; ***PV*** adnexal tenderness
Risk factors developmental abnormalities, early pregnancy, women undergoing hormonal stimulation for IVF
Differential diagnosis appendicitis, diverticulitis, ectopic pregnancy, urinary tract infection
Investigations MSU, urine pregnancy test; ***blds*** FBC, β-hCG, USS
Management IV access for fluids, analgesia, laparoscopy
Complications infection, peritonitis, adhesions, infertility (rare)

Ectopic pregnancy (*OHCS7* p262)

Consider this in every woman of child-bearing age presenting with collapse, acute abdominal pain ±PV bleeding; it is a surgical emergency. It usually presents at 6–9wk gestation.
Symptoms abdominal pain, shoulder tip/back pain, PV bleeding, history of amenorrhoea, dizziness; ***ruptured ectopic*** collapse, shock, peritonism
Risk factors ↑maternal age, previous ectopic, tubal surgery, previous STIs/PID, IUCD, assisted conception techniques
Signs ↑HR ±↓BP; ***abdo*** unilateral iliac fossa pain, guarding *PV* extreme cervical pain
Investigations β-hCG (serum and urine), FBC, G+S/X-match, transvaginal USS (look for fetal sac/pole in the adnexae, free fluid)
Differentials miscarriage, appendicitis, pelvic infection, ovarian cyst
Management IV access (14–16G), IV fluids and urgent referral to gynae; ***conservative*** if haemodynamically stable, monitor β-hCG; if doubling every 48h, likely IUP; ***surgical*** laparoscopic/open salpingectomy/salpingostomy or oophorectomy; send sample for histology; ***medical*** methotrexate sometimes used for small <3.5mm early ectopics in stable patients

Endometriosis

Endometrial tissue found outside the endometrial cavity that bleeds with the menstrual period; called adenomyosis if in the uterine muscle wall.
Symptoms often asymptomatic, painful periods, pelvic pain before/with periods or constantly (adhesions), deep dyspareunia, infertility, rectal pain
Signs generalised pelvic tenderness, fixed (retroverted) uterus, palpable nodule on uterosacral ligaments, large uterus in adenomyosis
Investigation laparoscopy (though it is a common incidental finding)
Management ***medical*** preventing cyclical hormone changes can shrink the ectopic tissue: continuous combined oral contraceptive pill, GnRH agonists eg goserelin, leuprorelin; ***surgery*** laparoscopic laser ablation of ectopic tissue and division of adhesions, removal of ovaries and fallopian tubes ±uterus

GI bleeding emergency

Airway	Check airway is patent; consider manoeuvres/adjuncts
Breathing	If no respiratory effort – **CALL ARREST TEAM**
Circulation	If no palpable pulse – **CALL ARREST TEAM**

Call for **senior help** early if patient deteriorating

- Lay the patient **on their side** if vomiting
- **15l/min O_2** in all patients
- **Monitor** pulse oximeter, BP, defibrillator's ECG leads if unwell
- Obtain a full set of **observations** including temp
- Two good (large) sites of **venous access**, take bloods:
  - FBC, U+E, LFT, clotting, urgent 4–8u X-match
- **0.9% saline** 1l IV or O –ve blood (call a senior before giving blood)
- Take brief **history** if possible/check **notes**/ask ward staff
- **Examine patient**: condensed CVS, RS and abdo exam
- **Correct clotting** abnormalities if present (p344)
- **Arterial blood gas**, but don't leave the patient alone
- Initiate **further treatment**, see following pages
- Consider **serious causes** (below) and treat if present
- Seniors may consider giving Glypressin® 2mg IV over 5min if **oesophageal varices** suspected

If bleeding is severe and the patient haemodynamically unstable:

- Call for **senior help**
- Request **urgent O –ve blood**
- Contact the on-call endoscopist and alert **surgeons**
- ***Reassess***, starting with A, B, C …

Life-threatening causes

- Gastroduodenal ulcer
- Gastroduodenal erosions
- Vascular malformations
- Oesophageal varices
- Mallory-Weiss tears
- Upper GI malignancy

Upper GI bleeds *(OHAM2 p608)*

Worrying features ↓GCS, postural BP drop, ↑HR, ↓BP, ↓urine output, continuous haematemesis, frank PR bleeding, chest pain, clotting abnormality, liver disease

Think about ***common*** gastroduodenal ulcer (NSAIDs, *H. pylori*), oesophagitis, oesophageal varices, Mallory–Weiss tear, swallowed blood (eg epistaxis); ***other*** oesophageal or gastric cancer, coagulation abnormalities, vascular malformation
Ask about colour, quantity, mixed in or throughout vomit, frequency, onset, stool colour, pain on vomiting, chest pain, abdominal pain, pain on eating, palpitations, dizziness, fainting, sweating, SOB, weight loss, dysphagia; ***PMH*** clotting problems, liver problems (?varices), gastroduodenal ulcers, heartburn; ***DH*** NSAIDs, warfarin, iron, steroids; ***SH*** alcohol
Obs HR, BP, postural BP, GCS, RR, sats
Look for continued bleeding, colour of vomit, cold extremities, sweating, pulse volume, bruises, other bleeding (nose, mouth), abdominal tenderness, ±peritonitic, masses, signs of chronic liver disease (see p263); ***PR*** fresh blood/melaena
Investigations ***blds*** FBC, U+E, LFT, clotting, G+S or 4–8u X-match; ***CXR***, ***ECG*** for ischaemia; ***OGD*** within 4h if severe bleeding and shocked, diagnosis, biopsy, ±treatment

- ***Initial bloods*** may show a normal Hb, reticulocyte count and urea, despite a significant bleed. Check HR, BP and postural BP

Rockall risk scoring system for GI bleeds

≤2 = low risk, ≥9 = high risk

Feature	0	1	2	3
Age	<60yr	60–79yr	≥80yr	
Shock: systolic BP and HR	>100mmHg <100/min	>100mmHg >100/min	<100mmHg >100/min	
Comorbidity	Nil major	Heart failure, IHD	Renal/liver failure	Metastatic disease
Diagnosis	Mallory–Weiss/ none	Other	Upper GI malignancy	
Bleeding on OGD	Nil recent		Recent	

Management NBM for 24h, O_2, two good (≥green) sites of IV access, blood/colloids/fluids IV, regular obs (HR, BP, postural BP, urine output), consider catheterisation, CVP line and HDU/ITU, admit for OGD

- ***Young patients*** with a postural drop and a pulse >90 may have lost a lot of blood
- ***Do not give a PPI*** unless the patient has had an OGD and cautery of a bleeding ulcer (usually requires 72h omeprazole infusion)

	History	Examination	Investigations
Gastroduo-denal ulcers	Epigastric/chest pain, heartburn, melaena, previous ulcers, NSAIDs, alcohol	Epigastric tenderness, may be peritonitic if perforated	Ulcer on OGD, CLO test may be +ve
Oesophagitis/ gastritis	Heartburn, NSAIDs, alcohol, hiatus hernia	Epigastric tenderness	Inflammation/erosions on OGD, CLO test may be +ve
Oesophageal varices	Frank haematemesis previous liver disease, alcohol	Epigastric tenderness, signs of chronic liver disease	↑INR, deranged LFT, varices on OGD
Mallory–Weiss tear	Normal coloured forceful vomit then bloodstained vomit	Epigastric tenderness	Tear seen on OGD if not resolving

Clotting abnormalities - see p344

Oesophageal varices (*OHCM*7 p246, *OHAM*2 p618)

Symptoms of chronic liver failure (p263), known liver disease, excess alcohol, varices are asymptomatic until they bleed
Signs of chronic liver failure (p263)
Investigations varices seen on OGD
Acute bleed resuscitate according to p244 then:
- ***Glypressin®*** 2mg/over 5min IV if not already given
- ***OGD*** (in <4h if shock) for sclerotherapy/banding
- ***Bleeding still uncontrolled*** consider a Sengstaken–Blakemore tube and transjugular intrahepatic portosystemic shunting (TIPS)
- ***Antibiotics*** (eg ciprofloxacin 400mg/12h IV or cefuroxime 1.5g/8h IV) in all variceal bleeds

Once bleeding controlled Glypressin® 2mg/over 5min IV, 1–2mg/4h for up to 3d, propranolol, treat cause of liver failure, TIPS

Giving Glypressin®

Glypressin® is vasopressin (ADH); it must be given by a doctor though there is little scientific basis for this. The perceived risk is of arterial spasm leading to arrhythmia, angina, MI and acute limb ischaemia. Give slowly over 5min to reduce the risk.

Mallory–Weiss tear (*OHAM*2 p622)

Symptoms repeated forceful vomiting, initially bloodless, then bright red blood streaks or throughout vomit, often follows binge drinking
Acute bleed management as on p244, usually resolves spontaneously, may need an OGD ±oversewing of the bleeding mucosa; a PPI may be used after OGD

Oesophagitis and gastritis

Symptoms as for GORD (p239) or gastroduodenal ulcer
Signs epigastric tenderness
Investigations OGD to identify inflammation and CLO test for *H. pylori*, 24h oesophageal pH study
Acute bleed management as on p244, PPI (PO or IV) after OGD
Treatment weight loss, stop smoking, reduce alcohol, *H. pylori* eradication if present (below), long-term PPI

Gastroduodenal ulcers and erosions (*OHCM*7 p234)

Causes *H. pylori*, NSAIDs, alcohol, smoking, stress
Symptoms epigastric pain related to eating, heartburn, chest pain, improves with antacids, bloating, melaena
Signs epigastric tenderness
Investigations ↓Hb, ↑urea (if bleeding), urea breath test for *H. pylori* (does not need OGD), ulcer on OGD, normal biopsy, CLO test on OGD for *H. pylori*
Acute bleed management as on p244, PPI (PO or IV) after OGD
Treatment treat *H. pylori* infection (below), PPI (eg lansoprazole, omeprazole), avoid NSAIDs, stop smoking, weight loss, reduce alcohol intake, avoid spicy food
Follow-up continue PPI and repeat OGD in 6–8wk

H. pylori infection and eradication

- Diagnosed by urea breath test (no OGD), CLO test (OGD) or serology
- Treat with triple therapy for 1wk, eg lansoprazole 30mg/12h PO, amoxicillin 1g/12h PO, clarithromycin 500mg/12h PO

Lower GI bleeds

> Worrying features continuous bright-red PR bleeding, postural drop, ↑HR, ↓BP, dizziness, ↓GCS, abdominal pain, weight loss, abdominal swelling, vomiting

Think about ***common*** polyps, diverticular disease, angiodysplasia, haemorrhoids, anal fissure, IBD, colon cancer, upper GI bleed (p245); ***other*** aorto-enteric fistulae, ischaemic colitis, Meckel's diverticulum

Ask about onset, quantity, colour (red, black, clots), type of blood (fresh, mixed with stool, streaks on toilet paper), abdominal pain, pain on eating, vomiting (colour), pain on opening bowels, straining, constipation, diarrhoea, change in bowel habit, anorexia, weight loss, bloating, palpitations, chest pain, dizziness, SOB, tiredness; ***PMH*** gastric ulcer, heartburn, liver disease, previous bleeding, IBD, aortic surgery; ***DH*** NSAIDs, warfarin, steroids, iron; ***FH*** IBD, bowel cancer; ***SH*** alcohol

Obs HR, BP, postural BP, GCS, RR, sats

Look for pale and cold extremities, sweating, pulse volume, bruises, other sources of bleeding (nose, mouth), abdominal tenderness, ±peritonitic, masses, signs of chronic liver disease (see p263), distension, absent/tinkling bowel sounds; ***PR*** blood, melaena, palpable mass; ***proctoscopy*** haemorrhoids

Investigations ***blds*** FBC, clotting, U+E, LFT, glucose, G+S or X-match 4–8units; ***ABG*** if unwell; ***OGD*** to exclude upper GI bleed, urgent if shocked; ***ECG*** if age >50yr; ***sigmoidoscopy/colonoscopy*** for investigation, biopsy and treatment, may require ***mesenteric angiography*** if bleeding source cannot be identified

Management lower GI bleeding is usually treated by surgeons whilst upper GI bleeding is usually a medical condition. Some patients' bowels do not realise this and upper GI bleeding may present with PR bleeding.

- ***Diagnosis*** it is rarely possible to tell the cause of significant lower GI bleeds from history and examination alone, investigations are essential
- ***Fresh blood on toilet paper*** or streaking stool only and patient well, treat as haemorrhoids/anal fissure but refer to surgeons for flexible sigmoidoscopy ±barium enema to rule out bowel cancer
- ***Mild bleeding*** (no evidence of shock) NBM for 24h, O_2, two good (≥green) sites of IV access, IV fluids, regular obs (HR, BP, urine output), reassess if further bleeding
- ***Moderate bleeding*** (postural drop, ↑HR) transfuse blood/colloids until haemodynamically stable, catheterise, hourly fluid balance, senior review, may need urgent OGD
- ***Severe bleeding*** (fresh bleeding/clots, ↓BP) treat as upper GI bleed, fast bleep senior, transfuse O –ve blood, call anaesthetist, on-call endoscopist and surgical registrar

	History	Examination	Investigations
Upper GI bleed	Fresh PR bleeding, clots or melaena,epigastric pain	Liver disease, epigastric tenderness, PR blood or melaena	↓Hb, ↑urea, lesion on OGD
GI cancer or polyps	Change in bowel habit, weight loss, abdominal pain	PR blood or melaena, mucus, palpable mass	↓Hb, lesion on sigmoidoscopy or colonoscopy
Inflammatory bowel disease	Abdominal pain, diarrhoea, weight loss, mouth ulcers	↑temp, abdo tender ±peritonitic, PR blood, mucus, melaena	↓Hb, ↑WCC, ↑CRP, lesions on sigmoidoscopy or colonoscopy
Diverticular disease	Abdominal pain, fever, change in bowel habit	Tenderness, ±peritonism, PR blood, mucus	↓Hb, diverticulae on colonoscopy
Bowel ischaemia	Abdo pain, previous arterial disease	Shock, generalised tenderness	↑WCC, acidotic, ±AF or previous MI on ECG
Angio-dysplasia	Often asymptomatic, old age, recurrent fresh blood or melaena	PR blood or melaena	↓Hb, lesion on colonoscopy, consider angiography
Haemorrhoids	Painless, fresh red blood on toilet paper, perianal itch, constipation	Often not palpable on PR, perianal tags, may have rectal prolapse	Lesions seen on proctoscopy
Anal fissure	Pain on defaecating, fresh blood on toilet paper, constipation	Posterior/anterior PR tear, perianal tags, tenderness	Proctoscopy to visualise lesions

Chronic gastrointestinal blood loss

Causes oesophagitis, gastric erosions, gastritis, drugs, gastroduodenal ulcer, gastric/bowel cancer, polyps, lymphoma, IBD, angiodysplasia (also see weight loss p418)

Symptoms unexplained anaemia, melaena, anorexia, weight loss, tired, change in bowel habit, vague intermittent abdo pain

Signs pale, cachexic, mild abdo tenderness; ***PR*** blood, mass

Investigations stool for faecal occult blood (FOB), ova, cysts and parasites, bloods for FBC (↓Hb, ↓MCV), iron, ferritin, B_{12}, folate, U+E, LFT, OGD, sigmoidoscopy, colonoscopy/barium enema, may need a barium follow-through if small bowel disease suspected

Treatment investigate and treat the cause, treat anaemia with ferrous sulphate 200mg/8h PO, consider admission for transfusion if Hb <8g/dl or if symptomatic with anaemia

Colorectal polyps (*OHCM*7 p612)

Causes sporadic, familial, genetic syndromes
Symptoms intermittent abdo pain, altered bowel habit, blood or melaena in stool, tenesmus, weight loss
Signs abdo tenderness; ***PR*** palpable mass, blood, mucus
Investigations ↓Hb, lesion on colonoscopy/barium enema
Treatment polypectomy (send for histology), multiple polyps may need colonic resection or regular colonoscopy follow-up

Haemorrhoids (*OHCM*7 p628)

Dilated and displaced perianal vascular tissue (anal cushions).
Symptoms painless, recurrent fresh red blood on toilet paper or streaking stools, pruritus ani, constipation
Risk factors, constipation with straining, multiple vaginal deliveries
Signs not palpable unless prolapsed; ***PR*** blood, otherwise normal
Investigations proctoscopy to visualise haemorrhoids, sigmoidoscopy to identify other pathology (eg malignancy)
Treatment high-fibre diet, topical Anusol®, injection of sclerosants, band ligation, coagulation, cryotherapy, may need haemorrhoidectomy
Strangulated haemorrhoids painful, tender mass, unable to sit down, treat with ice packs, stool softeners, regular analgesia and bed rest. Once stable, inject piles and consider elective haemorrhoidectomy

Anal fissure (*OHCM*7 p628)

Symptoms new onset pain on opening bowels, fresh red blood on toilet paper, history of constipation and straining, may be Crohn's or cancer
Signs anal tear visible posteriorly on the anal margin (10% anterior), perianal ulcers, fistulae; ***PR*** blood, tender
Investigations sigmoidoscopy if suspicious of cancer
Treatment ***conservative*** high-fibre diet, 5% lidocaine ointment, 0.2–0.3% GTN ointment, botox injection, internal sphincterotomy

Angiodysplasia (*OHCM*7 p588)

Submucosal arteriovenous malformation, often ascending colon.
Symptoms elderly, recurrent blood in the stool, abdo pain is rare
Signs may be normal, pallor; ***PR*** blood
Investigations faecal occult blood, barium enema/colonoscopy, mesenteric angiography
Treatment embolisation (via angiography), electrocoagulation (via endoscopy), resection, treat anaemia eg ferrous sulphate

Inflammatory bowel disease	p259	Upper GI bleed	p245
Bowel ischaemia	p239	Diverticular disease	p240
GI cancers	p424	Colorectal cancer	p424

Nausea and vomiting

Worrying features ↑HR, ↓BP, ↓GCS, recurrent vomiting, severe pain (head, chest, abdomen), head injury, constipation, blood/coffee grounds, risk of inhalation

Think about *life-threatening* raised intracranial pressure (ICP), meningitis, MI, bowel obstruction, acute abdomen, DKA; ***common*** post-op, pain, drug induced (opioids), gastroenteritis, other infection, alcohol; ***other*** paralytic ileus, pregnancy, electrolyte imbalance (Ca^{2+}, Na^{+}), migraine, labyrinthitis, Ménière's, chemotherapy, Addison's, bulimia
Ask about frequency, timing, relation to food or medications, content, colour, blood, coffee grounds, melaena, dizziness, diarrhoea, constipation, flatus, abdo pain, chest pain, other pain, headaches, head trauma, visual problems, weight loss, altered bowel habit; ***PMH*** previous surgery, migraines, DM; ***DH*** opioids, chemotherapy, digoxin; ***SH*** alcohol.
Obs temp, fluid balance, HR, BP, blood glucose, GCS
Look for and assess volume status (p319), respiratory creps, SOB, distended abdomen, tender abdomen, peritonitis, tinkling bowel sounds, hernias, scars from previous operations, mouth ulcers, neck stiffness, rash, photophobia
Investigations vomiting without the worrying features usually does not require urgent investigation. If vomiting is recurrent check ***U+E*** for signs of dehydration or electrolyte imbalance and ***AXR*** if bowel obstruction suspected. Otherwise investigate according to related symptoms, consider: ***blds*** FBC, U+E, LFT, glucose, amylase, Ca^{2+}, bld cultures; ***CXR*** aspiration; ***ABGs*** if acutely unwell; ***CT brain*** if head trauma, p358

Common anti-emetic drugs

Drug	Indications	Contraindications	Dose
Cyclizine (Antihistamine)	Most causes	Low GCS, severe heart failure	50mg/8h PO/IM/IV
Prochlorperazine (Phenothiazine – Stemetil®)	Post-op or drug induced	Low GCS, severe COPD	5–10mg/8h PO or 10–20mg PO/buccal one-off dose
Metoclopramide	Gastroenteritis, hepatobiliary disease, drug induced	<25yr, GI obstruction/ perforation/ haemorrhage, <4d post-GI surgery	10mg/8h PO/IM/IV
Domperidone	Drug induced, less sedating	Prolactinoma, liver failure. Not ideal post-op or for chronic use.	10–20mg/6h PO, 30–60mg/6h PR
Ondansetron ($5HT_3$ antagonist)	Post-op, severe vomiting, chemotherapy	Tight budget	4mg/4–8h IM/IV

	History	Examination	Investigations
Raised ICP/ meningitis	Headache, blurred vision, dizzy, feels ill, drowsy	Febrile, stiff neck, photophobia, rash, Cushing's reflex or shock, low GCS	↑WCC/NØ/CRP, abnormal CT brain or CSF results
Bowel obstruction	Colicky abdo pain, constipation, no flatus, brown vomit	Distended tender abdomen, tinkling bowel sounds, empty rectum	Distended bowel loops on AXR, see p626
Paralytic ileus	Constipation, absence of flatus	Distended abdomen, absent bowel sounds	Distended bowel loops on AXR, see p626
Acute abdomen	Severe abdo pain, feels ill	Tender, rigid, guarding, rebound, shock	Pneumoperitoneum on CXR
Upper GI bleed	Fresh blood or coffee-ground vomit	Tender abdomen, PR melaena	↓Hb, ↑urea
Gastro-enteritis	Vomiting after eating, diarrhoea, feels better after vomiting	Febrile, epigastric tenderness, not peritonitic	↑WBC, ↑LØ or NØ, positive stool culture
Labyrinthitis/ Ménière's	Dizziness is main feature, difficulty standing, tinnitus	Unable to stand	Acute investigations normal, see p302
Migraine	Visual aura, headache	Photophobia, visual field defects	Acute investigations normal
Hyperemesis gravidarum	Usually between 7-12 weeks of pregnancy	Normal	TFTs often raised, ↑urea if dehydrated
Drug induced	Many medications can induce vomiting, particularly opioids, chemotherapy and digoxin toxicity		

Treatment vomiting should be seen as a marker of disease severity and the diagnosis comes mostly from the associated symptoms; investigate and treat the underlying disease (see diagram on next page). Vomiting is very distressing for patients so try to relieve the symptoms with anti-emetics. In pregnancy, always check the *BNF* for which anti-emetics are safe to use.

Causes of nausea and vomiting and appropriate anti-emetics

Drugs with anti-emetic activity and their site(s) of action
Not all of these are **regularly** used as anti-emetics

Histamine antagonists	Cyclizine Promethazine
Muscarinic antagonists	Hyoscine Atropine
Dopamine antagonists	Prochlorperazine Metoclopramide Domperidone
Cannabinoids	Nabilone
Benzodiazepines	Midazolam Temazepam
$5HT_3$ antagonists	Ondansetron
Gastroprokinetic agents	Metoclopramide Erythromycin

Headache	p254	Pregnancy	p436
Abdominal pain	p234	Electrolyte imbalance	p327
Upper GI bleed	p245	Dizziness	p302

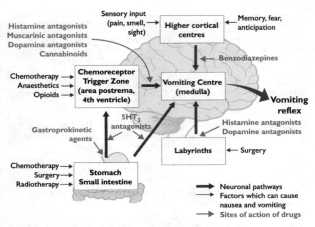

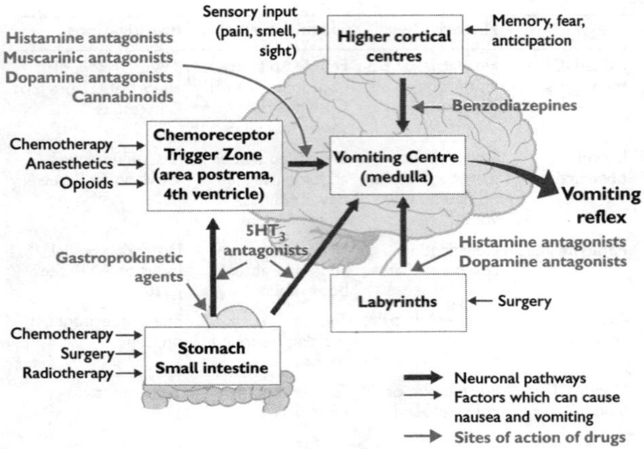

Diarrhoea

Worrying features ↑HR, ↓BP, low urine output, PR blood, weight loss, abdo pain

Think about ***acute*** gastroenteritis, antibiotics, laxatives, drugs, pseudomembranous colitis (see p258/157), overflow diarrhoea (2° to constipation), post-chemotherapy; ***chronic*** IBD, IBS, colorectal cancer, diverticular disease, chronic pancreatitis, alcoholism, malabsorption disorders (eg coeliac), thyrotoxicosis, bowel resection, bowel ischaemia, parasitic/fungal infections, autonomic neuropathy, carcinoid, ischaemic colitis, Addison's disease

Traveller's diarrhoea *E. coli, Salmonella, Shigella, Campylobacter species,* giardiasis, amoebic dysentery, cholera, tropical sprue

Ask about normal bowel habit and frequency, onset/frequency of diarrhoea, recent constipation, stool character (floating, greasy, bloody, mucus), colour, abdominal pain, pain better/worse on opening bowels, nausea, vomiting, flatus, fluid intake, weight loss, mouth ulcers; ***PMH*** colorectal cancer, IBD, diverticular disease, IBS, surgery; ***DH*** recent ABx, immunosuppression; ***SH*** travel abroad, occupation (food, healthcare), alcohol

Medications causing diarrhoea: antibiotics, laxatives, colchicine, digoxin, iron, NSAIDs, ranitidine, thiazide diuretics, propranolol, PPIs

Obs temp, HR, BP, postural BP, RR, sats, fluid balance

Look for volume status (p319), cachexia, mouth ulcers, clubbing, jaundice, rashes, pale conjunctiva, thyroid mass, abdomen tenderness, ±peritonitis, masses, distension, surgical scars; ***PR*** faecal impaction, pain, masses, stool colour, consistency

Investigations ***stool*** M,C+S x3, *C. diff.* toxin, ova, cysts and parasites; ***blds*** FBC, U+E, glucose, LFT, Ca^{2+}, TFT, CRP, bld cultures; ***AXR*** obstruction, ±faecal impaction; ***sigmoidoscopy*** if not improving; ***colonoscopy/barium enema*** if cancer suspected

General treatment

- ***Conservative*** increase fluid intake, avoid dairy products, review drugs: consider alternatives without GI side-effects
- ***Infective*** isolation, barrier nurse, ABx if systemically unwell
- ***Medical*** anti-diarrhoeal drugs should be avoided in infective diarrhoea, acute ulcerative colitis or pseudomembranous colitis

Anti-diarrhoeal drug	Dose
Loperamide	2mg/loose stool PO, max16mg/d
Codeine	30mg/6h PO, max 240mg/d
Colestyramine	4g/6h PO, max 36g/d

Inflammatory bowel disease – IBD

Ulcerative colitis (*OHCM*7 p264), **Crohn's disease** (*OHCM*7 p266)
Symptoms recurrent diarrhoea, ±blood, ±mucus associated with abdo pain, malaise, tiredness, anorexia and weight loss
Signs ↑temp, ↑HR, ±↓BP, pale, abdo pain, ±peritonitic, abdo swelling (toxic megacolon), malnourished, fistulae, fissures

Extra-intestinal signs clubbing, mouth ulcers, erythema nodusum, pyoderma gangrenosum, conjunctivitis, episcleritis, iritis, large joint arthritis, sacroiliitis, ankylosing spondylitis, fatty liver change, primary sclerosing cholangitis, cholangiocarcinoma

Investigations ↑WCC, ↑CRP, ±abnormal LFT, ↓Ca^{2+}, ↓iron, ↓folate, ↓B_{12} (terminal ileal disease), bld cultures; *AXR* toxic megacolon >6cm; ***sigmoidoscopy*** cobblestone appearance, ulcers, thick bowel wall; ***barium enema*** (never during acute episode) rose thorn ulcers, strictures, loss of haustra

Differentiating factors between ulcerative colitis and Crohn's

Feature	Ulcerative colitis (UC)	Crohn's
Symptoms	Diarrhoea and PR blood/ mucus prominent	Diarrhoea, abdo pain and weight loss prominent
GI involvement	Rectal involvement, may extend along the colon only	Anywhere along GI tract, most commonly terminal ileum
Sigmoidoscopy	Inflamed mucosa, continuous lesions	Inflamed, thickened mucosa, skip lesions
Histology	Mucosal and submucosal inflammation, crypt abscesses, reduced goblet cells	Inflammation extends beyond the submucosa, granulomas present
Treatment – **mild:** <4 motions a day, patient well	Prednisolone 30mg/24h PO + Pentasa® 500mg/6h PO both for 1-2wk then tail off steroids, consider steroid enema	Prednisolone 30mg/24h PO for 1wk then 20mg/24h for 1mth
Treatment – **moderate:** 4–6 motions a day, patient well	Prednisolone 40mg/24h PO for 1wk then 20mg/24h for 1mth + Pentasa® (mesalazine) 500mg/6h PO, steroid enema	Prednisolone 40mg/24h PO for 1wk then 30mg/24h for 1mth and tail off gradually, steroid enema
Treatment – **severe:** ≥6 motions a day, systemically unwell, marked PR bleeding, HR>100	NBM, IV fluids, hydrocortisone 100mg/6h IV, if ↑temp cefuroxime 1.5mg/6h IV and metronidazole 500mg/8h IV, frequent abdo exam, daily FBC, U+E, ESR, CRP, ±AXR, ±transfusion, discuss with senior	NBM, IV fluids, hydrocortisone 100mg/6h IV, metronidazole 500mg/8h IV, rectal steroids, frequent abdo exam, daily FBC, U+E, ESR, CRP, ±AXR, ±transfusion, discuss with senior – may need surgical intervention

Other therapies elemental diet, immunosuppressive drugs, surgery
Complications toxic megacolon, bowel obstruction, perforation, malabsorption, fistulae, fissures, strictures, malignancy

Overflow diarrhoea

Symptoms and signs elderly, immobility, poor diet, recent constipation, nausea, vomiting, bloating, abdo pain and tenderness, indentable stool-filled bowel palpable; ***PR*** hard, palpable stool, liquid stool in lower rectum
Treatment treat as constipation (p260)

Constipation

Worrying features abdominal pain, distension, nausea/vomiting, ↑HR, ↓BP, absent/tinkling bowel sounds, weight loss, PR bleeding

Think about ***serious*** bowel obstruction, bowel cancer; ***common*** opiates, poor diet, paralytic ileus, dehydration; ***other*** anal fissure/stricture, pelvic mass, immobility, spinal nerve injury, hypothyroid

Ask about abdo pain, nausea, vomiting, date bowels last opened, normal bowel habit and frequency, stool consistency and colour, blood in stools, pain on opening bowels, straining, bloating, flatus, fluid intake, weight loss, tenesmus, recent surgery; ***PMH*** IBD, diverticulosis, hernias, previous surgery, colon cancer, hypothyroidism; ***DH*** opiates, TCAs, iron ***SH*** mobility, diet

Obs temp, HR, BP, fluid balance

Look for volume status (p319), tenderness, ±peritonism, distension, masses, absent/tinkling bowel sounds, hernias, scars; ***PR*** anal fissures, rectal masses, faecal impaction, melaena/blood

Investigations ***blds*** FBC, U+E, TFT, Ca^{2+}; ***AXR*** to exclude obstruction ***sigmoidoscopy*** ±biopsy if sub-acute onset; ***colonoscopy/barium enema*** if cancer suspected

Common laxative agents – drugs with different mechanisms can be prescribed together

Mechanism	Name	Dose
Bulking agents	Fybogel®	1 sachet/12h PO
	Normacol®	1 sachet/12h PO
Stimulants	Senna	2 tablets/24h (at night) PO
	Bisacodyl	5–10mg/24h (at night) PO
	Glycerol suppositories	Single suppository PR
Softener/stimulant	Sodium docusate	200mg/8h PO
Osmotic	Lactulose	15ml/12h PO
	Movicol®	1–3 sachet/24h PO
	Phosphate enema	Single enema PR

Common choices of laxatives according to degree of constipation

Mild	Senna or lactulose
Moderate	Senna and sodium docusate
Severe	Senna and sodium docusate and Movicol®/glycerol suppositories
Very severe	Phosphate enema, consider Picolax® bowel prep after discussion with your senior

	History	Examination	Investigation
Bowel obstruction	Pain, distension, nausea, vomiting, constipation	Distension, tenderness, absent/tinkling bowel sounds	Dilated loops of bowel on AXR
Paralytic ileus	Absence of flatus, recent operation	Distended abdomen, absent bowel sounds	Distended bowel loops on AXR, ↓K^+
Bowel cancer	Abdo pain, weight loss, fresh blood or melaena	PR blood or melaena, mucus/ palpable mass	↓Hb, lesion on sigmoidoscopy/ colonoscopy
Recto-anal pathology	Fresh red blood on toilet paper, ±pain	Perianal tags, may have a tear or tenderness	Proctoscopy or sigmoidoscopy
Poor diet	Anorexia (eg post-op), low-fibre diet	Cachexia	↓Hb, ↓MCV, ↓Ca^{2+}
Drugs	Opiates, diuretics, aluminium/Ca^{2+} based drugs, iron, Ca^{2+} channel blockers, tricyclic antidepressants and anticholinergics		

Treatment

- ***Conservative*** good fluid intake, high-fibre diet, encourage mobilisation, review drugs – are there alternatives that do not affect bowel habit?
- ***Medical*** see laxatives opposite
- ***Surgical disimpaction*** literally scooping the hard faeces out of the rectum, should only be performed if requested by a senior

Poor diet

Aim for regular high-fibre meals, with good fluid intake
Symptoms nausea, vomiting, alcohol excess, malabsorption
Signs thin, dehydrated, post-op
Investigations FBC, U+E, TFT, Ca^{2+}
Treatment review diet, refer to dietician

Hints and tips

- Prescribe prophylactic laxatives for patients at risk of developing constipation (eg regular opiates, post-op)
- Exclude obstruction before prescribing a laxative
- Reassess if constipation does not resolve
- Consider malignancy in all patients >40yr presenting with altered bowel habit (see p421)

Anal fissures/haemorrhoids	p250	Bowel obstruction	p238
Inflammatory bowel disease	p259	Polyps	p250
Irritable bowel syndrome	p258	GI cancer	p424

Liver failure emergency

Airway	Check airway is patent; consider manoeuvres/adjuncts
Breathing	If no respiratory effort – **CALL ARREST TEAM**
Circulation	If no palpable pulse – **CALL ARREST TEAM**
Disability	If GCS ≤8 – **CALL ANAESTHETIST/ITU**

- Altered mental state and coagulopathy in the presence of jaundice
- Call for **senior help** early if patient deteriorating

Airway
- **Look** inside the mouth, wide-bore **suction** if secretions present
- **Jaw thrust**/head tilt/chin lift; **oro/nasopharyngeal** airway if tolerated

Breathing
- **15l/min** O_2 in all patients
- **Monitor** O_2 sats and RR

Circulation
- **Venous access**, take bloods:
  - FBC, U+E, LFT, INR, CRP, glucose, amylase, Ca^{2+}, Mg^{2+}, PO_4^{3-}, bld cultures, paracetamol levels, viral serology
- Start **IV fluids** 1l of 5% glucose over 4–6h
- **Monitor** HR, cardiac trace and BP

Disability
- Check blood **glucose** treat if <3.5mmol/l (p271)
- **Check** GCS, pupil reflexes, limb tone, plantar responses

Exposure
- Check **temp**
- Ask ward staff for a brief **history** or check notes
  - previous liver disease, likely causes
- **Examine** patient brief RS, CVS, abdo and neuro exam
  - signs of chronic liver disease
- **ECG, ABG** and urgent portable **CXR**
- **Stabilise** and treat, see following pages
- Call for **senior help** and arrange transfer to HDU/ITU
- **Reassess**, starting with A, B, C …

Causes of liver failure

Acute liver failure	Paracetamol overdose, drugs, toxins, viral hepatitis, autoimmune hepatitis, malignancy, ischaemic hepatitis (heart failure and shock), Budd–Chiari
Acute decompensated chronic liver disease	Alcohol excess, infection, GI bleeds, metabolic disturbances, sedatives, diuretics, acute illness, surgery, infection (spontaneous peritonitis)

Liver failure

Worrying features ↑HR, ↓BP, drowsiness, ↓GCS, bleeding, slurred speech, any neurology symptoms/signs, tremor/flap, renal failure

Think about *emergencies* acute liver failure, decompensated chronic liver disease, hepatic encephalopathy; ***acute liver failure*** paracetamol overdose (p306), viral hepatitis (A, B, C, E, CMV, EMV), pregnancy, medications (see below), toxins (eg poisonous mushrooms), vascular (eg Budd–Chiari), sepsis, Weil's disease, abscess, right heart failure; ***chronic liver failure*** alcohol, idiopathic, autoimmune, hepatitis (B±D, C), malignancy, Wilson's disease, haemochromatosis, α_1-antitrypsin deficiency

Drug-induced jaundice Antibiotics (co-amoxiclav, flucloxacillin, minocycline), NSAIDs, psych drugs (chlorpromazine, SSRIs), anti-epileptics (phenytoin, valproate), methyldopa, anti-TB drugs (isoniazid), statins, oestrogens

Ask about tiredness, jaundice (+onset), abdo pain, drowsiness, ±confusion, bruising, bleeding (skin, nose, bowel, urine), distension, ankle swelling, vomiting, rashes, recent infections (sore throat), weight loss, hair loss, darkening skin; ***PMH*** previous jaundice, gallstones, breathing problems, transfusions; ***DH*** paracetamol; ***FH*** liver disease, recent jaundice; ***SH*** alcohol, IVDU, tattoos, piercings, foreign travel, sexual activity (?abroad)

Obs temp, HR, BP, RR, O_2 sats, GCS, blood glucose, urine output

Look for volume status p319; ***acute liver failure*** drowsiness, confusion, slurred speech, jaundice, flapping tremor (asterixis), poor co-ordination, bruising, foetor hepaticus (sweet, faecal smell), lymphadenopathy, abdominal tenderness, hepatomegaly, ascites; ***chronic liver disease*** cachexia, palmar erythema, clubbing, xanthelasma, spider naevi, caput medusa, gynaecomastia, muscle wasting, splenomegaly, genital atrophy, track marks (IVDU), pneumonia/chronic lung disease, darkened skin

Investigations ***urine*** MSU; ***blds*** FBC, clotting, iron, ferritin, U+E, LFT, hepatitis serology (A, B+C), EBV and CMV serology, caeruloplasmin (if <50yr), autoimmune screen (antimitochondrial, antinuclear and anti-smooth muscle antibodies, p266), bld cultures; ***urgent USS abdo*** looking for metastases and dilated ducts; ***ascitic tap*** (p590) if ascites present; ***liver biopsy*** (percutaneous or transjugular) and ***CT abdo***

Grading of hepatic encephalopathy (West Haven criteria)

No detectable personality change	Grade 0
Altered mood or behaviour	Grade I
Mild drowsiness, confusion, slurred speech	Grade II
Stupor, very confused and restlessness, incoherent	Grade III
Coma	Grade IV

	History	Examination	Investigations
Hepatic jaundice	New jaundice	Jaundiced, ±RUQ pain and hepatomegaly	↑mixed bilirubin, ↑ALT/AST
Acute liver failure	New jaundice, drowsy, unwell	Signs of acute liver failure, altered mental state	↑mixed bilirubin, deranged ALT, ↑INR
Chronic liver failure	Previous liver problems, excess alcohol	Signs of chronic liver disease	Deranged LFT

Acute liver failure (*OHAM*2 p658)

Hepatic encephalopathy and coagulopathy in the presence of jaundice:

Types of acute liver failure	
Liver failure <7d of disease onset	Hyperacute fulminant hepatic failure
Liver failure 1–4wk of disease onset	Acute fulminant hepatic failure
Liver failure 4–12wk of disease onset	Subacute fulminant hepatic failure
Liver failure 12–26wk of disease onset	Late-onset hepatic failure

Symptoms jaundice, bruising/bleeding, drowsy, ±confusion, abdo pain

Signs ↑HR, ↓BP, ↓O_2 sats, ↓blood glucose, ↓urine output, signs of acute liver failure (p263)

Results ↑INR, deranged LFT, ↑bilirubin, ↑WCC, ↓glucose, ↓Mg^{2+}, ↓PO_4^{3-}, respiratory alkalosis, metabolic acidosis (bad sign), abnormal results specific to cause of liver failure

Treatment discuss with a senior early, often needs ITU/HDU with invasive monitoring, may need transfer to a specialist liver centre. Monitor blood glucose every 2h; insert a catheter and monitor fluid balance.

- *Raised INR* give one-off dose of vitamin K 10mg IV:
  - never give FFP without discussing with a senior because INR is used to monitor disease progress; it may be indicated if the patient is bleeding or needs invasive procedure
- *Stop* aspirin, NSAIDs and hepatotoxic drugs (see p263) and check other drugs in Appendix 2 of the *BNF*
- *Antibiotic* prophylaxis in all patients (eg cefotaxime) ±antifungals
- *Daily bloods* (FBC, U+E, LFT, INR)
- *Lactulose* 30–50ml/8h in all patients (helps remove ammonia)
- *Hypotensive* IV fluids, avoid Na^+ if chronic liver disease/ascites – salt-poor albumin is often used, contact blood bank
- *Hypoglycaemia* IV glucose, see p271

Complications cerebral oedema, bleeding, sepsis, renal failure, respiratory failure, ↓glucose, ↑Na^+, ↓K^+

Vascular liver disease

Diagnosed by Doppler USS; these diseases can cause hepatic jaundice or acute liver failure, often treated by endovascular methods:

- ***Budd–Chiari*** hepatic vein obstruction
- ***Portal vein** obstruction*
- ***Liver ischaemia*** due to hypotension and/or hepatic artery stenosis

Glandular fever (infectious mononucleosis, Epstein–Barr virus, EBV)

Symptoms usually young (10–30yr), sore throat >1wk, fever, lethargy, malaise, rash, lumps in the neck, anorexia

Signs red tonsils ±white exudate, tender lymphadenopathy, splenomegaly, rash (especially with amoxicillin/ampicillin), palatal petechiae, jaundice

Results ↑lymphocytes (atypical on film), ↑ALT, +ve Monospot/Paul Burnell, +ve IgM for EBV

Management rest, rehydration, analgesia, gargle with warm saline/aspirin, avoid amoxicillin/ampicillin, avoid alcohol, consider short course of oral steroids if very severe (eg hepatic encephalopathy)

Complications hepatitis, liver failure, thrombocytopenia, splenic rupture, haemolysis, encephalitis

Acute viral hepatitis (*OHCM*7 p394)

Causes hepatitis A,B,C and E, cytomegalovirus (CMV) and EBV

Symptoms jaundice, rash, diarrhoea, abdo pain, flu-like symptoms (eg fever, malaise, anorexia, fatigue, nausea, vomiting, arthralgia, sore throat)

Signs may have no signs, ↑temp, urticarial rash, jaundice, hepatomegaly, splenomegaly, lymphadenopathy

Results ↑WCC, ↑bilirubin, ↑AST/ALT, ±↑INR, +ve hepatitis serology

Management avoid alcohol, supportive treatment, monitor for progression to acute liver failure (opposite) which may need interferon-α

Complications acute liver failure, chronic disease

Chronic viral hepatitis (*OHCM*7 p394)

Lasts >6mth, ***causes*** hepatitis B (±D) and C

Symptoms and signs usually asymptomatic, signs of chronic liver disease

Results deranged LFT, ±↑INR, USS shows cirrhotic change, persistent raised viral serology

Treatment avoid alcohol, consider interferon-α therapy and ribavirin

Complications cirrhosis, hepatocellular carcinoma

Serology in hepatitis B

Surface antigen (HBsAg)	Active virus replication – acute or chronic disease
Anti-core (Anti-HBc) IgM	Acute infection
Anti-core (Anti-HBc) IgG	Chronic infection (or previous infection if HBsAg –ve)
'e' antigen (HBeAg)	High infectivity
Anti-e (Anti-HBe)	Low infectivity

Decompensated cirrhosis (chronic liver failure) (*OHCM*7 p252)

Symptoms jaundice, abdominal distension, itching, haematemesis, melaena; may be asymptomatic

Signs signs of chronic liver disease (p263), cachexic

Investigations LFT, FBC, clotting profile, immunoglobulins, autoantibodies, ferritin, transferrin saturation and α1-antitrypsin, ultrasound abdomen, ascitic tap, liver biopsy

Treatment avoid alcohol, NSAIDs, sedatives and opioids, refer to gastroenterologist and dietician, may need liver transplant

Ascites low salt diet, daily weights, spironolactone 100mg/24h PO increasing dose every 48h to 400mg/24h, may need furosemide, ascitic tap for diagnosis (p590) and to exclude spontaneous bacterial peritonitis, may need therapeutic paracentesis

Complications portal hypertension, bleeding varices, encephalopathy, hepatocellular carcinoma

Spontaneous bacterial peritonitis

Symptoms abdominal pain in the presence of ascites, associated with confusion, unwell, fever

Signs fever, ↑HR, ±↓BP, abdo tenderness, ± peritonitic

Results ↑WCC, ↑CRP, >250 white cells/mm^3 on ascitic tap (p590)

Treatment cefuroxime or ciprofloxacin

Autoimmune liver disease (*OHCM*7 p260)

Causes primary biliary cirrhosis, primary sclerosing cholangitis, autoimmune hepatitis (type I and II); primary biliary cirrhosis and type I autoimmune hepatitis may overlap

Symptoms often asymptomatic, may have fever, malaise, rash, joint pain or symptoms of chronic liver disease

Signs of chronic liver disease

Results deranged LFT, ±↑INR, USS and liver biopsy, autoantibodies (see table below)

Treatment ***autoimmune hepatitis*** prednisolone 30mg/24h PO initially then azathioprine; ***other diseases*** see p631

Complications acute liver failure, cirrhosis, hepatocellular carcinoma

Autoantibodies and HLA tests in autoimmune liver disease

Primary biliary cirrhosis	Anti-mitochondrial (AMA)
Primary sclerosing cholangitis	Anti-smooth muscle (SMA), antinuclear (ANA), p-ANCA
Autoimmune hepatitis type I	Anti-smooth muscle (SMA), antinuclear (ANA)
Autoimmune hepatitis type II (children only)	Anti-liver/kidney microsomal type 1 (LKM1)

Haemochromatosis (*OHCM*7 p254)

Autosomal-recessive disease causing excess iron absorption.

Symptoms fatigue, lethargy, arthralgia, hyperpigmentation, DM, family history of haemochromatosis

Signs arthralgia, hepatomegaly, signs of chronic liver disease, cardiac failure, osteoporosis, tanned skin

Results ↑AST/ALT, ↑glucose, ↑↑ferritin, ↑transferrin saturation, cardiomyopathy on ECG/echo, liver biopsy (diagnosis, severity), genetic test

Treatment venesection (1unit/wk) until ferritin normalises then every 3–6mth. Transferrin saturation can be used to screen relatives.

α_1-Antitrypsin deficiency (*OHCM*7 p256)

Genetic disease with complex inheritance causing liver and lung damage.

Symptoms breathlessness, liver failure, family history

Signs emphysema, signs of chronic liver disease

Results ↓α_1-antitrypsin levels, liver biopsy, genetic test

Treatment stop smoking, may need liver transplant, COPD treatment

Wilson's disease (*OHCM*7 p257)

Autosomal-recessive disease; copper accumulates in the liver and CNS.

Symptoms tremor, slurred speech, abnormal movements, clumsiness, depression, personality change, psychosis, liver failure, family history

Signs Kaiser–Fleischer rings in eyes, signs of liver failure

Results ↓caeruloplasmin, ↓total serum copper, ↑serum free copper, ↑24h urinary copper excretion (especially if a dose of penicillamine is given), copper on liver biopsy, positive genetic test

Treatment lifelong penicillamine, may need liver transplant, screen relatives

Weil's disease (leptospirosis)

Bacterial infection transmitted via rat urine, often via water and skin cuts.

Symptoms recent contact with water, flu-like symptoms: fever, malaise, anorexia, fatigue, nausea, vomiting, arthralgia, sore throat followed by neck pain, photophobia, jaundice, bleeding and kidney failure

Signs acute liver failure, meningism, bruising, tender RUQ, conjunctivitis, myocarditis

Results haematuria (dipstick), ↓Hb (haemolytic), ↑urea, ↑creatinine, ↑bilirubin, ↑ALT, positive serology or urine culture

Treatment doxycycline 100mg/12h PO or benzylpenicillin 600mg/6h IV and supportive care of renal/liver failure

Jaundice

Worrying features ↑HR, ↓BP, drowsiness, ↓GCS, bleeding, slurred speech, poor coordination, tremor/flap, renal failure, weight loss

Think about

- ***Pre-hepatic*** Gilbert's syndrome, haemolysis, malaria
- ***Hepatic*** paracetamol overdose, viral hepatitis, alcohol, chronic liver disease, pregnancy, medications (p263), toxins (eg poisonous mushrooms), vascular disease (eg ischaemia, Budd–Chiari), sepsis
- ***Cholestatic*** choledocholithiasis (gallstones in common bile duct), ascending cholangitis, pancreatic cancer, cholangiocarcinoma, primary biliary cirrhosis, primary sclerosing cholangitis

Ask about tiredness, jaundice (+onset), abdo pain, itching, dark urine, pale stools, drowsiness, confusion, bruising, bleeding (skin, nose, bowel, urine), bloating, vomiting, rashes, recent infections (sore throat), weight loss, generalised aching, hair loss, darkening skin, joint pain; ***PMH*** previous jaundice, gallstones, breathing problems, transfusions; ***DH*** paracetamol and medications on p263; ***FH*** liver disease, recent jaundice; ***SH*** alcohol, IVDU, tattoos, piercings, foreign travel, sexual activity (?abroad)

Obs temp, RR, HR, BP, urine output, O_2 sats, glucose, GCS

Look for volume status p319, bruising, evidence of bleeding, drowsiness, confusion:

- ***Pre-hepatic*** splenomegaly, pale conjunctiva, breathlessness
- ***Hepatic*** signs of acute or chronic liver failure p263
- ***Cholestatic*** abdominal tenderness, ±peritonism, Charcot's triad (fever, jaundice and RUQ pain = cholangitis), palpable gallbladder

Initial investigations ***urine*** MSU, bilirubin, urobilinogen; ***blds*** FBC, reticulocytes, blood film, clotting, U+E, LFT, amylase, lipase, LDH, paracetamol levels, hepatitis serology (A, B, C), EBV and CMV serology, bld cultures; ***urgent USS abdo*** dilated bile ducts, cirrhosis, metastases

	Urine	Liver tests	Other tests
Pre-hepatic jaundice	Urobilinogen	↑unconjugated bilirubin	↓Hb, ↔MCV, ↓haptoglobulin, ↑reticulocytes
Hepatic jaundice	Urobilinogen	↑mixed bilirubin, ↑ALT/AST	May have positive hepatitis serology or iparacetamol levels
Obstructive jaundice	Bilirubin, dark urine	↑conjugated bilirubin, ↑ALP, ↑γGT	Dilated biliary ducts on USS
Cholangitis	Bilirubin, dark urine	↑conjugated bilirubin, ↑ALP, ↑γGT	↑WCC, ↑CRP, dilated biliary ducts

Haemolysis	p334	Hepatic jaundice	p263
Acute liver failure	p264		

Gilbert's syndrome

Common genetic disease causing a rise in unconjugated bilirubin with acute illness, no progression to liver failure.

Choledocholithiasis

Gallstone in common bile duct, ±causing obstructive jaundice
Risk factors female, pregnant, DM, obesity
Symptoms often none, preceding biliary colic, dark urine, pale stool
Signs jaundice, mild RUQ tenderness
Results ↑ALP, ↑bilirubin, dilated bile duct on USS, ERCP, MRCP
Treatment maintain hydration, exclude pancreatitis and cholangitis, prophylactic antibiotics (eg cefuroxime 1.5g/8h IV and metronidazole 500mg/8h IV), urgent ERCP (diagnosis and stone removal), cholecystectomy once jaundice resolved
Complications pancreatitis, cholangitis, hepatitis, clotting defects

Cholangitis

Infection of the bile duct with Charcot's triad: fever, jaundice, RUQ pain
Symptoms unwell, abdo pain, rigors, jaundice
Signs ↑temp, ↑HR, ±↓BP, RUQ tenderness
Results ↑WCC, ↑CRP, ↑bilirubin, urgent USS
Treatment cefuroxime 1.5g/8h IV and metronidazole 500mg/8h IV, may need an urgent ERCP if gallstones are in the common bile duct

Primary biliary cirrhosis (*OHCM*7 p258)

Inflammation and damage of the interlobular bile ducts.
Symptoms and signs fatigue, itching, cholestatic jaundice, cirrhosis, IBD
Results ↑ALP, ↑γGT, ±↑bilirubin, anti-mitochondrial antibodies (AMA), ↑IgM, USS, ERCP, liver biopsy shows granulomas
Treatment ursodeoxycholic acid, replace fat-soluble vitamins (A, D, E, K) colestyramine 4–8g/24h PO for itching, may need liver transplant

Primary sclerosing cholangitis (*OHCM*7 p259)

Inflammation and fibrosis of intra- and extrahepatic bile ducts.
Symptoms and signs chronic biliary obstruction leading to cirrhosis, IBD
Results ↑ALP, ±↑bilirubin, ↑immunoglobulin levels, anti-smooth muscle antibodies (SMA), antinuclear antibodies (ANA), p-ANCA, HLA-A1, B8 + DR3, ERCP shows multiple strictures, fibrosis on liver biopsy
Treatment steroids, ursodeoxycholic acid may help symptoms, may need stenting or liver transplant

Cholangiocarcinoma (*OHCM*7 p262)

Tumour of the bile duct.
Symptoms and signs fever, weight loss, malaise, abdominal pain, jaundice; *Courvoisier's law* an enlarged gallbladder in the presence of jaundice is not caused by gallstones (suggests pancreatic or biliary cancer)
Investigations ↑ALP, ↑bilirubin, LFT, CA19.9, USS, ERCP, ±biopsy
Treatment surgery, palliative stenting by ERCP

Hypoglycaemia emergency

Airway	Check airway is patent; consider manoeuvres/adjuncts
Breathing	If no respiratory effort – **CALL ARREST TEAM**
Circulation	If no palpable pulse – **CALL ARREST TEAM**
Disability	If GCS ≤8 – **CALL ANAESTHETIST**

- Call for senior help early if patient deteriorating
- Blood glucose is normally >3.5mmol/l
- Poorly controlled diabetics can have symptoms of hypoglycaemia with a glucose >3.5mmol/l

Coma or low GCS with low glucose

- Protect airway
- **15l/min O_2** in all patients
- Establish **venous access** unless already present
- Give **IV glucose** stat (50ml of 50%, 100ml of 20% or 200ml of 10%)
- For large insulin overdoses give 1mg **glucagon** SC/IM/IV
- Begin to follow **emergency protocol** on **p280** (low GCS)
- If hypoglycaemia is responsible, GCS should return to 15 in <10min
- Start **1l 10% glucose/4–8h IV**, adjust rate to keep glucose >5mmol/l
- **Monitor finger-prick glucose** every 30min–1h until patient stable
- Attempt to determine the **cause** of the hypoglycaemia
- Call for **senior help**
- **Reassess**, starting with A, B, C; if no improvement see p162

GCS 15/15 with low glucose

- Give at least 120ml Lucozade® or a single dose of **Hypostop®** gel (**GlucoGel®**) orally (this will only last up to an hour, so give a sandwich too)
- **Monitor finger-prick glucose** 1–2h until stable, aim for >5mmol/l
- For persistent hypoglycaemia give **1l 10% glucose/6–8h IV**
- Attempt to determine the **cause** of the hypoglycaemia

Life-threatening causes

- Insulin overdose
- Oral hypoglycaemia overdose
- Sepsis
- Alcohol excess
- Acute liver failure

Hypoglycaemia

> **Worrying features** Worrying features unconscious, low GCS, recurrent, not diabetic

Think about ***most likely*** excess insulin or oral hypoglycaemics in a diabetic or accidental dose in non-diabetic, alcohol; ***other*** dumping syndrome (post-gastric surgery), liver failure, adrenal failure (Addison's), pituitary insufficiency, sepsis, insulinomas, other neoplasia, malaria

Ask about sweating, hunger, exercise, recent food, previous hypos, usual blood sugars, seizures, weight loss, tiredness, anxiety, palpitations; ***PMH*** DM, gastric surgery, liver or endocrine disease; ***DH*** insulin dose, oral hypoglycaemic dose; ***SH*** alcohol

Obs HR, BP, RR, temp, GCS, recent and current blood glucose

Look for pale, sweating, tremor, slurred speech, focal neurology (can be severe, eg hemiplegia), low GCS, abdo scars, pigmented scars, jaundice, spider naevi, hepatomegaly

Investigations ***finger-prick glucose*** – if the result is unexpected (eg non-diabetic) ask for a repeat on a different machine and send a blood sample in a fluoride oxalate (p557) tube for a laboratory glucose result. If the patient is ***not diabetic*** send samples for FBC, U+E, LFT, glucose, insulin and C-peptide prior to correcting hypoglycaemia, but do not let this delay your treatment; consider thick and thin films for malaria.

Further investigations hypoglycaemia is very rare in a non-diabetic in the absence of alcohol. The investigation of choice is glucose, insulin and C-peptide levels after a 72h observed fast. Gut hormones may also be requested. See *OHCM*7 p198.

Treatment follow the treatment plans on the opposite page.

DM A single episode of mild hypoglycaemia should not prompt a change of medication. If the patient is having regular hypos then consider a dose reduction. Reduce insulin doses by 20%, consult *BNF* to reduce the doses of oral hypoglycaemics. Ensure the patient is aware of the sick day rules (p276).

Alcohol hypoglycaemia following alcohol should not be recurrent unless alcohol consumption is recurrent. Once the patient's blood sugars are stable they can be discharged unless other problems.

Dumping syndrome fast passage of food into the small intestine following gastric surgery can cause fluid shifts and rapid glucose absorption. Excessive insulin secretion results in rebound hypoglycaemia 1–3h after a meal. A diet low in glucose and high in fibre will improve the condition.

Neoplasia refer to surgeons

Addison's/pituitary failure	p421/117
Sepsis	p392
Acute liver failure	p264

Hyperglycaemia emergency

Airway	Check airway is patent; consider manoeuvres/adjuncts
Breathing	If no respiratory effort – **CALL ARREST TEAM**
Circulation	If no palpable pulse – **CALL ARREST TEAM**
Disability	If GCS ≤8 – **CALL ANAESTHETIST**

Call for **senior help** early if patient deteriorating

Diabetic ketoacidosis (DKA) – type 1 DM, pH <7.3, ketonuria

- **15l/min O_2** in all patients
- Establish **venous access**, take bloods:
  - FBC, U+E, glucose, osmolality, HCO_3^-, bld cultures
- Give **1l 0.9% saline IV** stat
- Check **finger-prick glucose** and dipstick **urine** for ketones
- Start a **sliding scale**, see p275
- **Arterial blood gas;** if pH <7.0 get senior help
- **Monitor** U+E, glucose and venous HCO_3^- hourly, K^+ will fall unless replaced
- Further management, p274; attempt to **determine the cause**
- Call for **senior help**
- **Reassess**, starting with A, B, C …

HONK – type 2 DM, plasma osmolality >340 mosmol/kg, glucose >35mmol/l

- **15l/min O_2** in all patients
- Establish **venous access**, take bloods:
  - FBC, U+E, glucose, osmolality, bld cultures
- Give **1l 0.9% saline IV** over 30min
- Check **finger-prick glucose**
- Start a **sliding scale** if glucose still raised after 1h of fluids, see p275
- **Monitor** U+E and glucose
- Further management, p274; attempt to **determine the cause**
- Call for **senior help**
- **Reassess**, starting with A, B, C …

Life-threatening precipitants of DKA/HONK

- Sepsis
- MI
- Trauma/surgery
- Other acute illness

Hyperglycaemia

Worrying features ↓GCS, ketones in urine, acidosis, vomiting

Think about *emergencies* diabetic ketoacidosis (DKA), hyperglycaemic hyperosmolar non-ketosis (HONK); ***common*** after sugary food, steroids, non-compliance with diabetic treatment, infection or acute illness in diabetics, severe illness

Ask about tiredness, thirst, polyuria, frequency, dysuria, urgency, weight loss, vomiting, breathlessness, rashes, lumps, teeth problems, cough, sputum, chest pain, abdo pain, recent surgery; ***PMH*** DM; ***DH*** insulin dose, oral hypoglycaemic dose, steroids; ***SH*** alcohol

Obs temp, RR, GCS, recent and current blood glucose, fluid balance

Look for volume status (p319), signs of infection, check skin thoroughly (including perineum) for abscesses or rashes, look in mouth for dental infection, sweet-smelling breath, chest for poor air entry or creps, abdominal tenderness

Investigations ***finger-prick glucose*** repeat if result unexpected; ***urine dipstick*** ketones, evidence of infection; ***blds*** send if patient is unwell, has persistent hyperglycaemia (over 48h) or has urinary ketones (type 1 DM), request FBC, U+E, LFT, osmolality, HCO_3^- (venous), blood cultures; ***ABGs*** if the patient is unwell, look for pH <7.3 in type 1 DM; ***ECG/CXR*** if treatment has been required

Treatment a single episode of mild hyperglycaemia in an otherwise well patient is unlikely to suggest underlying pathology. DKA takes hours to days to develop whilst HONK takes days to weeks.

Type 1 diabetic Check finger-prick glucose and urine. Glucose is usually high in DKA but may be transiently normal soon after a dose of insulin. Assess volume status (p319) and check if the urine contains ketones. If unwell proceed with the treatment plan for DKA. Otherwise send a venous sample for pH/HCO_3^-; if normal this excludes DKA. Persistent hyperglycaemia should prompt a change to the insulin regime by ↑ doses by 20% and monitoring of blood glucose.

Type 2 diabetic Check finger-prick glucose and urine. The glucose must be raised for a diagnosis of HONK. If unwell follow the treatment plan for HONK initially. Otherwise monitor glucose levels every 6h for 48h, increase oral/IV fluid intake and reassess. DKA can occur in type 2 diabetics on insulin but it is very unusual (a small amount of insulin inhibits ketone production). For persistent hyperglycaemia increase the dose of hypoglycaemic medication or insulin with frequent finger-prick glucose checks.

Non-diabetic patients New diabetics often present with DKA/HONK; have a low threshold for starting the treatment plans opposite. Hyperglycaemia can also be precipitated by steroids and stress, eg severe illness or surgery.

DKA post-emergency (*OHAM*7 p814)

Stabilise the patient as shown on the treatment plan, p272:

- Continue IV fluids, see regime below or ask a senior
- Monitor U+E every 1–2h and add 20mmol/l KCl after the first litre of fluid even if the plasma K^+ is normal, the patient is likely to be K^+ depleted from their illness. Use 40mmol/l KCl if ↓K^+.
- Monitor glucose, osmolality and HCO_3^- every 1–2h
- Check venous pH if not improving
- If severely ill: catheterise, consider admission to HDU or ITU and an arterial and/or central line
- NG tube if GCS <15
- Nil by mouth for at least 12h
- Infection is common and patient may be asymptomatic, check blood cultures, MSU and CXR; have a low threshold for starting antibiotics (p156)
- Check an ECG to exclude MI as a precipitant
- Give prophylactic LMWH SC (p346)
- Convert to SC insulin once eating and urinary ketones ≤1

Excess or excessively fast fluid replacement can lead to potentially fatal cerebral oedema

DKA fluids 1l stat, 1l over 1h, 1l over 2h, 1l over 4h and 1l over 6h; tailor to the patient according to volume status and weight. Initially use 0.9% saline and convert to dextrose saline or 5% glucose if glucose <15mmol/l. Add 20–40mmol/l KCl to second and following bags as determined by U+E, ↓K^+ will develop otherwise. Monitor fluid balance and assess volume status (p319) for signs of overload.

Precipitants of DKA/HONK poor compliance/incorrect insulin dose, alcohol, infections (chest, UTI, abscesses, dental problems), MI, CVA, surgery, trauma, acute illness

HONK post-emergency (*OHAM*7 p816)

Stabilise the patient as shown on the treatment plan, p272:

- Continue IV fluid replacement at half the rate used in DKA
- Monitor U+E, glucose and osmolality every 2h
- May have spurious hyponatraemia due to excess glucose, call senior help if ↑Na^+ at any stage
- If severely ill: catheterise, consider admission to HDU or ITU and an arterial and/or central line
- NG tube if GCS <15
- Nil by mouth for at least 12h
- Septic screen and antibiotics as indicated
- ECG and look for an underlying cause (see box)
- Give prophylactic LMWH SC (p346)
- Convert to insulin/oral hypoglycaemics when glucose <12mmol/l

Sliding scales

These give strict monitoring and control of a diabetic patient's glucose levels. They are used in the treatment of DKA, HONK and for surgery on diabetics (see below). They are also used when serious illness disrupts diabetic control, eg post-MI.

You need to prescribe both the insulin infusion with appropriate IV fluids on the infusions section of the drug card. Use 5–10% glucose with 20mmol/l KCl, unless you are treating DKA or HONK in which case 0.9% saline is used until the glucose is <15mmol/l. Further IV fluids can be prescribed alongside a sliding scale at a slower rate to allow for the extra IV fluid infusion (p323).

Date	Route	Fluid	Additives	Vol	Rate	Signature
18.9.08	*IV*	*0.9% saline*	*50unit Actrapid*	*50ml*	*Sliding Scale*	*Dr C J Flint*
18.9.08	*IV*	*5% glucose*	*20mmol KCl*	*1l*	*8h*	*Dr C J Flint*

Example of sliding scale regime, check local policy

Insulin	Date	Start time	BM (mmol/l)	Rate (ml/h)
Actrapid	*18.09.08*	*13:45*	<4	*Stop – call doctor*
Dose	**Route**	**Check BM**	4–7	*1*
1unit/ml	*IV*	*1h*	7.1–11	*2*
	Signature		11.1–20	*4*
	Dr C J Flint		>20	*7 – call doctor*

If the sliding scale is not controlling blood glucose levels then check the infusion pump and cannula; if no problems found double the doses and check venous bicarbonate (type 1) or osmolality (type 2). If the finger-prick glucose is <4mmol/l check that there is 5–10% glucose running, increase the fluid rate and/or glucose concentration (up to 10%); recheck glucose in 30min. If persistently <4mmol/l consider halving the doses. If glucose <2 see p271.

Prescribing insulin

Most hospitals have separate drug cards for prescribing insulin. Check the patient's usual doses and write up accordingly, for example:

Breakfast	Insulin	Dose	Route	Start
	Mixtard 30	*18unit*	*SC*	*18.9.08*
Night	Insulin	Dose	Route	Start
	Mixtard 30	*10unit*	*SC*	*18.9.08*

Diabetes mellitus

- ***Type 1*** (insulin dependent – IDDM) an autoimmune disease that can occur at any age – always needs lifelong insulin
- ***Type 2*** (non-insulin dependent – NIDDM) caused by insulin resistance or hyposecretion – tends to occur in the elderly and overweight
- ***Impaired glucose tolerance (IGT)*** abnormal glucose tolerance test but below diabetic criteria – DM often develops
- ***Impaired fasting glucose (IFG)*** raised glucose levels after an overnight fast, but below criteria for DM – may develop into DM
- ***Gestational*** transient insulin resistance during pregnancy (p439)

Acute type 1 DM *(OHCM7 p190)*

Symptoms tiredness, weight loss, thirst, polyuria, abdo pain, vomiting
Signs cachexia, sweet-smelling breath, shock, acute abdomen
Investigations random glucose >11.1mmol/l, fasting blood glucose ≥7mmol/l (after an overnight fast). Check plasma HCO_3^-, venous pH and urine (glucose, ketones) to exclude DKA. Islet cell antibodies and HbA_{1C}.
Treatment resuscitate and investigate for DKA initially; monitor finger-prick glucose ≥4 times a day after starting a suitable insulin regime (discuss with a senior). Refer to a diabetic nurse specialist and arrange outpatient follow-up.

Properties of common subcutaneous insulins

Name	Type of insulin	Onset	Peak	Duration
Short-acting				
NovoRapid®	Aspart	15min	0.5–1.5h	5h
Humalog®	Lispro	15min	0.5–1.5h	5h
Actrapid®	Soluble	30min	2–4h	8h
Intermediate and long-acting				
Insulatard®	Isophane	2h	6–12h	24h
Lantus®	Glargine	1h	1–24h	24h
Levemir®	Detemir	1h	1–24h	24h
Mixtures (biphasic)				
Mixtard 30®	30% soluble 70% isophane	30min	2–12h	24h

Sick day rules

Educate diabetic patients what to do if they are feeling unwell:

- Never stop taking your insulin or tablets (may need to increase dose)
- Test your blood for glucose at least 4 times a day
- Test your urine for glucose (and ketones if on insulin)
- Drink plenty of fluids
- If not eating try milk, soup, fruit juice or fizzy drinks instead
- Contact your GP if you cannot keep fluids down

Acute type 2 DM (*OHCM*7 p190)

Symptoms as for type 1, but can also present with diabetic complications, eg visual problems, neuropathy, MI, claudication, confusion, coma
Signs foot ulcers, infections, peripheral neuropathy, poor visual acuity and retinopathy, evidence of cardiovascular disease
Investigations suspect if a random glucose is >11.1mmol/l or glycosuria. Confirm with a fasting blood glucose ≥7mmol/l (eg after an overnight fast); an HbA_{1C} >7% makes DM very likely. If there is doubt or fasting glucose is ≥6.1–7mmol/l perform an oral glucose tolerance test.
Oral glucose tolerance test check fasting blood glucose after an overnight fast; give 75g glucose in 300ml water then repeat glucose after 2h

Interpretation of oral glucose tolerance test

Fasting glucose	Glucose after 2h	Diagnosis
Any	≥11.1mmol/l	DM
≥7mmol/l	Any	DM
<7mmol/l	7.8–11.0mmol/l	Impaired glucose tolerance (IGT)
6.1–6.9mmol/l	≤7.7mmol/l	Impaired fasting glucose (IFG)
<6.1mmol/l	≤7.7mmol/l	Normal

Treatment type 2 DM may initially be controlled by a healthy diet with minimal rapid-release carbohydrates (eg sugary drinks, sweets) and weight loss. Oral tablets and insulin may be required.

Chronic management p471 and *OHCM*7 p192

Common oral hypoglycaemics for type 2 DM

Class	Examples	Comment
Biguanides	Metformin	Increase glucose uptake and reduce appetite; avoid if any renal failure
Sulphonylureas	Gliclazide	Stimulate remaining cells but cause weight gain
Thiazolidinediones	Pioglitazone	Reduces insulin resistance

Treatment options in IGT and IFG and DM

	IGT and IFG	Type 2			Type 1
		Step 1	Step 2	Step 3	
Insulin				✓	✓
Oral hypoglycaemics			✓	✓	
Diet and exercise	✓	✓	✓	✓	✓

Complications of type 1 + 2 DM

DKA, HONK, atheroma (MI, limb ischaemia, bowel ischaemia), CVA, neuropathy, nephropathy, retinopathy, glaucoma, cataracts, retinal bleeds, leg ulcers, infections, hypoglycaemia

Coma and reduced GCS emergency

Airway	Check airway is patent; consider manoeuvres/adjuncts
Breathing	If no respiratory effort – **CALL ARREST TEAM**
Circulation	If no palpable pulse – **CALL ARREST TEAM**
Disability	If GCS ≤8 – **CALL ANAESTHETIST**

Call for **senior help** early if patient deteriorating

Airway and C-spine
- Stabilise **cervical spine** if there is any risk of injury (eg fall)
- **Look** inside the mouth, remove obvious objects/dentures
- Wide-bore **suction** under direct vision if secretions present
- **Jaw thrust**/chin lift; **oro/nasopharyngeal** airway if tolerated

Breathing
- **15l/min O_2** in all patients
- If hypoxic see p219
- **Monitor** O_2 sats and RR
- **Bag and mask** ventilation if poor/absent respiratory effort

Circulation
- **Venous access**, take bloods:
  - FBC, U+E, LFT, glucose, Ca^{2+}, cardiac markers, clotting, G+S, bld cultures, paracetamol, salicylate and alcohol levels
- **ECG** and treat arrhythmias (tachy p186, brady p194)
- Start **IV fluids** if shocked
- **Monitor** HR, cardiac trace and BP

Disability
- Check blood **glucose**
- Check **drug card** especially for opiates and benzodiazepines
- Control **seizures** (p286)
- **Check** GCS, pupil reflexes, limb tone, plantar responses
  - **Look for** brainstem, lateralising or meningeal signs (see opposite)
- Call **anaesthetist** for intubation if GCS ≤8

Exposure
- Check **temp**
- **Look** over whole body for evidence of injury or rashes

- Ask ward staff for a brief **history** or check notes
- **Examine** patient brief RS, CVS, abdo and neuro exam
- **ABG,** but don't leave the patient alone
- Request urgent portable **CXR**
- **Stabilise** and treat, see following pages
- Call for **senior help**
- **Reassess,** starting with A, B, C …

Acute confusion

- ***Confusion*** acute deficit in thinking, memory, orientation or awareness
- ***Off-legs*** medical slang for acute inability to walk in the elderly
- ***Acopia*** medical slang for elderly patients no longer coping at home
- ***Dementia*** chronic deficit in thinking, memory and/or personality
- ***Delirium*** acute onset confusion with hallucinations or illusions
- ***Psychosis*** hallucinations or illusions without confusion

Think about *emergencies* ↓O_2, ↑CO_2, MI, sepsis, intracranial bleed, meningitis, encephalitis, ↑ICP, CVA, arrhythmia; ***common*** infection, metabolic (glucose, Na^+, Ca^{2+}, kidney/liver failure), drug toxicity (opioids, benzodiazepines, post-GA), heart failure, head injury, alcohol withdrawal or intoxication, endocrine, malignancy, post-ictal, B_{12} deficiency, Korsakoff's (amnesia due to ↓thiamine/B_1); ***chronic*** dementia
Ask about use direct questions about how they are at the moment; further history from the ward staff, relatives, notes or residential/nursing home: speed of onset, chest pain, cough, sputum, dysuria, frequency, incontinence, head injury, headache, photophobia, vomiting, dizziness; ***PMH*** DM, heart, lung, liver or kidney problems, epilepsy, dementia, psychiatric illness; ***DH*** benzodiazepines, opioids, steroids, NSAIDs, β-blockers, psychiatric drugs; ***SH*** alcohol, recreational drugs, usual mobility and state
Obs GCS, temp, HR, BP, RR, O_2 sats
Look for cyanosis, pulse (HR and rhythm), unequal air entry, bronchial breathing, creps, abdo pain, signs of head injury, neck stiffness, photophobia, focal neurology, pupil responses, papilloedema, tone and reflexes, record score on abbreviated mental test score
Investigations ***urine*** dipstick, M,C+S; ***blds*** FBC, U+E, LFT, CRP, glucose, Ca^{2+}, cardiac markers, blood cultures, consider amylase, Mg^{2+}, TFT, B_{12}, folate; ***ABGs*** ↓O_2 or ↑CO_2; ***ECG*** arrhythmias; ***CXR*** infection or aspiration; ***CT*** if focal neurology or non-resolving confusion; ***LP*** if CT normal

Abbreviated Mental Test Score (AMTS) ≥8 is normal for an elderly patient

Age	1	Recognise two people (eg Dr, nurse)	1
Date of birth	1	Year World War Two ended (1945)	1
Repeat: '42 West Street'	0	Who is on the throne (Elizabeth II)	1
Year	1	Count backwards from 20 to 1	1
Time (nearest hour)	1	Recall: '42 West Street'	1
Name of hospital	1	Total:	10

Management

- Nurse in a well-lit, quiet environment visible from nurse's desk
- Ask relatives/friends to stay with them
- See p309 if sedation is required for investigation and treatment
- Investigate and treat the cause, infection is the most common

Chronic confusion and dementia

Worrying features rapid progression, <65yr

Think about ***common*** Alzheimer's, Lewy body disease, frontotemporal dementia (Pick's), vascular dementia, Parkinson's, normal pressure hydrocephalus, depression, subdural haematoma; ***rare*** HIV, syphilis, schizophrenia, space-occupying lesions, hypothyroid, B_{12} deficiency, malnutrition, renal failure, liver failure, excess alcohol
Ask about age of onset, progression, memory (short and long term), personality, thinking, planning, judgement, language, visuospatial skills, concentration, social behaviour, confusion, wandering, falls, head injury, tremor, mood, sleep quality, delusions, halluzcinations, constipation, cold intolerance, hearing, sight; ***PMH*** seizures, CVA/TIA; ***DH*** regular medications, sleeping tablets, anticholinergics; ***FH*** dementia, neurological problems; ***SH*** effect on work, effect on relationships, effect on social abilities, who do they live with, support, ability to cope with ADLs (food, cleaning, washing, dressing, toilet), finances, alcohol intake
Obs GCS, HR, BP, glucose
Look for Mini-Mental State Examination (opposite), Abbreviated Mental Test Score (p281), full systems exam and careful neurological exam including general appearance, tremor, gait, cog-wheeling, dysphasia
Investigations FBC, ESR, U+E, LFT, Ca^{2+}, TFT, B_{12}, folate, CT/MRI brain, consider HIV, VDRL/THPA, CXR, ECG, LP, EEG

Management

- Refer to a psychogeriatrician for diagnosis and management
- Aim of investigations is to rule out reversible causes

Dementia

Progressive cognitive impairment with normal consciousness.
Causes Alzheimer's, Lewy body disease, frontotemporal dementia (Pick's), vascular dementia
Symptoms memory impairment (short term>long term), behavioural and personality changes (wandering, aggression, disinhibition), clumsiness, unawareness of problems, poor concentration
Signs neglect, score <25 on the MMSE p283
Results MRI may show characteristic features of specific dementia
Management multi-disciplinary team approach to ensure that the patient has appropriate accommodation and is able to cope with activities of daily living (ADLs). Anticholinesterase drugs eg donepezil help to slow Alzheimer's; there is NICE guidance available.

Normal pressure hydrocephalus

Symptoms and signs apraxic gait (inability to lift legs despite normal power, 'stuck to the floor'), dementia, urinary/faecal incontinence
Management enlarged ventricles seen on CT/MRI, normal pressure on LP, walking speed improves with removing CSF, treated with a ventricular peritoneal (VP) shunt

Mini-Mental State Examination (MMSE)

This is a standardised means of assessing the memory and cognition of a patient and can be used over time to monitor changes. Results are unreliable if the patient is delirious or has an affective disorder. An abbreviated (10 point) version is often used (p281).

The maximum score is 30, though ≥28 is regarded as 'normal', assuming the patient has been taught to read and write in English. Scores of 25–27 are borderline and <25 suggests dementia.

What day of the week is it?	1 point
What is the date today?	1 point
What is the month?	1 point
What is the year?	1 point
Which season of the year is it?	1 point
What country are we in?	1 point
What town/city are we in?	1 point
What are the two main streets nearby?	1 point
What floor of the building are we on?	1 point
What is the name of this place?	1 point
Read the following. Then offer the paper: 'I am going to give you a piece of paper. Take it in your right hand, fold it in half and place it on your lap.'	1 point for each of three actions
Show a pencil and ask what it is called	1 point
Show a wrist-watch and ask what it is called	1 point
Say: 'Repeat after me. No ifs, ands, or buts.'	1 point
Say: 'Read what is written here and do as it says.' Show them a card which reads 'CLOSE YOUR EYES'	1 point
Say: 'Write a complete sentence on this sheet of paper.'	1 point
Say: 'Here is a drawing, please copy it.' [See drawing at bottom of page]	1 point
Say: 'I am going to name three objects. When I have finished repeat them back to me, and remember them as I am going to ask you to say them again in a few minutes. Apple, penny, table.'	1 point for each object repeated
Say: 'I want you to take 7 away from 100. Take 7 away from that number and keep subtracting until I say stop.' [100, 93, 86, 79, 72, 65]	1 point for each of 5 subtractions
What were the objects I asked you to remember? [Apple, penny, table]	1 point for each object

Close your eyes

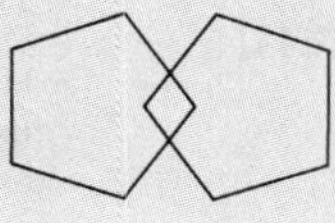

Adult seizures emergency

Airway	Check airway is patent; consider manoeuvres/adjuncts
Breathing	If no respiratory effort – **CALL ARREST TEAM**
Circulation	If no palpable pulse – **CALL ARREST TEAM**
Disability	If GCS ≤8 – **CALL ANAESTHETIST**

Call for **senior help** if seizure >5min

0–5min

- Start **timing**; this is very important and easy to forget
- Insert a **Guedel** or nasopharyngeal airway
- **15l/min O_2** in all patients
- Keep patient safe and put into **recovery position** if possible
- **Monitor** HR, O_2 sats, BP, cardiac trace, temp
- **Venous access** (after 3–4min). Take bloods:
  - FBC, U+E, LFT, Ca^{2+}, glucose, bld cultures, anticonvulsant levels
- **Check GLUCOSE**: if <3.5mmol/l give 100ml of 20% dextrose stat

5–20min

- Call for **senior help** and attach a cardiac monitor
- If IV access: **lorazepam** 4mg IV over 2min, repeat at 10min if no effect
- If no IV access: diazepam 10mg PR, repeat up to 30mg if no effect
- Ask ward staff about **history**/check notes
- If alcoholism/malnourished give **Pabrinex®** 2 pairs IV over 10min if not already given this admission

20–40min

- Call for **anaesthetist** and senior help
- If not taking phenytoin: **phenytoin** 15mg/kg IV at 50mg/min
- If taking phenytoin: phenobarbital 10mg/kg IV over 10min
- **Monitor** ECG, BP and temp

>40min

- **Thiopental** or propofol on ITU/HDU
- Transfer to **ITU** for general anaesthetic and EEG monitoring

Life-threatening causes

- Hypoxia/cardiac disease
- Hypoglycaemia
- Metabolic (↓Ca^{2+}, ↑↓Na^{+})
- Trauma
- Meningitis, encephalitis, malaria
- ↑ICP and CVA
- Drug overdose
- Hypertension/eclampsia (pregnancy)

Paediatric seizures emergency

Airway	Check airway is patent; consider manoeuvres/adjuncts
Breathing	If no respiratory effort – **CALL ARREST TEAM**
Circulation	If no palpable pulse – **CALL ARREST TEAM**
Disability	If GCS ≤8 – **CALL ANAESTHETIST**

Call for **senior help** in all children having a seizure

Step 1
- Start **timing**; this is very important and easy to forget
- Maintain **airway**, assess ABC, check pupil size, posture, neck stiffness, fontanelle, temp and for rashes
- **15l/min O_2** in all patients
- Check **GLUCOSE**: if <3.5mmol/l give 5ml/kg of 10% dextrose stat
  - take 10ml of clotted blood and one fluoride bottle (p557) prior to giving dextrose, but don't let this delay treatment
- Keep patient safe, be alert for vomiting occluding the airway
- **Monitor** HR, O_2 sats, BP, cardiac trace, temp
- **Venous access,** take bloods:
  - FBC, U+E, LFT, CRP, Ca^{2+}, Mg^{2+}, glucose, bld cultures, anticonvulsant levels (if on anticonvulsants), venous blood gas
- If IV access: **lorazepam** 0.1mg/kg IV (max 4mg)
- If no IV access: diazepam 0.5mg/kg PR (max 10mg)
- Ask parents or ward staff about **history**/check notes

Step 2 (10min after either lorazepam/diazepam)
- If IV access: **lorazepam** 0.1mg/kg IV (max 4mg)
- If no IV access: paraldehyde 0.4ml/kg PR with 0.4ml/kg olive oil or 0.8ml/kg of a preprepared 50:50 solution (max 20ml of mixture)

Step 3 (10min after either lorazepam/paraldehyde)
- Call for **anaesthetist** and senior help
- **Paraldehyde** 0.4ml/kg PR as above unless already given
- If not on phenytoin: **phenytoin** 18mg/kg IV/IO over 20min
- If on phenytoin: phenobarbital 15-20mg/kg IV/IO over 10min

Step 4 (20min after either phenytoin/phenobarbital)
- Rapid sequence **intubation**
- **Consider** mannitol, pyridoxine, paracetamol, diclofenac

Life-threatening causes
- Meningitis, encephalitis, malaria
- Hypoglycaemia
- Metabolic (↓Ca^{2+}, ↑↓Na^{+})
- Trauma/non-accidental injury
- Hypoxia
- ↑ICP and CVA
- Drug overdose
- Hypertension

Seizures and fits

Worrying features preceding headache or head injury, recent depression (overdose), duration >5min, prolonged post-ictal phase, adult onset

Think about *life-threatening* see box on emergency page; ***most likely*** idiopathic (>50%), epilepsy, alcohol withdrawal, hypoglycaemia, hypoxia, trauma; ***other*** kidney or liver failure, pseudoseizures, overdose of tricyclics, phenothiazines, amphetamines; ***non-seizure*** brief limb jerking during a faint, rigors, syncope, arrhythmias

Ask about get a detailed description of the fit from anyone who witnessed the episode (see below), headache, chest pain, palpitations, SOB; ***PMH*** previous seizures, DM, alcoholism, cardiac, respiratory, renal or hepatic disease, pregnant; ***DH*** anticonvulsants, hypoglycaemics; ***SH*** alcohol intake, last drink, recreational drugs, recent travel; ***FH*** epilepsy

Obs GCS, temp, glucose (recheck), BP, O_2 sats

Look for sweating, tremor, head injury, tongue biting, neck stiffness, papilloedema, focal neurology, urinary or faecal incontinence, pregnancy, infection, limb trauma, posterior dislocation of shoulder

Investigations if a known epileptic or acute withdrawal from excess alcohol it is often appropriate to do none, see below for investigation of a first fit. Consider: ***urine*** β-hCG if pre-menopausal female (urine can give false –ve after 20wk gestation); ***blds*** FBC, U+E, LFT, glucose, Ca^{2+}, Mg^{2+}, blood cultures, anticonvulsant levels; ***ABG*** if hypoxia or metabolic upset suspected; ***ECG*** to exclude arrhythmia; ***CT*** may show a focal lesion, ↑ICP, haemorrhage or infarction; ***MRI*** may be required to exclude small lesions ***LP*** if meningitis or encephalitis suspected; ***EEG*** may help to exclude encephalitis or outpatient EEG to investigate epilepsy

Witnessing/describing a seizure

- ***Onset*** position, activity, any warning, starting in one limb or all over, presence of tonic phase (arched back, muscle spasm)
- ***During*** reaction to voice and pain, limb movements, eye movements, jaw and lip movements, breathing, peripheral or central cyanosis, sounds (may scream as air forced out of lungs), incontinence (urinary and faecal), duration, HR and rhythm
- ***Afterwards*** tongue trauma, sleepy, limb weakness (Todd's paresis, p295), muscle pain, headache

First fit

History Detailed account from a first-hand witness

Investigations FBC, U+E, LFT, glucose, Ca^{2+}, Mg^{2+}, PO_4^{3-}, clotting, medication levels, urine and serum toxicology screen (including paracetamol and salicylate), CT, consider LP after CT, may need an MRI if a lesion is suspected

Management Admit for 24h unless GCS 15 and alert, decision regarding seizure status and driving (see p646, 1yr ban), follow up with neurology (first fit clinic)

	History	Examination	Investigations
Seizure	Sudden onset, muscle pain, post-ictal confusion	Often normal, may have tongue or limb trauma	Often normal, may have focal lesion or metabolic cause
Alcohol withdrawal	>50units/wk alcohol consumption, last drink >24h ago	Anxious, sweating, tachycardic, tremor, liver disease	↑MCV and γGT, may have a mild anaemia
Pseudo-seizures	Unusual features, short duration of active movements, memory of event	Responsive to pain, normal respiration, no injuries	Normal investigation
Meningitis or encephalitis	Drowsy, confused, irritable, vomiting, headache	Febrile, ±septic, neck stiffness, photophobia, non-blanching rash, focal neurology	Abnormal CSF, see p630
Trauma, raised ICP and CVA	Prolonged drowsiness/confusion, headache, vomiting, blurred vision, dizzy, weakness	Falling/↓GCS, focal neurology, papilloedema, neck stiffness, head injury	Abnormal CT
Eclampsia	Pregnant, may be unaware	↑BP, proteinuria, palpable uterus	Fetal heart on Doppler
Transient arrhythmia/ Stokes–Adams	Sudden LOC, any posture, palpitations, pale, ±limb jerking, rapid full recovery with flushing	Evidence of cardiac disease, injury following fall, weak/ irregular/absent pulse during attack	Arrhythmia or heart block on ECG, 24h ECG and BP monitoring
Rigors	Coarse shaking, felt cold/hot, no LOC, symptoms of infection	Febrile, source of infection eg UTI, pneumonia, viral illness, no injury	↑WBC, NØ or LØ and CRP, +ve urine dipstick
Syncope	Rare lying down, ±fine limb jerking, ±urinary incontinence, rapid recovery, no postictal phase	Bradycardia and hypotension during episode, GCS 15/15 within min, no focal neurology	Postural drop (systolic drop of 20mmHg or more)

Treatment

General Stop the seizure using the treatment outlined on p286. Correct any metabolic upset (glucose, Ca^{2+}, Na^{+}) and exclude life-threatening causes, try to establish the cause. Get an ***urgent CT*** if the patient has a persistent GCS <15 post-fit, focal neurology or if the seizure was <4d post-trauma. Secure airway if still fitting or GCS ≤8.

Partial seizures are more likely to have a focal source. Diagnosing limb jerking as a seizure could prevent the patient driving for one year. If in doubt write a detailed description and allow senior staff to decide.

Epilepsy (*OHCM*7 p482)

Symptoms diagnosis is mainly from the history. There are many types:

- ***Partial*** seizure that involves only one cerebral hemisphere, only one side of the body will be affected. Can be motor, sensory or both:
  - *simple* partial seizure without altered consciousness, eg jerking/ spasm of left side or spreading of jerking (Jacksonian)
  - *complex* partial seizure with altered consciousness, eg temporal lobe epilepsy (altered mood, hallucinations, stereotyped movements)
- ***Generalised*** seizure involving both cerebral hemispheres:
  - *tonic–clonic* initial muscle spasm of whole body (tonic) followed by jerking phase (clonic); LOC throughout
  - *absences* sudden stopping of activity with staring or eye rolling, lasts <45s, most common in children
- ***Secondary generalised*** partial seizure that spreads to both hemispheres

Signs ↓GCS, tongue trauma, limb weakness, incontinence

Investigations often normal, may have an abnormal CT or EEG if there is a focal lesion

Treatment follow the treatment plan on p286. There is no specific treatment required post-seizure. Do not alter the patient's regular medication yourself, but make sure the patient is able to take their medication (consider NG medications) and is doing so. See *OHCM*7 p484 for ongoing management.

Alcohol withdrawal (*OHAM*2 p500)

Symptoms anxiety, shaking, sweating, vomiting, seizures *3–4d post-alcohol* confusion, delusions, hallucinations, amnesia, encephalopathy

Signs hypertension, tachycardia, pale, sweaty, tremor *3–4d post-alcohol* pyrexia, nystagmus, past pointing, ataxia, hypoglycaemia

Investigations may have ↓Mg^{2+} or ↓PO_4^{3-}

Treatment any patient who consumes >50units a week needs a reducing dose of chlordiazepoxide (see p116) with thiamine 25mg/24h PO and multivitamins one tablet/24h PO.

If >100units a week replace the thiamine with Pabrinex® 2 pairs/8h IV infusion over 10min for 5d, this is a high-potency combination vitamin B and C that may rarely cause an anaphylactic reaction. Monitor BP and blood glucose.

Complications seizures, coma, encephalopathy, hypoglycaemia

Post-traumatic

Urgent CT scan. If haematoma seen (p358), contact a neurosurgeon, otherwise hourly neuro obs and reassess if GCS falling.

Raised ICP	p300	Hypertension	p199
Hypoglycaemia	p271	Syncope	p350
Hypocalcaemia	p331	Tachy/bradyarrhythmias	p186/194
Hyper/hyponatraemia	p328/329	Hypoxia	p219
Eclampsia	p438	Meningitis/encephalitis	p300

Stroke/CVA/TIA emergency

Airway	Check airway is patent; consider manoeuvres/adjuncts
Breathing	If no respiratory effort – **CALL ARREST TEAM**
Circulation	If no palpable pulse – **CALL ARREST TEAM**
Disability	If GCS ≤8 – **CALL ANAESTHETIST**

Call for **senior help** early if patient deteriorating

If **GCS is reduced** see p280

- **15l/min O_2** in all patients
- Check blood **glucose**; treat if too low (p271) or high (p273)
- Check **temp**; treat if too low (blankets) or high (rectal paracetamol)
- **Monitor** O_2 sats, RR, HR, cardiac trace, temp and BP
- **Venous access**, take bloods:
  - FBC, ESR, U+E, LFT, lipids, glucose, cardiac markers, clotting, G+S
- **NBM** and start **IV fluids** for hydration (eg 0.9% saline at 100ml/h)
- **ECG** looking for atrial fibrillation or arrhythmia
- Take a focused **history** particularly:
  - when did the symptoms start (get an exact time)?
  - are symptoms worsening, static or improving?
  - intracranial pathology, clotting problems, bleeding (eg GI/PV), pregnancy, recent trauma/invasive procedures/surgery/thrombolysis
- **Examine** patient: RS, CVS, abdo and neuro exam
  - Document exact neurological deficits
- Request urgent **CT** scan
- Consider thrombolysis (see box) **OR** aspirin 300mg PO stat after CT

Consider thrombolysis with t-PA in CVA if:

- ≤3 hours from start of symptoms
- Non-haemorrhagic stroke (excluded by CT)
- Significant symptoms and not improving

Contraindications as for cardiac thrombolysis p576

- Call for **senior help**
- **Reassess**, starting with A, B, C …

Key differentials

Hypo/hyperglycaemia	p271	Other intracranial pathology	p291
Encephalitis/meningitis	p300	Seizure/Todd's paresis	p286
Overdose	p304	Severe liver/renal failure	p236/316
Bell's palsy	p295	Hypertensive encephalopathy	p199

Focal neurology

Worrying features ↓HR, ↑BP, ↓BP, ↓GCS, severe headache, pyrexia, neck stiffness, photophobia, vomiting, papilloedema

Think about see p292; varies with lesion location

Ask about weakness, clumsiness, tingling, pain, numbness, double vision, blurred vision, talking problems, swallowing problems, balance problems, speed of onset, weight loss, fever, cough, headache, nausea, vomiting (early morning), photophobia, neck stiffness, rashes, recent infections, behavioural change, tiredness; ***PMH*** previous neurology, migraines, epilepsy, eye problems, ↑BP, irregular heart, DM, psychiatric disorder (eg conversion disorder) ***DH*** antipsychotics, isoniazid; ***SH*** alcohol and cocaine; ***FH*** nerve or muscle problems

Obs BP, HR, GCS (see p280 if low), glucose

Neuro obs GCS, limb movements, pupil size and reactivity, HR, BP, RR, temp

Look for perform a complete neuro exam (p508) including cerebellar signs (p302), CVS exam for AF and carotid bruit

Investigations these should be determined by the location of the lesion determined by clinical examination. Investigations include ***blood tests*** and autoimmune markers, ***nerve conduction studies, CT/MRI*** imaging and ***LP*** (procedure p592, interpretation p630)

Urgent CT brainstem or cerebral (lateralising) signs, persistent ↓GCS, sudden onset headache lasting >2h, head injury with loss of consciousness and recurrent vomiting or seizures

Lesion location the aim is to determine which region of the nervous system is affected to allow further investigation and diagnosis. With motor symptoms there are three main areas:

- ***Lower motor neurone (LMN)*** peripheral nervous system; wasting, fasciculations, reduced reflexes and tone, forehead involved if CN VII
- ***Upper motor neurone (UMN)*** central nervous system; increased tone and reflexes with upgoing plantars, forehead spared if CN VII
- ***Mixed*** consider cord compression of the conus, motor neurone disease, Friedreich's ataxia, syphilis (taboparesis), subacute combined degeneration of the cord

The following table offers a simplified guide to locating the lesion in patients with focal neurology. Due to the complexity of the nervous system, diseases can present with atypical features that do not fit these patterns. Acute intracranial pathology may present with decreased tone and reflexes before the characteristic UMN signs develop.

	Motor	Sensory	Reflexes and tone	Features
Cerebrum	Whole leg/ arm/face	Whole leg/ arm/face	↑	Unilateral, dysphasia/ inattention
Cerebellum	Normal	Normal	Normal/↓	Ataxia, nystagmus, intention tremor
Brainstem	Whole leg/ arm/face	Whole leg/ arm/face	↑	Crossed, cranial nerve lesion (not II)
Myelopathy	Distal > proximal	↓ Below sensory level	↑	Bilateral, urinary retention
Radiculopathy	Distal > proximal	Painful with tingling or numbness	Normal/↓	Unilateral, painful, atrophy and fasciculations
Neuropathy	Distal > proximal	Tingling or numbness	Normal/↓	Unilateral or glove and stocking, atrophy and fasciculations
NMJ	Proximal > distal	Normal	Normal/↓	Bilateral, fatigability (or re-enforcement)
Myopathy	Proximal > distal	Normal	Normal/↓	Bilateral

Common causes

- ***Cerebrum*** CVA, neoplasia, multiple sclerosis, migraine, abscess, encephalitis, meningitis, subdural/epidural haematoma
- ***Cerebellum*** CVA, neoplasia, multiple sclerosis, alcohol, abscess
- ***Brainstem*** CVA, neoplasia, multiple sclerosis, abscess
- ***Myelopathy (spinal cord)*** multiple sclerosis, infection, neoplasia, epidural haematoma, syringomyelia, spinal stenosis, spondylosis, central disc herniation, note cord compression is an emergency
- ***Radiculopathy (nerve root)*** disc protrusion (usually L4, L5, S1), spondylosis, spinal stenosis, NB sciatica is a radiculopathy affecting the sciatic nerve (L4, L5, S1); cauda equina syndrome is a radiculopathy affecting all the cauda equina nerves and is an emergency
- ***Peripheral neuropathy (nerve)*** DM, trauma, vitamin B_{12}/folate deficiency, alcohol, renal failure, inflammatory (eg Guillain–Barré, SLE), hypothyroid, carcinoma, motor neurone disease, Bell's palsy, nerve entrapment syndromes (p407)
- ***Neuromuscular junction (NMJ)*** myasthenia gravis (fatigability) or Lambert–Eaton (reinforcement), botulism toxin
- ***Myopathy (muscle)*** alcohol, hypothyroid, inflammatory (eg polymyositis), medication (eg statins), muscular dystrophy, myotonic dystrophy
- ***Also consider*** hypoglycaemia, hyponatraemia, meningitis, encephalitis, ↑ICP, focal seizure, autoimmune

Stroke

Causes haemorrhage (15%) or ischaemia (85%, eg AF, carotid stenosis)
Symptoms sudden onset focal neurology though onset can be stuttering
Signs Check for irregular heartbeat and carotid bruit. Determine region:

- *Total anterior circulation* (TACS); all three features shown in the table
- *Lacunar* (LACS); affects the internal capsule causing profound weakness and/or anaesthesia without other defects
- *Partial anterior circulation* (PACS); similar features to TACS or LACS, but not fulfilling the full criteria
- *Posterior circulation* (POCS); affects the brainstem or cerebellum

	TACS	**LACS**	**PACS**	**POCS**
	All of following	**Any abnormality listed**		
Motor and/or sensory defect	Unilateral in ≥2 out of face, arm and leg	Face with arm and/or leg	Unilateral, <TACS or LACS criteria	Bilateral or associated with cranial nerve defect on opposite side
Eyes	Homonymous hemianopia[1]	Normal	Variable	Homonymous hemianopia or new diplopia
Ataxia	Absent	Ataxic hemiparesis[2]	Absent	Present, other cerebellar signs
Higher cerebral[3]	Present	Normal	Present	Normal or ↓GCS

[1] Visual field defect on same side in both eyes, eg right-sided vision in right and left eyes for a left side of brain stroke (p509)

[2] Unilateral weak and ataxic arm and leg without other cerebellar signs

[3] Higher cerebral dysfunction includes dysphasia (right side of brain) or visuospatial disorder, eg inattention (left side)

Prognosis LACS, PACS and POCS have a similar prognosis with 15% mortality by 1yr while 60% live independently; TACS are worse with a mortality of 60% at 1yr with only 5% living independently
Investigations FBC, U+E, LFT, glucose, ESR, lipids, clotting, ECG, CXR, urgent CT head if GCS persistently low or evidence of ↑ICP; otherwise within 48h, consider non-urgent echo and carotid Doppler
Treatment see emergency treatment p290, aim to get the patient scanned and thrombolysed before the 3h deadline. Otherwise: aspirin 300mg/24h PO/PR for 14d unless high suspicion of haemorrhage (severe headache, meningism, persistent ↓GCS). Nil by mouth with IV fluids unless swallow is safe (requires SALT assessment). Monitor BP, but do not try to lower BP without discussing with a senior. Admit to stroke ward for rehabilitation with multidisciplinary team.
Prevention aspirin (75mg/24h PO) and dipyridamole MR 200mg/12h PO, control BP, statin, stop smoking, exercise, warfarin (AF) or carotid endarterectomy (stenosis)
Complications aspiration pneumonia, dependent lifestyle, further CVA

Transient ischaemic attack (TIA)

Symptoms/signs as for stroke but resolve completely within 24h
Management if <3h since symptoms began see p290; if risk of stroke is very high (see ABCD score) consider admission; otherwise give aspirin 300mg PO followed by daily aspirin (75mg/24h PO), BP control, statins, anticoagulation if atrial fibrillation present, stop smoking, exercise

ABCD score to calculate 7day stroke risk

Age	≥60yr	1 point
BP	Systolic >140mmHg and/or diastolic ≥90mmHg	1 point
Clinical features	Unilateral weakness	2 points
	Speech disturbance without weakness	1 point
	Other signs	0 points
Duration	≥60min	2 points
	10–59min	1 point
	<10min	0 points

Add up the points to get a total out of 6

Score	7d risk	Management
0–4	0.4%	Urgent outpatient follow up (1–2wk)
5	12%	Urgent investigation
6	31%	Admit for monitoring and urgent investigation

Parkinson's (*OHCM*7 p486)

Symptoms shaking, difficulty getting up, slow walking, depression
Signs resting tremor (pill rolling), rigidity, bradykinesis (slow movement), monotonous voice, expressionless face, altered handwriting
Investigations clinical diagnosis, MRI and CT not usually required
Treatment levodopa (reduced effectiveness after 5yr, start if symptoms interfere with life), peripheral dopa-decarboxylase inhibitor eg carbidopa, dopamine agonists eg cabergoline, anticholinergics eg benzatropine
Complications depression, dementia

Causes of dystonia Parkinson's, Wilson's, multiple sclerosis, CVA, trauma, antipsychotics, levodopa, metoclopramide, anticonvulsants, Huntington's chorea, Sydenham's chorea, ataxia telangiectasia, syphilis, AIDS, CJD

Multiple sclerosis (*OHCM*7 p488)

Symptoms recurrent focal neurology that varies between locations, weakness, numbness, tingling, vision loss, ataxia, urinary incontinence or retention; dysphasia and seizures are rare
Signs any focal neurology, especially spastic limb paralysis and vision loss
Investigations areas of inflammation and demyelination on MRI, slowed nerve conduction, CSF may show oligoclonal bands (p630)
Treatment ***acute*** steroids, baclofen, diazepam or botulinum toxin to relieve spasticity; ***disease-modifying drugs*** β-interferon, glatiramer
Complications incontinence, relapse, pain

Space-occupying lesion (*OHCM*7 p490)

Causes tumour, aneurysm, abscess, chronic subdural haematoma
Symptoms focal neurology, seizures, behavioural change, early morning headache, vomiting, visual disturbance
Signs focal neurology, papilloedema
Investigations CT, MRI (brainstem/cerebellum), do not perform an LP
Treatment for ↑ICP see p300, surgical removal of tumour/lesion

Todd's paresis transient focal neurological symptoms following a seizure, typically limb weakness; lasts minutes to hours so mimics a TIA.

Syringomyelia central tubular spinal cord cavities seen on MRI; weakness and loss of pain/temp sensation in the arms.

Cervical/thoracic spinal stenosis caused by degenerative changes or spondylosis resulting in a radiculopathy or myelopathy.

Motor neurone disease (*OHCM*7 p498)
Symptoms stumbling, poor grip, muscles quivering, speech and swallowing problems, aspiration pneumonia
Signs mixture of LMN and UMN signs, normal sensation, fasciculations
Investigations electromyography (EMG)
Treatment mostly symptomatic, life expectancy is usually 3–5yr
Complications aspiration pneumonia, respiratory failure, spasticity

Myasthenia gravis (*OHCM*7 p504)

Symptoms weakness, diplopia, dysarthria, worse in evening than morning
Signs muscle fatiguability, especially on upward gaze, normal reflexes
Investigations antibodies to ACh receptor, improvement with edrophonium (perform in resuscitation area only), CT of thymus
Treatment anticholinesterase (eg pyridostigmine), immunosuppression, removal of thymus gland, plasmapheresis, immunoglobulins
Myasthenic crisis can be triggered by illness, surgery and medications; severe fatigue can affect the diaphragm causing respiratory failure requiring ventilation; assess with spirometry (FVC). Treat as above.

Guillain–Barré post-infectious proximal neuropathy that can rapidly progress to respiratory failure; use spirometry (FVC) to assess severity and progression; treat with immunoglobulins ±ventilation if worsening.

Mononeuropathy

Bell's palsy rapid onset mononeuropathy of the facial nerve (VII). Treat with prednisolone and aciclovir, taping the affected eye closed at night, using artificial tears and sunglasses.

Peripheral neuropathy (polyneuropathy)
Causes see p292
Symptoms/signs clumsiness, weakness, tingling, numbness
Signs usually glove and stocking distribution
Investigations urine dipstick, FBC, B_{12}, folate, U+E, LFT, glucose, TFT, ESR, serum electrophoresis, ANCA, ANA, CXR, nerve conduction studies
Treatment treat or remove the cause if possible
Complications wounds, ulcers, joint abnormalities eg Charcot joint

Back pain (*OHCS7* p670)

Worrying features bladder/bowel changes, progressive/night pain, weight loss, age <20yr or >55yr, steroids, thoracic or non-mechanical pain, previous cancer, bilateral leg neurology or pain, altered perianal sensation, expansile mass

Think about *serious* cord compression, cauda equina syndrome, metastases, myeloma, infection, fracture, aortic aneurysm; ***common*** mechanical back pain (see table), bruising, sprain, renal colic
Ask about trauma/lifting (mechanism), location of pain, pain character, duration, aggravating/relieving factors, radiation, pain in joints, pain or tingling in legs, leg weakness, bladder (retention or incontinence), faecal incontinence, altered sensation on passing stool, weight loss; ***PMH*** previous back/joint pain, neurological problems, osteoporosis, anaemia; ***DH*** steroids, allergies, analgesia; ***FH*** joint or back problems; ***SH*** occupation (lifting, prolonged sitting)
Look for scoliosis, kyphosis, bony tenderness, tenderness next to spine, reduced range of movement (especially flexion), tenderness on compressing pelvis, pain on straight leg raise (p505), leg weakness, reduced sensation, tendon and plantar reflexes, expansile abdominal mass; ***PR*** reduced sensation or tone
Investigations usually none if no worrying features are present and diagnosis fits mechanical trauma; otherwise consider: FBC, ESR, CRP, Ca^{2+}, ALP, PSA, CXR, spinal X-ray if centrally tender post-trauma or risk of pathological fracture, urgent MRI spine if cord compression or cauda equina suspected, DEXA bone scan

	History	Examination	Investigations
Cord compression	Weakness, numbness, pain below lesion, incontinence	Sharp dermatome, UMN below lesion, LMN at lesion	Lesion seen on urgent MRI
Cauda equina syndrome	Leg weakness and pain (often bilateral), urinary and/or faecal incontinence	↓perianal sensation, ↓anal tone, ↓leg power, sensation and reflexes	Lesion seen on urgent MRI
Mechanical back pain	Pain, worse on movement, brought on my lifting/ trauma	Pain reproduced by straight leg raise, unilateral neurology	Rarely needed, MRI may show the injury
Spondylitis	Chronic pain, joint pain, rashes, no trauma, family history	Reduced lumbar flexion, pain on squeezing pelvis	RhF –ve, ↑ESR, sacroilitis on X-ray
Vertebral collapse fracture	Sudden onset pain associated with a specific action in elderly patient	Pain over central vertebrae, reduced range of movement	Fracture seen on X-ray

Mechanical back pain including disc prolapse

Symptoms low back pain, worse on coughing/moving, may radiate to leg
Signs pain brought on by straight leg raise (p505), tenderness next to the vertebrae, may have unilateral numbness with reduced reflexes (radiculopathy) on side of the pain, normal sensation and tone on PR
Investigations urgent MRI spine especially if rapidly progressing
Treatment early mobilisation, avoid lifting, maintain good posture, analgesia (p428), diazepam 2mg/8h PO for muscular spasm, hot/cold packs, refer if symptoms not improving at 6wk; reassess urgently if bilateral symptoms or urinary/faecal incontinence

Types of mechanical back pain	
Sprain	Muscular pain and spasm without neurology
Disc prolapse	'Slipped disc', may compress the nerve root causing a unilateral radiculopathy (sciatica)
Spondylosis	Degenerative changes of the spine eg osteoarthritis
Spondylolysis	Recurrent stress fracture leading to a defect in the vertebrae
Spondylolisthesis	Slippage of lumbar vertebrae usually in young patients
Lumbar spinal stenosis	Narrowing of the spinal canal due to osteoarthritis, causes leg aching and heaviness on walking (spinal claudication)

Cord compression

Causes tumour, abscess/TB, trauma, haematoma, central disc prolapse
Symptoms weakness and/or numbness of legs, continuous/shooting pains, urinary retention or incontinence, faecal incontinence
Signs LMN signs at the level of the lesion, UMN signs below, normal above, sharp boundary of reduced sensation, spinal shock (p217)
Investigations urgent MRI spine, look for cause
Treatment refer immediately to orthopaedics/neurosurgeons for surgery
Complications weakness, reduced sensation, incontinence, impotence

Cauda equina syndrome

Causes central disc prolapse, tumour, abscess/TB, haematoma, trauma
Symptoms urinary incontinence or retention (may be painless), faecal incontinence, bilateral leg weakness and pain
Signs bilateral reduced power (LMN) and sensation, reduced perianal (saddle) sensation, reduced anal tone, bilateral absent ankle reflexes
Investigations urgent MRI spine
Treatment refer immediately to orthopaedics/neurosurgeons for surgery
Complications weakness, reduced sensation, incontinence, impotence

Vertebral collapse fracture

Causes trauma, osteoporosis, tumour
Symptoms sudden onset back pain, may be mild trauma if pathological
Signs central vertebral tenderness, reduced mobility
Investigations spinal X-ray
Treatment analgesia, assess ability to cope, treat osteoporosis p475

Headache

Worrying features ↓GCS, rapid onset, severe, recurrent vomiting, photophobia, rash, neck stiffness, focal neurology, seizures, papilloedema, ↓HR, ↑BP

Think about ***emergencies*** intracranial haemorrhage (subarachnoid, subdural, extradural), meningitis, encephalitis, ↑intracranial pressure (ICP), temporal arteritis, acute glaucoma, hypertension; ***common*** dehydration, tension, infection, migraine, trauma, post-LP, post-nitrates, extracranial (sinuses, eyes, ears, teeth); ***other*** cluster, hypoglycaemic, hyponatraemic
Ask about severity, location, bilateral vs. unilateral, speed of onset, character, change with coughing, nausea and vomiting, rashes, trauma, visual changes (before or currently), dizziness, seizures, joint pain, recent LP, sweating, malaise; ***PMH*** previous headaches, migraines (and usual symptoms); ***DH*** nitrates, antihypertensives, insulin, oral hypoglycaemics; ***SH*** recent stressors
Obs temp, GCS, glucose, HR, BP, fluid balance
- ***Cushing's reflex*** is a late sign of ↑ICP: ↓HR and ↑BP

Neuro obs GCS, limb movements, pupil size and reactivity, HR, BP, RR, temp

Look for volume status (p319), neck stiffness, photophobia, Kernig's (fully flex hip and passively extend knee, +ve if painful in head or neck), visual and eye problems including tenderness (press on closed lid) and papilloedema, focal neurology, temporal artery tenderness and pulsatility, tender over sinuses, head trauma, dental hygiene, ear pathology, non-blanching rash (check whole body)
Investigations in the absence of worrying features it is appropriate to give pain relief without investigations; otherwise secure IV access and send ***blood*** for FBC, ESR, U+E, LFT, glucose, CRP, clotting and bld cultures; ***ABG*** especially if GCS is reduced. Discuss with a senior whether a ***CT head***, ±***LP*** are required (LP procedure and contraindications p592). An ***EEG*** may help diagnose encephalitis
Treatment exclude emergencies and treat other causes with simple analgesia (p428); ask to be contacted if symptoms fail to improve or worsen:
- ***New onset GCS <15*** see p280
- ***New onset focal neurology*** treat as meningitis, encephalitis or ↑ICP, p300: 15l/min O_2, consider antibiotics – call a senior urgently
- ***Sudden (<2min), severe and constant*** treat as subarachnoid p300: 15l/min O_2, lie flat – call a senior urgently
- ***Unwell, deranged obs*** could be meningitis/sepsis p300, classic symptoms in <30%: 15l/min O_2, IV fluids, antibiotics – call a senior urgently
- ***Red, painful eye, ↓acuity*** acute glaucoma p387, urgent ophthalmology
- ***Temporal tenderness*** temporal arteritis p301: 15l/min O_2, high-dose prednisolone, ESR and urine dipstick – call a senior urgently
- ***Hypertensive*** (BP >200/120mmHg) see p199

	History	Examination	Investigations
Subarachnoid or warning bleed	Rapid onset, severe pain, vomiting, ↓GCS if severe	May be normal, neck stiffness, photophobia, focal neurology	Bleed seen on CT or red cells and xanthochromia in CSF
Subdural or extradural haematoma	Trauma, confusion, vomiting	Reduced/fluctuating GCS, may be signs or ↑ICP	Blood seen on CT
Meningitis ±septicaemia	Unwell, irritable, drowsy, feels ill, ±rash	Febrile, ±septic, neck stiffness, photophobia, ±non-blanching rash	↑WCC, ↑CRP, neutrophils in CSF
Raised ICP	Vomiting, progressive, blurred vision, dizzy, drowsy, seizures, worse on coughing/bending	Small or big pupils, focal neurology, papilloedema and Cushing's reflex are late signs	Abnormal CT, large ventricles, may have a focal lesion
Encephalitis	Drowsy, confused, vomiting, seizures, preceding flu-like illness, non-specific symptoms	Pyrexia, may have focal neurology, neck stiffness, photophobia and papilloedema	↑LØ and protein in CSF, ±RBCs, cerebral oedema on CT or MRI
Temporal arteritis	Age >55yr, visual disturbances, ill, weight loss, polymyalgia, jaw pain when eating	Tender, palpable, non-pulsatile temporal artery, tender scalp	↑CRP, ↑↑↑ESR with anaemia, ↑plts and ↑ALP
Migraine	Previous migraines, visual aura, usually unilateral, throbbing, nausea, ±vomiting	Photophobia, visual field defects, may have focal neurology	None
Cluster	Recurrent daily headaches, unilateral	Agitated	None
Tension	Bilateral, band-like pressure, worse when stressed	May have scalp tenderness, otherwise normal	None
Sinusitis	Frontal pain, blocked/runny nose	Tender above or below eyes	May have ↑LØ, NØ or EØ
Acute glaucoma	Age >50yr, blurred vision, pain in one eye, often occurs at night	↓visual acuity, dilated, ±oval pupil, red around cornea, tender	↑Intraocular pressure
Drug induced	Many medications can induce headaches, particularly nitrates, Ca^{2+} channel antagonists and metronidazole with alcohol		

Subdural haematoma	p358	Extradural haematoma	p358
Acute glaucoma	p387	Sepsis	p214

Subarachnoid haemorrhage (*OHAM7* p466)

Suspect if over 40yr with recurrent vomiting and severe headaches.
Symptoms rapid onset (<2min), severe and continuous (>2h) headache, often occipital, vomiting, dizziness, may have seizures
Signs neck stiffness, drowsy, focal neurology, ↓GCS, photophobia
Investigations urgent CT head; if normal, LP to exclude small bleeds
Treatment 15l/min O_2, analgesia (codeine 60mg PO or 5–10mg morphine IV) and anti-emetic, eg metoclopramide 10mg IV/IM. Reassess often and request neuro obs. Lie the patient flat and advise not to get up or eat. If GCS is low or diagnosis confirmed involve an anaesthetist and neurosurgeon early and consider transfer to HDU/ITU. Use fluids to keep systolic >100mmHg, but try to avoid sudden increases in BP. Focal neurology or ↓GCS carry a worse prognosis.
Complications cerebral ischaemia, rebleeding, hydrocephalus

Meningitis (*OHAM2* p432, *OHAM7* p806)

Symptoms headache, neck pain, photophobia, seizures, unwell
Signs ↑HR, ±↓BP, ↑temp, ↓GCS or abnormal mood, neck stiffness, ±rash, focal neurology
Investigations ↑WCC, ↑CRP, CT scan then LP (p592), treat first
Treatment resuscitate as needed (p214). 15l/min O_2, IV fluids and contact a senior. Start cefotaxime/ceftriaxone 2g IV immediately if you have a clinical suspicion of bacterial meningitis. Contact public health regarding contact tracing. See also septicaemia p214.
Complications ↑ICP, hydrocephalus, seizures, focal neurology

Encephalitis (*OHAM7* p442)

An uncommon disease with non-specific symptoms that is hard to diagnose. It is caused by numerous viruses including herpes.
Symptoms not acting as normal, seizures, drowsy, headache, neck pain
Signs altered personality, ↓GCS, focal neurology, neck stiffness, ↑temp
Investigations CT followed by LP (p592), send CSF for viral PCR, EEG may show temporal lobe changes
Treatment aciclovir 10mg/kg/8h IV (10d) and antibiotics as for meningitis
Complications ↑ICP, seizures

Raised intracranial pressure – ICP (*OHAM7* p452)

Causes CVA, tumours, trauma, infection (including abscess), cerebral oedema (eg post-hypoxia), electrolyte imbalance, benign
Symptoms headache and vomiting (worse in morning and coughing/bending over), tiredness, visual problems, seizures
Signs altered GCS, papilloedema (late sign), focal neurology, Cushing's reflex (late sign, ↓HR, ↑BP)
Investigations urgent CT head to assess cause and severity
Treatment elevate the head end of the bed to 40° and correct hypotension with 0.9% saline. Discuss with a senior before giving mannitol or dexamethasone (tumours only) to reduce the ICP. Involve a neurosurgeon/neurologist early.
Complications herniation of the brain (coning)

Temporal arteritis (*OHAM2* p760)
Symptoms headache, jaw pain on eating, visual problems, aching muscles
Signs temporal artery and scalp tenderness, pulseless or nodular temporal artery
Investigations ↑↑ESR (>50mm), ↑CRP, ↑plts, ↓Hb
Treatment start 60mg/24h prednisolone PO and strong analgesia. Discuss with on-call surgeon to arrange a temporal artery biopsy within 5d (signs will resolve); alternatively a Doppler USS of the artery may be diagnostic. Refer to a rheumatologist for follow up and reducing steroids; liaise with an ophthalmologist to exclude visual complications.
Complications blindness, stroke, MI

Migraine (*OHCM7* p450)
New migraines are uncommon >40yr, exclude underlying pathology (CT).
Symptoms visual aura (flashing lights, zigzag, loss of visual field) followed by throbbing one-sided headache (worse on exertion), nausea, vomiting, pain from light and sound
Signs visual field defects, focal neurology
Investigations normal
Treatment treat with simple analgesia (see p428), ±anti-emetic and rest. If attack is severe consider triptan or ergotamine (see *BNF*). Ask nurses to contact you if symptoms worsen; consider other diagnoses.

Sinusitis
Symptoms blocked nose, runny nose (clear/yellow/green), headache worse on bending, unable to smell
Signs tender over sinuses (above medial eyebrows, bridge of nose, below eyes), ↑temp
Treatment try a mixture of saline nebs 5ml/2–4h, beclometasone nasal spray 2 sprays to each nostril/12h and/or ephedrine nasal drops 1–2 drops in each nostril/6h (7d max). If severe (eg purulent mucus, systemically unwell) prescribe amoxicillin 500mg/8h PO.
Complications local spread of infection, chronic sinusitis

Cluster headaches
Symptoms recurrent severe one-sided headaches often at night
Signs unable to lie still
Treatment sumatriptan nasal spray or 15l/min O_2 for 20min for headaches; verapamil started during an attack cluster to prevent recurrence, this is stopped once the cluster has finished

Acute glaucoma see p387, needs urgent ophthalmology review.

Post-dural puncture (eg LP) usually <48h of LP, epidural or spinal anaesthetic, but up to 7d; advise the patient to lie flat, treat with analgesia and increased fluid intake. Contact anaesthetist if severe or persistent.

Other headaches prescribe simple analgesia, see p428. If the patient is dehydrated prescribe appropriate fluids (p323); if hypoglycaemic see p271; if profoundly hypertensive see p199.

Dizziness

Worrying features ↑HR, irregular HR, hypoxia, ↓BP, ↓glucose, chest pain, sudden onset, unable to stand

Think about ***faint*** shock, arrhythmia, MI, postural hypotension, anxiety, hyperventilation, syncope, epilepsy, hypoglycaemia, reaction to pain, numerous medications; ***vertigo*** labyrinthitis, vestibular neuronitis, benign positional vertigo, trauma, ototoxic drugs, Ménière's, CVA, multiple sclerosis, acoustic neuroma; ***imbalance*** alcohol intoxication, Wernicke's encephalopathy, CVA, cerebellar space-occupying lesion, intracranial infection, B_{12} deficiency, coeliac disease, normal pressure hydrocephalus
Ask about world moving or spinning, sudden or gradual, duration, position when attack came on, ringing in the ears, new hearing problems, blacking out, loss of consciousness, nausea/vomiting, falling, head injury; ***PMH*** previous dizziness, ↑BP, DM, MS, epilepsy; ***DH*** antihypertensives, diuretics, aminoglycosides; ***SH*** alcohol.
Obs temp, HR, lying and standing BP, glucose, GCS
Look for ability to stand, standing with eyes shut (Romberg's, +ve if falls with eyes shut), ability to walk, change with position, cerebellar signs (DANISH – dysdiadochokinesia, ataxia, nystagmus, intention tremor and past pointing, slurred speech, hypotonia; nystagmus is found with many peripheral and central causes of vertigo), focal neurology, appearance of ear through an otoscope (effusion, perforation).
Investigations the type of dizziness (vertigo, imbalance, fainting) should be determined from history alone; beyond ***postural BPs*** acute investigation is rarely required. In the long term a ***tilt table test*** and ***audiometry*** may be considered and a ***CT scan*** if a CVA or tumour is suspected or there are cerebellar signs

	History	Lesion
Fainting	Light-headed, no sensation of movement, anxious, palpitations, sweating, may have loss of consciousness	Shock, arrhythmia, MI, postural hypotension, anxiety, syncope, epilepsy, ↓glucose, reaction to pain; see p350 (falls)
Vertigo	Sensation of the world or patient moving, better when still, no loss of consciousness	Labyrinth, vestibular nerve, central connections of vestibular nerve, eg brainstem
Vertigo and hearing change	As above with either tinnitus (ringing/buzzing) or hearing loss	Labyrinth or vestibular nerve (VIII)
Imbalance	Inability to stand or walk straight, no sensation of movement, may have cerebellar signs (above)	Peripheral nerve, dorsal/posterior columns, cerebellum; may be Romberg +ve

Syncope/fainting p351 CVA p290

Vertigo (*OHCS7* p554)

Worrying features focal neurology, multidirectional or non-fatiguing nystagmus

The sensation of vertigo can be treated with the same drugs used for nausea and vomiting (p252) eg cyclizine 50mg/8h PO or betahistine 16mg/8h PO; the underlying cause should be determined.

Benign positional vertigo Sudden onset vertigo lasting seconds following specific head movements. Treated with Epley Manoeuvre (a series of movements to dislodge the vestibular debris causing the symptoms *OHCS7* p555) and referral to physiotherapy for vestibular exercises.

Inner ear inflammation causes sudden onset vertigo without focal neurology. Reassure and treat with the medications above.

- ***Vestibular neuronitis*** viral infection of the vestibular nerve; improves within 1wk but can take 2–3mth to fully resolve
- ***Labyrinthitis*** as for vestibular neuronitis with hearing loss or tinnitus

Ménière's severe vertigo with tinnitus, nausea and vomiting lasting hours. Treat with cyclizine/betahistine and refer to ENT.

Motion sickness rarely encountered in hospital, however cinnarizine 30mg PO 2h before journey is effective.

Causes of nystagmus labyrinthitis, vestibular neuronitis, benign positional vertigo, trauma, ototoxic drugs, Ménière's, alcohol intoxication, Wernicke's encephalopathy, CVA, multiple sclerosis, acoustic neuroma, space-occupying lesion, intracranial infection, B_{12} deficiency, coeliac disease, hydrocephalus, idiopathic, congenital

Imbalance/ataxia

Ataxia can be differentiated from vertigo on history; there are two types:

- ***Cerebellar*** Romberg's –ve, classic 'DANISH' signs (opposite)
- ***Sensory*** Romberg's +ve, loss of proprioception, preservation of fine co-ordination, stamping gait, spinal/neuropathy signs

Cerebellar ataxia

Causes CVA, multiple sclerosis, alcohol toxicity, Wernicke's encephalopathy, B_{12} deficiency, coeliac disease, normal pressure hydrocephalus, infection, space-occupying lesions, trauma, paraneoplastic

Management MRI is the most useful diagnostic test (consider CT if acute onset), neurology referral, some underlying causes are treatable

- ***Wernicke's encephalopathy*** thiamine (B_1) deficiency often as a result of chronic alcohol excess resulting in confusion, ataxia, short-term memory loss, ophthalmoplegia (defects to CN III, IV or VI) and peripheral neuropathy; treated with thiamine (oral or IV – Pabrinex) p288.

Sensory ataxia

Causes cervical spondylosis, MS, peripheral neuropathy, syringomyelia, spinal tumour, spinal infection, B_{12} deficiency, Friedreich's ataxia, syphilis

Management urgent MRI if acute onset, otherwise consider tests for peripheral neuropathy (p295), spinal X-rays, routine MRI, nerve conduction studies, neurology referral; often treated with B_{12}

Overdose emergency

Airway	Check airway is patent; consider manoeuvres/adjuncts
Breathing	If no respiratory effort – **CALL ARREST TEAM**
Circulation	If no palpable pulse – **CALL ARREST TEAM**
Disability	If GCS ≤8 – **CALL ANAESTHETIST**

Drug overdoses are often deliberate but can happen accidentally at home or in a hospital. The emergency management is the same.

Call for **senior help** early if patient deteriorating

- **Lie patient down** ask a colleague to observe for vomiting and be ready to turn them onto their side
- **Assess respiration** RR, O_2 sats, O_2 requirement, consider blood gas
  - call anaesthetist if poor respiratory effort, it will only get worse
- **Assess CVS** HR, BP, consider fluid resuscitation (p209)
- **Venous access**, take bloods:
  - FBC, U+E, LFT, salicylate, paracetamol, glucose, INR
- **Monitor** pulse oximeter, BP cuff, defibrillator ECG leads if unwell
- Take brief **history** to establish the medication(s), quantity and timing
- Ask a colleague to **contact Toxbase/Poisons service** (p305) about specific overdose
- Consider **gastric lavage** if <1h since overdose
- **Examine patient** condensed CVS, resp, abdo and neuro exam
- Repeat set of **observations** and **ECG**
- **Consider**
  - urine toxicology
  - urinary catheter
  - arterial blood gas
- **Follow management plan from Toxbase/Poisons service** (p305)
- If patient deteriorating:
  - call for senior help
  - **reassess** starting with A, B, C …

Life-threatening causes

Paracetamol	p306
Other overdoses	Check Toxbase/Poisons service (p305)

Overdose and deliberate self-harm

> Worrying features violent methods, intent to kill themselves, still wishing to kill themselves, previous attempts, preparation, concealment

Think about *emergency* psychosis, acute suicidal intent; ***common*** depression, grief, stressful situations, relationship breakdown
Ask about *medical* medications taken, dose, number of tablets, time-frame, source of medications, symptoms (vomiting, tinnitus, dizziness, abdo pain), mechanism of injuries; ***psychiatric*** events leading to overdose, expected outcome, intent (eg call for help, to kill themselves), suicide note, extent of planning/preparation (eg spontaneous), circumstances of seeking help, expectation of being found, current intent (eg still suicidal), alcohol intoxication prior to events, recent stresses (relationships, work, money, family, legal); ***PMH*** previous suicide attempts and methods, psychiatric care, chronic illness, HIV status (if paracetamol overdose); ***DH*** regular medications, alternative medicines (eg St John's Wort), tetanus status, allergies, alcohol intake, substance abuse; ***SH*** who do they live with? who is at home? relationships, family, friends, employment
Obs temp, HR, BP, RR, GCS, glucose
Look for *medical* orientation, conscious level, pupil size, reflexes, tone, tremor, sweating, agitated, abdo tenderness, sweating, nutritional state; ***psychiatric*** (see p535 for mental state examination) neglect, scars on wrist/forearms, eye contact, withdrawn, abnormal posture or movements, anxiety, paranoia, flat affect, speech form and content, thought form and content including delusions, perception including hallucinations, concentration, memory, insight into actions
Investigations paracetamol and salicylate levels in all overdoses (ideally 4h post-overdose), if unwell consider glucose, FBC, U+E, LFT, INR, ECG and ABG or tests for the specific drug

Management

Severe overdose stabilise the patient according to the emergency page opposite and get senior help early
Severe trauma call the trauma team and see p168
Other overdose for paracetamol see p306 otherwise check a poisons service eg Toxbase (www.spib.axl.co.uk, needs ED registration details) or National Poisons Information Service (0870 600 6266)
Other trauma see p352–362
Risk assessment (p307) this determines the psychiatric management of the patient. Once the medical issues are resolved the patient must be discussed with the on-call psychiatrist. They will either review the patient or recommend discharge home in the care of a responsible and sober adult with psychiatric follow up.
Acutely suicidal patients must not leave the hospital without psychiatric assessment. If necessary they can be restrained or sedated (p309) under the Mental Capacity Act (2005); always seek senior help.

	Symptoms and signs	Investigations
Salicylates (aspirin)	Vomiting, ↑RR, tinnitus, vertigo, sweating	Respiratory alkalosis then metabolic acidosis, ↑↓glucose, ↑salicylate levels
Tricyclic antidepressants (TCAs)	Dilated pupils, blurred vision, seizures, ↓GCS, arrhythmia, tachycardia	Acidosis, prolonged PR, QRS and QT, heart block, ventricular arrhythmias
Digoxin	Nausea, confusion, hallucinations, yellow halos roundlights, anorexia	Arrhythmias, ST depression (tick shaped), ↑↓K^+
Opioids	Pinpoint pupils, ↓RR, ↓GCS	Respiratory acidosis, opioids on urine toxicology
Benzodiazepines, barbiturates, alcohol	↓GCS, ↓BP, ↓tone, ↓reflexes	Respiratory acidosis, maybe mixed if excess alcohol
Ecstasy,amphet-amines,cocaine	Thirst, confusion, agitation, tremor, dilated pupils ↑HR, ↑temp	Substance may be seen on urine toxicology

Paracetamol overdose

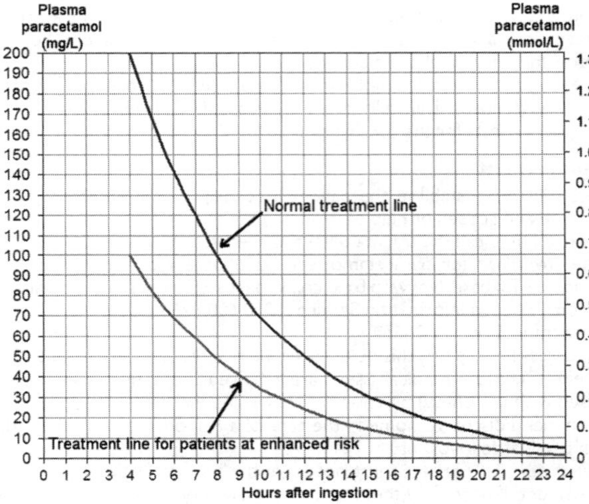

National Poisons Information Service guidelines 2003
Reproduced by kind permission of the Paracetamol Information Centre.

Paracetamol overdose causes minimal symptoms or signs initially but can result in liver failure and death. Take a blood sample for paracetamol and salicylate levels 4h after the overdose or as soon as possible if over 4h. The level should be plotted on the graph opposite and treatment started if the level is above the relevant line (see high-risk line below). Treatment is with N-acetylcysteine (Parvolex®); in adults three doses are given:

- 150mg/kg IV infusion in 200ml 5% dextrose over 15min
- 50mg/kg IV infusion in 500ml 5% dextrose over 4h
- 100mg/kg IV infusion in 1000ml 5% dextrose over 16h

High-risk line this is used for the following patients: malnourished, HIV +ve, eating disorder, excess alcohol or regularly taking carbamazepine, phenytoin, phenobarbitoal, primidone, St John's Wort or rifampicin.

Assessing risk

This is a difficult judgement that requires experience; making the wrong decision could result in a preventable death. All cases should be discussed with the on-call psychiatrist. ED often use a modified 'sad person scale' to assess risk of suicide. It is by no means foolproof; trust your instinct and ask for help if you are in any doubt.

Modified SAD PERSONS, score	
Sex: Male	Score 1
Age <19yr or >45yr	Score 1
Depressed or hopeless	Score 2
Previous suicide attempts or psychiatric care	Score 1
Excessive alcohol or drug use	Score 1
Rational thinking loss: psychotic or organic illness	Score 2
Separated, widowed or divorced	Score 1
Organised or serious attempt at suicide	Score 2
No social support	Score 1
State future intent (determined to repeat or ambivalent)	Score 2

Interpreting the score	
Score <6	may be safe to discharge, depending upon circumstances
Score 6–8	probably requires psychiatric services assessment
Score >8	likely to need admission and urgent psychiatric services assessment

Other important risk factors include stressful life-events, unemployment or retirement, identifying with others who have committed suicide, chronic illness (medical or psychiatric) and availability of lethal weapons.

Aggressive behaviour emergency

Safety	• Stay between the patient/relative and the exit • Get extra help from other staff and/or security • Consider phoning the police

Call for **senior help/security** early if the situation is deteriorating

- **Assess the safety** is anyone at acute risk?
- **Emergency sedation** if they are a risk to themselves or others[1]
  - lorazepam 1–2mg (1mg elderly/renal failure) PO/IM/IV stat
  - haloperidol 5–10mg (2mg elderly) PO/IM/IV stat
  - can be used together or separately
- Try to **establish the precipitant** from staff/relatives
- Ask a **member of staff** who knows the patient to accompany you
- Invite the patient to **sit down** with you and discuss the problem
- **Listen** until they feel they have explained the problem
- **Assess** the patient for signs of psychosis or acute confusion
- **Apologise** and/or offer sympathy as appropriate
- **Address any concerns** raised by the patient
- **Ask** specifically about pain or worry
- Consider offering **oral sedation** or **analgesia**
- Attempt to **defuse the situation**
- If unsuccessful **contact a senior** for help

Common causes

- Acute confusion (delirium) p281
- Intoxication (drugs/alcohol) p116
- Psychosis due to an underlying psychiatric disorder p310–2
- Anger/frustration/poor communication p125
- Pain p428

1 If a patient poses a risk to themselves or others any doctor can give emergency sedation, against the patient's consent and with restraint, under the Mental Capacity Act (2005)

Mood disturbance/psychosis

Worrying features delusions, hallucinations, suicidal intent

Think about *emergency* acutely suicidal, psychosis; ***psychosis*** schizophrenia, depression, bipolar disorder, postpartum, substance abuse, alcoholism or withdrawal; ***low mood*** depression, bipolar disorder, schizophrenia, anxiety disorder, personality disorder, eating disorder, seasonal affective disorder, postpartum, grief, alcoholism or withdrawal, substance abuse; ***high mood*** bipolar disorder, cyclothymia, substance abuse; ***organic*** endocrine (hypo/hyperthyroid, Cushing's, Addison's), neurological (epilepsy, CVA, dementia, MS, Parkinson's, head injury, brain tumour), infections (HIV, Lyme disease, syphilis, EBV), inflammatory disease (eg rheumatoid, SLE), electrolyte imbalance (eg Na^+, Ca^{2+}), metabolic problems (eg porphyria, Wilson's), malnutrition, anaemia, sleep apnoea, chronic disease, malignancy, medications (p310)

Ask about (see psychiatric history p534) ***medical*** bowel habit, weight change, appetite, cold/heat intolerance, tremor, previous head trauma, changes in vision, headaches, unusual sensations, weakness, seizures, sleeping problems, sexually transmitted illnesses and risk, rashes, joint pain, exercise tolerance; ***psychiatric*** early morning waking, concentration, energy levels, lack of pleasure, appetite, recent stresses, mood, change in personality, suicidal ideation, childhood, employment history, relationship history, legal problems; ***PMH*** previous psychiatric problems or care, previous mania, previous suicide attempts, chronic illness; ***DH*** regular medications, alternative medicines, contraception, allergies; ***FH*** psychiatric problems, thyroid, liver or brain problems, occupations; ***SH*** who do they live with, relationships, family, friends, employment, alcohol intake, smoking, illicit substance abuse

Obs GCS, temp, HR, BP, RR, glucose

Look for (see mental state examination p535) ***medical*** full systems exam and careful neurological exam including tremor, eye reflexes, papilloedema, tendon reflexes; ***psychiatric*** general appearance, signs of neglect or flamboyancy, unusual posture or movements, aggression, affect, speech (form and content), thought (form and content including delusions), perception including hallucinations, cognition (concentration, memory, orientation), risk (to selves or others), insight

Investigations it is important to consider organic causes of mental disturbance. If history and examination are unremarkable it may not be necessary to investigate further. If there are further concerns the following may be considered: FBC, U+E, LFT, Ca^{2+}, TFT, ESR, ANA, B_{12}, folate, cortisol, HIV (p426), EBV and Lyme disease serology, VDRL/THPA, urine toxicology screen, LP, EEG, CT/MRI brain.

Management

- Is the patient manic, psychotic (delusions or hallucinations, p308) or acutely suicidal? If so they need urgent psychiatric referral.
- Could there be an organic cause for their symptoms (see above)?
- For milder symptoms would referral to their GP be sufficient?

	History	Examination	Investigations
Depression	Low mood, tearful, loss of interests, sleep disturbance	Poor eye contact, neglect, low mood and affect, ±psychosis	Usually normal
Bipolar disorder	Mixture of low and high mood events	Signs of high or low mood, ±psychosis	Usually normal
Schizophrenia	Delusions, auditory hallucinations, apathy	Neglect, poverty of speech/thought	Usually normal
Anxiety	Worry, sweating, dizziness, palpitations	Fearful, tense or normal	Usually normal
Personality disorder	Longstanding difficulties	Evidence of self-harm, usually normal	Usually normal
Dementia	Reduced concentration, memory, cognition	Neglect, poor cognition with normal consciousness	May have abnormal CT/MRI brain
Organic cause	Weight loss, seizures, rapid onset, visual hallucinations	Neurological signs, rashes, wasting	Usually abnormal

Examples of medications with psychiatric side-effects

NSAIDs, antihypertensives, β-blockers, digoxin, oral contraceptive pill, antiepileptics, corticosteroids, antibiotics, cytotoxics, L-dopa, anticholinergics, sedatives

Bipolar disorder

Recurrent episodes of low or high mood, with low mood being more common. High mood may be mania (impairs job or social life and may have psychotic features) or hypomania (no impairment to job or social life). If the patient has ever had an episode of mania it is called 'bipolar I'; if they have only had hypomanic episodes it is called 'bipolar II'. Recurrent swings between mild depression and hypomania are called 'cyclothymia'.

Mania symptoms high mood, hyperactive, reduced sleep, reckless behaviour, impulsive, irritable, increased energy, over-familiar, increased sex drive, distractible, loss of insight, disorganised thoughts, flight of ideas

Psychotic symptoms delusions, hallucinations

Mania signs flamboyant dress/appearance, excess/rapid speech, restless

Investigations if first manic episode: CT head, EEG and urine toxicology

Treatment consider admission based on severity of episode and risk to self (suicide or reputation), job, assets, relationships. Mania is treated acutely with antipsychotics (particularly olanzapine) and benzodiazepines. Antidepressants are used for depressive episodes but may precipitate mania. Preventive treatment is with lithium, carbamazepine, valproate or lamotrigine.

Complications suicide, unemployment, relationship breakdown

Depression

Depression is low mood that is not usual and persists for over two weeks. It can be a symptom of other psychiatric disorders (eg bipolar disorder, personality disorders) or a disease in its own right: unipolar depression. Unipolar depression can be classified as mild or major and may be associated with somatic symptoms or psychotic symptoms.

Symptoms low mood, low energy, feeling worthless or guilty, poor concentration, indecisive, thoughts of suicide or death, low self-esteem, tearfulness, loss of interests, loss of pleasure (anhedonia) **somatic symptoms** weight/ appetite loss, sleep problems (early morning wakening, insomnia or excess sleeping), loss of sex drive, psychomotor agitation or retardation (agitated or slowed speech and movement), change in mood with time of day **psychotic symptoms** delusions, hallucinations

Signs neglect, agitation, slowed speech or movement, poor eye contact

Investigations often none; consider an organic cause and investigate if suspected, otherwise initiate treatment and review if not working

Treatment

- Psychotherapy usually cognitive–behavioural therapy (CBT) but interpersonal therapy (IPT) may also be effective; can be used with or without medications
- Antidepressants:
  - first line: selective serotonin reuptake inhibitors (SSRIs) eg citalopram, fluoxetine
  - if a patient does not respond to SSRIs liaise with a psychiatrist about which medications to recommend; this may be second-line antidepressants, eg venlafaxine, mirtazepine or augmentation with lithium
- Electroconvulsive therapy (ECT) is considered if the patient is at high risk (eg not eating or drinking) and/or has failed to respond to medications

Prognosis outcome is generally good with the following: young, somatic symptoms, reactive depression (due to a life-event) and acute onset

Complications suicide, deliberate self-harm, unemployment, relationship breakdown, recurrence

Starting an antidepressant medication

Antidepressants generally start to work by 2–3wk but they can take up to 6wk to have an effect

Suicide risk may increase over the first few weeks

Antidepressants are generally well tolerated; side-effects are usually mild
Treatment should continue for at least 6mth after the symptoms have resolved

Antidepressants should be gradually weaned rather than stopped abruptly

Schizophrenia

A chronic illness characterised by psychotic symptoms lasting over a month. Acute presentations are often characterised by positive symptoms; negative symptoms can persist despite treatment.

Positive symptoms delusions, hallucinations (often auditory), see first-rank symptoms below *Negative symptoms* blunted affect, apathy, loss of drive, social withdrawal, social inappropriateness, poverty of thought/speech, cognitive impairment

Signs neglect, disorganised behaviour, paranoia

Investigations FBC, U+E, LFT, Ca^{2+}, glucose, urine toxicology consider TFT, VDRL, cortisol, EEG, CT/MRI

Treatment consider admission based on severity of episode, including risk to self (suicide, job, assets, relationships) and others. Antipsychotic medications (neuroleptics) are the mainstay of acute and chronic treatment, there are two types:

- ***Atypical antipsychotics*** have less extrapyramidal side-effects and a better effect on negative symptoms eg amisulpride, clozapine, olanzapine, risperidone, quetiapine, zotepine
- ***Conventional antipsychotics*** eg chlorpromazine, haloperidol, trifluoperazine, flupentixol

Clozapine is a 3rd line antipsychotic; it is used in treatment-resistant schizophrenia. It can cause potentially fatal agranulocytosis so the patient needs weekly FBC for the first 18wk of treatment.

Side-effects of antipsychotics include sedation, anticholinergic effects (eg dry mouth, blurred vision, constipation), extrapyramidal side-effects (eg parkinsonism) and tardive dyskinesia (late onset oral grimacing and upper limb writhing). Procyclidine may be used to reduce parkinsonism symptoms.

Complications suicide, deliberate self-harm, unemployment, relationship breakdown, recurrence, tardive dyskinesia

First-rank symptoms

Delusions	**Passivity**
Delusional perception	Passivity of thought, feelings or actions
Hallucinations	**Thought flow and possession**
Thought echo (audible thoughts)	Thought withdrawal
Third-person auditory hallucinations	Thought insertion
Running commentary	Thought broadcasting

Anxiety disorders/neurosis

It is normal to have a degree of worry or fear, however if this causes distress or interferes with life then it is considered abnormal. There are several types of anxiety- and stress-related disorders:

- *Specific phobic* fear of a specific situation or object eg flying, spiders
- *Social phobia* fear in social situations eg public speaking
- *Panic attack* excessive fear associated with symptoms of autonomic arousal eg sweating, dizziness, nausea, palpitations, breathlessness; they usually last less than 30min
- *Panic disorder* recurrent panic attacks with fear of having another
- *Generalised anxiety disorder* (GAD) excessive worry in everyday life
- *Obsessive–compulsive disorder* (OCD) obsessive thoughts eg hands are dirty leading to compulsions eg washing hands

Symptoms worry, irritability, fear, avoidance of feared situations, checking, seeking reassurance, tight chest, shortness of breath, palpitations, 'butterflies', tremor, tingling of fingers, aches, pain

Signs tremor, ↑HR, ↑RR; be careful to exclude any organic causes of symptoms such as breathlessness, chest pain or palpitations

Investigations consider FBC, U+E, LFT, Ca^{2+}, troponins, TFT, glucose, urinary VMA, ECG to exclude organic causes of symptoms

Treatment careful explanation of the cause of their problems, teaching relaxation techniques, psychological therapies eg cognitive–behavioural therapy, medications eg antidepressants, try to avoid using benzodiazepines as these have poor long-term benefits and carry a risk of dependence

Relaxation techniques

Breathing exercises (silently counting breaths up to 10)
Visualisation techniques (imagining a place, colour or image that is calming)
Progressive muscle relaxation (tensing and relaxing muscle groups in turn)
Relaxation CDs
Yoga

Personality disorders

An abnormality of personality that causes either the patient and/or others to suffer[1]; the diagnosis is avoided in adolescents when the personality is developing.

Classification ICD-10 divides personality disorders into 9 categories:

- Paranoid, schizoid, dissocial, emotionally unstable (borderline and impulsive subtypes), histrionic, anankastic, anxious, dependent, other

Investigations usually none, but they require careful assessment over multiple occasions and the exclusion of other psychiatric diagnoses

Treatment personality disorders are challenging to treat. Psychotherapies may be useful, including dialectical behaviour therapy, cognitive–analytical therapy, cognitive–behavioural therapy (CBT) and psychodynamic psychotherapy. Antidepressants, mood stabilisers and antipsychotics are also used though the evidence of benefit is limited.

Complications suicide, self-harm, social isolation

1 Schneider, K. 1958 *Clinical Psychopathology*, 5th edn, Grune and Stratton.

Haematuria

Worrying features ↑BP, weight loss, frank blood, clots, proteinuria

Think about ***macroscopic*** UTI, tumours, stones; ***microscopic with red cells*** UTI, bladder tumour, renal tumour, stones, recent catheterisation, prostate hypertrophy/tumour, clotting abnormality, glomerulonephritis, nephritis, hypertension, endocarditis, sickle-cell, TB, schistosomiasis, trauma, strenuous exercise, PV bleeding (p432); ***microscopic without red cells*** (haemoglobinuria) haemolytic anaemia, myositis, rhabdomyolysis, trauma, ischaemia; ***red discolouration*** rifampicin, beetroot

Ask about urine colour, clots, dysuria, frequency, urgency, fever, vomiting, abdominal pain, hesitancy, poor stream, urine output, recent falls/lying on floor, recent catheterisation, weight loss, malaise, lethargy, joint pain, beetroot, exercise, menstruation; ***PMH*** kidney disease, stones, prostate disease, cancer, hypertension, heart disease, clotting disorders, sickle cell; **DH** nephrotoxic drugs (eg NSAIDs, gentamicin), rifampicin

Obs BP, HR, temp, fluid balance

Look for BP is very important, look at the urine, suprapubic tenderness, loin tenderness, masses, rashes, bruises, enlarged prostate, PV bleeding, arthritis/arthralgia, lymphadenopathy

Investigations ***urine dipstick*** many cannot distinguish red cells and haemoglobin; ***urine*** microscopy and culture; ***blds*** FBC, U+E, LFT, Ca^{2+}, ESR, CRP, consider G+S, clotting, autoantibodies, complement, PSA

Management

Macroscopic (red/pink urine) resuscitate (p209), if heavy consider inserting a large three-lumen catheter for bladder wash-out, discuss urgently with urology to exclude malignancy (IVU, cystoscopy, CT)

Microscopic (urine looks normal, red cells on microscopy):

- ***With nitrites/white cells*** treat as a UTI/pyelonephritis (p394), check urine once infection has cleared to be sure haematuria has resolved
- ***Without proteinuria*** suggests tumour (below) or stones (p240), refer to urology (urgently if >50yr) for IVU ±cystoscopy
- ***With proteinuria*** suggests glomerular pathology, refer to nephrology and check BP, urinary output, urine casts, autoantibodies, complement, urine protein:creatinine, 24h urine collection for protein, renal USS

Haemoglobinuria (blood on dipstick but no red cells seen) haemolytic anaemia (p334), rhabdomyolysis (p320)

Renal cancer

Symptoms/signs haematuria, weight loss, mass, flank pain, bone pain
Management IVP/renal USS; treated by nephrectomy ±radiotherapy
Prognosis 50% 5yr survival overall

Bladder cancer

Symptoms/signs haematuria, dysuria, frequency, recurrent/male UTI
Management IVU, cystoscopy and biopsy; treated with intravesicular BCG (carcinoma-in-situ), transurethral resection, radiotherapy, cystectomy
Prognosis 60% 5yr survival overall

Proteinuria

Worrying features ↑BP, oliguria, haematuria, ↑↑proteinuria, oedema

Think about fever, postural/orthostatic, UTI, glomerulonephritis, nephritis, nephrotic syndrome, myeloma, pregnancy (pre-eclampsia), DM, ↑BP, heart failure, exercise, vaginal mucus

Ask about dysuria, frequency, urgency, fever, blood in urine, urine output, swelling, bone pain, abdominal pain, weight loss, malaise, lethargy, joint pain, rashes, exercise, vaginal discharge, pregnancy, vomiting, orthopnoea, breathlessness recent URTI/tonsillitis; ***PMH*** kidney disease, ↑BP, heart disease, cholesterol, DM; ***DH*** nephrotoxic drugs (eg NSAIDs, gentamicin), contraception.

Obs BP, HR, RR, temp, fluid balance, glucose

Look for BP is very important, look at the urine, oedema, suprapubic tenderness, loin tenderness, palpable kidneys, palpable uterus, rashes, arthritis/arthralgia, bone tenderness, basal creps, ↑JVP

Investigations most patients will simply require repeat urine dipstick, if unwell or concerning features other tests may be indicated; ***urine dipstick*** protein, blood, nitrites, leucocytes; repeat early in morning to exclude postural proteinuria, check β-hCG; ***urine*** M,C+S, protein:creatinine ratio, 24h protein, urine electrophoresis; ***blds*** FBC, U+E, LFT, triglycerides, ESR, CRP, autoantibodies (ANA, ANCA, anti-DNA), complement, cryoglobulins, serum electrophoresis; ***renal USS***

Management

- ***Fever/exercise/transient*** repeat urine dipstick normal, no treatment
- ***Orthostatic*** age <30yr, no protein in early morning, no treatment
- ***UTI*** (p394) dysuria, frequency, urine nitrites/leucocytes, culture +ve
- ***Pre-eclampsia*** (p438) NB urine β-hCG negative after 20wk
- ***Myeloma*** (p330) >60yr, bone pain, Bence-Jones protein (urine), ↑Ca^{2+}
- ***Glomerulonephritis*** (p321) oliguria, ↑BP, haematuria
- ***Nephrotic*** (below) oedema, ↓albumin, ↑triglycerides

The following require referral to a nephrologist for renal biopsy:

- Protein:creatinine ratio >100mg/mmol
- Protein:creatinine ratio >45mg/mmol and microscopic haematuria
- Protein:creatinine ratio >45mg/mmol and estimated GFR <60ml/min

GFR can easily be estimated from the patient's age, weight and plasma creatinine, see p321.

Nephrotic syndrome

Definition oedema, proteinuria (>3g/24h) and ↓albumin (<30g/l)
Causes DM, glomerulonephritis, SLE, amyloidosis, malignancy
Symptoms swelling of ankles and legs, frothy urine, vomiting, infection
Signs dependent pitting oedema, ascites, pleural effusions, hypovolaemia
Results proteinuria, ↓albumin, ↑triglycerides
Treatment nephrology referral, fluid restrict (<1.5l/24h), ↓Na^+, furosemide, prophylactic LMWH (p346), monitor fluid balance, aggressive treatment of infections, treat underlying condition
Complications thromboembolism, infection, hypovolaemia, renal failure

Acute renal failure

Airway	Check airway is patent; consider manoeuvres/adjuncts
Breathing	If no respiratory effort – **CALL ARREST TEAM**
Circulation	If no palpable pulse – **CALL ARREST TEAM**

Call for ***senior help*** early

Acute rise in urea and creatinine ±oliguria; there are four types:

- ***Prerenal hypoperfusion*** reversible failure caused by ↓BP (often hypovolaemia) progresses to acute tubular necrosis if untreated
- ***Acute tubular necrosis*** caused by prolonged hypoperfusion, rhabdomyolysis or nephrotoxic drugs (NSAIDs, gentamicin, amphotericin)
- ***Renal*** glomerulonephritis, nephritis, vascular emboli/thrombosis
- ***Obstructed*** enlarged prostate, single kidney with stones, pelvic surgery

Features of different types of renal failure	
Prerenal hypoperfusion	Oliguria, urine osmolality >500mosmol/kg, urine Na^+ <20mmol/l
Acute tubular necrosis	Oliguria/normal/polyuria, urine osmolality <350mosmol/kg, urine Na^+ >40mmol/l
Renal	Oliguria, haematuria, ↑BP
Obstructed	Painful, anuria, palpable bladder
Chronic renal failure	Small kidneys, previous abnormal urea/creatinine, under a nephrologist, ↓Hb, ↓Ca^{2+}, ↑PO_4^{3-}

History kidney problems, urine output, fluid intake, other medical problems, medications (?nephrotoxic), rashes, bleeding

Examination volume status (p319), BP, HR, JVP, basal creps, gallop rhythm, oedema, palpable bladder

Investigations ***urine*** colour, dipstick, M,C+S, osmolality and Na^+(p628); ***blds*** FBC, U+E, LFT, CK, CRP, osmolality, ESR, clotting; ***ABG*** expect acidosis, check K^+; *urgent ECG* ↑K^+ causes flat P waves, wide QRS and tall, peaked T waves; ***CXR, bladder USS, renal USS***

Treatment assess and treat for serious complications:

- ***Obstructed*** palpable bladder, bladder USS; insert catheter p586
- ***Shocked*** ↑HR, ↓BP, absent JVP; fluid resuscitate p209
- ***Overloaded*** oedema, basal creps, ↑JVP, CXR; O_2, furosemide p226
- ***Hyperkalaemia*** ECG, bld gas; salbutamol, Ca^{2+} gluconate p326

Indications for urgent dialysis persistent hyperkalaemia (>7mmol/l), severe metabolic acidosis (pH <7.2, be <–10), unresolving pulmonary oedema, uraemic encephalopathy (falling GCS or seizures), uraemic pericarditis (chest pain)

Continue IV fluids unless overloaded (no KCl), stop nephrotoxic drugs (p148), refer to HDU/ITU for CVP monitoring, monitor urine output

Low urine output

> **Worrying features** prolonged low urine output <0.5ml/kg//h, ↑HR, systolic BP <100mmHg, ↑K^+, ↑creatinine

Remember it is easier to treat fluid overload than acute renal failure.

	Volume in 24h	Volume in 1h
Normal urine output	>1,600ml	>60ml
Low urine output	<800ml	<30ml (0.5ml/kg)
Oliguria	<400ml	<17ml
Anuria	<100ml	<4ml
Absolute anuria	None	None

Think about ***severe*** acute renal failure, shock; ***most likely*** hypovolaemia, urinary retention, blocked catheter, prostatic hypertrophy; ***other*** rhabdomyolysis, chronic renal failure, renal vascular problems (eg thrombosis, emboli), urethral trauma

Ask about abdominal pain, hesitancy, poor stream, oral intake, vomiting, diarrhoea, stoma output, leaking wounds, sweating, breathlessness, orthopnoea, tiredness, recent falls/lying on floor; ***PMH*** kidney disease, number of kidneys, prostate disease, ↑BP, heart disease, DM; ***DH*** nephrotoxic drugs (eg NSAIDs, gentamicin, ACEi)

Obs BP, HR, fluid balance, CVP if possible

Look for volume status (p319), oedema, palpable bladder, suprapubic pain, evidence of infection or haemorrhage, unrecorded leakage from wounds, loin pain, enlarged prostate, extensive bruising

Investigations urine colour, dipstick, M,C+S. If not responding to fluid challenges send urine for osmolality (p628) and Na^+; ***blds*** FBC, U+E, CK, osmolality; ***bladder scan*** if urinary retention or a blocked catheter is suspected; this may be available on the wards; ***USS abdo*** if urine output is persistently low; request a Doppler USS if renal artery stenosis is suspected

Treatment insert a urinary catheter (some nurses are able to female catheters, ±male) and ask the nurses to keep an hourly fluid balance including any diarrhoea, vomiting and fluid loss from wounds. Consider asking for a catheter flush if already catheterised. Assess the patient and if in doubt treat as hypovolaemia (p212) and review in 1–2h

If urine output is still low despite treatment It can take up to 2h for a fluid bolus to work. If there is still no improvement send a urine sample and bloods as described above. Ask for a bladder scan. Get senior advice. ***Do not ignore patients with very low urine output.***

	History	Examination	Investigations
Hypovolaemia	Low fluid input, excess losses, post-op	Negative fluid balance, ↑HR, absent JVP	↑urea, concentrated urine, ↑osmolality
Septic shock	Feels ill, symptoms of infection, acute illness or blood loss	↑HR, ↓BP, may be septic, exclude haemorrhage	May have ↓Hb, ↑WCC and ↑CRP
Acute renal failure	Severe illness, untreated low urine output	May be dehydrated or shocked	New onset ↑urea and creatinine, ↑CK if rhabdo-myolysis
Chronic renal failure	DM, ↑BP, tired, previous kidney problems	Pale, anaemic, oedema, bruising, peripheral neuropathy	Persistent ↑urea and creatinine, small kidneys on USS
Urinary retention	Lower abdominal pain, previous prostate problems	Palpable bladder, often anuric, enlarged prostate	Full bladder on scan
Fluid overload	Cardiac history, excess fluids, SOB	↑JVP, basal creps, cold hands/feet, oedema	CXR shows pulmonary oedema

Hypovolaemia

This is by far the most common cause of low urine output.
Symptoms, signs, investigations see opposite
Treatment increase fluid input; the rate of rehydration depends on the patient. If urine output is >0.5ml/kg/h simply increase the rate of current IV fluids. If <0.5ml/kg/h consider a fluid challenge (p210) and prescribe some quick fluids to follow, eg 0.9% saline 1l/4h; review the patient in 2h.
Complications acute renal failure

Fluid overload

This is a rare cause of low urine output.
Symptoms, signs, investigations see opposite
Treatment see p209 'pulmonary oedema'. For mild overload reduce the speed of IV fluids and review in a few hours; ask the nurses to weigh the patient, record hourly obs and contact you if the patient's RR rises. If you are certain they are overloaded try 20–40mg furosemide PO or IV. This will cause a diuresis in all patients and potentially cause acute renal failure if the patient was hypovolaemic.
Complications pulmonary oedema

Hypotension/shock	p226	Pulmonary oedema	p620

Assessing volume status

HR, postural hypotension and low urine output (<0.5ml/kg/h) are sensitive signs of hypovolaemia while orthopnoea suggests overload.

Ask about ***hypovolaemia*** urine output, headache; ***fluid overload*** shortness of breath, orthopnoea, cough, sputum (white/pink frothy), swelling

Obs ***early hypovolaemia*** ↑HR (including upper range of normal, ie >90/min – NB remains slow if taking β-blockers), postural BP (a drop of more than 20mmHg on standing is significant), urine output <0.5ml/kg/h; ***late hypovolaemia*** urine output <17ml/h, ↓BP; ***fluid overload*** ↑RR, ↓O_2 sats

Look for ***early hypovolaemia*** dry mucous membranes (lips, mouth, nose), prolonged central capillary refill (normal <2s), absent JVP on lying flat; ***late hypovolaemia*** sunken eyes, increased skin turgor; ***fluid overload*** ↑JVP, bilateral basal crackles, pitting oedema (ankles if sitting, sacrum if in bed), gallop rhythm (3rd heart sound), cold hands and feet

Investigations ***early hypovolaemia*** *urine* dark, ↑osmolality; ***blds*** may be normal, ↑urea, ↑packed cell volume (PCV, also called haematocrit), ↑albumin, ↑osmolality, look for trends; ***late hypovolaemia*** ↑creatinine ***fluid overload*** pulmonary oedema on CXR (p620), abnormal ECG (p610 – LVH, MI), ↑CVP

Fluid balance is calculated by measuring a patient's urine output and fluid input along with any losses from vomit, diarrhoea or drains. The patient must be catheterised for accurate measurement.

Insensible losses these are unrecordable fluid losses, eg sweating and breathing. 500–1000ml is usually lost each day, but this increases with pyrexia (from sweating), breathing rapidly and burns; this loss will not be apparent from the fluid chart. Litres of fluid can be lost from burns and wound seepage which is missed unless the bandages are weighed.

Third–space fluids Also called 'fluid sequestration'; inflammation and injury causes capillary permeability to increase so that fluid and protein leak from the blood vessels (intravascular space) causing oedema. The patient is intravascularly hypovolaemic despite normal fluid balance and fluid should be replaced according to clinical signs, especially urine output. It is common with sepsis, pancreatitis and after major operations.

CVP lines Central venous pressure measurements are used primarily in ITU and HDU since they require a central line (p574). By recording the pressure in the line at the level of the right atrium an estimate of blood volume is obtained. The normal range is 2–5mmHg (5–10cmH_2O); high pressure suggests fluid overload or heart failure while a low CVP suggests hypovolaemia. Trends are more important than absolute values; the CVP should rise with a fluid challenge; hypovolaemia has been corrected once this rise persists after the challenge has finished.

Acute urinary retention

Causes enlarged prostate, post-operative, pain, anticholinergics, spinal pathology/MS (painless), pregnancy, urethral strictures, constipation
Symptoms suprapubic pain, severe urge to urinate, anuria, oliguria
Signs palpable distended bladder (dull to percussion and tender), check leg power/reflexes and tone, perianal sensation and prostate on PR
Investigations bladder scan if unsure or simply pass a catheter
Management urgent catheterisation (p586), record volume of urine (normal bladder size is 400–500ml, consider acute-on-chronic retention if >1l), urine dipstick and send for M,C+S, refer to urology (may need admission in case of secondary diuresis), note that PSA will be falsely elevated; within 48h attempt a trial without catheter (TWOC), if retention recurs the catheter will need reinserting and treat as chronic retention
Complications acute renal failure, chronic obstruction

Chronic urinary retention

Causes obstruction (prostate), DM, MS, dysfunctional bladder
Symptoms incontinence, dribbling, poor stream, recurrent UTI
Signs palpable distended bladder (usually non-tender), enlarged prostate
Investigations FBC, U+E, PSA, Ca^{2+}, PO_4^{3-}
Management do not catheterise unless in pain, refer to urology to investigate cause, catheterisation will probably lead to diuresis, may need TURP, recurrent self-catheterisation or finasteride
Complications chronic renal failure, acute-on-chronic retention, UTI

Rhabdomyolysis

Causes lying on a hard surface for prolonged periods, crush injuries, strenuous exercise, burns
Symptoms and signs extensive bruising or damaged tissue, dark urine
Investigations ↑↑↑CK with normal troponins; ↑urea, ±↑creatinine, ↑K^+, blood on urine dipstick, no red cells on microscopy (myoglobin), ↑urate
Treatment treat as for acute renal failure (p316), may need Na^+ bicarbonate or surgical removal of damaged tissue
Complications acute renal failure, ↑K^+

Tumour lysis

The destruction of malignant cells during chemotherapy can cause acute renal failure and metabolic derangement.
Risk factors leukaemia, high-grade tumours, renal impairment, ↑LDH
Symptoms occurs within 3d of chemotherapy, oliguria, swelling, vomiting, muscle cramps, seizures, tingling, syncope
Signs tetany, spasm, weakness
Results ↑K^+, ↑PO_4^{3-}, ↓Ca^{2+}, ↑urate, ↑urea, ↑creatinine
Treatment hyperhydration with IV fluids, allopurinol, bicarbonate, K^+ restriction, PO_4^{3-} binding, dialysis
Prevention allopurinol 24–48h and IV hydration started prior to therapy, careful monitoring of U+E, Ca^{2+}, urate, LDH during chemotherapy
Complications acute renal failure, hyperkalaemia, arrhythmia, congestive cardiac failure

Chronic renal failure

A long-standing and irreversible reduction in GFR.
Causes DM, ↑BP, chronic urinary retention, glomerulonephritis, nephritis, pyelonephritis, polycystic kidneys, vasculitis
Symptoms initially none, tiredness, weight loss, nausea
Signs initially none, may have signs of causative disease eg DM
Results persistent haematuria and/or proteinuria, ↑urea, ↑creatinine, ↓GFR (see below), ↓Hb, ↓Ca^{2+}, ↑PO_4^{3-}, abnormal or small kidneys on USS, glomerulonephritis on biopsy
Treatment regular review by a nephrologist, ACEi, control BP, treat underlying condition, avoid nephrotoxins; disease progression may require fluid restriction, salt restriction, dialysis, renal transplant
Complications ↑BP, anaemia, ↓Ca^{2+}, renal osteodystrophy, ↑K^+, fluid overload
Prescribing use Appendix 3 of the *BNF*; try to avoid nephrotoxic drugs, eg NSAIDs, gentamicin and reduce doses of many others, eg opioids, benzodiazepines, cephalosporins and digoxin; do not prescribe metformin
Fluid and electrolytes see p323
Radiology avoid all types of IV contrast imaging, this is nephrotoxic

Estimating the glomerular filtration rate (GFR) – Cockcroft and Gault formula

Estimated GFR (ml/min)
(also called Creatinine clearance)

$$= C \times \frac{(140\text{–age in years}) \times \text{weight (kg)}}{\text{Plasma creatinine } (\mu\text{mol/l})}$$

Replace 'C' with 1.23 for men and 1.04 for women

Estimated GFR (ml/min)	Plasma creatinine (μmol/l)	Interpretation
>75	70–120	No serious damage
40–75	110–200	Mild renal impairment
15–40	175–350	Chronic renal failure
<15	>300	Severe renal failure

Glomerulonephritis

Inflammation of the glomeruli in the kidney; there are many histological types and they may be idiopathic or caused by systemic disease eg SLE.
Symptoms/signs nephritic/nephrotic syndrome, renal failure, ↑BP
Investigations renal biopsy gives the diagnosis, autoantibodies may help
Treatment often immunosuppression, varies with type
Complications acute/chronic renal failure

Nephritic syndrome

A presentation of glomerulonephritis with haematuria, ↑urea, oedema.
Symptoms/signs ↑BP, low urine output, facial oedema
Results haematuria, ±proteinuria
Management refer to nephrologist for renal biopsy; do not give steroids

Diabetes insipidus

Deficiency of antidiuretic hormone (ADH).
Causes ***neurogenic*** brain tumour, pituitary tumour, head trauma, cranial surgery; ***nephrogenic*** renal disease, renal failure, ↑Ca^{2+}, ↓K^+
Symptoms polyuria, thirst
Signs dilute urine, clinically dehydrated (p319)
Investigations ↓urine osmolality (<400mOsmol/kg), ↑plasma osmolality and Na^+, 8h water deprivation test (measuring urine and plasma osmolality and weight over 8h without fluids), desmopressin (an ADH analogue) is given to determine if the cause is neurogenic (urine osmolality increases >50%) or nephrogenic (osmolality increase <45%)
Neurogenic treatment treat the cause, intranasal desmopressin
Nephrogenic treatment treat the cause, bendroflumethiazide and restrict salt and protein intake
Severe dehydration Rapid rehydration – match input to output, do not attempt to reverse hypernatraemia rapidly (see p328). Give desmopressin 1µg IM (neurogenic) or indometacin 75mg PO (nephrogenic) or both if source unknown

Female incontinence

Types of incontinence:
- ***Stress*** leakage on exercise/coughing/laughing
- ***Urge*** severe and sudden urgency (often due to detrusor instability)
- ***Overflow*** amount of urine exceeds the bladder size
- ***Functional*** restricted mobility so unable to get to toilet in time

Causes detrusor instability, prolapse, weak pelvic muscles, UTI, neurological problem (eg MS, DM), pelvic mass, age, diuretics
Ask about fluid intake, urgency, frequency, dysuria, poor stream, haematuria, leg weakness, urine leakage, faecal incontinence, effects on lifestyle, number or pregnancies with type of deliveries and birthweight, previous spinal/pelvic surgery, trauma, DM, chronic cough
Look for abdo/pelvic masses, bladder distension, prolapse (p379), effect of coughing with a full bladder
Investigations MSU, glucose, urinary diary, urodynamics studies
Treatment ***general*** weight loss, less caffeine, stop smoking, treat prolapse; ***stress incontinence*** fluid restriction, pelvic floor exercises, transvaginal tape; ***detrusor instability*** behavioural therapy (bladder drill), tolterodine 2mg/12h PO; ***overflow*** see chronic retention p320; ***functional*** aid mobility

Male incontinence

Causes UTI, neurological problem (eg MS, DM), detrusor instability, chronic urine retention, post-TURP, age, diuretics
History, examination and investigation as for female incontinence along with checking the size of the prostate and sending a PSA sample before performing the PR or inserting a catheter
Treatment ***general*** weight loss, less caffeine, stop smoking; ***stress incontinence*** fluid restriction, pelvic floor exercises, sling tape, artificial sphincter; ***detrusor instability*** behavioural therapy (bladder drill), α-blockers, antispasmodics, 5α-reductase inhibitors; ***overflow*** see chronic retention p320; ***functional*** aid mobility

Simple fluids

Who needs fluids?

Hypovolaemic shock, dehydration, low urine output, excess fluid loss, third-space losses (see opposite); ***reduced intake*** nil-by-mouth (pre-op and post-op), reduced oral fluids, reduced consciousness, vomiting, acutely ill.

Rate and type

Situation	Rate	Type of fluid
Resuscitation/acute shock	1l/stat–1h	Blood, 0.9% saline, Hartmann's, ±colloid
Hypovolaemic/acutely ill	1l/4–6h	0.9% saline, ±colloid
Maintenance	1l/8–10h	0.9% saline, dextrose saline or 5% dextrose
Elderly/mild overload	1l/10–18h	0.9% saline, dextrose saline or 5% dextrose

Maintenance fluids

The majority of hospital patients receive bags of fluid over 8h. A common regime, is shown below:

Date	Route	Fluid	Additives	Vol	Rate	Signature
19.9.08	*IV*	*5% dextrose*	*20mmol KCl*	*1l*	*8h*	*Dr C J Flint*
19.9.08	*IV*	*0.9% saline*	*Nil*	*1l*	*8h*	*Dr C J Flint*
19.9.08	*IV*	*5% dextrose*	*20mmol KCl*	*1l*	*8h*	*Dr C J Flint*

Children's maintenance fluids

Milk volume babies >5d require 150ml/kg milk each day (1fl = 30ml)
Maintenance calculate daily fluid (oral/IV) requirements from this table; 500ml bags of 0.45% saline 5% dextrose ±10mmol KCl are often used

Weight	Fluids/kg/24h	Fluids/kg/h	Expected 24h volume
first 10kg	100ml/kg/24h	4ml/kg/h	0–1000ml
10–20kg	50ml/kg/24h	2ml/kg/h	1000–1500ml
above 20kg	20ml/kg/24h	1ml/kg/h	1500–3000ml

Example 23kg child: (10 x 100ml) + (10 x 50ml) + (3 x 20ml) = 1560ml/24h

Fluid challenge

Patients in shock or with low urine output are often prescribed a fluid challenge. A bolus of 500ml (250ml if frail or heart problems) 0.9% saline IV is infused over 30min. In children use 10–20ml/kg of 0.9% saline. If the patient's urine output improves it suggests that hypovolaemia was the cause and the rate of IV infusion can be increased.

Date	Route	Fluid	Additives	Vol	Rate	Signature
19.9.08	*IV*	*0.9% saline*	*Nil*	*500ml*	*30min*	*Dr C J Flint*

Further fluids

Maintenance requirements On average per adults require 30–35ml of water/kg/24h to cover their urine output and insensible losses (sweat, respiration, stool). This equals about 2–2.5l per day for a 70kg adult; paediatric fluid requirements are on p323.

Excess losses Illness may cause patients to lose excess fluid. This may be:
- *Recordable* polyuria, NG aspirate, diarrhoea, vomiting, drains
- *Insensible* wound leakage, pyrexia, tachypnoea, burns
- *Third space* (p212), eg pancreatitis, post-op

Fluid deficit significant loss of fluid without adequate intake may be apparent on the fluid chart or from the history. The following table should act as a guide for fluid deficit in acute situations.

Fluid deficit	<750ml	750–1500ml	1500–2000ml
HR	<100	>100	>120
BP	Normal	Normal	Reduced
Urine output	>30ml/h	<30ml/h	<17ml/h

Fluid requirements

No fluid chart The patient's 24h requirements are estimated from three components:
- Estimate of maintenance requirement from weight (30ml/kg/24h)
- Additional fluids if significant insensible losses are expected (0.5–1.5l/24h)
- Estimate of fluid deficit (from history, examination, obs)

The following groups of patients may need less fluids than estimated:
- Small/elderly/frail, heart problems, renal failure, partial oral intake

Fluid balance recorded The 24h requirement can be calculated more accurately if a patient's fluid balance has been recorded. This is especially important in patients at risk of fluid overload. Again three components need to be considered:
- Recorded losses over last 24h (from fluid chart)
- Estimate of insensible losses (usually 0.5–1.5l/24h)
- Estimate of fluid deficit (from history, examination, obs and fluid chart)

Prescribing Once the 24h fluid requirement is known it can be converted into litre bags at appropriate rates. If there is a deficit the initial bags should be run more quickly to correct hypovolaemia. Prescribe the fluids so that they run out during the normal working day to reduce work for those on-call and ensure continuity of care.

Electrolyte requirements

Estimation of electrolyte requirements should take into account U+E, medications (especially diuretics and supplements) and fluid loss. Average maintenance requirements are:
- ***Na^+*** 2mmol/kg/24h – about 140mmol a day
- ***K^+*** 0.5–1mmol/kg/24h – about 40–60mmol a day

The table below shows the electrolyte content of the commonly used IV fluids. All these are isotonic (the same osmolality as plasma).

Electrolyte constituents of common IV fluids

	Na^+ (mmol/l)	K^+ (mmol/l)	Cl^- (mmol/l)
5% Dextrose	0	0/20/40	0
Dextrose saline	30	0/20/40	30
0.9% Saline	150	0/20/40	150
Hartmann's	131	5	111
Gelofusine® (colloid)	154	0	120
Packed red cells:			
Fresh	15	0.3	150
At expiry date	10	6.0	150

Special cases

Post-op Patients often leave surgery with hypovolaemia due to blood loss and oedema (third space); they may require more fluids to make up this deficit. Despite lysis of cells during surgery causing a release of K^+, most post-operative patients who remain NBM will still require supplementary KCl in their post-operative fluid replacement after 24h.

Intestinal fluid losses Most intestinal fluids have a composition similar to 0.9% saline with 20mmol/l of KCl and should be replaced with this. For the exact composition of different intestinal fluids see Section 9.2 of the *BNF*.

Heart problems Patients with previous heart disease are more prone to fluid overload and pulmonary oedema. Simple attention to fluid balance prevents problems in the majority of patients. If fluid overload develops the patient may require a ↓Na^+ diet, daily weights and fluid restriction (eg 1.5l/24h). Try to avoid furosemide if possible.

Chronic liver failure Excess Na^+ causes ascites in chronic liver failure. Restrict Na^+ by using 5% dextrose; fluid restriction is rarely required. If fluid resuscitation is required use salt-poor albumin (a blood product).

Acute renal failure Initially give rapid infusions of a colloid or 0.9% saline and avoid K^+. Further IV fluids should be determined by fluid balance and CVP in ITU or HDU.

Chronic renal failure A reduction in glomerular filtration rate (GFR) means that the kidney cannot excrete as much water, Na^+ or K^+. In mild renal failure excess fluids and Na^+ should be avoided though acute deterioration in renal function is usually a sign of hypovolaemia. In severe renal failure restriction of Na^+, K^+ and fluid (eg 1.5l/24h) is required.

Potassium emergencies

Airway	Check airway is patent; consider manoeuvres/adjuncts
Breathing	If no respiratory effort – **CALL ARREST TEAM**
Circulation	If no palpable pulse – **CALL ARREST TEAM**

Call for senior help early if patient deteriorating

Hyperkalaemia (K^+ ≥7mmol/l or >5.6mmol/l with ECG changes)
- **ECG changes:** arrhythmias, flat P waves, wide QRS, tall/tented T waves
- **15l/min O_2** in all patients
- **Monitor** defibrillator's ECG leads, BP, pulse oximeter
- **Venous access**, take bloods for urgent repeat U+E
- If **ECG changes** seen or K^+ ≥7mmol/l (arrhythmias, p186):
  - 10ml of 10% calcium gluconate IV over 2min, repeat every 15min up to 50ml (five doses) until ECG normal
  - 10units Actrapid® in 50ml of 50% glucose over 10min
  - salbutamol 5mg nebuliser
- **Arterial blood gas** to exclude severe acidosis
- Consider **calcium resonium** 15g PO or 30g PR
- Call for senior help
- Reassess, starting with A, B, C . . .

Hypokalaemia (K^+<2.5mmol/l or <3mmol/l with ECG changes)
- **ECG changes**: arrhythmias, prolonged PR interval, ST depression, small/inverted T waves, U waves (after T wave)
- **15l/min** O_2 in all patients
- **Monitor** defibrillator's ECG leads, BP, pulse oximeter
- **Venous access**, take bloods for urgent repeat U+E, Mg^{2+}
- **Replace K^+**, 40mmol/l KCl in 1l 0.9% saline IV unless oliguric
  - do not run fluids faster than 2hrly so that ≤20mmol KCl/h
  - never give KCl stat
- **Arterial blood gas** to exclude severe alkalosis
- Call for senior help
- Reassess, starting with A, B, C . . .

Life-threatening causes

Hyperkalaemia	Hypokalaemia
• Renal failure	• Hypovolaemia
• Acidosis	• Alkalosis
• Tissue necrosis	

Electrolyte imbalance

Hyperkalaemia (K^+ >5.3mmol/l)

Worrying features ↓GCS, chest pain, palpitations, abnormal ECG

Causes haemolysed blood samples, renal failure, diuretics (spironolactone, amiloride), ACE inhibitors, trauma, burns, excess K^+ (oral or IV), large blood transfusions, Addison's disease
Symptoms chest pain, palpitations, dizziness
Signs burns, dark urine, bruises, sudden death
Investigations ECG (tall tented T waves, broad QRS, flat P waves, VF), urgent repeat U+E; if K^+<7mmol/l with no new ECG changes or the sample is reported as haemolysed then await the repeat sample, otherwise follow the treatment plan opposite
Treatment calcium gluconate protects the heart against ↑K^+. Salbutamol and insulin move K^+ into cells to reduce plasma levels in the short term (1–2h) after which a rebound increase may occur. K^+ is only excreted by the action of calcium resonium (takes 24h, give with lactulose 30ml/6h PO) or by dialysis (p541).

Hypokalaemia (K^+<3.5mmol/l)

Worrying features ↓GCS, chest pain, palpitations, abnormal ECG

Causes vomiting, diarrhoea, most diuretics, steroids and Cushing's, inadequate replacement in fluids, alkalosis, renal disease, Conn's syndrome
Symptoms weakness, cramps, spasms, chest pain, palpitations, dizziness
Signs muscle weakness, hypotonia, arrhythmias
Investigations ECG (small T wave, U waves, ↑PR interval, ST depression), Mg^{2+} (often low making hypokalaemia resistant to treatment), arterial blood gas if unwell, repeat U+E
Treatment if K^+ ≥2.5mmol/l with no ECG changes add 20–40mmol KCl to IV fluids or give Sando-K® 2 tablets/8h PO and monitor U+E, consider writing up Sando-K® only for 3–5d to prevent continuous unmonitored treatment. If K^+ <2.5mmol/l or ECG changes see treatment plan opposite

Hypernatraemia (Na^+ >145mmol/l)

Worrying features ↓GCS, ↑HR, ↓BP

Causes fluid loss (diarrhoea, burns, fever, sweating, glycosuria eg DM, diabetes insipidus) or excess Na^+ (excess 0.9% saline, Conn's syndrome)
Symptoms thirst, weakness, tiredness, confusion, coma
Signs assess fluid balance, urine output, volume status p319
Investigations plasma osmolality (this is likely to be raised for both causes), urine osmolality (>400mosmol/kg if fluid loss, <400mosmol/kg if excess Na^+, normal range 350–1000mosmol/kg)
Treatment fluid replacement with slow correction of Na^+. If hypovolaemic give 0.9% saline 1l/6h (prevents sudden Na^+ shifts) until normovolaemic; if normovolaemic encourage oral fluids or 5% glucose 1l/6h. Monitor fluid balance and plasma Na^+; consider a urinary catheter.

Hyponatraemia (Na^+ <135mmol/l)

Worrying features ↓GCS, irritable, seizures, ↑HR, ↓BP

↓Na^+ is usually asymptomatic initially. As plasma Na^+ falls below 120mmol/l the patient may become irritable or confused, below 110mmol/l there may be seizures or coma.
Causes
- ***Hypovolaemic*** diarrhoea, vomiting, burns, fluid sequestration (peritonitis/pancreatitis), insufficient fluid intake or due to renal loss (diuretics, Addison's, salt-losing nephropathy)
- ***Normovolaemic or mild overload*** excess 5% glucose or oral fluids, hypothyroidism, SIADH (cancer, chest infections, stroke, trauma, opiates, antipsychotics), liver failure
- ***Oedematous*** heart failure, renal failure and nephrotic syndrome, liver failure

Ask about diarrhoea, vomiting, abdo pain, tiredness, urine frequency, quantity and colour, thirst, constipation, SOB, cough, chest pain, weakness, head trauma; ***PMH*** heart, liver or kidney problems; ***DH*** diuretics, opiates, antipsychotics
Look for assess fluid balance and volume status p319, air entry and basal creps, oedema (legs and sacrum), ascites, focal neurology
Investigations FBC, U+E, LFT, CRP, plasma osmolality, urine osmolality, Na^+ and dipstick, try to establish the underlying cause
Spurious ↓Na^+ can be caused by taking blood from an arm with IV fluids running, a lipaemic sample (labs should detect this) or osmotically active substances in the blood, eg glucose. Discuss with lab if unsure.

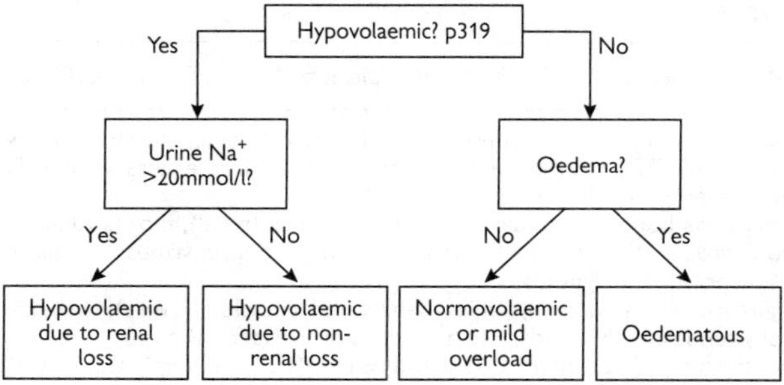

Treatment get senior help if Na^+<120mmol/l, seizures or coma; may need hypertonic saline. Chronic hyponatraemia should be corrected slowly to prevent fluid overload or osmotic demyelination (this is very rare). In all patients monitor fluid balance closely with catheter, regular obs and possibly CVP. Repeat U+E daily.

- ***Hypovolaemic*** replace lost fluid with 0.9% saline according to degree of dehydration, see p319; severe hypovolaemia should be corrected according to p212 and takes precedence over hyponatraemia. Try to establish the cause of fluid loss and treat accordingly. Stop diuretics.
- ***Normovolaemic or mild overload*** slow 0.9% saline IV eg 8–10h, Na^+ levels should rise over a few days (max 15mmol/l per day). If urine osmolality >500mosmol/kg consider SIADH.
- ***SIADH plasma*** Na^+ <125mmol/kg, osmolality <260mosmol/kg; ***urine*** Na^+ >20mmol/l, osmolality >500mosmol/kg in the absence of oedema, diuretics, hypovolaemia or abnormal thyroid/adrenal function. Fluid restrict to 500ml/24h and establish the cause, consider CXR, CT head.
- ***Oedematous*** urine Na^+ usually <10mmol/l, treat the underlying cause (see relevant chapter)

Heart failure	p226	Renal failure	p316
Liver failure	p263	Nephrotic syndrome	p315

Hypercalcaemia (Ca^{2+} >2.65mmol/l)

> Worrying features ↓GCS, chest pain, palpitations, ↑HR, ↓BP, abnormal ECG

Causes primary/tertiary hyperparathyroidism, malignancy (myeloma, bone metastases, PTH-related peptide secreting tumours), excess vitamin D supplements, sarcoidosis

Symptoms bones (bone pain ±fractures), stones (renal), moans (depression), groans (abdo pain). Also vomiting, constipation, weakness, tiredness, thirst, polyuria, weight loss.

Signs hypertension, arrhythmias, dehydrated (shock if severe), cachexia, bony tenderness secondary to a local lesion – especially along spine

Investigations ECG (short QT, arrhythmias), FBC, U+E, Mg^{2+}, Ca^{2+}, PO_4^{3-}, ALP, consider ESR, serum and urine electrophoresis, CXR, bone scan. Suspect malignancy if ↓albumin, ↓Cl^- and alkalosis.

Treatment continuous 0.9% saline 1l/4–8h for 4–5 days depending on degree of dehydration and coexistent heart disease. Consider catheterisation and CVP monitoring to assess fluid balance; monitor U+E, Ca^{2+} and Mg^{2+} daily. To further lower Ca^{2+} add furosemide 40mg/12h PO or IV in a well-hydrated patient (monitor fluid balance) and pamidronate eg 30mg in 300ml 0.9% saline over 3h. Investigate and treat the cause of ↑Ca^{2+}.

Complications renal failure, arrhythmias, osteopenia, renal stones, peptic ulcers, pancreatitis

Primary hyperparathyroidism ↑PTH from parathyroid tumour

- *Investigations* ↑PTH, ↑ Ca^{2+}, ↑ALP, ↓PO_4^{3-}
- *Treatment* correct ↑Ca^{2+} then parathyroidectomy
- ***Secondary hyperparathyroidism*** ↑PTH caused by ↓Ca^{2+}; treat the underlying cause of ↓Ca^{2+} (p331)
- ***Tertiary hyperparathyroidism*** Same presentation and treatment as primary, but caused by a parathyroid adenoma due to prolonged secondary hyperparathyroidism. Consider if renal failure.

Myeloma Plasma-cell cancer secreting monoclonal immunoglobulins

- *Investigations* ↑ESR, ↑Ca^{2+}, normal ALP, often a degree of renal failure, monoclonal immunoglobulin band in urine or plasma
- *Treatment* correct ↑Ca^{2+} as above and with pamidronate IV; give adequate analgesia. Lesions can be treated palliatively with radiotherapy or chemotherapy.
- *Complications* infection, renal failure, haemorrhage

Paget's disease Metabolic bone disorder with excessive bone resorption and formation

- *Features* ↑ALP, Ca^{2+} normal, lytic lesions and coarse trabeculations on X-ray
- *Treatment* analgesia, bisphosphonates, surgery for fractures and nerve entrapment
- *Complications* fractures, osteoarthritis, osteosarcoma (rare), cranial nerve compression (eg visual deficit)

> ***Bone mets*** five cancers commonly metastasise to bone – these can be remembered as the five 'Bs': • Breast • Bronchus • Bidney (kidney) • Byroid (thyroid) • Brostate (prostate)

Hypocalcaemia (Ca^{2+}<2.12mmol/l)

Worrying features ↓GCS, chest pain, palpitations, ↓BP, abnormal ECG

Causes vitamin D deficiency (Asians, Africans, chronic renal failure), hypoparathyroid, acute pancreatitis, alkalosis, ↓Mg^{2+}

Symptoms spasm of hands and feet (carpopedal), twitching muscles, tingling around the mouth, bone fractures, depression

Signs hyperreflexia, tetany, Trousseau's (spasm of hand from inflated BP cuff) and Chvostek's (unilateral twitching of face from tapping facial nerve 2cm anterior to ear lobe), ↓BP, bradycardia, arrhythmias

Investigations ECG (prolonged QT, arrhythmias), U+E, Ca^{2+}, PO_4^{3-}, Mg^{2+}, albumin, PTH

Treatment treat arrhythmias according to p186. If tetany is severe give 10ml 10% Ca^{2+} gluconate IV over 10min. Monitor if deficit is mild and the patient is asymptomatic. Prolonged ↓Ca^{2+}will need vitamin D replacement and Ca^{2+} supplements, eg Calcichew D3® one tablet/24h PO

Complications arrhythmias, seizures, cataracts, bone fractures

Primary hypoparathyroidism ↓PTH, despite ↓Ca^{2+}
- *Causes* iatrogenic (neck surgery), infection, metastases, idiopathic
- *Investigations* ↓Ca^{2+}, ↓PTH, ↑ PO_4^{3-}
- *Treatment* vitamin D, eg calciferol 1–2.5mg/24h PO

Pseudohypoparathyroidism Genetic resistance to PTH, presents with ↓Ca^{2+} but high PTH and dysmorphic features (short stature, strabismus, short 4/5th metacarpals, low IQ, obesity); treat as hypoparathyroid

Pseudopseudohypoparathyroidism Patients with the morphological appearance of pseudohypoparathyroidism but normal Ca^{2+} and PTH

Rickets/osteomalacia Rickets is the childhood equivalent of osteomalacia, both characterised by vitamin D deficiency or defect in metabolism.
- *Features* ↓Ca^{2+}, ↓PO_4^{3-}, ↑ALP, decreased urine Ca^{2+}, crush fractures, spontaneous fractures (eg of ribs), rickets rosary (prominent costochondral junctions), long bone bowing and Looser's zones (pseudofractures, perpendicular to cortex, common in femoral/humeral necks) on X-ray
- *Treatment* depends on cause, but usually simply by intake of adequate diet (egg yolk, milk, some fortified cereals); may require calciferol and Ca^{2+} supplements (eg Calcichew-D3® one tablet/24h PO)

Anaemia (↓Hb, ♂<13g/dl, ♀<11.5g/dl)

Worrying features Hb<8g/dl, SOB, ↑HR, ↓BP, dizziness, fainting, lethargy, palpitations, weakness, chest pain, ↓GCS/restlessness

Think about ***most likely*** acute/chronic blood loss, iron-deficiency anaemia, anaemia of chronic disease, alcoholic liver disease, malignancy; ***other*** folate/B_{12} deficiency, haemoglobinopathy (sickle cell, thalassaemia), haemolysis, inadequate dietary intake (elderly, alcoholism, vegan diet); ***medical*** hypothyroidism, coeliac disease, Crohn's disease, partial gastrectomy, pregnancy, lymphoma, rheumatoid arthritis, tropical sprue

Ask about any bleeding? (site (eg nose, rectum, vaginal), quantity, frequency) SOB (exertional/at rest), tiredness, dizziness, lethargy, weight loss, tinnitus, chest pain, palpitations, abdominal cramps, reflux, change in bowel habit, blood in stool, menorrhagia, pregnancy, recent surgery, haemoglobinopathy; ***DH*** trimethoprim, anticonvulsants, atypical antipsychotics, NSAIDs; ***SH*** alcohol, diet (vegan)

Obs HR, BP, postural BP, sats, RR, GCS

Look for pallor (conjunctiva, nail beds, tongue), bruising, glossitis, mouth ulcers, hepatomegaly, splenomegaly, jaundice, ascites; ***CVS*** palpitations, bruits, signs of active bleeding, signs of heart failure, new onset heart murmurs, lymphadenopathy; ***PNS*** peripheral neuropathy; ***CNS*** optic atrophy; ***PR*** blood in stool

Investigations ***blds*** FBC (with MCV), blood film, iron, ferritin and TIBC, serum B_{12} and folate, reticulocyte count, direct antiglobulin test (see below), CRP, ESR, U+E, LFT, TFT; ***ECG*** if CVS symptoms; ***CXR*** if suspicion of cancer and to help explain SOB; ***other*** LDH, urine and serum electrophoresis, autoantibodies screen, bone marrow biopsy

Treatment

Asymptomatic anaemia

- Look for a cause; aim to exclude malignancy in patients >40yr (p421)
- Note that Hb may be normal immediately after a large acute bleed
- Assess diet (refer to dietician)
- Consider oral iron and folate supplements

Symptomatic anaemia or Hb <8g/dl

Consider blood transfusion (see p340) and identify precipitating cause

Direct antiglobulin test (Coomb's test)

The ***direct*** antiglobulin test (direct AGT) is used to identify if the patient has developed antibodies against their own red blood cells, and as such is part of a haemolysis screen. The ***indirect*** antiglobulin test is used primarily in transfusion medicine to investigate if a recipient patient is likely to experience an antibody–antigen reaction after receiving blood from a given donor.

Mean cell volume (MCV) in different forms of anaemia

MCV < 76fl	MCV 77-95fl	MCV > 96fl
Iron deficiency	Pregnancy	B_{12}/folate deficiency
Thalassaemia	Haemorrhage	Alcohol
Haemoglobinopathies	Haemolysis	Liver disease
Sideroblastic anaemia	Renal failure	Thyroid disease
	Malignancy	Myelodysplasia
	Anaemia of chronic disease	Anti-folate drugs (eg methotrexate)
	Bone marrow failure	

Laboratory findings in different forms of anaemia

	Iron	TIBC	Ferritin	MCV
Iron deficiency	↓	↑	↓	↓
Chronic disease	↓	↓	↔ or ↑	↔
Haemolysis	↑	↓	↑	↔
Pregnancy	↑	↑	↔	↔

Abnormalities on the peripheral blood film (*OHCM*7 p314)

Acanthocytes	Irregularly shaped RBCs (liver disease)
Anisocytosis	RBCs of various sizes (megaloblastic anaemia/thalassaemia)
Blast cells	Nucleated precursor cells (myelofibrosis/leukaemia)
Echinocytes	Spiculated RBCs seen in renal failure
Howell–Jolly bodies	Nuclear remnants in RBCs (post-splenectomy)
Hypochromic	Pale RBCs (iron-deficiency anaemia)
Left shift	Immature white cells (infection or marrow infiltration)
Leukaemoid reaction	Reactive leucocytosis (infection/burns/haemolysis)
Poikilocytes	Variably shaped cells (iron or B_{12} deficiency)
Reticulocytes	Immature RBCs (haemorrhage/haemolysis)
Right shift	Hypersegmented neutrophils (megaloblastic anaemia and liver disease)
Rouleaux	Clumping of RBCs (infection/inflammation)
Schistocytes	Fragmented RBCs (microangiopathic haemolytic anaemia)
Spherocytes	Spherical RBCs (autoimmune or hereditary)
Target cells	RBCs with central staining and outer pallor (liver disease/haemoglobinopathy)

Anaemia secondary to blood loss (p212)

Symptoms epistaxis, haematemesis, blood in stool (melaena), PV bleeding, chest pain, palpitations, gastroduodenal ulcer, recent surgery, trauma
Signs ↑HR, ↓BP, postural BP drop, ↑RR, ↓GCS/restlessness, shock, pallor, sweating, cold, clammy; look at the wound site if post-op, PR
Investigations ***acute*** may be normal; repeat Hb, MCV, U+E, LFT, clotting, G+S/crossmatch, send stool sample for FOB; ***long-term*** recheck Hb, reticulocytes, OGD/sigmoidoscopy if bleeding source not apparent
Acute treatment *(p212)*

- Lay flat, elevate legs if hypotensive; give O_2
- IV access, take bloods, give rapid IV infusion (1l 0.9% saline stat)
- If bleeding site is obvious, apply firm pressure and elevate

Contact your senior – treat the cause (eg return to theatre if bleeding from operation site)

Acute blood loss

Measurement of haemoglobin does not accurately estimate the volume of blood loss in the first few hours after haemorrhage.

Acute	Hb concentration may be normal as volume of blood lost is compensated for by rise in heart rate and vasoconstriction. Only when IV fluids or normal haemodilution occurs will a fall in Hb become evident.
Intermediate	During IV fluid resuscitation Hb is diluted, unmasking loss of RBCs. Even in the absence of IV therapy the body retains salt and water in this circumstance, resulting in a natural haemodilution.
Late	Homeostasis regulates the volume of fluid in the intravascular compartment and the Hb often rises as the 'clear' fluid (colloids/crystalloids) is eliminated. Without IV therapy Hb may remain low and rise slowly over the following weeks as erythropoeisis generates more RBCs.

Anaemia of chronic disease

Causes infection (eg TB, endocarditis), rheumatoid arthritis, chronic renal failure, malignancy, collagen vasculitides, liver failure
Symptoms fatigue, SOBOE, lethargy; may have very few symptoms/signs
Investigations ↓MCV, ↓TIBC/serum iron, ↔/↑ferritin
Treatment treat the underlying disease; consider EPO in renal failure

Haemolytic anaemia

Causes ***acquired*** autoimmune, microangiopathic (TTP, HUS, DIC, HELLP, mechanical heart valves, extracorporeal circuit), blood transfusion incompatibility, drugs, toxins, burns; ***hereditary*** haemoglobinopathy, G6PD deficiency, red cell membrane disorder (eg spherocytosis)
Signs mild jaundice, murmurs, lymphadenopathy, hepatosplenomegaly
Investigations ↑bilirubin (unconjugated), reticulocyte count >85 × 10^9/l (or >2%), ↑LDH, ↓haptoglobin, ↑urobilinogen
Treatment depends upon the cause. Often steroids, immunosuppression ±splenectomy if autoimmune, treat precipitating cause if acquired.

Iron-deficiency anaemia

Iron found in red meat, kidney beans, spinach
Causes GI loss (gastroduodenal ulcer, oesophageal varices, colitis, haemorrhoids, malignancy), menorrhagia, poor diet, malabsorption syndromes, tropical infections
Symptoms abdominal pain, blood in stool, dysphagia, haemoptysis, haematemesis, menorrhagia, pregnancy, diet, diarrhoea, epistaxis
Signs pallor, koilonychia, glossitis, angular stomatitis; **PR** blood in stool
Investigations ***blood*** film (microcytic, hypochromic with anisocytosis and poikilocytosis), ↓serum iron, ↓ferritin, ↑TIBC; ***stool*** check for FOB; ***other*** upper/lower GI endoscopy, contrast enema
Treatment treat the anaemia with oral iron supplements (ferrous sulphate 200mg/8h PO for 2wk, then 200mg/12h PO) though warn about side-effects: change in bowel habit (constipation or diarrhoea), black stools, nausea, epigastric pain. Admit if anaemia is severe enough to warrant transfusion (p340), find and treat the cause. If the patient has been prescribed oral iron tablets, make sure they have been taking them.

> Treatment with oral iron raises the Hb by ~1g/dl per week at best

Folate/folic acid (vitamin B_9) deficiency

Folate found in liver, yeast, spinach, nuts, green vegetables
Causes ***malabsorption*** alcohol, coeliac disease, Crohn's disease, tropical sprue; ↑***requirement*** pregnancy, DM, lymphoma, malignancy; ***drugs*** anticonvulsants, trimethoprim, methotrexate
Symptoms breathlessness, fatigue, headaches
Signs glossitis, other features of anaemia
Investigations B_{12}/folate, ↑MCV, investigate for malabsorption
Treatment treat the cause; folic acid 5mg/24h PO for 4mth. For chronic haemolysis give long-term, but exclude and treat any concurrent B_{12} deficiency as this will worsen B_{12} deficiency neuropathy

> If planning pregnancy, folate should be taken 0.4mg/24h until 12/40

Vitamin B_{12} deficiency

Vitamin B_{12} found in liver, kidney, fish, chicken, dairy products
Causes poor dietary intake, pernicious anaemia, malabsorption (as for folate deficiency), stomach/bowel resection, Crohn's disease
Symptoms sensory neurological deficit, autoimmune disorders (eg vitiligo, infectious mononucleosis, Addison's disease), dementia
Signs sore mouth (glossitis, angular cheilosis, mouth ulcers), neurological defects (peripheral neuropathy, optic atrophy), jaundice
Investigations B_{12}/folate, ↑MCV, blood film, ↑methylmalonic acid (MMA), intrinsic factor/gastric parietal cell antibodies (↑ in pernicious anaemia)
Treatment dietary advice, hydroxocobalamin 1mg/72h IM for 2wk, then 1mg/3mth IM as maintenance dose

Leukaemia (*OHCM*7 p336)

Type		Patient	Prognosis
Acute	Lymphoblastic (ALL)	2–4yr or >60yr	Children 85% cure Elderly <20% cure
	Myeloid (AML)	Old>young, post-chemo	30% 5yr survival
Chronic	Lymphocytic (CLL)	>40yr, often male	60% 5yr survival
	Myeloid (CML)	Middle aged	90% 5yr survival

Symptoms recurrent/unusual infection, easy bruising, bleeding, joint pain, bone pain, malaise, weakness, abdo pain, weight loss, sweats
Signs pale, petechiae, bruises, bleeding (check gums), lymphadenopathy, signs of infection, hepatosplenomegaly, focal neurology
Investigations FBC (anaemia, ↑WCC, look at differential), blood film, U+E, LFT, LDH, urate, clotting, bone marrow biopsy
Treatment ***acute*** antibiotics, blood and platelet transfusions; ***chronic*** chemotherapy, radiotherapy, bone marrow transplant
Complications infection, bleeding (DIC), hyperviscosity, cell lysis

Lymphoma (*OHCM*7 p344)

Type	Patient	Prognosis
Hodgkin's	Young adults or elderly, often male	60–90% 5yr survival
Non-Hodgkin's	Any age, especially the elderly	50% overall survival

Symptoms enlarged non-tender lumps, fever, night sweats, infection, itching, tiredness, weight loss, malaise, weakness, rarely pain with alcohol
Signs pale, lymphadenopathy, hepatosplenomegaly
Investigations FBC, blood film, U+E, LFT, Ca^{2+}, LDH, urate, CXR, CT/MRI of thorax, abdo and pelvis, lymph node biopsy (Reed–Sternberg cell seen in Hodgkin's) and bone marrow biopsy
Treatment chemotherapy, radiotherapy, bone marrow transplant
Complications infection, bone marrow failure, SVC obstruction

Paraproteinaemia Several diseases can cause an excess of a single (clonal) immunoglobulin including **myeloma** (see p330). Elderly patients may get a benign monoclonal gammopathy that causes a mild but stable increase in IgG, IgM or IgA, often mistaken for myeloma. A raised IgM can also be caused by lymphoplasmocytic lymphoma (Waldenström's).

Myeloproliferative disease (*OHCM*7 p350)

A group of neoplastic diseases including:
- Polycythaemia [rubra] vera (↑Hct; angina, focal neurology)
- Essential thrombocytosis (↑platelets; bleeding or thrombosis)
- Myelofibrosis (marrow fibrosis; marrow failure, splenomegaly)

Causes of lymphadenopathy

Infection local infection, EBV, CMV, hepatitis, HIV, TB, syphilis, toxoplasmosis, bartonella 'cat-scratch', fungal; **malignancy** lymphoma, leukaemia, metastases; **autoimmune** SLE, rheumatoid; **other** sarcoidosis, amyloidosis, drugs

Pancytopenia – ↓Hb, ↓plts and ↓WCC (*OHCM*7 p348)
Marrow failure aplastic anaemia, malignancy, myelodysplasia, fibrosis
Other hypersplenism, SLE, infection (eg TB, AIDS), B_{12}/folate deficiency
Investigations FBC, blood film, bone marrow biopsy, B_{12}/folate
Treatment treat the underlying cause, blood and platelet transfusions

Sickle-cell disease and trait (*OHCM*7 p326)
Common genetic disease in African and Caribbean populations; all patients with an Afro-Caribbean background must be screened pre-op.
Homozygote haemolytic anaemia (Hb 6–8g/dl), reticulocytes, bilirubin
Heterozygote (trait) normal Hb, usually healthy
Complications thrombosis, severe haemolysis, cerebral infarction, priaprism, gallstones, avascular necrosis, sickle crisis (below)
Sickle crisis precipitated by hypoxia, hypothermia, acidaemia and dehydration (common in homozygotes, uncommon in heterozygotes). RBCs sickle, causing infarctions and severe pain (long bones, back, ribs, sternum, chest). Chest symptoms (pleuritic pain and SOB) may warrant ITU.
Treatment Warm, O_2, IV fluids, analgesia (often strong opioids), folic acid, ±antibiotics, avoid acidosis. May need an exchange transfusion.

Thalassaemia (*OHCM*7 p328)
These are common genetic diseases in Mediterranean, Arabian and Asian populations. ***β-thalassaemia major*** (homozygote) and ***α-thalassaemia*** cause severe anaemia that requires treatment (see below). ***β-thalassaemia minor*** (heterozygote) causes a mild anaemia (>9g/dl, MCV<75fl) that rarely requires treatment.
Treatment repeated transfusions, iron chelation (protection against iron overload), folate, may need splenectomy

Bone marrow aspiration and biopsy A common investigation of haematological disease. The sample is taken from the iliac crest or sternum under local anaesthetic. The needle is pushed through the bone cortex and 2–3ml of marrow is aspirated; a marrow trephine biopsy may be taken with another needle. Complications include bleeding, infection and pain. Often performed under a GA in children.

Graft vs. host disease Rashes, vomiting, diarrhoea and deranged LFTs following allogeneic (donated) bone marrow transplants. Discuss with transplant centre and treat with high-dose steroids.

Splenomegaly See p468

Post-splenectomy See p119

Transfusion of blood products

Blood product transfusions carry risks as well as benefits. Ensure the benefits outweigh the risks before commencing a transfusion and consider alternatives to transfusion. Risks and types of transfusion-related reactions are shown on p341 and p342.

When taking blood for blood bank samples it is essential to **hand-label** the blood bottle at the bedside and check them against the patient's identification wristband. Errors here would be disastrous.

Group and save (G+S) blood is analysed for ABO and Rh(D) grouping (see below) and for common red cell antibodies which are documented in the notes and recorded on the pathology computer system.

Crossmatch (X-match) blood is analysed to establish the patient's ABO and Rh(D) grouping, for common red cell antibodies and then paired with a stored blood product which is compatible.

Ordering blood products for elective use depend upon the type of surgery planned or the severity of anaemia. Most hospitals have guidelines instructing juniors on pre-operative blood bank requests to prevent excess crossmatching which results ultimately in products becoming out of date and being wasted. A G+S is sufficient for many procedures – check your local guidelines. Ensure blood bottle and form are labelled fully and clearly and indicate when the blood products are required.

Ordering blood products for emergency use is a daily occurrence in most hospitals. In extreme emergencies blood can be issued without a full crossmatch (group-specific, p340), but this carries a greater risk of transfusion reactions. Ensure blood bottle and form are labelled fully and clearly, and indicate the quantity and type of blood product(s) needed as well as where they are needed. Speak to the haematology technician and arrange a porter to collect and deliver the blood products.

How many units to transfuse depends upon the clinical situation and following advice from a haematologist (where appropriate). In adults it is seldom necessary to transfuse just one unit of packed red cells, even for elective transfusions for chronic anaemia as the risks in this situation would likely outweigh the benefits. Seek senior/specialist advice.

Checking blood products before they are given to a patient requires two people. Ask the patient their name, DoB and check against the form supplied with the blood product or check the form against their identification band. Next check the name, DoB, hospital number and blood product number, blood group and expiry date on each bag and the form; initial and time against each unit on the form once checked.

ABO blood groups

Blood group	Serum antibodies	UK frequency	Comment
O	Anti-A, anti-B	44%	Universal donor
A	Anti-B	45%	
B	Anti-A	8%	
AB	None	3%	Universal recipient

Packed red cells*

Indication	Symptomatic/severe anaemia or severe haemorrhage
Immunology	Needs ABO and Rh(D) compatibility between donor and recipient
Volume	220–320ml
Donor	Each unit from one donor
Shelf life	35d at 4°C; must be used within 4h once removed from fridge
Cost	~£130 per unit

* Whole blood seldom used and all blood is now leucocyte-depleted

Platelets

Indication	Symptomatic/severe thrombocytopenia, platelet dysfunction
Immunology	Rh(D) compatibility more important than ABO, but not crucial[1]
Volume	~300ml (adult dose is 300ml; one unit, ~300 x 10^9 platelets)
Donor	Usually pooled from four donors
Shelf life	5d at room temperature – must be kept agitated
Cost	~£210 per unit

Fresh frozen plasma (FFP)

Indication	Replacement of coagulation factor deficiency (if no safe single factor concentrate available), multiple coagulation deficiencies (associated with severe bleeding), disseminated intravascular coagulation (DIC)
Immunology	Rh(D) compatibility more important than ABO, but not crucial[1]
Volume	~250ml (adult dose is 10–15ml/kg (usually three to four units))
Donor	Each unit from one donor
Shelf life	1–2yr at –30°C; must be used within 4h once thawed
Cost	~£30 per unit (~£120 per adult dose)

Cryoprecipitate (cryo)

Indication	Fibrinogen replacement and factors VIII, XIII, von Willebrand's factor
Immunology	Rh(D) compatibility more important than ABO, but not crucial[1]
Volume	250ml (adult dose 500ml; two units)
Donor	Each (250ml) unit from five donors
Shelf life	1–2yr at –30°C; must be used within 4h once thawed
Cost	~£165 per unit (~£330 per adult dose)

[1] ABO compatibility is reversed for non-red cell blood products so AB becomes the universal donor and O the universal recipient. Rh(D) status is unaffected, Rh(D) –ve recipients should receive Rh(D) –ve blood products if possible.

Red cell transfusion

Indications To correct symptomatic or severe anaemia, to replace blood loss in haemorrhage. Trigger factors for transfusion are illustrated opposite. Generally a unit of packed cells raises the Hb by 1g/dl in the adult.
Contraindications absolute patient refusal (eg Jehovah's Witness) relative pernicious anaemia/macrocytic anaemia, CRF/fluid overload.
Prescribing Blood should be prescribed on the fluid part of the drug chart. If the patient is hypovolaemic from haemorrhage then each unit of blood should be infused quickly (stat-30min), though for more elective transfusions each unit can be administered at 3–4h. In elective transfusions it may be necessary to give furosemide 20–40mg/stat PO/IV with alternate units (starting with the second unit) to prevent fluid overload in patients with LV dysfunction.
In acute haemorrhage it may be necessary to obtain blood quickly. The table below illustrates options available in this situation:

Options for crossmatching of packed red cells

O-negative	Universal donor. Often stored in the ED, theatres or blood bank. Does not first require a specimen from patient.
Group-specific	ABO and Rh(D) status-specific. Takes ~15min.
Full crossmatch	ABO, Rh(D) status and antibody-tested. Takes ~45min.

Transfused blood should be given through at least an 18G cannula (green); larger bore cannula in the emergency setting. Blood should not be left unrefrigerated for more than 4h and cannot be returned to blood bank if it has been unrefrigerated for >30min.

Monitoring of the patient should be undertaken regularly in the initial stages of a transfusion, paying special attention to HR, BP, RR and temp. A small rise in temp and HR are common. See p342 for transfusion reactions.

Example of an elective transfusion

Date	Route	Fluid	Additives	Vol	Rate	Signature
19/9/08	*IV*	*Red cells*	*Nil*	*1 unit*	*4h*	*CJFlint*
19/9/08	*IV*	*Red cells*	*20mg furosemide PO*	*1 unit*	*4h*	*CJFlint*
20/9/08	*IV*	*Red cells*	*Nil*	*1 unit*	*4h*	*CJFlint*
20/9/08	*IV*	*Red cells*	*20mg furosemide PO*	*1 unit*	*4h*	*CJFlint*

Example of an emergency transfusion

Date	Route	Fluid	Additives	Vol	Rate	Signature
19/9/08	*IV*	*Red cells*	*Nil*	*1 unit*	*stat*	*CJFlint*
19/9/08	*IV*	*Red cells*	*Nil*	*1 unit*	*stat*	*CJFlint*
19/9/08	*IV*	*Red cells*	*Nil*	*1 unit*	*30min*	*CJFlint*

When to transfuse

While consumption of blood products has remained pretty constant over the last few years, the size of the donor pool has shrunk, making blood and blood products more scarce. Up-to-date information on blood stocks in the UK can be viewed on the National Blood Service website[1].

Why not transfuse? Besides the fact that blood products are expensive and have limited availability, they carry significant risks (see below).

Transfusion triggers have been used previously to aid doctors in deciding when to transfuse (Hb values of 8g/dl are commonly quoted as a transfusion trigger). The problem with these is that many patients are asymptomatic at these values and have sufficient haemoglobin to provide tissue oxygenation. In an otherwise fit and healthy patient (say a young man who has undergone repair of an open femoral fracture), transfusion is often not required for an Hb 8g/dl, though a frail arteriopath may suffer with SOB or anginal symptoms with a Hb of 9g/dl and require a slow transfusion to rectify this.

If in doubt speak to your senior after assessing the patient for signs or symptoms relating to anaemia.

Always ensure the cause for the anaemia is known and that appropriate treatment for this is being undertaken.

Complications of blood and blood product transfusion

Immunological	Non-immunological
Anaphylaxis	Transmission of infection:
Urticaria	• Viruses (HIV, HCV, CMV etc)
Alloimmunisation	• Parasites (malaria etc)
Incompatibility	• Bacteria (staph/strep)
Haemolytic transfusion reactions	• Prion (vCJD)
Non-haemolytic transfusion reactions	Fluid overload/heart failure
Transfusion-associated lung injury	Iron overload (repeated transfusions)
	Hypothermia

Massive blood transfusion

This is defined as replacement of one or more circulating volumes (usually >10units) within a 24h period.

Consider that platelets, clotting factors and fibrinogen will have been lost/diluted and that these should also be transfused, as well as electrolytes and minerals. Speak to a haematologist who will advise appropriately.

Ensure that steps are being taken to prevent further blood loss and that senior members of the team have a transfusion ceiling if appropriate.

1 www.blood.co.uk

Following a blood transfusion

It takes ~6–12h after a transfusion for the concentration of the RBCs to settle; FBC measurement before this is likely to give an inaccurate value.

Transfusion reactions

- These are potentially fatal, so must be managed urgently
- ABO incompatibility is the most serious complication; reactions are seen within minutes of starting the transfusion
- Low-grade pyrexia is common during a transfusion, though a rapid rise in temp at the start is worrying

Signs ↑temp, ↑HR, ↓BP, cyanosis, dyspnoea, pain, rigors, urticaria, signs of heart failure

Investigations blds FBC, U+E, bilirubin, LDH, blood film, direct antiglobulin test, clotting, regroup and save (check blood group), antibody screen, blood cultures (if pyrexia persists); ***urine*** free haemoglobin; ***CXR*** if signs of heart failure

Treatment

- As outlined below
- Inform senior/haematologist early
- Re-check labelling on blood products and return bags to laboratory

Acute transfusion reactions (*OHCM7* p571)

Features	**Management**
≥2 of: • Temp >40°C • Chest/abdo pain • ↑HR/↓BP • Agitation • Flushing	Likely haemolytic transfusion reaction (ABO incompatibility – potentially life-threatening) Stop transfusion. **Call senior help.** 15l/min O_2, 1l 0.9% saline stat, hydrocortisone 200mg/stat IV, chlorphenamine 10mg/stat IV. Monitor BP, urine output. Check ECG, U+E (↑K^+), clotting/fibrinogen.
• Temp <40°C • Shivering	Likely **non-haemolytic transfusion reaction** Slow transfusion. Give paracetamol 1g/6h PO. Monitor obs (HR, BP, temp). **Call senior help** if no improvement or worsening.
• ↑HR/↓BP • Bronchospasm • Cyanosis • Oedema	Likely **anaphylaxis** (p206) Stop transfusion. **Call senior help**. 15l/min O_2, adrenaline (epinephrine) 0.5mg (1:1000) IM, 1l 0.9% saline stat, hydrocortisone 200mg/stat IV, chlorphenamine 10mg/stat IV.
• Urticaria • ±↑temp <40°C • ±itch	Likely **allergic reaction** Observe closely to exclude anaphylaxis. Slow transfusion. **Inform senior.** Monitor obs (HR, BP, temp). Hydrocortisone 200mg/stat IV, chlorphenamine 10mg/stat IV.
• Fluid overload	Slow transfusion. 15l/min O_2 and sit upright. Consider furosemide 40mg/stat IV. Catheterise. See p226. **Call senior help** if no improvement or worsening.

The Jehovah's Witness and blood products

Healthcare professionals must not be frightened to talk to any patient about sensitive matters if it may affect their care, and patients who are Jehovah's Witnesses are no different. You might feel uncomfortable talking to a Jehovah's Witness about what they regard as acceptable practice, but they will welcome the fact you are open and addressing an issue which is an important part of their religion. You are also likely to learn a great deal about their religion and about the person inside. Most Jehovah's Witnesses carry an advanced directive stating their requests with regards blood products.

Acceptable treatments includes non-blood volume expanders (saline, Hartmann's, glucose, gelatins (Gelofusine®), starches (Voluven®), dextrans), agents which control haemorrhage (recombinant factor VIIa (NovoSeven®), tranexamic acid, aprotinin) and agents which stimulate red cell production (recombinant erythropoietin (check preparation is free from human albumin), intravenous iron).

Unacceptable treatments are those which involve the transfusion of donor whole blood, packed red cells, white cells, fresh frozen plasma and platelets. Pre-operative autologous (self-donated) blood is also not acceptable.

Treatments which individuals may consider include blood salvage (intra-operative and post-operative), haemodilution, haemodialysis and cardiac bypass (pumps must be primed with non-blood fluids). Some fractions of plasma or cellular components may be considered acceptable by some individuals (cryoprecipitate, albumin, immunoglobulins, clotting factors, and haemoglobin-based O_2 carriers). Transplants including solid organ (heart, liver) as well as bone and tissue may also be accepted.

For further information the Hospital Liaison Committee for Jehovah's Witnesses, which is a national organisation, has several centres all over the country run by Jehovah's Witnesses. Hospital switchboard will have contact details of your local representatives though there is also a 24-hour contact service for urgent advice for patients and Healthcare professionals (0208 906 2211); non-urgent enquiries can be sent via email to his@wtbts.org.uk.

The paediatric patient who is a Jehovah's Witness

If the parents refuse life-saving treatment this can be a complex issue. In an immediately life-threatening situation blood products can be given under common law, but always involve the most senior member of the team available (eg consultant). If the requirement is less than immediate (eg ≥2h) then the most senior member of the medical team should seek legal advice, which might involve approaching the High Court.

Clotting emergencies

Airway	Check airway is patent; consider manoeuvres/adjuncts
Breathing	If no respiratory effort – **CALL ARREST TEAM**
Circulation	If no palpable pulse – **CALL ARREST TEAM**

↑INR *(OHAM2 p686)*

Most likely over-anticoagulation with warfarin (see below), consider DIC (see opposite).

For other causes of ↑INR see p605.

Patient not bleeding	Patient bleeding

INR 5–8
• Withhold warfarin until INR <5
• Identify cause of ↑INR
	Medical emergency
	• Seek senior help urgently
	• Discuss with haematologist
	• Vitamin K 5mg/stat IV
	• Consider factors II, VII, IX or X
	  • Octaplex®
	  • or FFP 4units/stat
	• Withhold warfarin until INR <5
	• Identify cause of ↑INR

INR 8–12 • Withhold warfarin until INR <5 • Vitamin K 2mg/stat PO/IV • Daily INR – consider admission • Identify cause of ↑INR	
INR >12 • Withhold warfarin until INR <5 • Vitamin K 5mg/stat PO/IV • Admit for daily INR • Identify cause of ↑INR	

↑APTTr *(OHAM2 p686)*

Most likely over-anticoagulation with heparin (p347), consider DIC (see opposite).

For other causes of ↑APTTr see p348.

Bleeding

Disseminated intravascular coagulation (*OHAM*2 p702)

Mechanism Clotting cascade triggered pathologically resulting in consumption of fibrinogen, platelets and clotting factors. Microthrombi form in small vessels causing end-organ damage and RBC lysis in fibrin meshwork. Results in ↑bleeding tendency.
Signs bruising, bleeding, signs of triggering pathology (see below)
Investigations ↓platelets, ↑PT/INR, ↑APTTr, ↓fibrinogen, ↑↑D-dimer
General treatment request urgent senior help and discuss with haematologist. Treat underlying cause (most commonly sepsis), supportive measures for BP, acidosis, hypoxaemia and maintain normothermia. Blood transfusion to compensate for anaemia (may exacerbate coagulopathy).
Correction of coagulopathy give FFP (15ml/kg, ie 3–4 units) if PT or APTT >1.5 x control (ie INR or APTTr >1.5). Platelets and cryoprecipitate (rich in fibrinogen) may be recommended by haematologist.
Complications massive haemorrhage, end-organ failure, death (severe DIC carries significant mortality)

Common precipitants of DIC

- Septicaemia (Gram –ve > Gram +ve)
- Disseminated malignancy
- Incompatible blood transfusion reactions
- Profound hypoxia
- Liver failure
- Severe trauma/burns

Thrombocytopenia (*OHAM*2 p690)

Often an incidental finding on the FBC, but patients can present with bleeding (gums, epistaxis) or easy bruising. Often it does not cause problems, but if surgery or a procedure which could result in bleeding is planned then it is an important finding. Reduced production (eg aplastic anaemia, leukaemia), increased consumption (eg idiopathic thrombocytopenia (ITP), haemolytic-uraemic syndrome), and drug-induced (eg heparin, valproate) forms are all recognised. Treatment includes identification and reversal of cause, usually by a haematologist. Heparin-induced thrombocytopenia (HIT) must be considered if ↓plt >50% of baseline 5–10d after commencing heparin/LMWH.

Bleeding disorders (*OHCM*7 p330)

Haemophilia A factor VIII deficiency; X-linked recessive, but 30% of cases have no FH due to new mutation. ***Presents*** with bleeding in childhood, usually haemarthrosis. ***Investigations*** ↑APTTr and ↓factor VIII. ***Treatment*** avoid NSAIDs and IM injections. Seek senior help early, and ensure team speaks to haematologist on-call if patient is bleeding.

Haemophilia B (Christmas disease) factor IX deficiency; X-linked recessive. Clinically treat in the same fashion as haemophilia A.

von Willebrand's disease absent or ineffective von Willebrand's factor (vWF). Over 22 inherited and acquired types. ***Presents*** with mucocutaneous bleeding and menorrhagia. ***Investigations*** ↑APTTr, ↓factor VIII, INR and platelets normal. ***Treatment*** avoid NSAIDs and IM injections. Seek senior help early, and ensure team speaks to haematologist on-call if patient is bleeding.

Anticoagulation

Anticoagulant drugs are used to prevent primary thrombotic events or to prevent clot propagation after a thrombotic event has occurred. The two main types of anticoagulants used are:

- **Heparin** (LMWH/unfractionated) – used acutely or in the short term
- **Warfarin** – used for long-term prophylaxis/treatment

Indications and contraindications for anticoagulants

	Indications	Contraindications (absolute and relative)
Heparin	Venous thromboembolism (treatment and prophylaxis), PE, MI, ACS, unstable angina, acute peripheral arterial occlusion, haemodialysis, pre/post-op, AF[1]	Haemorrhage, haemophilia, active gastroduodenal ulcer, thrombocytopenia, allergy, recent major trauma/ haemorrhagic CVA
Warfarin	Venous thromboembolism, PE, prosthetic heart valves, AF[1]	Recent haemorrhagic CVA, severely ↑BP, pregnancy, active gastroduodenal ulcer, cerebral artery thrombosis, endocarditis, liver failure, risk of falls or non-compliance

[1] NICE guidelines, June 2006, *Atrial fibrillation*.

Thromboprophylaxis in *medical* patients

Consider if age >40yr, obese, known malignancy, prolonged immobility, oedema, inflammatory bowel disease, pregnant, on COC/HRT, recent surgery or trauma (within 2wk), long distance travel (within 1wk).

- Treat with LMWH, eg:
  - enoxaparin 20mg/24h SC until mobile
  - enoxaparin 40mg/24h SC, if **high risk**[2], until mobile
- TED stockings

If the patient has thromboembolic event whilst on anticoagulation:

- Contact haematologist
- Check clotting
- Check compliance with medication; review other medications

Thromboprophylaxis in pre-operative *surgical* patients

Generally, all surgical patients are given thromboprophylaxis unless they are day cases or actively bleeding. Those who are on long-term warfarin should stop taking this at least 3d pre-operatively. The INR should be <1.5 for most operations and lower if spinal or epidural anaesthetic techniques are to be employed; **warn the anaesthetist**. Patients who have prosthetic heart values will need IV heparin whilst warfarin is omitted (p347). See p348 for restarting warfarin post-operatively.

2 Previous DVT/PE, obesity, thrombophilia (*OHCM*7 p358)

Starting heparin (*OHCM*7 p334)
LMWH DVT/PE prophylaxis or therapeutic for ACS/MI or DVT/PE.
- ***Prophylaxis*** eg enoxaparin 20–40mg/24h SC
- ***Therapeutic for ACS/MI*** eg enoxaparin 1mg/kg/12h SC
- ***Therapeutic for DVT/PE*** eg enoxaparin 1.5mg/kg/24h SC

Monitor platelets if long term (risk of heparin-induced thrombocytopenia)

Unfractionated heparin (check local policy)
Anticoagulation for prosthetic heart valves or in acute limb ischaemia.
- Check baseline clotting (INR and APTTr)
    - If APTTr <1.3 and patient weighs 50–100kg and <80yr give a bolus dose of heparin 5000units IV. Start an infusion at 30,000units/24h IV.
    - If APTTr <1.3 and patient weighs <50kg or >100kg give a bolus of 80units/kg and infuse at 25units/kg/h IV.
    - If APTTr <1.3 and patient aged >80yr give an initial bolus dose of 2500units/stat IV and infuse at 20,000units/24h IV; if weight <50kg or >100kg d/w haematologist
    - If APTTr >1.3 omit bolus dose and commence infusion as above
- Check the APTT ratio 6h after starting treatment and then every 12–24h Adjust the dose according to the APTTr (see table below), rechecking the APTTr 6h after each dose change
- For heparin use in obstetric or paediatric patients discuss with the consultant obstetrician or haematologist, respectively
- If planning to discharge patient on anticoagulant therapy, start warfarin (see opposite) whilst still on heparin and monitor using the INR. Discontinue the heparin once the INR is therapeutic.

Dose changes to unfractionated IV heparin

APTTr	Next dose	Retest time
<1.3	Bolus dose of 5000u; ↑infusion by 5000units/24h	6h
1.3–1.4	↑infusion by 5000units/24h	6h
1.5–2.4	No change	12–24h
2.5–3.0	Stop infusion for 30min; ↓infusion by 5000units/24h	6h
3.1–4.0	Stop infusion for 60min; ↓infusion by 5000units/24h	6h
4.1-5.0	Stop infusion for 60min; ↓infusion by 7500units/24h	6h
>5.1	Stop infusion for 60min; ↓infusion by 12000units/24h	3h

Over-anticoagulation with unfractionated heparin

The elimination half-life of unfractionated heparin is 0.5–2.5h (longer in hypothermia), so stopping an infusion rapidly normalises the APTTr. Reversal of anticoagulant effect can be achieved with protamine. Protamine 1mg over 10min IV neutralises ~100units unfractionated heparin within 15min. Maximum dose of 50mg; higher doses have anticoagulant effects. Protamine can cause allergic reaction in patients who have allergies to fish.

Starting warfarin (*OHCM*7 p334)

Day 1 – warfarin 10mg/PO at 1800h; use 5mg if elderly or liver disease
Day 2 – measure INR at 0900h

- If INR <1.8 warfarin 10mg/PO at 1800h
- If INR >1.8 warfarin 5mg/PO at 1800h

Day 3 – measure INR at 0900h; use table below to guide further dosing

Warfarin dosing – can be written up for three days unless ↑INR or poorly controlled

INR	<2.0	2.0–2.4	2.5–2.8	2.9–3.2	3.3–3.5	3.6–4.0	≥4.1
Day 3 dose	8mg	5mg	4mg	3mg	2mg	0.5mg	Omit[2]
Further doses[1]	≥6mg	5.5mg	4.5mg	4mg	3.5mg	3mg	Omit[2]

[1] Day 4 dose and likely maintenance dose.
[2] Omit this dose, give 1mg the next day at 1800h and recheck INR the following day.

Check INR daily for 5d, then alternate days until stable, then weekly if inpatient or hand care over to anticoagulation clinic or GP.

Target INR and duration of therapy for warfarin

Indication	Duration of therapy	Target INR range
DVT/PE prophylaxis	Whilst at high risk only	2–3
Treatment of DVT/PE	6mth (life if recurrent)	2–3
AF	Until in sinus rhythm	2–3
Prosthetic heart valve	Lifelong	3–4

Restarting warfarin post-operatively

Confirm with seniors that warfarin therapy is to be recommenced. Load with warfarin as described above or in accordance with local policy.

Discharging patients on warfarin

- Explain to patient why compliance is crucial and need for INR checks
- Ensure suitable follow-up with either anticoagulation clinic or GP
  - speak to these directly and arrange patient's first appointment
- Issue yellow warfarin book
  - prescribe enough warfarin to last until next INR check
- Tablet colours – white (0.5mg), brown (1mg), blue (3mg), pink (5mg)

Drugs interacting with warfarin – consult Appendix 1 of *BNF*

Drugs which ↑INR	Alcohol, amiodarone, cimetidine, simvastatin, NSAIDs
Drugs which ↓INR	Carbamazepine, phenytoin, rifampicin, oestrogens

Over-anticoagulation with warfarin see p344

Falls and collapse

> Worrying features ↑HR, ↓BP, chest pain, palpitations, head injury, loss of consciousness, recurrent vomiting, incomplete recovery, focal neurology, long time spent on hard surface, hypothermia

Think about *serious* MI, arrhythmias, shock, sepsis, CVA, seizure, hypoglycaemia, hypoxia, PE; ***common*** postural hypotension, mechanical fall (eg tripping), syncope (vasovagal, situational, cardiac), ataxia

Ask about symptoms and activity before falling (aura, dizziness, chest pain, palpitations), speed of onset, visual changes, loss of consciousness (can you remember: falling, being on the floor, getting up), incontinence, recovery, head injury, other injuries, mechanism of injury, length of time spent immobile; ***PMH*** previous falls (and investigations), heart problems, DM, parkinsonism; ***DH*** warfarin, antihypertensives, diuretics, nitrates; ***SH*** usual mobility and aids, ability to eat and drink independently, alcohol

Obs temp, HR, lying and standing BP, glucose, GCS, sats, RR

Look for pulse volume, HR and regularity, carotid bruit, volume status (p319), heart murmurs (aortic stenosis), focal neurology, ability to stand, ability to walk, bruising, lacerations or haematomas on the head or body, movement of all limbs, sites of tenderness

Investigations simple mechanical falls only need investigation for injuries, otherwise ***ECG*** arrhythmia or MI (consider cardiac monitor); ***blds*** FBC, U+E, CRP, cardiac markers (repeat at 12h, CK often raised if there is significant bruising); ***CT*** if focal neurology, persistent ↓GCS or post-head injury (p358); ***X-ray*** clinical suspicion of a fracture

Treatment ABC. Give all patients 15l/min O_2 and lie flat or with legs up initially. Exclude serious conditions (HR, ECG, BP, glucose) and establish IV access. Treat according to diagnosis. See also trauma p352.

History	Examination	Investigations	
Vasovagal syncope	Onset in seconds, precipitated by fear, stress, pain or standing	±Postural drop, otherwise normal	Normal
Cardiac syncope	Sudden onset and recovery, chest pain, palpitations, SOB	Fast, slow or irregular pulse	Arrhythmia or MI on ECG, ±↑cardiac markers
Neurological	Rapid onset, headache, ↓GCS, weakness, altered sensation	Focal neurology, persistent ↓GCS, ataxia	CVA or intracranial haemorrhage on CT; check glucose
Seizure	±Aura, no memory, limb movements, tongue biting, post-ictal phase, incontinence	Drowsy, injuries, ±Todd's paresis	Initial investigations often normal, check glucose

Please review this patient who has fallen . . .

If a patient falls whilst in hospital the nurses should fill out an incident form (p76) which requires the patient to have been reviewed by a doctor. You should exclude serious causes of falls (opposite) and post-fall injuries (particularly head and hip).

Ask the nurse for a **full set of obs** including blood glucose, ±postural BP.

In the **notes** document the circumstances and symptoms, specifically mention chest pain, palpitations, head injury, loss of consciousness, vomiting and confusion.

Examination A brief cardiovascular and neurological examination is essential. Look over the head for signs of injury, feel for midline c-spine tenderness and check for reduced movement or pain in the shoulders, elbows, wrists, hips, knees and ankles.

Investigations Have a low threshold for an ECG. See p352 for management of trauma and p358 for head injury. Other investigations as indicated.

Review Ask the nurses to record regular neuro obs (pupils and GCS) and bleep you again if concerned.

Seizures	p286	Hypoglycaemia	p271
Focal neurology	p291	Pyrexia	p392
GCS + confusion	p280	Chest pain	p177
Head injuries	p358	Tachyarrhythmias	p186
Postural drop	p217	Bradyarrhythmias	p194
Joint examination	p496	Hypoxia	p219
Vertigo	p302	Ataxia	p302

Vasovagal syncope (faint)

Syncope is a transient loss of consciousness with complete recovery.
Symptoms brought on by stress, pain or fear, usually whilst standing, onset over seconds, feeling faint, nausea, blurred vision, spontaneous and full recovery within minutes, clammy, cold
Signs may have a postural drop (p217), pale, flushing, sweating, eyes rolling, twitching whilst unconscious, rapid recovery, otherwise well
Investigations normal ECG, consider a tilt table test if recurrent
Treatment 15l/min O_2 (until serious diagnoses excluded), lay flat with legs elevated, remove stimulus (eg needle, blood), gradually sit up once symptoms have passed

Situational syncope

Similar to vasovagal syncope, but brought on by a specific action:

- ***Micturation*** middle-aged men; advise to sit down to urinate
- ***Carotid sensitivity*** can be brought on by shaving
- ***Cough*** brought on by coughing fits

Causes of recurrent falls old age, confusion/dementia, inappropriate use of aids (sticks, frames), poor sight, peripheral neuropathy, Parkinson's, cerebellar disease, multiple sclerosis, alcoholism, foot drop, vertigo, incontinence/diuretics, arthritis

Trauma

Worrying features shock, breathlessness, ↓GCS, significant mechanism

Think about *emergency* severe trauma see p168; ***common*** head injury, neck injury, fractures, dislocations, sprains, strains, bruises, incisional wounds, lacerations, abrasions, foreign bodies

Ask about location at time of injury, activity prior to injury, cause/mechanism of injury, direction of injury, ability to walk/move immediately and now, exacerbating/relieving actions, pain, severity, associated symptoms, time of last meal; ***PMH*** all medical problems, asthma (and previous use of NSAIDs), clotting abnormalities, kidney problems, stomach problems, surgery, admissions, psychiatric problems; ***DH*** NSAID reactions, tetanus status, allergies; ***SH*** occupation, dominant hand, normal mobility, help at home

Important questions to assess RTAs

Speed, seatbelt, airbag, driver/passenger, front/back, type of impact, what stopped the car, was the car written off, was the car drivable, did the doors open

Obs HR, BP, RR, GCS, temp

Look for see p496–506 for specific joint examinations; resting position, bruising, swelling, deformity, skin changes, active range of movement, tenderness (bony vs. soft tissue), passive range of movement, stability of joint, ability to use joint eg walking, always check:
- Joints directly above and below the site of injury
- Distal sensation and circulation (HR, capillary refill) of affected limb

Investigations *X-ray* if fracture/dislocation is possible or to exclude a radio-opaque foreign body (eg glass, metal), see p632 for interpretation

Treatment Analgesia (p428) can be given prior to examination and investigation to give the medication time to act. Treatment depends on the injury:

Wounds	p356	Neck injury	p360
Head injury	p358	Nosebleeds	p357

The following injuries need senior review or referral:
- Wounds with involvement of deep structures eg tendons
- Wounds in cosmetically sensitive areas eg face
- Wounds with loss of skin tissue
- Displaced fractures
- Unstable fractures
- Open fractures
- Fractures with skin tenting or dislocation
- Dislocation of major joints

Soft tissue injuries (sprains, strains)

A sprain is minor damage to a ligament while a strain is caused by minor damage to a muscle. Both are managed the same way:

- ***Rest*** initially, but weight-bear or exercise as soon as symptoms allow
- ***Ice*** to reduce swelling over the first 48h; keep the ice away from the skin (eg use a tea towel) and apply for 10–15min at a time
- ***Elevation*** reduces both swelling and pain

Prescribe adequate analgesia (eg regular paracetamol 1g/6h PO and ibuprofen 400mg/8h PO) and give reassurance. Compression is not recommended as it can delay regaining full mobility.

Natural history symptoms often worsen over 24-48h then start to improve; they may take up to 6wk to resolve completely. Most heal completely, otherwise physiotherapy strengthening exercises can help.

Dislocations

- Provide adequate analgesia
- Document deficits in distal circulation and sensation and at-risk nerves
- X-ray to confirm dislocation and exclude coexisting fracture (except ankle dislocation which should be reduced urgently p355)
- Relocate with adequate analgesia or sedation
- Strap/dress to hold in place
- Recheck and document any deficits in distal circulation and sensation and at-risk nerves
- Repeat X-ray to confirm relocation
- Discharge with analgesia and orthopaedic follow-up

Natural history symptoms improve dramatically with relocation though some discomfort may be present for days/weeks. Further dislocation is common and may need physiotherapy or orthopaedic treatment.

Fractures

Types **hairline** very small fracture, no bony displacement; **simple** 2 bone sections; **comminuted** ≥3 bone sections; **open/compound** bone is has pierced the skin or overlying wound exposes bone.

You should suspect a fracture if there is a history of high forces, bony tenderness, swelling or reduced range of movement (ROM)

Treatment

- ***Analgesia only*** eg single ribs or coccyx fractures, these do not need X-raying unless a complication is suspected (eg pneumothorax)
- ***Immobilisation*** (eg backslab, sling) analgesia, fracture clinic follow-up for fractures that do not need an urgent orthopaedic review
- ***Orthopaedic referral*** if unstable, compound (open) or neurovascular involvement

Natural history pain worst after the injury with little improvement by day 3–5. Simple fractures should heal over 6wk with minimal complications; serious fractures may reduce range of movement permanently.

Open/compound fractures resuscitate (p168), get immediate senior help if distal sensation/circulation are impaired or coexisting dislocation. Give analgesia (eg IV morphine), take a digital/polaroid photo, cover the wound with saline-soaked swabs, backslab under gentle traction, start IV antibiotics (cefuroxime 1.5g/8h IV and metronidazole 500mg/6h IV), review tetanus status, X-ray, refer urgently to orthopaedics.

Hands (examination p504)

Crushed fingertip (subungual haematoma) fingertip is bruised and tender with a blood clot under the nail; should be X-rayed to exclude a tuft fracture (comminuted fracture of the distal phalanx).

- *Trephining* pain can be relieved by using a heated element to burn through the nail and relieve the pressure
- *Nail bed repair* if the nail is displaced there will be a nail bed laceration; this needs to be sutured to prevent abnormal nail growth which can severely impair finger function. Repair with absorbable sutures by removing the entire nail under a ring block or GA; replace the nail and use non-adherent dressing

If a tuft fracture was present then antibiotics should be prescribed after either procedure since the fracture is now effectively open.

Finger dislocation (distal/proximal interphalangeal joint) finger is flexed and swollen at the DIPJ/PIPJ. Relocate with Entonox® or digital nerve block by pulling the distal finger dorsally then straight; neighbour strap.

Punch injury (fractured ring or little metacarpal) swelling and tenderness over lateral knuckles; exclude rotational deformity by looking at the line of the nails (viewed end-on) with the fingers extended and flexed. Analgesia, X-ray, orthopaedic referral if grossly displaced/unstable otherwise volar splint and hand clinic follow-up. If they punched a face treat any cut as a bite (co-amoxiclav 375mg/8h PO and check tetanus status).

Wrist (examination p503)

Colles' fracture distal radial, ±ulna fracture, distal segment displaced dorsally (dinner fork). Manipulate with Bier's/haematoma block.

Smith's fracture similar to a Colles' fracture but with the distal segment displaced towards the palmar surface and unstable; refer to orthopaedics.

Scaphoid fractures tender over the anatomical snuff-box, palmar or dorsal aspect of scaphoid, pain on loading the thumb or stressing scaphoid by flexing and ulnar deviating the wrist. Fracture usually not visible on X-rays immediately so apply scaphoid splint and review in 10–14d.

Elbow (examination p502)

Radial head fractures reduced forearm supination and pronation with pain; raised anterior fat pad on X-ray (p632), collar and cuff.

Shoulder (examination p501)

Dislocation (anterior) unable to flex shoulder forwards, anterior bulge under clavicle, gap below the acromion. Check axillary nerve sensation (50p-sized patch over the deltoid insertion), use IV analgesia/sedation, reduce by manipulation (eg Kocher's) under senior supervision, recheck X-ray, pulses, sensation post-reduction and apply collar and cuff sling.

Head of humerus fracture upper arm swelling and bruising in elderly patient, check radial and axillary nerve sensation (above), collar and cuff.

Clavicle fracture tender clavicle ±deformity, exclude pneumothorax clinically, broad arm sling, urgent orthopaedics referral if skin tenting.

Nose

Fracture X-ray does not help with assessment, feel for tenderness and swelling over nasal bridge, exclude septal haematoma (cherry in septum, get senior help immediately if present), provide analgesia and offer ENT review in 1–2wk for assessment ±reduction once swelling has resolved.

Chest

Rib fracture X-ray if suspected pneumothorax or flail chest (eg sharp trauma, breathlessness, examination findings), otherwise discharge with analgesia, teach breathing exercises (regular deep breaths) and advise not to smoke.

Hip (examination p497)

Fracture pain on external and internal rotation or loading, shortened and externally rotated if displaced, FBC, U+E, glucose, G+S, ECG, CXR and hip X-ray, exclude medical cause of fall (eg MI), refer to orthopaedics.

Knee (examination p498)

Sprain may be unable to weight-bear or allow adequate examination of the knee. Make sure the knee is stable (ligaments), X-ray to exclude fractures (check tibial plateau) and discharge with analgesia, Thackery splint and crutches, review in 1wk.

Dislocation (patella) knee is half flexed with patella away from midline. Relocate with Entonox® by gently straightening the knee and pressing on the patella to move it to the midline.

Ankle (examination p499)

Sprain the Ottowa ankle rules are used to decide if an ankle X-ray is required (see below). Ankle sprains require analgesia, rest, ice and elevation; in extreme cases crutches may be needed for 48h.

Ottowa ankle rules (see p500 for bones of the foot)

If all the following are present there is usually no need to X-ray an ankle:

- Can weight-bear 2 steps or was able to weight-bear immediately after injury
- No tenderness over the posterior surface or the tip of the lateral malleolus
- No tenderness over the posterior surface or the tip of the medial malleolus
- No tenderness over the calcaneum, navicular or base of 5th metatarsal
- No tenderness over the proximal fibula

Fracture (lateral malleoli) check for medial malleolar tenderness and talar shift (gap between the medial malleolus and talus of >4mm on X-ray), refer to orthopaedics if the fracture is above the joint line or talar shift is present; otherwise backslab and fracture clinic.

Ankle dislocation (posterior fracture dislocation) this is an emergency. Deformed ankle, skin tenting, peripheral circulation and sensation often reduced. Get a senior immediately, give Entonox® and/or IV analgesia/sedation; grip the calf and pull the heel forward with the other hand then hold whilst plaster is applied. Check pulses, sensation and X-ray.

Wounds

Ask about mechanism of injury, paying particular attention to bites (animal or human), foreign bodies (broken glass), contamination with soil or manure and when the wound occurred. Always ask about and document tetanus status.

Look for record the site, size (measure) and type of the wound, check distal sensation, pulse/cap refill and movement, look and feel inside the wound (possibly with local anaesthetic) to assess depth, presence of foreign bodies and involvement of deep structures (eg tendons).

Types of wound	
Puncture	Deep wound with a small skin defect, eg cat bite, nail
Incisional wound	Wound caused by sharp objects, eg knife/broken glass, often have straight edges and can be deep
Laceration	Wound following blunt trauma, eg banging head on pavement, edges are often ragged and bruised
Abrasion	Graze
Full thickness	Wound that fully penetrates the skin (epidermis and dermis) so that subcutaneous fat is visible
Superficial	Wound that does not fully penetrate the skin

Cleaning all wounds should be thoroughly cleaned with water or 0.9% saline. Abrasions may need to be scrubbed and deeper wounds may need cleaning with high-pressure 0.9% saline (use a syringe and green needle hub with the needle broken off). Cleaning can be done under anaesthetic.

Important rules

- X-ray all wounds involving broken glass or metal foreign bodies
- Wounds should not be closed if:
  - older than 12h (unless facial)
  - very dirty or infected
  - foreign bodies present
  - bites
- Refer wounds that involve tendons, joints, arteries or nerves

Primary closure is closing the wound in ED. There are several options:

- ***Glue*** for faces, children and small wounds (<2cm) if the edges are not gaping. The glue should just hold the edges together, not enter the wound. Be very careful not to get the glue in the eye.
- ***Steristrips*** for fingertips, pretibial lacerations and small wounds.
- ***Sutures*** (p600) for wounds which are large, deep or over joints. Simple, interrupted stitches of mono-filament, non-absorbable suture are used for the vast majority. A layered closure with absorbable sutures may be required if the wound is especially deep; seek senior help. Do not close wounds under tension unless under senior supervision.

Delayed primary closure the wound is left open for 3–5d then reviewed and closed if no infection is evident.

Secondary closure allowing the wound to heal without intervention.

Tetanus status should be documented for all wounds. Ensure adequate prevention and remember that patients over 50yr and immigrants may have received no previous tetanus vaccinations.

Tetanus prophylaxis

Immunisation status	Clean wound	Tetanus-prone wound[1]
Full course (5 injections) **or** booster <10yr ago	No prophylaxis needed	HATI[2] only if contaminated with manure
Partial course **and** booster ≥10yr ago	Tetanus booster	Tetanus booster and HATI[2]
Not immunised or unknown	Start tetanus course	Start tetanus course and give HATI[2]

[1] Tetanus-prone wounds:
- Heavy contamination especially with soil or manure (remember gardeners)
- Infection or wounds >6h old
- Puncture wounds (eg cat bites, nails)
- Devitalised tissue

[2] HATI – human anti-tetanus immunoglobulin

Antibiotics amoxicillin 500mg/8h PO and flucloxacillin 500mg/6h PO for 5d for puncture wounds, wounds involving bones (eg crushed fingertips) and patients with valvular heart disease; consider antibiotics for wounds >6h old that have not been cleaned. Co-amoxiclav 625 mg/8h PO for 5d for heavily contaminated wounds.

Animal/human bites treat with co-amoxiclav 625mg/8h PO for 5d.

Assaults the notes you make may be used in a legal case many years from now so think carefully about what you write. For example:
- Distinguish facts from hearsay; make it clear where information came from, eg 'Patient alleges assault with an iron bar, witnesses describe LOC for 3min'.
- Document injuries accurately including location, size (measure) and type of wound (see table previous page); use simple line diagrams. Do not interpret what caused the wound.
- Write your notes imagining them being read out in public by someone wishing to make you appear stupid.

Epistaxis (nosebleeds)

Ask about onset, duration, severity, previous episodes, frequency, trauma, ↑BP, NSAID/anticoagulation therapy, bleeding tendency, alcohol
Look for postural BP change, shock, site of bleeding, fracture
Investigations if persistent/recurrent: FBC, clotting/INR, LFT, G+S
Management resuscitate if needed; try the following to stop bleeding:
- Tilt head down and apply pressure to the soft fleshy part of the nose just below the bone for 15min
- Pack with nasal tampons for 48h making sure the attached ribbon is visible to aid removal; if bleeding continues refer immediately to ENT
- If severe and persistent review resuscitation and refer urgently to ENT

Head injury

Worrying features ↓GCS, vomiting, seizures, basal skull fracture, amnesia

Think about *emergency* unconscious, ↑ICP, extradural haematoma, subdural haematoma; ***common*** concussion

Ask about mechanism of injury, time of injury, loss of consciousness, seizures, memory (before, during and after), blood/fluid from nose or ears, vomiting, weakness/tingling/numbness in limbs, time of last meal, dizziness, visual changes, headache; ***PMH*** clotting abnormalities, all previous medical, surgical or psychiatric problems; ***DH*** warfarin, tetanus status, allergies; ***SH*** occupation, normal mobility, help at home

Obs GCS, HR, BP, RR, glucose

Look for GCS (p280), orientation, CSF leaking from ears (otorrhoea) or nose (rhinorrhoea), Battle's sign (bruising over the mastoid processes, a late sign), blood behind eardrum (haemotympanium), 'panda' eyes, (bruising around the eyes), focal neurology (eg weakness or numbness)

Investigations *CT* if indicated (opposite), skull X-rays are rarely used

Treatment

Unconscious bleep an anaesthetist immediately and see p280
CT head according to the CT criteria opposite ±admission

- *Admit* for 12h observation with 30–60min neuro obs if unwell but do not meet the CT criteria or if they live alone
- *Discharge* if well, acting their normal selves, GCS 15 and CT not required, discharge into care of a responsible sober adult with head injury advice sheet and analgesia; they do not need to be kept awake

Head injury discharge advice
Reattend if: severe headache, vomiting, fits, difficult to rouse, vision/balance changes
Do not: drink alcohol, be in a house alone or take sleeping tablets for next 24h
Do: take analgesia (eg paracetamol), take usual medications, rest

Subdural haematoma

Venous bleed into the skull; can be acute (↓GCS and ↑ICP post-trauma) or chronic (fluctuating conscious level over days in elderly, alcoholics, patients on anticoagulation).

Management CT diagnosis; drained by craniotomy or burr hole

Extradural haematoma

Arterial bleed into skull often from middle meningeal artery.
Symptoms/signs initially well but GCS falls over 6–8h as blood collects
Management CT diagnosis; drained by craniotomy or burr hole

Post-concussion syndrome

Patients may have concussion symptoms for months after a head injury eg headaches, dizziness, tiredness, depression, memory problems.

NICE head injury guidance

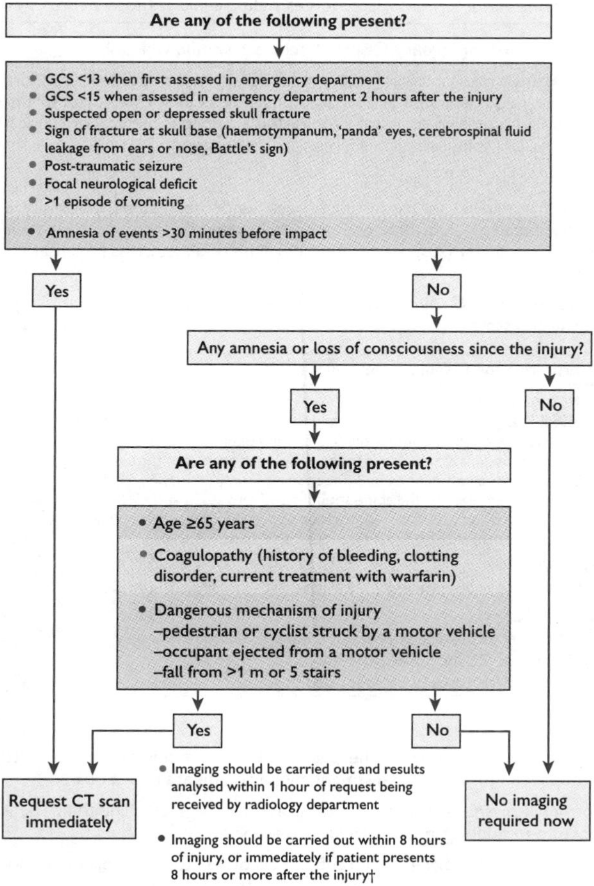

†If patient presents out of hours and is ≥65, has amnesia for events more than 30 minutes before impact or there was a dangerous mechanism of injury, it is acceptable to admit for overnight observation, with CT imaging the next morning, unless CT result is required within 1 hour because of the presence of additional clinical findings listed above.

Neck injury

Worrying features ↓GCS, large forces, multiple injuries, focal neurology

Think about *emergency* C-spine fracture; ***common*** whiplash

Ask about mechanism of injury, walking since the accident, comfort sitting up, neck pain, time of neck pain onset, head injury, weakness or tingling of limbs, time of last meal; ***PMH*** asthma, previous medical or surgical problems; *DH* tetanus status, allergies; ***SH*** occupation

Obs GCS, HR, BP, RR, glucose

Look for midline vs. paravetebral neck tenderness, steps, deformity, if appropriate (see algorithm opposite) test patient's ability to turn their neck 45° each way (stop if limbs tingling), limb weakness, loss of sensation, other injuries

Investigations ***C-spine X-rays*** if indicated (opposite); ***CT neck*** if **X**-rays difficult to assess or take

Interpreting the C-spine X-ray

Lateral view
- Should be able to see all of C1–7 and the top of T1 otherwise re-X-ray
- Check the smooth alignment of: ① anterior vertebral bodies ② posterior vertebral bodies ③ spinolaminar line ④ spinous processes (not including C1)
- Check each vertebral body and disc space is a similar size and shape
- Soft tissue anterior to the spine should be <5mm at C2 and <22mm at C6
- Gap between odontoid peg (bone seen above C2 vertebral body) and C1 (small bone anterior to the peg) should be <3mm

AP view
- Check the spinous processes are aligned with similar sized spaces

Odontoid peg view
- Entire peg and lateral borders of C1 and C2 should be visible
- Check that C1 and C2 are aligned
- Check for fractures of the odontoid peg

Treatment

Abnormal X-rays/CT leave the patient's neck immobilised and refer to orthopaedics for urgent assessment; monitor patient's neuro obs

Normal X-rays/CT remove neck collar and sandbags, examine the neck as above to exclude ligamentous injury, treat for sprain

No X-rays/CT if imaging is not required according to the algorithm opposite then remove neck collar and sandbags, treat for sprain

Neck sprain (if severe called 'whiplash')

Symptoms/signs gradual onset neck pain and stiffness getting worse over 48h before settling, tender over neck paravertebral>midline
Diagnosis normal imaging (if performed)
Treatment advise that symptoms are likely to worsen overnight, give paracetamol and regular NSAIDs, heat/ice may help initially, soft collars are not used, initial rest (≤48h) then gradual return to normal activity

NICE neck injury guidance

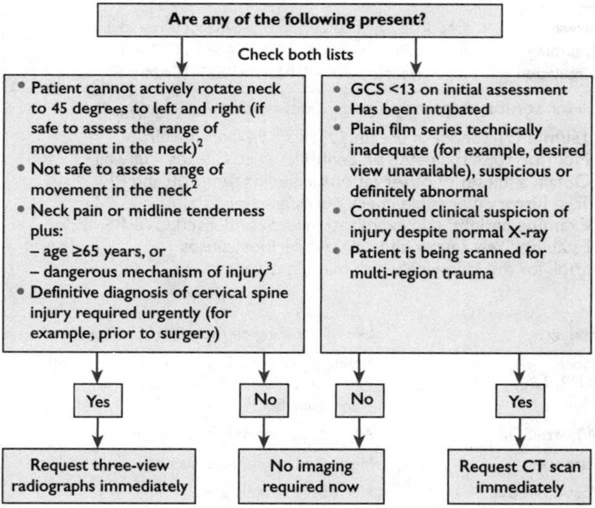

[2] Safe assesment can be carried out if patient: was involved in a simple rear-end motor vehicle collision; is comfortable in a sitting position in the emergency department; has been ambulatory at any time since injury and there is no midline cervical spine tenderness; or if the patient presents with delayed onset of neck pain.

[3] Dangerous mechanism of injury: fall from > 1m or 5 stairs; axial load to head – for example, diving; high-speed motor vehicle collision; rollover motor accident; ejection from a motor vehicle; accident involving motorised recreational vehicles; bicycle collision.

Children under 10 year

- Use anterior/posterior and lateral radiographs without an anterior/posterior peg view.
- Use CT imaging to clarify abnormalities or uncertainties.

Rash emergency

Airway	Check airway is patent; consider manoeuvres/adjuncts
Breathing	If no respiratory effort – **CALL ARREST TEAM**
Circulation	If no palpable pulse – **CALL ARREST TEAM**

Call for **senior help** early if patient unwell or deteriorating

- **15l/min O_2** if short of breath, O_2 sats <94% or unwell
- **Monitor** pulse oximeter, BP, defibrillator ECG leads if unwell
- Obtain a full set of **observations** including temp, BP and RR
- Take **history** if possible/check **notes**/ask ward staff
- **Examine patient**: skin examination and condensed CVS, RS, abdo
- Establish likely causes and rule out **serious causes**
- Look for the following which may aid diagnosis

Finding	Life-threatening diagnoses to consider
Shock (↑HR, ↓BP)	Meningococcal septicaemia p365 Allergic reaction/anaphylaxis p206 Necrotising fasciitis p365
Wheeze/SOB	Allergic reaction/anaphylaxis p206
Purpura	Meningococcal septicaemia p365
Post-operative	Necrotising fasciitis p365 Allergic reaction/anaphylaxis p206
Following drug administration	Allergic reaction/anaphylaxis p206 Erythema multiforme major p370
Mouth involvement	Allergic reaction/anaphylaxis p206 Erythema multiforme major p370 Meningococcal septicaemia p365

Shock	p209
Wheeze/SOB	p219

Rash

> **Worrying features** RR >30, sats <92%, wheeze, systolic <100mmHg, confusion, tachy/bradycardia, rapidly changing rash

Think about *life-threatening* meningococcal septicaemia, necrotising fasciitis, erythema multiforme major (Stevens–Johnson syndrome), urticaria (anaphylaxis), staphylococcal scalded skin syndrome; ***other*** cellulitis, viral rash (including chickenpox, shingles), fungal infections, Henoch–Schönlein purpura (HSP or anaphylactoid purpura), ecchymosis; ***chronic*** eczema, psoriasis, contact dermatitis, vasculitis, bullous disease

Ask about speed of onset, distribution of rash, associated symptoms, exacerbating and relieving factors, family history; ***PMH*** previous skin disease, GI disease, immunosuppression, weight loss; ***DH*** allergies, vaccinations, antibiotics, previous drugs to treat skin disease; ***SH*** occupation, exposure to irritants, pets, exposure to others with illness/skin disease

Obs temp, RR, BP, HR, O_2 sats

Look at hands and nails for pitting, Janeway lesions or Osler's nodes, splinter haemorrhages, and then affected area and rest of skin for purpura, petechiae, telangiectasia, urticaria, weals, erythema, target lesions, macules, papules, pustules, blisters, excoriation, fissures and cracks, lichenification, and ulcers noting distribution (extensor or flexor surfaces), size, shape, surface and edges. Also examine the scalp and mouth. Other examination as dictated by history.

Investigations are often not necessary as history and clinical examination often gives the diagnosis. Some specific investigations listed below.

Treatment depends upon cause of rash, see following pages.

Test	Use	Example
Blister fluid	Viral culture	Herpes simplex
Blood test	Autoantibodies	Discoid lupus erythematosus
	Serology	Streptococcal cellulitis
Nail clippings	Fungal culture	Onychomycosis
Patch testing	Allergy testing	Nickel allergy
Skin biopsy	Culture	Mycobacteria/fungi
	Histology	Microscopic diagnosis
	Immunohistochemistry	Cutaneous lymphoma
Skin scrapings	Fungal culture	Tinea
	Microscopy	Scabies
Skin swab	Bacterial culture	Impetigo
Wood's light	Fungal fluorescence	Scalp ringworm

Bacterial infections causing a rash

Cellulitis

Symptoms hot, sometimes tender area of erythematous skin which is spreading, usually on leg or face, but can occur anywhere especially if history of trauma to skin (insect bite, small cut, cannula site). May be systemic effects – fever, anorexia, N+V, diarrhoea.

Signs blanching warm spreading erythema (outline area with marker to observe response to treatment), ±mild oedema, break in the skin, serous discharge, lymphadenopathy in draining nodes, ↑temp, ↑HR, ↑RR

Investigations ***blds*** ↑WCC and NØ, ↑CRP/ESR; blood cultures if pyrexial; D-dimer likely to be raised in infection so not useful in differentiating cellulites from DVT; ***skin swabs*** not usually helpful; ***USS*** to exclude DVT or ruptured Baker's cyst

Treatment – check local guidelines
- If patient is systemically well and has no other significant comorbidities, oral antibiotics (flucloxacillin 500mg/6h PO or erythromycin 500mg/12h PO)
- If signs of systemic upset (↑temp, ↑HR, ↑RR) or coexisting disease (DM, IHD, PVD) admit for short stay for IV antibiotics (flucloxacillin 2g/6h IV or vancomycin 1g/12h IV)
- If profoundly unwell, request senior help immediately and consider necrotising fasciitis (p365)

Impetigo

Symptoms weeping, spreading erythema, highly contagious
Signs background of erythema with yellow crust and serous discharge, usually on face, but can occur anywhere. Occasionally blisters.
Investigations ***skin swabs*** show *Staphylococcus aureus* in >90% of cases, but group A streptococcus can sometimes be found
Treatment of localised disease can be achieved with topical fusidic acid (Fucidin®) 8h for 1wk. More extensive impetigo should be treated with oral antibiotics, flucloxacillin 500mg/8h PO (for staphylococci) and penicillin V 500mg/8h PO (for streptococci). Ensure close contacts are examined and treated if necessary, and encourage good hand hygiene and non-sharing of towels or flannels given its highly contagious nature.

Erythematous cannula site

Cannulae should be resited every 72h to prevent local inflammation/infection. If a cannula site is red and inflamed or pus is present, take a skin swab for C+S, remove cannula and **clean** and dress the site. Give oral flucloxacillin 500mg/6h PO or erythromycin 500mg/6h PO (if penicillin allergic) for 5d.

Necrotising fasciitis (*OHAM*2 p330)

Symptoms rapidly spreading eryhema sometimes from break in skin or operation site but may be no apparent skin trauma, usually disproportionately painful; features of systemic sepsis, fever, sweating, N+V, diarrhoea, anorexia, ↓GCS

Signs blanching warm spreading erythema (outline area with marker to observe rate of spreading), blisters, ±oedema, lymphadenopathy in draining nodes, sometimes crepitus over tissues, ↑temp, ↑HR, ↑RR, ↓BP – patient will rapidly become very sick

Investigations ***blds*** ↑WCC and NØ, ↑CRP/ESR; ***blood cultures and skin swabs/tissue aspiration*** may identify infective organism(s) but do not withhold treatment to do these tests if patient is systemically unwell; ***X-ray*** may reveal gas in subcutaneous tissues of affected area

Treatment – this is a medical emergency

- Seek senior help **immediately**
- Surgical debridement is the most important measure, **consult senior surgeon without delay**
- Likely to need a combination of IV flucloxacillin, metronidazole, ciprofloxacillin and clindamycin

Do not wait for investigations before starting antibiotic treatment

Pathogens is usually a group A streptococcus (type 2 necrotising fasciitis) or a combination of aerobic and anaerobic organisms typically seen following abdominal surgery or in diabetics (type 1 necrotising fasciitis)

Outcome depends upon speed of identification and initiation of treatment. Extensive tissue loss from surgery and tissue necrosis is common, and the disease has ~25% mortality rate.

Meningococcal septicaemia (*OHCM*7 p807)

Symptoms include fever, joint and muscle ache, non-blanching rash, N+V, diarrhoea, anorexia, malaise; if meningitis is present too, headache, neck stiffness and photophobia are also classical

Signs ↑temp, ↑HR, ↑RR, cap refill >2sec, ↓BP, non-blanching petechial or purpuric rash; **meningism/photophobia if meningitis also present** **(p300)**

Investigations ***blds*** ↑WCC and NØ, ↑CRP/ESR, meningococcal PCR, deranged clotting if severe sepsis (DIC); ***blood cultures*** do not withhold antibiotics before taking these if patient is systemically unwell

Treatment – this is a medical emergency

- **A**irway, **B**reathing (give O_2), **C**irculation (obtain IV access)
- Seek senior help immediately
- If patient is in shock (systolic BP <100), involve ITU team urgently
- 0.9% saline 1l/STAT IV
- Ceftriaxone 4g/STAT IV if septicaemia is suspected
- Inform public health consultant once patient is stable

Pathogen Neisseria meningitides, a Gram-negative diplococcus; groups B and C being the predominant strains in Europe and North America. A group C vaccine is available, but a group B is not

Outcome depends upon speed of identification and initiation of treatment. Loss of limbs is common in both children and adults. Mortality for meningococcal septicaemia is about 10% in the developed world.

Viral infections causing a rash

Chickenpox (varicella zoster virus (VZV)) (*OHCM*7 p388)

Symptoms begin with fever and malaise 14–21d after exposure to VZV. Typical rash then develops, flat lesions initially which eventually evolve into itchy scabs. In older children and adults, breathlessness or altered mental functioning or loss of balance can also occur.

Signs ↑temp, ↑HR, and presence of evolving rash; macules, papules, vesicles, pustules, scabs, in centripetal distribution (spreading out from the trunk). ↑RR and ↓O_2 sats may suggest respiratory involvement. Altered personality, ↓GCS or ataxia may suggest CNS involvement.

Investigations not usually undertaken but ***vesicular fluid*** can be examined under electron microscopy or cultured for viruses; ***serology*** viral antibody titres can be monitored but this is seldom necessary; ***CXR*** may show diffuse consolidation in chickenpox pneumonitis; ***CT brain*** to exclude other causes of neurology in chickenpox encephalitis

Treatment for simple cutaneous disease is symptomatic with antipyretics for fever and simple creams for itch. Pneumonitis will likely require ITU admission for respiratory support and CNS involvement will also require admission to hospital. Antiviral therapy is usually given to patients over the age of 16, aciclovir 800mg/5h PO. In patients with immunocompromise or with severe disease (pneumonitis, encephalitis) aciclovir 10mg/kg/8h IV. Pregnant woman who have not had chickenpox before but have been exposed to it should be considered for zoster immune immunoglobulin (ZIG) to prevent the onset of disease, and given aciclovir if the disease develops – discuss with microbiologist.

Shingles (herpes zoster)

Symptoms initially focal pain, followed by classical chickenpox rash in a dermatomal distribution which does not cross the midline, ±malaise and prodrome of chickenpox

Signs observations often normal and rash is the only obvious clinical sign; classical chickenpox rash usually one of the branches of the trigeminal nerve (often ophthalmic) or a thoracic dermatome. Presence of vesicles in external auditory canal with CN VII palsy is called Ramsay–Hunt syndrome (*OHCM*7 p388).

Investigations not usually undertaken but ***vesicular fluid*** can be examined under electron microscopy or cultured for viruses

Treatment antiviral therapy limits post-herpetic neuralgia, aciclovir 800mg/5h PO; in patients with immunocompromise, parenteral antivirals should be used, aciclovir 10mg/kg/8h IV. Pain should be treated with simple analgesia (paracetamol, NSAIDs) and amitriptyline 25mg/24h PO. If eye is involved, use 3% aciclovir ointment to affected eye/5h topically and **seek ophthalmic opinion**.

Chickenpox very rarely occurs in the same individual twice. **Shingles** only occurs in patients who have had chickenpox previously; the virus lies dormant in the dorsal root/cranial nerve ganglia. **Non-immune individuals** can catch chickenpox from patients who have either chickenpox or shingles.

Viral exanthema (the viral rash)

Symptoms non-itchy rash associated with prodromal symptoms of viral illness (fever, muscle/joint aches, fluey)
Signs widespread maculopapular rash, may be features of concurrent illness/infection (↑temp, ↑HR, pharyngitis etc). Rash associated with numerous viruses (echovirus, parvovirus, EBV, measles) so not diagnostic.
Investigations none required routinely
Treatment rash will subside over 7–10d, treat concurrent symptoms

Slapped cheek fever (Fifth disease)

Symptoms non-itchy rash on cheeks associated with mild viral illness, usually in children, can occur more than once
Signs dense erythematous rash on cheeks, and reticulate erythema (net-like rash) on proximal limbs, usually associated with coryzal symptoms (runny nose, sneezing). Caused by parvovirus B19.
Investigations none required routinely
Treatment rash will subside over 7–10d, treat concurrent symptoms

Herpes simplex virus (cold sore/genital herpes)

Symptoms small painful blisters usually around mouth or in genital area
Signs vesicles or pustules around mouth (usually HSV1) or in genital area (usually HSV2). Often resolve, but then return months or years later.
Investigations not usually undertaken but ***vesicular fluid*** can be examined under electron microscopy or cultured for viruses
Treatment consists of aciclovir 200mg/5h PO for primary HSV infections and painful genital infections. Treat facial and genital 'cold sores' with aciclovir 5% to affected area/4h topically.

Molluscum contagiosum (water blisters)

Symptoms small, non-itchy spots, occurring usually in childhood, and distributed anywhere on the body; highly contagious
Signs small translucent vesicles (1–3mm), which look fluid-filled, but are actually solid, often with the central depression (punctum). Caused by a poxvirus, and usually resolve spontaneously after 6–12mth.
Investigations none required routinely
Treatment cryotherapy can be used in older children and adults

Human papillomavirus (wart virus)

Common warts are papular lesions with a rough surface with black dots within them, often on the hands and feet. Spread is by direct contact.
Plantar warts (veruccas) are usually flat or inward growing with black dots ('heads'). Often painful if over pressure areas.
Plane warts are small, flesh-coloured, flat-topped lesions usually on the face or backs of the hands without black dots.
Anogenital warts are transmitted sexually and HPV subtypes 16 and 18 are potentially oncogenic.
Treating warts is often difficult. Topical keratolytic agents (such as salicylic acid or trichloracetic acid) is usually first-line treatment, and cryotherapy (freezing) is undertaken by many general practioners as well as in dermatology clinics. Often resolve spontaneously over 2–3yr.

Fungal infections causing a rash

Dermatophyte infections

Tinea corporis also known as 'ringworm', is mildly itchy, asymmetrical rash which spreads with a slightly raised, scaly edge, often leaving a clear centre. Can occur on the face, tinea faciei.

Tinea cruris is essentially ringworm in the groin, though this lesion is often red and more plaque-like with a well demarked border.

Tinea pedis also known as 'athlete's foot', is usually found in the web-spaces of the toes, resulting in itchy skin which is fissured and macerated. If found elsewhere on the foot it is often more diffuse and scaly, but just as itchy. Pustules are not uncommon in more aggressive disease.

Treatment of small focal areas of tinea can be achieved with topical anti-fungal creams (terbinafine, clotrimazole, miconazole etc); more wide-spread infections require oral therapy (terbinafine, itraconazole)

Candida albicans

Candida is a yeast, and thrives in warm moist areas, in children's nappies (nappy rash), in body folds (intertrigo) and also in interdigital webspaces, mimicking tinea pedis. The rash is erythematous with a ragged, peeling edge which may contains small pustules. The mouth and genital tract can also be affected and present with small white plaques/white discharge.

Treatment consists of removing predisposing factors (ensure skin remains clean and dry) and topical antifungal creams (as for tinea) or lozenges or pessaries for oral and genital tract infections respectively; see p691 for oral dose.

Infestations causing a rash

Scabies is an intensely itchy rash, often worse at night, caused by the scabies mite, *Sarcoptes scabiei*, and commoner in children and with social overcrowding. The rash is papular and usually in the interdigital web-spaces of the hands and feet, around the ankles, wrists, axillae and umbilicus. Linear skin burrows are pathognomonic but not always present. The diagnosis can be confirmed by microscopic examination of skin scrapings, looking for mites or their eggs. Highly contagious.

Treatment with a scabicide (malathion or permethrin) is only successful if the whole body is treated, if all close contacts are treated and if bedding and clothing are washed. Itching may last up to 4wk after treatment.

Lice are blood-sucking parasites. **Head lice** (pediculosis capitis) are commonest in children, spread by direct contact and can result in scalp excoriation. The presence of eggs ('nits') in the hair confirms the diagnosis. **Body lice** (pediculosis corporis) are associated with poverty and not often seen in the developed world; excoriations on the skin are often the only sign. **Pubic lice** (phthiriasis pubis or 'crabs') are transmitted by sexual contact and largely affect the coarse hairs of the pubic region, but can infest leg and body hair, as well as eyelashes and eyebrows.

Treatment is with malathion or permethrin, but resistance is common and close contacts should also be treated; clothing and bedding should be thoroughly washed.

Chronic inflammatory rashes (*OHCS*7 p594)

Eczema occurs in ~5% of the population, usually presenting in childhood. Exacerbations can be precipitated by detergents, chemicals, stress and anxiety, pet fur and potentially some dietary factors (eg dairy).
Symptoms include itchy, dry skin, or patches of infected skin
Signs erythematous patches on the flexures of the elbow, knees and around the neck, with excoriations from itching; vesicles and serous weeping may be a feature. Superimposed bacterial infections in open skin are common, as is infection with cutaneous viruses (warts, molluscum). Chronically lichenification and hyperpigmentation of affected skin occurs
Treatment is multifactorial. Avoidance of known irritants should be attempted in all patients. Triple therapy with topical steroids (p155), topical emollients and bath oil and soap substitutes are the mainstay for most cases. Second-line agents such as UVB/PUVA, ciclosporin and azathioprine should only be prescribed by a dermatologist.

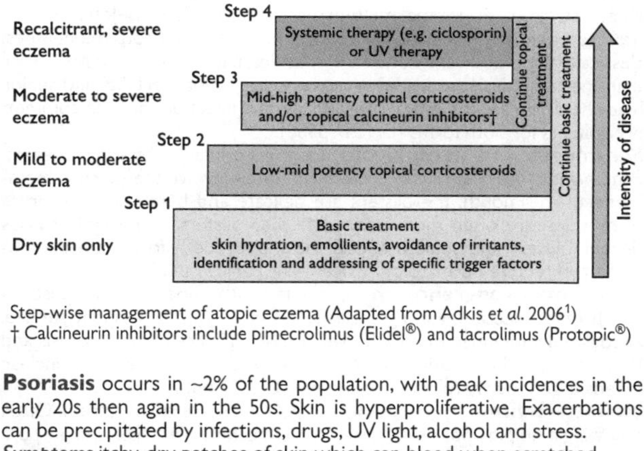

Step-wise management of atopic eczema (Adapted from Adkis *et al.* 2006[1])
† Calcineurin inhibitors include pimecrolimus (Elidel®) and tacrolimus (Protopic®)

Psoriasis occurs in ~2% of the population, with peak incidences in the early 20s then again in the 50s. Skin is hyperproliferative. Exacerbations can be precipitated by infections, drugs, UV light, alcohol and stress.
Symptoms itchy, dry patches of skin which can bleed when scratched
Signs of **chronic plaque psoriasis** are pink/red scaly plaques, especially on the extensor surfaces of elbows and knees, lower back and scalp; pitting of the nails is common; **pustular psoriasis** affects the palms and sole; **guttate psoriasis** occurs in the young, and causes numerous small oval plaques on the trunk; **flexural psoriasis** tends to occur in later life, and forms in the groins, natal cleft and sub-mammary area
Treatment is symptom-led and largely topical; emollients, mild to moderate topical steroids, vitamin D analogues, retinoids and purified coal tar are common topical treatments. Use of UVB/PUVA, methotrexate and ciclosporin therapy may be considered by a dermatologist.

1 Akdis *et al.* Diagnosis and treatment of atopic dermatitis in children and adults: European Academy of Allergology and Clinical Immunology/American Academy of Allergy, Asthma and Immunology PRACTALL Consensus Report. J Allergy Clin Immunol 2006; 118:152–69.

Other causes of rash

Urticaria also known as 'hives' or 'nettle rash' is characterised by the formation of prominent papules or plaques (the weal) which are pale initially but become erythematous with a surrounding rim of pale skin or erythema (the flare). Common in response to certain topical chemicals (such as nettle sting) but also in response to systemic drugs (sometimes part of anaphylaxis) or antigens (during a blood transfusion). Can also occur as part of the rare hereditary angio-oedema syndrome, due to deficiency in plasma C1 esterase inhibitor (*OHCS*7 p603).

Erythema nodosum is characterised by tender, erythematous nodules on the shins. Commoner associations include: infections (tuberculosis, streptococcal, *Mycoplasma pneumoniae* and EBV), sarcoidosis, inflammatory bowel disease, autoimmune disorders, pregnancy and drugs (sulphonamides and the oral contraceptive pill) (*OHCS*7 p588).

Erythema multiforme is a hypersensitivity rash and has two subtypes. **Erythema multiforme minor** produces target lesions, which have a red centre, a clear circular area, then an outer red ring, and look like their names suggests. **Erythema multiforme major** or Stevens–Johnson syndrome, is a more sinister rash involving two or more mucous membranes, classically the mouth, and consists of macules, papules and pustules rather than the target lesions; this form carries a significant mortality and senior help should be sought immediately. Drugs and infections are the common precipitants for both forms (*OHCS*7 p588).

Pemphigus and pemphigoid are rare primary blistering diseases. Pemphigus causes superficial blisters and often involve the mucous membrane of the mouth; the blisters are delicate and burst easily, so areas of raw skin are often more noticeable than blisters. Pemphigoid causes deeper blisters and seldom affects the mouth. Both forms are autoimmune and require dermatology assessment (*OHCS*7 p602).

Pyoderma gangrenosum presents with nodules or pustules which often ulcerate, leaving a blackened ulcer with a purulent surface. Associated with inflammatory bowel disease, primary biliary cirrhosis and rheumatoid arthritis amongst others, its exactly cause remains unclear. Needs urgent dermatologist assessment (*OHCS*7 p602).

Henoch–Schönlein purpura is largely a disease of childhood. Often following a simple upper respiratory tract infection, petechiae and purpura develop on the legs and buttocks and may be associated with abdominal pain, haematuria and an arthropathy. It usually resolve spontaneously (*OHCS*7 p197).

Vasculitis is a broad term applied to a myriad of diseases involving an inflammatory process of blood vessels. Skin lesions vary from small telangiectasia (spider naevi) to urticaria, purpura and skin necrosis. The commoner autoantibodies used to aid in the diagnosis of these can be found on p631. A dermatologist should be consulted if a complex vasculitic rash is suspected.

Granuloma annulare occurs most often in children and younger adults, and initially presents as a cluster of papules which often merge into a ring. It is commoner on the hands and feet, and as associated with DM. Often resolves spontaneously.

Rashes in systemic disease

Common skin manifestations in systemic disease	
Diabetes mellitus (DM)	Candidiasis, necrobiosis lipoidica (non-itchy yellow maculopapular lesions on the shins), folliculitis (infected hair follicles), skin infections
Coeliac disease	Dermatitis herpetiformis (itchy papules and vesicles on knees, elbows, back and buttocks)
IBD	Erythema nodosum (red nodules, classically on the shins), pyoderma gangrenosum (papular lesions which become ulcerated)
Rheumatoid arthritis	Rheumatoid nodules (firm nodules either loose or attached to deep structures over extensor surfaces), vasculitis, pyoderma gangrenosum (papular lesions which become ulcerated)
SLE	Facial butterfly rash, photosensitivity, red scaly rashes, diffuse alopecia (hair loss)
Hyperthyroidism	Pre-tibial myxoedema (non-pitting plaques and nodules, classically on the shins), clubbing, diffuse alopecia
Hypothyroidism	Sparse coarse hair, dry skin, eczema craquelé (asteatotic)
Neoplasia	Acanthosis nigricans (velvety, brown pigmented plaques, often around the neck), dermatomyositis, ichthyosis (scaly skin), pruritus
Drug eruptions (*OHCS7* p601)	Erythema multiforme (target lesions, Stevens–Johnson syndrome), urticaria, exfoliative dermatitis, toxic epidermal necrolysis (skin necrosis and detachment)
HIV	Infections (thrush, molluscum contagiosum, herpes simplex, varicella zoster), inflammatory conditions

Lumps

Worrying features weight loss, night sweats, hard irregular lump, progression

Think about *serious* skin cancer, sarcoma, TB; ***common*** lipoma, sebaceous cyst, abscess, boil, carbuncle, ganglion, fibroma, lymph node, naevi, skin tags, keratocanthoma, keloid scaring

Ask about location, speed and duration of onset, change with time, pain, other lumps, trauma, bites, infections, skin changes, systemic symptoms (eg weight loss, vomiting, fever); ***PMH*** previous lumps, cancer, radiotherapy; ***SH*** foreign travel, sun exposure; ***FH*** skin cancer

Look for site, size, shape, consistency (hard, firm, soft, fluctuant), tenderness, temperature, surface, association with skin (moves with skin – intradermal, skin moves over it – subcutaneous), overlying skin (colour, punctum, ulcerated), edges, mobility/tethering, pulsatility, transillumination, relationship to nearby structures, lymphadenopathy, splenomegaly

Investigations ***blds*** consider FBC, U+E, LFT, CRP, ESR; ***imaging*** CXR, USS, CT/MRI; ***biopsy*** fine needle aspiration (FNA), skin biopsy, USS guided biopsy, excision biopsy

Skin cancer	p385	TB	p427
Lymphadenopathy	p336	Lymphoma	p336

Lipoma

Benign swelling of fatty tissue.

Symptoms single or multiple, non-painful, can cause pressure effects, common on the trunk and neck, never found on palms/soles of feet

Signs smooth, well-defined, soft, subcutaneous, mobile, no skin changes

Management can be surgically excised if causing distress

Sebaceous cyst (epidermal cyst)

Overgrowth of epidermal cells often as a result of blocked follicles.

Symptoms single or multiple, painful if infected, common on the trunk, neck and face, almost never found on palms/soles of feet

Signs firm, well-defined, Smartie® shaped, intradermal, mobile, overlying punctum is common, may drain white material, may be inflamed

Management consider flucloxacillin 500mg/6h PO if inflamed/tender, may also require incision and drainage; surgical excision once non-inflamed

Reactive lymph node

Worrying signs non-tender, >3wk, >1cm, hard, irregular surface, tethering, no infection, weight loss, night sweats, tiredness

Causes ***isolated*** local/regional infection; ***multiple*** see p336

Symptoms lump usually in the neck, axilla or groin

Signs firm, subcutaneous, mobile, well-defined, smooth surface

Management enlarged lymph nodes can often be treated by 'watchful waiting' however investigation may be necessary if worrying signs are present

Abscess

Suppurative infection causing build up of pus.
Symptoms single, painful, onset over days, may be febrile/unwell
Signs fluctuant, well-defined, under the skin, tender, inflamed (red, hot), may spontaneously discharge, common on neck, axilla, groin, perineum
Management requires incision and drainage ±antibiotics eg flucloxacillin 500mg/6h PO and penicillin V 500mg/6h PO

Boil (furuncle)

Inflamed hair follicle that develops into an abscess.
Symptoms single, painful, common on neck, axilla, groin, perineum
Signs red, tender, hot, central punctum, may discharge pus
Management often discharges spontaneously, otherwise treat as abscess

Carbuncle

Infection of multiple hair follicles.
Symptoms multiple, painful, may be febrile/unwell, common on neck
Signs fluctuant, subcutaneous, tender, inflamed (red, hot), discharges pus
Management requires incision and drainage and antibiotics eg flucloxacillin 500mg/6h PO

Naevi (moles)

Benign proliferation of skin cells.
Worrying signs enlargement, change in pigmentation, irregular outline, bleeding, itching, inflammation, crusting
Symptoms and signs there are many types of moles; the most common are acquired naevi that develop during childhood as small, flat pigmented areas and may progress to pale, raised, fleshy naevi with age
Management refer to specialist if worrying signs are present

Ganglion

Cystic lesion of joint or synovial sheath of tendon.
Symptoms single, non-painful, common at wrist
Signs smooth, well-defined, subcutaneous, transilluminable
Management may spontaneously disappear; can be drained, often recurs

Fibroma

Benign tumour of connective tissue.
Symptoms and signs vary according to tissue affected, usually slow growing with no overlying skin changes
Management biopsy/imaging; surgical excision often possible

Sarcoma

Malignant tumour of connective tissue; they are rare but often have a poor prognosis. It is important to biopsy if there is diagnostic doubt.
Symptoms single, painful, progressive enlargement, weight loss
Signs firm/hard, tethered, regional lymphadenopathy
Management combination of surgery, radiotherapy and chemotherapy

Neck lumps

> Worrying features >45yr, weight loss, night sweats, hard irregular lump

Think about *serious* malignancy (primary, metastases, lymphoma); ***common*** many of the lumps discussed on p372 can be present in the neck, however the following causes are only found in the neck:

Location	Causes
Midline	Goitre, thyroid isthmus mass, dermoid cyst, thyroglossal cyst
Anterior triangle	Lymph node, thyroid mass, salivary gland mass, branchial cyst, carotid artery aneurysm
Posterior triangle	Lymph node, cervical rib, pharyngeal pouch

Ask about location, speed and duration of onset, change with time, pain, other lumps, trauma, bites, infections, skin changes, systemic symptoms (eg weight loss, vomiting, fever), sore throat, cough, hoarse voice; ***PMH*** previous lumps, cancer, radiotherapy, thyroid problems; ***SH*** foreign travel, smoking, alcohol intake; ***FH*** cancer

Look for assess as for other lumps (p372) along with the following: movement on swallowing, movement on protruding the tongue, dentition, mouth ulcers, lumps inside the mouth, lumps in the tongue, appearance of the tonsils (?asymmetry), ear examination, facial nerve palsies

Investigation blds consider FBC, U+E, LFT, TFT, CRP, ESR; ***imaging*** CXR, USS, CT/MRI; ***biopsy*** fine needle aspiration (FNA) especially for thyroid or salivary gland lumps, USS-guided biopsy, excision biopsy

Management a neck lump should always be taken seriously and referred to ENT (p462) unless it is clearly a reactive lymph node

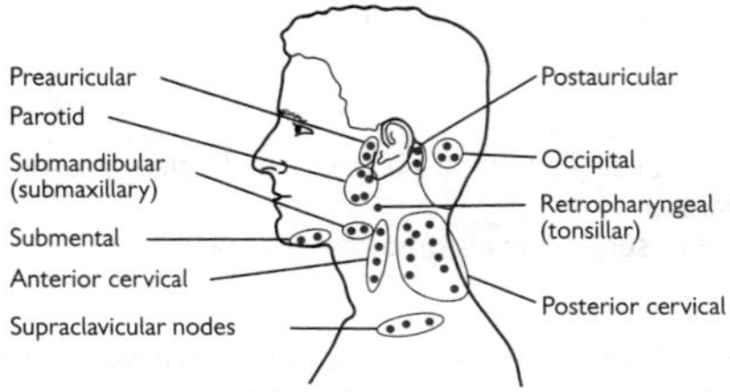

Lymph nodes of the head and neck

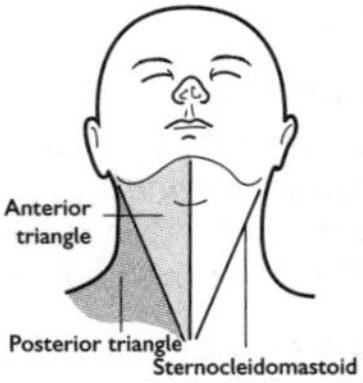

Anatomical triangles of the neck

Thyroid lump/goitre

Symptoms and signs midline or anterior triangle mass, moves with swallowing but not with protruding tongue, may be hypo/eu/hyperthyroid
Management TFT, refer to ENT for fine needle aspiration, high risk of malignancy with increasing age

Salivary gland lump

Causes stone, gland inflammation, malignancy
Symptoms and signs lump in sublingual, submandibular or parotid gland
Management refer to ENT for fine needle aspiration, high risk of malignancy with increasing age

Thyroglossal cyst

Embryological remnant from the descent of the thyroid gland.
Symptoms and signs young patient (<40yr) with single lump by the hyoid which moves with swallowing and protruding tongue, may be inflamed
Management refer to ENT for removal, may be the only thyroid tissue

Dermoid cyst

A benign teratoma which may contain fat or hair.
Symptoms and signs single subcutaneous lump, found in the midline of the neck or next to the eye in young patients (<20yr)
Management refer to ENT for removal, can recur

Branchial cyst

Embryological defect of the second branchial arch.
Symptoms and signs young patient (<20yr), smooth mass, anterior border of the upper sternocleidomastoid, may be tender, may follow URTI
Management refer to ENT for surgical excision, may recur

Pharyngeal pouch

Symptoms and signs elderly patient with dysphagia that rapidly worsens during the meal, coughing, regurgitated food, mass only after eating
Management confirmed by contrast swallow, treated by surgical excision

Cervical rib

An extra rib attached to C7.
Symptoms and signs hard lump palpable in the posterior triangle, often unilateral, may have Raynaud's, distal muscle weakness or pain
Management may require physiotherapy or excision if causing problems

Breast lumps

Worrying features >50yr, fixed, hard, skin tethering, enlarging, previous breast cancer, breast eczema, new nipple inversion, bloody nipple discharge

Think about *serious* breast cancer (p422); ***common*** fibroadenoma, fibroadenosis, abscess, isolated cyst, seroma, trauma (fat necrosis)

Ask about speed and duration of onset, change since detected, change with menstrual cycle, pain, other lumps, trauma, skin changes, nipple changes, nipple discharge; ***PMH*** previous lumps, breast cancer; ***GH/OH*** breastfeeding, pregnancy; ***DH*** contraceptive pills, HRT; ***FH*** breast cancer

Look for see p448 for breast examination

Management breast lumps require a triple assessment of ***clinical examination***, ***imaging*** (USS if <35yr, mammography and USS if >35yr) and ***histology*** (fine needle aspiration (FNA) or trucut biopsy); breast cancer is common so all solid lumps must have histological analysis

Breast cancer	p422

Fibroadenoma

Symptoms and signs young women (<40yr) with highly mobile, non-tender, well-defined and small lump (breast mouse), otherwise well
Management refer to breast surgeon; usually not excised unless >40yr, suspicious USS appearance or >4cm

Fibroadenosis (fibrocystic change)

Symptoms and signs 35–50yr, single or multiple, painful and tender lumps, size and pain vary with menstrual cycle
Management refer to breast surgeon; often assessed with USS and aspiration, but may require mammography and excision

Abscess

Risk factors breast feeding, DM, rheumatoid arthritis, smoking, steroids, trauma, obesity, poor hygiene
Symptoms and signs single, red, hot, tender lump, fluctuant, may discharge pus from the nipple, fever
Management refer to surgeon for incision and drainage with antibiotics

Breast seromas

Collections of serous fluid; common after breast surgery.
Symptoms and signs may discharge fluid, non-tender, fluctuant
Management Using a 20ml syringe and green/white (21/19G) needle:

- Clean the skin over the seroma (eg chlorhexidine, iodine)
- Insert needle and syringe almost parallel to the skin, aspirating until straw-coloured/bloody fluid is obtained; local anaesthetic is not required
- Aspirate all the fluid; use a 3-way tap for large seromas

Complications iatrogenic pneumothorax, bleeding, infection, recurrence

Groin lumps

> **Worrying features** testicular mass, painful lump, tenderness, vomiting, constipation

Think about *serious* testicular cancer, testicular torsion, strangulated hernia; ***common*** lymph node, inguinal hernia, femoral hernia, hydrocele, varicocele, spermatocele, epididymitis/orchitis, ectopic testis, urogenital prolapse, saphena varix, psoas abscess
Ask about location, speed and duration of onset, change with time, pain, reducibility, other lumps, trauma, skin changes, coughing, lifting, nausea, vomiting, constipation, weight loss, urinary incontinence; ***PMH*** previous lumps, cancer; ***GH/OH*** number of pregnancies, type of delivery; ***SH*** foreign travel, recent intercourse; ***FH*** cancer
Look for see p487 for female genital examination, p545 for male
Management most lumps can be identified from history and examination; painful lumps need immediate referral to surgeons to exclude testicular torsion or strangulated hernias. Testicular lumps need urgent (2wk) referral

Lymph node	p372	Testicular torsion	p242

Differential diagnosis of a scrotal lump

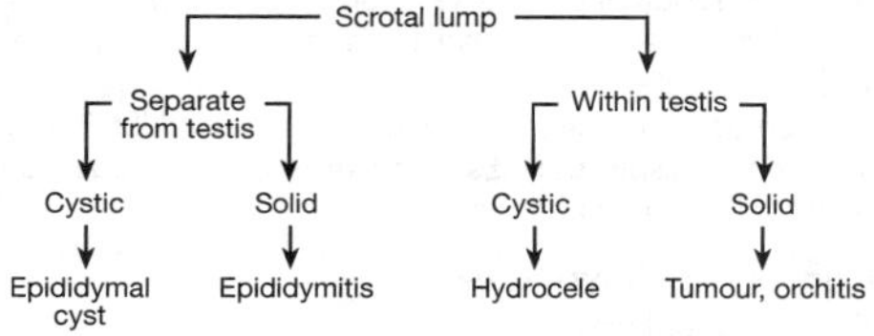

Strangulated hernia

An irreducible hernia where the blood supply has been compromised.
Symptoms irreducible, painful lump near a hernial orifice (usually inguinal or femoral); may have nausea, vomiting, absolute constipation, abdo pain
Signs tender, red, hot lump, ±abdominal distension, ±peritonism
Investigations ***blds*** FBC, U+E, glucose, amylase, CRP, G+S; ***AXR*** (exclude bowel obstruction); ***erect CXR*** (exclude bowel perforation)
Management NBM, analgesia (eg morphine 5mg/1h IV with cyclizine 50mg/8h IV), IV access, 0.9% saline 1l/4h IV, call for immediate senior review, book emergency theatre

Inguinal hernia

Risk factors male, increasing age, chronic cough, constipation, heavy lifting, previous abdominal surgery, ascites, obesity
Symptoms often asymptomatic apart from lump
Signs examine with the patient lying, then repeat standing up: scars, external genitalia, tenderness, reducibility (by patient and yourself), cough impulse, check other side; only 'indirect' hernias extend into the scrotum
Management ***conservative*** weight loss, truss, high-fibre diet, stop smoking, treat lung disease; ***surgery*** day surgery, either open or laparoscopic
Complications irreducible hernia, strangulation

Femoral hernia

As for inguinal hernia but more common in women and greater risk of irreducibility and strangulation; surgical repair at earliest opportunity.

Testicular cancer

Symptoms painless lump felt within testicle, difference in size of testicles
Signs hard, non-transilluminable, irregular surface to testicle, may have a secondary hydrocele
Investigation ***blds*** FBC, LFT, α-FP, β-hCG, LDH; ***imaging*** scrotal USS, CXR and CT for staging; ***biopsy***
Management surgical removal with radiotherapy and/or chemotherapy
Prognosis 98% 5yr survival

Hydrocele

Fluid in the sack surrounding the testis (tunica vaginalis).
Symptoms and signs enlarged 'testicle', soft, non-tender, smooth, well-defined, transilluminable
Investigation can be secondary to a testicular tumour, USS if in doubt
Management none, aspiration ±sclerosant, surgical repair; the testicle should feel entirely normal after aspiration

Spermatocele (epididymal cyst)

A cyst within the epididymis.
Symptoms and signs soft, small, well-defined, spherical, transilluminable, separate (superior) to the testicle, may be uncomfortable
Management surgical removal if symptomatic

Varicocele

Varicose veins within the spermatic cord, associated with subfertility.
Symptoms and signs soft, tubular lumps like a 'bag of worms' above the testicle, resolves on lying, cough impulse present, may be uncomfortable
Management usually none, can be surgically repaired

Ectopic testis

Failure of testicle to descend through inguinal canal.
Symptoms and signs usually diagnosed in childhood, smooth, well-defined, spherical mass between inguinal ring and scrotum, empty scrotal sac on the same side
Management surgical orchidoplexy to reduce cancer risk

Epididymitis/orchitis

Infection of the epididymis and/or testes following UTI or STI; may be indistinguishable from testicular torsion.
Causes Chlamydia species, *N. gonorrhoea*, *E. coli*, viral eg mumps
Symptoms and signs acute testicular swelling and pain, tender, enlarged testicle, ±urethral discharge, fever
Management if unsure treat as testicular torsion (p246), otherwise doxycycline 100mg/12h PO and analgesia; exclude STI (p485) and UTI (urine dipstick/M,C+S)

Saphena varix

Dilated proximal long saphenous vein due to incompetent valves.
Symptoms and signs single, soft, compressible, bluish lump below the inguinal ligament, disappears on lying, cough impulse present
Management high saphenous vein ligation

Psoas abscess

Symptoms and signs painless lump below inguinal ligament, back/flank pain, limp, fever
Investigation ↑WCC, ↑CRP, ↑ESR, seen on CT
Management abscess drainage (surgical or percutaneous CT-guided), appropriate antibiotics

Urogenital prolapse

Risk factors multiple childbirth, vaginal deliveries, large babies, heavy lifting, age, chronic cough, constipation, obesity
Symptoms vaginal lump, dragging sensation, urinary frequency/urgency, urinary incontinence, constipation, intercourse problems
Signs exclude masses, prolapse can be seen using Sim's speculum
Treatment weight loss, stop smoking, treat constipation, pelvic floor exercises; ***interventional*** ring pessaries; ***surgery*** hysterectomy, pelvic floor repair
Ring pessary review every 6mth to replace, check for bleeding/ulceration and symptoms. Prescribe topical oestrogen to reduce the risk of ulceration.

Types of urogenital prolapse

Uterine prolapse	**First degree**	cervix remains within vagina
	Second degree	cervix visible at introitus
	Third degree	procidentia; uterus protruding from vagina
Vault prolapse	Prolapse of the vaginal wall after hysterectomy; may contain small intestine or omentum	
Urethrocele	Urethra bulges onto the lower anterior vaginal wall	
Cystocele	Bladder wall bulges on the anterior vaginal wall	
Rectocele	Rectal wall bulges into the middle posterior vaginal wall	
Enterocele	Intestinal loops herniate into the upper posterior vaginal wall	

Swelling

Worrying features weight loss, night sweats, pain, hard irregular lump, vomiting

Think about causes depend on site:

One leg (pitting)	DVT, cellulitis, ruptured Baker's cyst, trauma, compartment syndrome, lymphatic obstruction, thrombophlebitis, ischaemia
Both legs (pitting)	Venous insufficiency, heart failure, renal failure, nephrotic syndrome, cirrhosis, malnutrition, pre-eclampsia, myxoedema
Any limb (non-pitting)	Lymphoedema: congenital, lymph node excision, post-radiotherapy, malignancy, filariasis, abscess
Face	SVC obstruction, anaphylaxis, allergic reaction, angioedema, steroid use, mumps (unilateral parotid swelling)
Trunk	The five 'Fs' – fat, fluid (ascites), flatus, fetus (pregnancy), faeces; others: malignancy, bowel obstruction, hernia, fibroids, abscess, urinary retention, AAA

Ask about location of swelling, duration, onset, nature of pain (constant, colicky, changes with eating/vomiting/bowels), severity, radiation, nausea and vomiting, pyrexia, sweating, redness of swelling, warmth of swelling, stool colour, change in bowel habit, urinary symptoms, prostatism, dysmenorrhoea, intermenstrual bleeding, post-coital bleeding, last period, pregnancy, headache, weight loss, cough, breathlessness, itching, thirst, rashes, lumps, weight loss, dietary intake, foreign travel, insect stings/bites, breaks in skin; ***PMH*** recent operations, cancer (±radiotherapy?), DM, AF, IBD, IHD, ↑lipids, mitral stenosis, polycythaemia, thrombocytosis, thyroid disease, hepatitis B/C; ***DH*** COCP, steroids, methotrexate, amiodarone, drug allergies; ***SH*** alcohol, smoking

Obs temp, HR, BP, RR, sats, urine output

Look for site, size, shape, colour, tenderness and temperature of swelling, evidence of trauma, skin breaks between toes (for leg cellulitis), nail condition, skin colour and texture, sweating, tortuous veins, scars, fetal movements (in ♀), clubbing, lymphadenopathy (Virchow's node), abdominal scars, ascites, visible peristalsis, hepatomegaly, splenomegaly, masses (?expansile/pulsatile), palpable bladder, check hernial orifices, femoral pulses, bowel sounds; ***PR*** tenderness, masses, prostate hypertrophy, stool, check glove for blood, mucus, melaena and stool colour; ***PV*** tenderness, palpable masses

Investigations depend on site of swelling and suspicion of likely cause (see following page)

Deep vein thrombosis (*OHCM7* p564)

Symptoms unilateral pain, worse when lowered, improved with elevation
Signs warm, red, tender, swollen limb (measure both sides with a tape measure), pitting oedema
Risk factors age, obesity, recent surgery/immobility/travel, oestrogen (pregnancy, HRT, the pill), previous PE/DVT, malignancy, recent stroke or MI, thrombophilia
Investigations FBC, U+E, D-dimer, ECG, consider ABG. A negative D-dimer excludes DVT in 95% if there is low clinical risk, however a positive D-dimer is present with many conditions. Doppler USS of limb.
Treatment Treat PE if present (p225). Otherwise elevate affected limb, analgesia and LMWH, eg enoxaparin 1.5mg/kg/24h SC. Start warfarin at the same time (p348) for 3–6mth.
Complications PE

Well's score for determining the pre-test probability of first DVT

The following measures each score 1 point:

- Active cancer (or treatment within past 6mths)
- Leg paralysed or in plaster
- Recent bed rest >3d or surgery within 4wk
- Collateral veins (non-varicose)
- Pitting oedema
- Tenderness along veins
- Whole leg swollen
- >3cm calf swelling

Minus 2 points if there is another diagnosis that is as likely (eg cellulitis)

Score	Risk of DVT	Management
≤0	Low (3%)	D-dimer test, if +ve USS, if –ve unlikely to be DVT
1 or 2	Moderate (17%)	Treat as DVT, ±treating other possible diagnoses
≥3	High (75%)	Treat as DVT, ±treating other possible diagnoses

Lymphoedema (*OHGP2* p1013)

Symptoms limb swelling, difficulty walking if legs affected, loss of finger and toe flexion
Signs firm swollen limbs, tense skin, non-pitting, may be bilateral
Risk factors female sex, malignancy, breast cancer surgery, radiotherapy, poor nutritional status, obesity
Treatment elevation of the limb, compression bandages, massage of the limb in a proximal direction (to aid fluid return), exercise, antibiotics if secondary skin infection present. No evidence for use of diuretics.
Complications cellulitis, ulcers, psychological issues, pain

Venous insufficiency

Symptoms bursting/throbbing leg pain, relieved by elevating legs, worse on standing, previous DVT or thrombophlebitis
Signs pain ↓ by lifting legs, red discolouration, swelling, varicose veins
Investigations Duplex ultrasound, D-dimer if DVT suspected
Treatment compression bandages (if ABPI >0.8), varicose vein surgery
Complications varicose veins, thrombophlebitis, ulcers, cellulitis

Angioedema

Symptoms colicky abdominal pain, shortness of breath (due to laryngeal oedema), dysphagia, vomiting, weakness, watery diarrhoea, rash, decreased sensation of affected areas

Signs stridor, swelling of the hands/feet/face, tongue swelling, urticaria

Investigation diagnosis made clinically; mast-cell tryptase may be elevated if reaction was in response to anaphylaxis, complement levels help confirm diagnosis (see anaphylaxis p206)

Treatment urgent intubation if laryngeal oedema and airway compromise, stop likely precipitant (eg new ACEi) and avoid in future, antihistamines may help, androgens, tranexamic acid; seek specialist advice

Post-cannula swelling

Tissuing is where an intravenous cannula has not been inserted correctly and is sited only partially in the vein or outside the vein altogether, meaning that fluid or drugs cannot be infused/injected

Treatment remove cannula and re-site if required, elevate the affected limb and give simple analgesia for pain

Infection of intravenous cannula sites used to be a common problem with localised erythema, pain and swelling around the site of insertion. It is less frequent now due to new infection control guidelines stating that IV cannulas should be replaced every 72h. Sites should be inspected daily Treatment remove cannula and re-site (ideally in other arm) if still required, swab site if any purulent discharge and send for M,C+S, analgesia, cold compresses, may require short course of flucloxacillin 250mg/6h PO.

If no improvement consider blood cultures, USS of swelling to rule out a collection - if present, you will need to discuss drainage with surgeons and consider IV ABx

Baker's cyst

Symptoms pain and swelling behind the knee, may radiate to calf, similar to symptoms of DVT, common in osteoarthritis

Signs fluctuant swelling in the popliteal fossa, can also have calf swelling

Investigation distinguishable from DVT by USS

Treatment aimed at underlying cause, joint aspiration and intra-articular injection of steroids may help

Cellulitis	p364	Renal failure	p321
Compartment syndrome	p405	Nephrotic syndrome	p315
Heart failure	p226	Cirrhosis	p253
Pre-eclampsia	p438	SVC obstruction	p231
Anaphylaxis	p206	Hernias	p378
Fibroids	p434	Bowel obstruction	p238

Limb ulcers

Causes venous insufficiency, peripheral vascular disease, neuropathic (eg DM), pressure ulcers, trauma, infection, pyoderma gangrenosum (eg rheumatoid arthritis), vasculitides, skin cancer, steroids
Ask about onset, duration, pain, trauma, claudication; ***PMH*** peripheral vascular disease, ↑BP, CVA, MI, angina, varicose veins, DVT, DM; ***DH*** steroids; ***SH*** smoking, alcohol
Look for number, site, size, base, edge, depth, sensation, shape, colour, discharge, lymphadenopathy, oedema, eczema, peripheral pulses
Investigations ankle brachial pressure index (ABPI), FBC, ESR and fasting glucose; duplex USS, wound swab, CRP, complement, RhF, ANA, ANCA, serology, X-ray (if ulcer overlies bone), biopsy and histology

	Venous	Arterial	Neuropathic
History	Varicose veins, DVT	Intermittent claudication, MI, angina	Numbness, DM, family history
Leg	Pigmented, varicose veins, swollen, hot	Shiny, hairless, cold	Joint destruction
Site	Medial aspect of legs	Toes, bony prominences and pressure points	Heel, metatarsal head, lateral malleolus
Size	Can be very large	Usually small	Usually small
Base	Usually superficial with sloughy exudate	Deep with a dark, dry base, few signs of healing	Can be very deep and extend to bone
Edge	Irregular, areas of repeated healing and exacerbation	Well defined, often circular	Surrounded by thickened skin
Sensation	Painful	Painful	Relatively painless

Treatment Ensure good nutrition and treat the cause, 80% of leg ulcers are due to venous insufficiency. Healing often takes weeks to months and is commonly managed by community nurses:

- ***Venous*** so long as the ABPI is >0.8 compression bandaging should be used (eg 4-layer 'Charing Cross') with absorbable dressings to dry out the slough. Emollients and steroid creams also help; may need surgery.
- ***Arterial*** as for peripheral vascular disease with referral to a vascular surgeon. Do not use compression bandages
- ***Neuropathic*** avoid repeated injury, often needs surgical debridement and antibiotics, osteomyelitis is common
- ***Infection*** ulcers usually have bacteria present; infection or cellulitis should be suspected if there is pus, excessive pain, surrounding erythema or pyrexia. Swab the ulcer and treat as for cellulitis (p364).

No improvement consider other diagnoses (including TB and cancer) or dermatitis from therapeutic agents. Swab the ulcer and consider biopsy. Discuss with dermatology, may need curettage or skin grafting.

Basal-cell carcinomas (BCC)

These are the most common form of skin cancer, accounting for approximately 75% of diagnoses.
Risk factors high exposure to UV light (sunlight and sunbeds), family history of BCC, exposure to arsenic
Appearance usually on face and neck but can be anywhere on body. Body BCC are usually flat, red, scaly patches; facial BCC typically tend to be a firm nodule with central telangiectasia, rolled pearly edges and central ulceration ('rodent ulcer').
Investigation biopsy and histology if large, followed by surgical excision, usually fully excised initially if small and sent for histological analysis
Treatment excision (including Mohs' surgery), topical chemotherapy, radiotherapy, cryosurgery
Prognosis BCC rarely metastasise but can cause local tissue destruction (eg ear, lip) and very occasionally cause death

Mohs' surgery involves surgical removal of the obvious tumour and a thin layer of tissue from the site. This layer is frozen and stained then examined under a microscope. If there are tumour cells present, a further (deeper) layer of tissue is removed, and the process is repeated until the layer is tumour-free. This procedure minimises the need for large skin excisions and gives the best cosmetic outcome.

Squamous-cell carcinomas (SCC)

These account for approximately 25% of skin cancers.
Risk factors high exposure to UV light (sunlight and sunbeds), chronic exposure to industrial carcinogens (eg arsenic, soot), chronic ulcer inflammation, immunosuppression, premalignant conditions (eg Bowen's disease)
Appearance usually appear on sun-exposed skin, approximately half of lesions on head and neck, rapidly growing painless nodule, may bleed or have exudates, often has 'cauliflower' appearance
Investigation usually none, may be biopsied
Treatment surgical excision or radiotherapy, chemotherapy may be used in widespread disseminated disease
Prognosis if localised disease, excision gives 90% cure rate but SCC can metastasise rapidly via local lymph nodes with poor outcome

Malignant melanoma

- Accounts for <1% of all skin cancers
- *Risk factors* pale-skin, sun exposure, sunburn
- *Symptoms/signs* mole with abnormal features see p373
- *Management* surgical excision, ±lymph node removal, ±chemotherapy
- *Prognosis* 5yr survival 85%; worse if male, elderly or delayed diagnosis

Acute red eye emergency

Airway	Check airway is patent; consider manoeuvres/adjuncts
Breathing	If no respiratory effort – **CALL ARREST TEAM**
Circulation	If no palpable pulse – **CALL ARREST TEAM**

Call for **senior help or speak to on-call ophthalmologist** urgently if patient has new onset ↓visual acuity (VA) in affected eye.

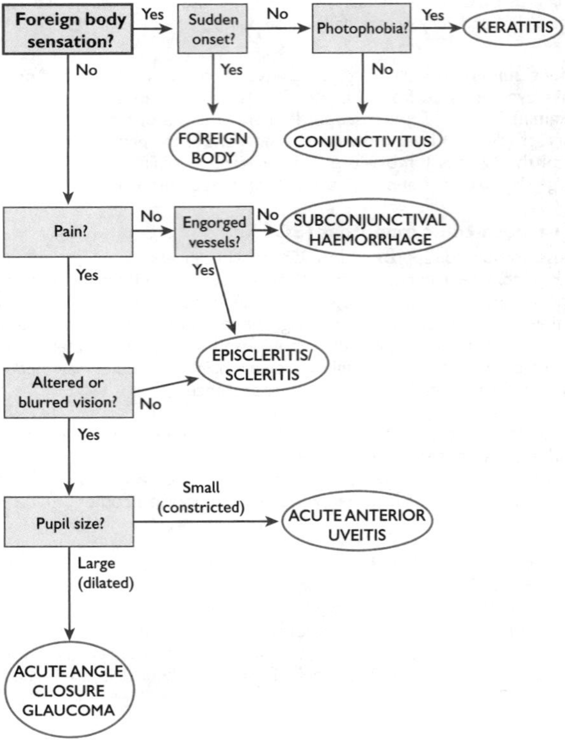

Keratitis (*OHCS7* p432)

Symptoms eye irritation/foreign body sensation often on background of chronic gritty/irritated eyes or in a contact lens wearers. Pain and altered visual acuity are uncommon; photophobia may feature in more severe disease.

Signs mild localised redness, often only in one sector of the cornea (unlike conjunctivitis which is usually bilateral with a discharge and with diffuse corneal inflammation), normal visual acuity. Fluorescein with a blue light may show corneal ulceration with corneal haze.

Management refer urgently for ophthalmologist to exclude infectious or autoimmune causes and for definitive care

Likely ophthalmic management topical antibiotic and steroid drops under close supervision ±lid scrubs for blepharitis

Episcleritis and scleritis (*OHCS7* p432)

Symptoms mild eye irritation and redness; pain, photophobia and altered visual acuity are uncommon in episcleritis, but may feature in **scleritis**

Signs mild localised redness (often involving just one sector, but occasionally diffuse), normal visual acuity; otherwise normal examination in episcleritis. In **scleritis** the globe may be tender to touch and there may be ↓visual acuity.

Management speak to ophthalmologist urgently as this may be **scleritis**

Likely ophthalmic management topical steroids or non-steroidal agents for episcleritis, potentially oral immunosuppressants for **scleritis**

Acute anterior uveitis (iritis) (*OHCS7* p430)

Symptoms blurred vision, photophobia, and pain if severe; sometimes a history of autoimmune disease (IBD, ankylosing spondylitis)

Signs red eye, ↓visual acuity, cornea usually clear, pupil may be irregular and small, ±hypopyon (pus in the anterior chamber)

Management refer urgently to ophthalmologist

Likely ophthalmic management exclude inflammation at the back of the eye, intensive topical steroids and dilating agents ±immunosuppressants

Acute angle closure glaucoma (*OHCS7* p430)

Symptoms aching eye pain (may be severe), often associated with N+V; blurred vision and haloes around lights are common

Signs red eye, ↓visual acuity, hazy cornea (if severe), pupil often mid-dilated, can be unreactive to light and oval shaped (rugby ball-like); globe tender and firm to touch. ↑intraocular pressure; usually >40 mmHg.

Management refer urgently to ophthalmologist; antiemetics and IV opiates may be needed for symptoms but should not delay referral

Likely ophthalmic management constrict the pupil (miosis) with pilocarpine drops, and reduce aqueous formation with acetazolamide PO/IV. Mannitol IV is also sometimes used to reduce intraocular pressure. Definitive care achieved with peripheral iridectomy to allow constant drainage of aqueous even when pupil dilated.

Superficial foreign body (FB) and corneal abrasions

Symptoms usually sudden onset discomfort/foreign body sensation and usually occurs when chance of foreign body entering the eye is high (windy day on the beach or whilst hammering or chiselling without eye protection), or following minor trauma to the eye. Eye watering and redness are also common. A contact lens may sometimes have been 'lost' and cause foreign body sensation.
Signs red, watering eye, FB may be visible. Always evert both top and bottom lids to check for FBs here as well. Visual acuity is usually normal. Fluorescein with a blue light may show corneal ulceration abrasion(s).
Treatment may need to anaesthetise the eye with topical local anaesthetic (proxymetacaine, tetracaine or oxybuprocaine) to allow examination and treatment. Gently pick up FB with cotton bud, or irrigate lavishly with sterile 0.9% saline. Re-examine eye afterwards to ensure all FBs have gone. Protect the eye with an eye shield until local anaesthetic has worn off and give chloramphenicol eye drops 0.5% 4h/topical or ointment 1% 6h/topical for 3d. **If unable to remove FB or evidence of corneal abrasion speak to senior, or on-call ophthalmologist.**

Conjunctivitis

Symptoms eye discharge, ±FB sensation, itch, concurrent cold, hayfever
Signs red eye, discharge, normal visual acuity, clear cornea
Treatment **bacterial and viral conjunctivitis are highly contagious so care should be taken not to share towels and for thorough hand-washing.** ***Bacterial*** topical antibiotics (eg chloramphenicol drops 0.5%) to both eyes every 2h whilst awake for 2d, then 6h for 1wk; ***viral*** may need topical antibiotics to prevent secondary infections, but usually self-limiting; ***allergic*** identify allergen if possible and encourage avoidance, topical mast-cell inhibitors (cromoglicate) may offer relief but can take several days to work; artificial tears (eg Viscotears®) may help if dry eyes are a problem.

	Bacterial	Viral	Allergic
Discharge	Sticky, pus-like	Watery	Watery
Itch	+/–	+/–	++++
Recurrent	+/–	+/–	Often seasonal
Contagious	Yes	Yes	No
Uni- or bilateral	One, then both	One, then both	Both
Other symptoms	Often none	Common cold	Hay fever

Subconjunctival haemorrhage

Symptoms often an incidental finding by the patient and usually benign; can sometimes initially cause mild FB sensation. Pain, photophobia or altered vision should suggest an alternative diagnosis.
Signs diffuse area of bright red blood under the conjunctiva, very different to inflamed blood vessels seen in other forms of red eye; normal VA
Treatment check BP, and if recurrent check FBC and clotting. **Speak to on-call ophthalmologist if recurrent or severe.**

Sudden visual loss

Worrying features sudden loss, additional neurological deficits, scalp pain

Causes retinal artery occlusion, giant-cell arteritis, retinal vein occlusion, retinal detachment, ischaemic optic neuropathy, optic neuritis, bleeding within the globe (traumatic or spontaneous)
Symptoms often painless loss of vision
Signs ↓visual acuity or no vision in affected eye, pupil unresponsive to light (suggest optic nerve disorder), abnormal retina on fundoscopy. Check for other neurological signs, for scalp pain/tenderness and ECG for AF.
Management immediate referral to on-call ophthalmologist

Giant-cell (temporal) arteritis (*OHAM*2 p760)

Symptoms usually unilateral sudden visual loss, malaise, jaw claudication (chewing pain), scalp pain when brushing hair
Signs ↓visual acuity in affected eye, may be retinal splinter haemorrhages or disc oedema, tender and hard temporal arteries
Investigations ↑ESR (>50mm), ↑CRP, ↑plts, ↓Hb, transcranial Doppler for microemboli, temporal artery biopsy for histological confirmation
Treatment Medical emergency. Prednisolone 60mg/24h PO. Seek urgent ophthalmic opinion. Discuss with surgeons for consideration of temporal artery biopsy or radiologists for Doppler assessment (p301).

Gradual visual loss

Causes refractive error, cataracts, macular degeneration, chronic glaucoma, diabetic retinopathy, optic atrophy, inherited disease, drug toxicity, optic neuroma and brain tumour
Symptoms often painless loss of vision, symptoms of underlying disease
Signs ↓visual acuity or no vision in affected eye, pupil unresponsive to light (suggest optic nerve disorder), abnormal cornea, lens, retina and optic disc on fundoscopy
Treatment needs full ophthalmic assessment. If inpatient see if they can been seen in a clinic prior to their discharge, or refer back to GP.

Cataracts (*OHCS*7 p442)

Causes congenital, DM, steroids, trauma, eye surgery
Symptoms blurred vision (bilateral), poor distance judgement (unilateral)
Signs ↓visual acuity, cataract visible in lens; retina and red reflex visible unless cataract is dense
Treatment cataract surgery is performed on a single eye at a time if the cataract(s) are interfering with lifestyle (eg reading or driving). They are usually done as a day-case procedure under local anaesthetic; the lens is removed (phaecoemulsion) and an artificial lens implanted. The posterior capsule may become cloudy after the operation and may require laser treatment as an outpatient.

Age-related macular degeneration (*OHCS*7 p438)

Causes age related
Symptoms deterioration of central vision
Signs ↓visual acuity, but normal visual fields, normal disc, but macula often pigmented or bleeding upon fundoscopy
Treatment is aimed at reducing further visual loss. Laser photocoagulation can be used to destroy abnormal vessels overlying the macula and limit disease progression.

Blind registration

A consultant ophthalmologist can apply to register a patient as blind to the local authority; this is a voluntary not a statutory process. Registration entitles the individual to some tax allowances, benefits, and some concessions for public transport and other public facilities.

The Royal National Institute of Blind People advise on benefit entitlements, aids for the house and independent living, and for guide dogs:

Royal National Institute of Blind People
105 Judd Street, London, WC1E 9NE
020 7388 1266
www.rnib.org.uk

Other visual disturbances

Photophobia

Causes ***neurological*** meningitis, subarachnoid haemorrhage, migraine, encephalitis, hangover; ***ophthalmic*** glaucoma, scleritis, keratitis and corneal injury, iritis, cataracts
Symptoms bright light causes discomfort or exacerbates pain (especially painful having fundoscopy performed)
Signs dislike of light. Check for signs of meningism and for focal neurology; perform full eye examination.
Treatment treat for likely cause(s); **seek senior help urgently**

Diplopia – double vision

Causes extra-occular muscle palsy, cranial nerve palsy, myasthenia gravis, orbital fracture, multiple sclerosis
Symptoms double vision which is corrected by closing one eye or at extremes of gaze is called binocular diplopia; monocular diplopia is rarer and is not corrected by closing one eye, being caused by a structural abnormality within the eye
Signs double vision relieved or not by occluding vision in one eye, loss of conjugate gaze, ↓ROM of eye when testing all movements in turn, fatiguability of muscles, other evidence of associated disease (MS, CVA etc)
Treatment discuss with senior; refer to neurologist/ophthalmologist

Tunnel vision

Causes glaucoma, severe cataracts, alcohol consumption, retinitis pigmentosa, migraine
Symptoms loss of peripheral vision with preservation of central vision, as though looking through a tunnel
Signs check for visual field defect, ↓visual acuity, cataracts, or abnormal retina; check BP and palpate temporal arteries for tenderness
Treatment treat the cause

Haloes around lights

Causes glaucoma, cataracts, post-corrective surgery, idiopathic
Symptoms halos and glare from lights, often more obvious at night
Signs look for ↓visual acuity, cataracts
Treatment treat the cause

Floaters and flashing lights

Causes retinal detachment, vitreous detachment, migraine, idiopathic (non-sinister)
Symptoms dark flecks or webs which drift about in the line of vision; flashing lights, usually in the periphery of vision even when eye closed
Signs often very few signs if non-sinister cause. ↓visual acuity, visual field, or abnormal fundoscopy may feature in retinal or vitreous detachment
Treatment often not necessary. If lots of new floaters have appeared quickly or there are associated flashing lights, haloes or newly impaired visual acuity refer urgently to ophthalmologist.

Pyrexia

Worrying features ↑HR, ↓BP, ↓GCS, ≥40°C, swinging fever, headache

Think about *serious* septic shock (p214); ***most likely*** focus of infection including UTI, cellulitis/wound infection, URTI/pneumonia, endocarditis, internal abscesses, meningitis or septicaemia; ***other*** pulmonary embolism, iatrogenic (transfusion reaction/drug reaction, p342, infected lines), inflammatory conditions and malignancy; ***rare*** malignant hyperpyrexia (*OHA*2 p260), neuroleptic malignant syndrome (*OHCC*2 p522)

Ask about urinary symptoms (frequency, dysuria, pyuria), respiratory/ENT symptoms (cough, sputum production and colour, haemoptysis, breathlessness, chest pain, sore throat/ear, coryza, contact and immunisation to TB), joints/skin (arthropathy, rash, erythema/breaks to skin, eye symptoms), neurological (headache, photophobia, neck stiffness), general well-being (appetite, weight loss, night sweats); ***PMH*** previous UTI/URTI and previous TB, prosthetic heart valve or valvular lesion; ***DH*** immunosuppressive agents (including steroids), blood transfusions or new drugs commenced (antipsychotic or anti-emetic), allergies; ***SH*** any contacts with similar symptoms or known exposure to TB, smoking, recreational drug use (ecstasy)

Obs temp (?swinging), HR, BP, RR, sats, cap-refill, urine output

Look for pulse rate/rhythm/volume, warm peripheries, sweating, flushing, tachypnoea, tremor, splinter haemorrhages, break in skin, needle tracks in arms/feet/groin, focal skin/wound infection, bronchial breathing/crackles/reduced air entry, heart murmur, suprapubic/loin tenderness, red catheter/line sites, joint swelling

Investigations septic screen (p393); ***urine dipstix*** and C+S (p628); ***blds*** FBC, ↑NØ (bacterial), ↑LØ (viral), ↑EØ (parasites/allergy), blood film (may suggest haematological malignancy/malaria), U+E, LFT, inflammatory markers (CRP, ESR/PV), D-dimer if PE suspected (p225 for PE risk stratification), bld cultures (p555); ***sputum*** C+S, if active TB suspected request urgent 'smear' microscopy for acid-fast bacilli (AFB); ***stool culture, skin swabs; ABGs*** respiratory failure or metabolic acidosis (p622); ***CXR*** pneumonia/effusion; ***echo*** if you suspect bacterial endocarditis; transoesophageal is more sensitive than transthoracic (speak to cardiologist on-call); ***LP*** if meningitis suspected (CT first)

Treatment assess the severity of illness, have a low threshold for treatment as septic shock (p214). Septic screen again (p393) if new rise in temp >38°C even if already commenced on antibiotics (p156).

Symptom management paracetamol (1g/6h PO) ±ibuprofen (400mg/8h PO) for pyrexia, analgesia for pain, ensure adequate hydration (consider IV fluids if nauseous or NBM), supplementary O_2 if sats <95%. An electric fan may produce symptomatic relief for the patient. Review patient with results of septic screen to form a management plan.

Request early ***senior review*** if in doubt of diagnosis or patient unwell

The septic screen

In most patients the likely source of an infection/fever is obvious, and investigations and management can be tailored specifically towards that; in others it is less clear, and a more widespread approach is required

History a thorough history can sometimes shed new light on the potential cause or highlight the potential for immunocompromise

Examination of all the patient's systems and a top to toe examination of the skin and joints may reveal a source of infection. All line sites should be inspected and changed if old or inflamed – send the tips of removed lines to microbiology for culturing.

Investigations see box below:

Septic screen

- Full blood count (repeat every 2d)
- Inflammatory markers, ESR/PV, CRP (repeat every 2–4d)
- Urine culture
- Sputum culture, if indicated
- Blood cultures (3 sets at 6–8h intervals from different veins)
- Microbiology swabs of wounds/pressure areas/cannula or central line sites
- CXR if productive cough or abnormal clinical signs present

If infectious source not identified, consider:

- Stool for M,C+S
- Echocardiogram if new murmur or new stigmata of bacterial endocarditis
- Check sickle-cell status
- Blood film for parasites (if malaria is suspected)
- Lumbar puncture if CNS infection suspected or needs excluding (CT first)

Pyrexia of unknown origin (PUO)

This term specifically refers to a prolonged fever (>3wk) without obvious cause (*OHCM*7 p376). Causes include infection, malignancy, non-infectious inflammatory disease (connective tissue disease, vasculitis etc), drug reactions and in over ~25% of cases the cause is never found.

Iatrogenic causes of pyrexia

Transfusion reactions (p342)

- Infected lines:
  - cannula, central lines, arterial lines, urinary catheters, long-lines etc
- Malignant hyperthermia (*OHA*2 p260):
  - muscle relaxants/volatile anaesthetic agents
- Neuroleptic malignant syndrome (*OHCC*2 p522):
  - antipsychotic drugs
- Sulphonamides
- Isoniazid
- Aspirin
- Post-operative
  - atelectasis (often 24h post-op)

Urinary tract infection, including pyelonephritis (*OHCM*7 p282)

Worrying signs ↓BP/shock (p209), temp >40°C, new renal impairment. Elderly patients can be afebrile but heavily bacteraemic.

Symptoms ***cystitis*** urinary frequency, dysuria, urgency, pyuria, haematuria, suprapubic pain; ***pyelonephritis*** fever, rigors, vomiting, loin pain, pyuria, haematuria
Risk factors ♀, sexual intercourse, catheterisation, DM, immunosuppression, pregnancy, menopause, urinary tract strictures/stones, elderly
Signs warm peripheries, vasodilation, tachycardia, suprapubic/loin pain
Investigations ***Urine dipstix*** positive for two or more of blood, protein, leucocytes and nitrites suggests UTI (p628); *C+S* if high suspicion of UTI on dipstix and in all pyrexial/vomiting children; *blds* FBC (↑WCC, ↑Nø), U+E (↑urea, ↑creatinine if outflow tract obstruction p320), ↑inflammatory markers, ↑glucose (?DM/DKA); ***bld cultures*** if ↑temp (rigors) or systemically unwell; ***ultrasound/IVU/cystoscopy*** if recurrent infections, evidence of renal impairment or male (p321)
Acute treatment if ↓BP/shock treat as septic shock (p214), otherwise paracetamol ±ibuprofen (for fever), ensure investigations sent and consider commencing 'blind' antibiotic therapy (trimethoprim or nitrofurantoin if uncomplicated, or co-amoxiclav if complicated depending upon local guidelines) whilst awaiting sensitivities, ↑oral fluid intake, double voiding (half emptying bladder then emptying fully after 5min). Change to more appropriate antibiotic once sensitivity known and treat for 3d for simple infections and 10d if complicated (♂, renal disease, systemically unwell). Repeat urine C+S 1wk post-therapy to ensure resolution of infection.
Complications scarring of urinary tract including kidneys, CRF

Simple measures to prevent urinary tract infections

- Drink >2l fluid day
- Voiding at 2–3h intervals
- Double voiding
- Voiding before bedtime and after sexual intercourse
- Wipe front to back after micturition (♀)

Recurrent urinary tract infections

- Avoidance of constipation which may impair bladder emptying
- Avoidance of bubble bath and other irritants in bathwater
- Antibiotic prophylaxis (trimethoprim, nitrofurantoin)
- Drinking cranberry juice may have a protective action[1]

[1] Kontiokari 2001 *BMJ* **332**:1.

Endocarditis (*OHAM*2 p120)

Symptoms malaise, anorexia, weight loss, fever, rigors, night sweats, ±dyspnoea, oedema
Risk factors prosthetic valve, valvular lesion (aortic > mitral), congenital cardiac defect, pacemaker/central line, mural thrombus (post-MI), recurrent bacteraemia (IV drug users, severe dental disease), atrial myxoma
Signs new murmur, splinter haemorrhages, Janeway lesions, Osler's nodes, Roth spots, conjunctival haemorrhages, tachycardia, warm peripheries, CCF, poor teeth and oral hygiene, signs of intravenous drug abuse
Investigations for diagnostic criteria see below; ***blds*** FBC (↑WCC, ↑Nø, ↓Hb), U+E, LFT, ↑inflammatory markers; ***bld cultures*** take 3 sets (prior to commencing ABx) from different sites at intervals of >1h; ***ECG*** features of underlying valvular lesion, AV block, pericarditis; ***CXR*** pulmonary oedema, septic pulmonary emboli; ***echo*** (transoesophageal more sensitive than transthoracic) valvular lesion/vegetation (normal does not exclude endocarditis); ***V/Q scan*** if pulmonary emboli suspected; ***urine dipstix*** blood (often present in infective endocarditis cases), ±protein
Acute treatment try to obtain at least 3 sets of blood cultures prior to commencing antibiotics unless patient unwell. Blind treatment should include a penicillin (benzylpenicillin or flucloxacillin) and gentamicin, ±vancomycin if ?MRSA. O_2 if unwell, paracetamol ±ibuprofen and other supportive measures (anti-emetics, IV fluids if dehydrated or NBM).
Chronic treatment antibiotic therapy for at least 4–6wk. Surgical valve replacement indicated if heart failure evident or signs of aortic root abscess (lengthening PR interval, RBBB), prosthetic valve unstable, or infection uncontrolled.
Complications valve destruction, cardiac failure, AV block, intracardiac abscess, embolism (to brain, limbs, lungs), septicaemia, death

Diagnostic criteria for infective endocarditis (IE) – Duke classification

Definite IE – 2 major, or 1 major and 3 minor, or 5 minor criteria
Possible IE – findings fall short of 'definite' but not 'rejected'
Rejected IE – firm alternative diagnosis or resolution within <4d of therapy

Major criteria

- Positive blood cultures

Typical micro-organisms for IE on three separate blood cultures[1] and/or persistently positive blood cultures

- Evidence of endocardial involvement

Positive echocardiogram (vegetation, abscess, new regurgitation, or dehiscence of prosthetic valve)

Minor criteria

- Predisposing condition or drug use
- Fever >38°C
- Vascular phenomena (septic emboli anywhere)
- Immunologic phenomena (glomerulonephritis, rheumatoid factor)
- Microbiological evidence (non-major criteria positive blood cultures)
- Echocardiographic findings (consistent with IE but not meeting major criteria)

[1] Commonly Streptococci (esp *S. viridans*), Enterococci, Staphylococci (*S. aureus*, *S. epidermidis*); rare pathogens include gram negative bacilli, Diptheroids, fungi, multiple organisms.

Neutropenia (Nø <0.5 x 10^9/l, regardless of total WCC) management depends upon whether the patient is well and afebrile or sick/febrile (febrile neutropenia, see below).

Causes of neutropenia requiring hospital admission are usually related to marrow suppression from chemotherapy (usually 7–10 days later) for an underlying malignancy. Other causes of neutropenia present less often to hospital, but include viral infections, brucellosis, TB, drugs (carbimazole, sulphonamides), hypersplenism or anti-neutrophil antibodies and marrow failure secondary to either infiltration or B_{12}/folate deficiency.

Well neutropenic patients clearly are immunocompromised so will be prone to infections; question if hospital is appropriate as the patient may be 'safer' at home. If admission is necessary ensure a clean side-room is used and the patient should have reverse barrier nursing to prevent healthcare staff introducing infection to the patient (p117). Check cause of neutropenia and look at FBC and clotting to exclude a significant pancytopenia. Discuss with haematology and microbiology consultants if specialist prophylactic antibiotics or growth factors (encourage marrow activity) should be given. Regularly change cannula sites (every 48h).

Febrile neutropenia requires prompt medical action. A trigger temp of >38°C is usually taken as warranting urgent action, though severely ill or severely neutropenic patients may not be able to mount a febrile response to infection. The box below outlines assessment and management of febrile neutropenia:

Febrile neutropenia (*OHAM2* p718)

Pre-conditions	• Neutropenia • Pyrexia >38°C (though patient can be normo/hypothermic)
Source of infection	• Often not clear clinically; pyrexia of unknown origin (PUO) • Commonly: chest, Hickman/central line, urine, skin, perianal • Microbiological diagnosis made in only about 40% of cases
Investigations	• Monitor FBC and differential, ±clotting, U+E, LFT, glucose • Culture blood, urine, sputum, swab Hickman line and skin folds • CXR • Repetitive clinical examination to identify source of infection
Treatment	• Manage underlying pathology as usual (eg O_2 for pneumonia) • Commence antibiotics early in accordance with local policy • Common empirical regimens are shown below • Two or more drugs are usually necessary • Early involvement with haematologist and microbiologist • Consider antifungal prophylaxis

Empirical antibiotic therapy for febrile neutropenia

Early discussion with microbiologist is advised (check your local policy guidelines)

1st line	Tazocin® 4.5g/8h IV, ± gentamicin (if in septic shock, p214)
2nd line	Add in vancomycin 1g/12h IV or teicoplanin 400mg/24h IV
3rd line	Consider adding in amphotericin if fever not settling. Rediscuss with haematologist/microbiologist

Recurrent/unusual infections

Patients reattending with recurrent infections are more likely to be identified by the GP. In hospital, isolation of an unusual pathogen by microbiology staff will usually start alarm bells ringing, and a consultant microbiologist is likely to be the first to suggest further investigations, as well as suggest appropriate treatment.

Opportunistic infections are commonly seen in HIV and other immunocompromised states, a list of some are shown on page 398. Identification of an unusual pathogen doesn't infer immunocompromise, it merely makes it more likely. Equally, many immunocompromised patients develop 'standard' infections with 'standard' pathogens.

Causes of immunocompromise are diverse and diagnosis requires meticulous history taking, examination and investigation (mostly blood-based). Increasing age, steroids (p154) and immunosuppressants can cause a relative increase in susceptibility to infections, though less so than neutropenia (p396).

Opportunistic pathogens in the immunocompromised (*OHCM*7 p399)	
Candidiasis	Usually furry white oral plaques (thrush), though can form in skin folds, genitalia and oesophagus and in severe cases cause a septicaemia. Treated locally with nystatin or systemically with fluconazole or amphotericin B.
CMV retinitis	Most common in HIV patients. Reduction in visual acuity, ±blindness. 'Mozzarella pizza' appearance on fundoscopy. Treated with ganciclovir or foscarnet.
Cryptococcus	Can cause eye infections, but most commonly meningitis, often without neck stiffness. Amphotericin B and flucytosine are used.
Herpes virus	Cold sores/genital lesions. More seriously CNS infections (meningitis/encephalitis) require high-dose intravenous aciclovir.
***Pneumocystis jiroveci* (formerly *carinii*)**	Typically a severe pneumonia, most commonly in HIV, but also in patients with leukaemia and following bone marrow transplantation. Treat aggressively with co-trimoxazole (trimethoprim + sulfamethoxazole). HIV patients with ↓CD4+ counts should receive this in a lower dose as primary prophylaxis. Following PCP patients should remain on co-trimoxazole as secondary prophylaxis.
Tuberculosis (TB)	This is the commonest of the mycobacteria which present clinically. Frank pulmonary TB in the immunocompromised usually results from reactivation of a primary infection many years prior. Treatment should be aggressive and consist of triple or quadruple therapy (p427). Compliance is crucial and should be emphasised. Always consider MDR-TB (p427).
Tinea	Fungal skin infections are common in the healthy, but more so in the immunocompromised. Treat with topical agents (nystatin, clotrimazole, terbinafine) unless more invasive disease (p368).
Toxo-plasmosis	Usually associated with HIV. Causes meningitis/encephalitis or serious intracerebral abscesses. Treat aggressively with sulfadiazine and pyrimethamine. Secondary prophylaxis required.
Varicella-zoster virus	Cutaneous manifestations (chickenpox and shingles) and more seriously pneumonitis/encephalitis. Requires high-dose intravenous aciclovir. Seek ophthalmology input if ophthalmic shingles.

Notifiable diseases

Notification of a number of diseases (see box below) is mandatory under the Public Health (Infectious Diseases) 1988 Act and the Public Health (Control of Diseases) 1988 Act. Notification came about over 100 years ago to identify and stem the spread of certain infectious diseases, which remains its main purpose. If a patient has been diagnosed with a notifiable disease, or is strongly suspected of having a notifiable disease, the Consultant in Communicable Disease Control should be informed – they can usually be contacted via the hospital switchboard. Ensure you know the patient's address and home circumstances, any foreign travel and their clinical history before referring the case.

Disease surveillance is carried out nationally by the Health Protection Agency (HPA) who publish a very interesting and informative weekly report of the numbers and location of the various notifiable diseases. These reports can be found at:

www.hpa.org.uk/infections/topics_az/noids/menu.htm

HIV is not a notifiable disease, but it is often voluntarily reported to Communicable Disease Control (CDC). This should only be undertaken by a senior member of the team with the consultant's approval.

UK Notifiable diseases

- Anthrax
- Cholera
- Diphtheria
- Dysentery
- Encephalitis (acute)
- Food poisoning
- Leprosy
- Leptospirosis
- Malaria
- Measles
- Meningitis – all types
- Meningococcal septicaemia
- Mumps
- Ophthalmia neonatorum
- Paratyphoid fever
- Plague
- Poliomyelitis (acute)
- Rabies
- Relapsing fever
- Rubella
- Scarlet fever
- Smallpox
- Tetanus
- Tuberculosis
- Typhoid fever
- Typhus fever
- Viral haemorrhagic fever
- Viral hepatitis – all types
- Whooping cough
- Yellow fever

Malaria (*OHCM*7 p382)

Commonest cause of fever and illness in the tropics.

Suspect any foreign traveller who presents with fever or unexplained illness of having malaria within 2mth of travel to endemic areas regardless of prophylaxis

Plasmodium falciparum, vivax, ovale and *malariae*

Transmitted by the *Anopheles* mosquito

Incubation period between 7–40d

Non-specific flu-like illness, headache, malaise, myalgia, anorexia

Subsequently fever (classically peaking every 3d though this is rare in practice)

Diagnosis serial thick and thin blood films for malaria parasites

Treatment quinine-based drugs but resistance is common; discuss with infectious diseases

Prophylaxis combinations of: chloroquine, proguanil, doxycycline, mefloquine, Malarone®

Acutely painful limb emergency

Airway	Check airway is patent; consider manoeuvres/adjuncts
Breathing	If no respiratory effort – **CALL ARREST TEAM**
Circulation	If no palpable pulse – **CALL ARREST TEAM**

Call for **senior help** early if patient deteriorating

- **Sit patient up**, unless pain will not allow
- **15l/min O_2** in all patients
- **Monitor** O_2 sats, HR, BP, temp
  - is the patient shocked or febrile?
- Brief **history**/check notes/ask ward staff
  - arterial/cardiac problems or DM
  - recent trauma/surgery
- **Examine** patient: condensed RS, CVS and abdo exam
- **Examine all limbs**: vascular, neuro and joint exams
  - is the pain localised to a joint or specific area?
  - check distal sensation, pulses and cap refill ? ischaemia
- **Venous access**, take bloods:
  - FBC, ESR, U+E, CRP, ±cardiac markers, ±sickle-cell, D-dimer, clotting, G+S
- Check pulses with **Doppler** if available
- **ECG** to exclude acute MI, AF
- **ABG** if systemically unwell
- Analgesia, eg IV morphine titrated to pain
- **Consider** serious causes and treat if present:
  - **acute ischaemia** 15l/min O_2, analgesia, heparin, (vascular) surgeons
  - **compartment syndrome** 15l/min O_2, remove plaster, orthopaedics
  - **septic arthritis** 15l/min O_2, joint aspiration, orthopaedics
  - **necrotising fasciitis** 15l/min O_2, fluids, IV antibiotics, surgeons
  - **gangrene** 15l/min O_2, fluids, IV antibiotics, surgeons
- Call for **senior help**
- **Reassess**, starting with A, B, C . . .

Life and limb-threatening causes

Acute ischaemia	p404	Septic arthritis	p410
Compartment syndrome	p405	Necrotising fasciitis	p365
Myocardial infarction (arm)	p180	Gangrene	p405
Spinal cord compression	p297	Sickle-cell crisis	p337

Acute limb pain

See also joint pain p408 and trauma p352

> **Worrying features** sudden onset, severe pain, reduced sensation, tingling, pulselessness, cold, shock, pyrexia, recent surgery, concurrent chest pain

Think about *serious* acute ischaemia, septic arthritis, compartment syndrome, gangrene, necrotising fasciitis; ***most likely*** muscular, joint or bone pain, DVT, cellulitis, thrombophlebitis, sciatica; ***other*** osteomyelitis, Baker's cyst, vasculitides, myositis, peripheral neuropathy; ***chronic*** arthritis (osteo-, rheumatoid, gout), peripheral vascular disease, varicose veins, spinal stenosis, ulcers

Ask about location, trauma, speed of onset, change on moving and raising, recent surgery, back pain, chest pain, SOB, feeling unwell; ***PMH*** previous limb pain, DM, MI, CVA, DVT, PE; ***DH*** warfarin, heparin; ***SH*** exercise tolerance

Obs temp, BP, HR, O_2 sats, RR

Look for hot/cold, colour, mottling, skin trauma, swelling (distal, joint, calf), pulses (compare both sides), cap refill, power, sensation, reflexes, range of movement (active and passive), muscle, joint or bone tenderness, see p496–506 for specific joint examinations; resp exam if SOB

Investigations most limb pain can be diagnosed from clinical examination; consider the following investigations; ***blds*** FBC, U+E, ESR, CRP, D-dimer, blood cultures; ***Doppler*** for pulses to exclude ischaemia; ***ECG*** for AF; ***X-rays*** for joint disease or bone fractures; ***ABG*** if suspicion of PE

Management give everyone adequate analgesia, p428. Try to determine what structure is causing the pain (eg skin, muscle, joint, bone) or if there is no obvious structure consider arterial problems, infection or DVT

	History	Examination	Investigations
Acute ischaemia	Rapid onset, distal >proximal, worse with legs raised	Pulseless, cap refill >2s, pale, cold, weak, reduced sensation	↓or absent Doppler pulse, obstruction on angiography
Infection eg cellulitis	Gradual onset, feels unwell, history of trauma or bite	Pyrexia, red, tender, warm, swollen	↑WCC, ↑CRP, ↑ESR, often ↑D-dimer
DVT	Gradual onset, improved with legs raised	Red, swollen, hot, tender leg	↑D-dimer, thrombosis on Doppler USS
Compartment syndrome	Recent trauma or surgery ±POP	Severe pain on passive movement	Increased compartment pressure
Joint	Trauma, pain on movement, unableto bear load	Tender over joint, joint effusion, pain: active = passive	Arthritic changes on X-ray, abnormal synovial fluid
Muscle	Trauma, pain on movement	Tender, ±swelling on muscle/tendon insertion, pain: active >passive	Normal X-rays, may have a ↑CK
Bone	Trauma, pain on movement and at rest	Bony tenderness with swelling and reduced range of movement	Abnormal X-ray

Back pain/sciatica	p296	Joint pain	p408
Cellulitis	p364	Rashes	p363
Chronic limb pain	p407	Necrotising fasciitis	p365
DVT	p381	Trauma	p352

Acute limb ischaemia

This is an *emergency*, ischaemia is irreversible after 6h.

Worrying signs ↓sensation, purple mottling, non-blanching mottling

Causes emboli, thrombosis, dissecting aneurysm, trauma

Risk factors AF, prosthetic heart valves, recent MI, arterial graft, peripheral vascular disease, previous thrombo-emboli, dehydration, malignancy

Symptoms unilateral painful, tingling, weak limb, worse on raising limb

Signs absent pulses, slow cap refill compared with opposite limb, cold and pale (can be red if limb below heart), reduced power and sensation

Results Doppler will show a reduced or absent pulse; angiography will show an obstruction

Treatment ABC, 15l/min O_2 and analgesia (morphine). IV access with IV fluids if dehydrated and call a senior surgeon since this needs urgent surgery (embolectomy, intra-arterial thrombolysis, bypass or amputation). May require heparinisation (p347) pre or post-op.

Complications amputation, gangrene, ↑K^+, renal failure, sepsis

Gas (wet) gangrene

This is an *emergency*, clostridium infection causing necrosis and sepsis.
Symptoms unwell with painful extremities or wound
Signs pyrexia, shock, tender brown/black area with blistering and oedema, muscle necrosis, crepitus (from gas in tissue)
Risk factors ischaemia, DM, malignancy, surgery/trauma
Investigations FBC, U+E, LFT, CRP, CK, blood cultures, clotting, ABG (acidosis). Gram stain of pus or necrotic tissue. X-ray may show gas (dark patches in soft tissues).
Treatment ABC including 15l/min O_2 and fluids. Benzylpenicillin 2.4g/4h IV, clindamycin 600mg/6h IV, metronidazole 500mg/6–8h IV and surgical debridement.
Complications amputation, sepsis, death

Dry gangrene

Ischaemic muscle necrosis without infection.
Signs well-defined, painless, shrivelled brown/black area
Treatment requires debridement or amputation to prevent infection, may autoamputate if not treated
Complications wet gangrene

Compartment syndrome

This is an *emergency*, measure compartment pressure if suspected.
Symptoms excessive pain following an injury or fracture, distal tingling, numbness or weakness
Signs pain at rest, worse on passive stretching of a muscle, reduced sensation (loss of two point discrimination), redness, swelling, slow cap refill; absent pulse and pallor are late signs
Risk factors long bone fractures and plaster casts, significant injury, crush injury, vascular injury, warfarin or heparin, burns
Investigations measure compartment pressure by inserting a manometer through the skin (eg Wick catheter), >30mmHg requires urgent treatment, check FBC, U+E, CK, clotting and urine dipstick
Treatment ABC, 15l/min O_2, lie the patient flat, elevate limb, adequate analgesia, IV fluids if dehydrated, monitor urine output, remove plaster cast if present, discuss with orthopaedics regarding urgent fasciotomy
Complications rhabdomyolysis, ↑K^+, neurological damage, amputation

Osteomyelitis

Risk factors DM, immunocompromise, open fractures, prostheses
Symptoms fever, bone pain, malaise (or fever without focus)
Signs bony tenderness, warm, red, swollen
Investigations ↑WCC, ↑ESR, ↑CRP, blood cultures, X-ray (though there are rarely changes in the first 10d), USS may show periosteal lifting, bone scan is sensitive, MRI can also be useful
Culture a pus sample must be obtained prior to starting antibiotics; this is either by USS-guided aspiration or drilling in theatre
Treatment high-dose antibiotics (eg clindamycin IV) for at least 6wk often requiring central access; surgical drainage of abscess if present
Complications septic arthritis, fracture, chronic osteomyelitis, bone destruction, seeding to other sites

Superficial thrombophlebitis

Inflammation and thrombosis of a vein which can progress to DVT.
Symptoms gradual onset of tenderness over a vein
Signs red, tender area with hard palpable vein/varicosity
Risk factors IV cannulas, varicose veins, IVDU and DVT risk factors
Investigations no specific investigations but have a low threshold for blood and Doppler scans to exclude DVT which is common
Treatment resite/remove IV cannula, elevation, exercise, compression and NSAIDs eg ibuprofen, if suspicious of DVT start LMWH
Complications DVT, PE. If thrombophlebitis recurs or affects other sites (migratory) suspect malignancy or vasculitis.

Muscle pain

Causes trauma, strains, fibromyalgia, infection, rhabdomyolysis, drugs (statins, ACE inhibitors, steroids), inflammation (polymyalgia rheumatica, polymyositis, dermatomyositis, SLE), metabolic ↓Ca^{2+}, ↓K^+, ↓Na^+, alkalosis), endocrine (hypo/hyperthyroid, Cushing's), referred joint pain
Investigations often none; FBC, U+E, Ca^{2+}, CK, ESR, CRP, X-ray
Treatment simple analgesia including NSAIDs, rest for first 24h then gradually exercise the joint, ice packs, compression (eg tubigrip) and elevation. Consider physiotherapy referral if persists.

Other limb problems

Causes of red limbs

• Venous eczema (venous insufficiency) • DVT • burns • cellulitis • ringworm • psoriasis • eczema • vasculitis • porphyria • erythema nodosum (strep, fungi, TB, sarcoid, ulcerative colitis, OCP, antibiotics with sulphur) • pretibial myxo-edema (hyperthyroid) • necrobiosis lipoidica (type 1 DM) • skin cancer

Rashes	p363	Swelling	p380
Ulcers	p384	Lumps	p372

Chronic limb pain

Peripheral arterial disease (PAD)

Chronic limb ischaemia causes intermittent claudication/critical ischaemia.
Intermittent claudication cramp in calf, thigh or buttock on walking a fixed distance, worse uphill, relieved by stopping or rest
Critical ischaemia pain in limb extremity at night, relieved by hanging legs out of bed, ulcers, dry gangrene
Signs early cool, hairless, pulseless limbs; ***late*** pain and pallor on elevation
Investigations FBC, U+E, lipids, ESR, ECG, ankle brachial pressure index (ABPI see below), arteriography
Treatment exercise, stop smoking, treat DM, BP and cholesterol, aspirin 75mg/24h PO, may need angioplasty, stent or bypass graft. Avoid β-blockers; GTN rarely helps.
Complications acute ischaemia, gangrene, rest pain, ulcers

Ankle brachial pressure index (ABPI)			
Using a Doppler probe the systolic BP (ie lowest pressure at which the pulse cannot be detected) is measured at both brachial fossae and both ankles. The result is expressed as a ratio of the ankle pressure to the average brachial pressures.			
Example: ankle pressure of 126, brachial pressures of 138 and 142			
Average brachial pressure = (138 + 142) ÷ 2 = 140, ABPI = 126/140 = 0.9			
Normal	0.9–1.3	Moderate PVD	0.6–0.9
Severe PVD	<0.6	Calcification	>1.3

Nerve entrapment syndromes

Syndrome	Symptom
Carpal tunnel syndrome (median) thumb, index, middle, ±ring finger	Aching of wrist and forearm, tingling of
Ulnar entrapment (wrist or elbow)	Tingling of ring and little fingers, ±forearm
Radial tunnel syndrome or posterior interosseous syndrome	Weak extension of fingers and thumb
Meralgia parasthetica	Tingling lateral thigh
Common peroneal compression	Weak dorsiflexion of foot

Lumbar spinal stenosis (spinal claudication)

Symptoms cramp in thigh or leg on walking, worse on walking downhill or standing, associated back pain
Signs pain on straight leg raise/back extension, often no neuro symptoms
Investigations lumbar spine X-ray and MRI spine
Treatment exercise, NSAIDs, steroid injections, spinal decompression
Complications cord compression, cauda equina syndrome (p297)

Osteoarthritis	p410	Sciatica/radiculopathy	p292
Peripheral neuropathy	p295	Analgesia in chronic pain	p431

Joint pain

Worrying features fever, weight loss, severe pain, rashes

Think about ***emergency*** septic arthritis; ***polyarthritis*** rheumatoid, osteoarthritis, ankylosing spondylitis, psoriatic arthritis, connective tissue disease (eg SLE), reactive arthropathy (Reiter's), rheumatic fever (post-strep), polymyalgia rheumatica, IBD; ***monoarthritis*** septic arthritis, trauma, crystal arthropathy (gout, pseudo-gout), monoarthritic presentation of polyarticular disease, leukaemia, endocarditis, sickle cell, haemophilia

Ask about site of pain, relieving/exacerbating actions, duration of pain, pain in other joints, pain at night, stiffness, change in symptoms with time of day or activity, fever, night sweats, weight loss, nausea, sore throat, rashes, change with sunlight, chest pain, diarrhoea, constipation, abdominal pain, mouth ulcers, pain on urination, vision problems, dry eyes, dry mouth, trauma; ***PMH*** previous joint pain, previous trauma, clotting abnormalities, TB, heart problems; ***DH*** steroids, anticoagulants, thiazide diuretics, allergies; ***FH*** joint problems, psoriasis; ***SH*** occupation, mobility, help at home, change in lifestyle due to symptoms

Obs temp, HR, BP

Look for see p496–506 for specific joint examinations; always check the joint above and below; ***look*** resting position, swelling, erythema; ***feel*** warmth, tenderness, rashes, nodules, deformed joints; ***move*** reduced range of movement (passive and active), crepitus; ***systemic*** psoriasis (check nails and belly button), enthesitis (tenderness at tendon insertions eg Achilles), back flexion, sacroilitis (pain on pelvic squeeze), gait, ulcers, muscle tenderness, lymphadenopathy, hepatomegaly, splenomegaly

Investigations FBC, U+E, CK, CRP, ESR, RhF, ANA, urine dipstick, X-rays of affected joints, joint aspiration (M,C+S, crystals) consider: sickle-cell, clotting, urate, anti-Sm, anti-dsDNA, complement, antiphospholipid

Classification of rheumatological disease

Seronegative spondylarthritis (also called spondarthritis)

Causes of arthritis (eg ankylosing spondylitis, psoriatic arthritis, reactive arthritis (Reiter's), IBD arthropathy) which share the following features:

- *Negative rheumatoid factor*, hence the name seronegative
- *Spondylitis/sacrolilitis* inflammation of vertebrae or sacroiliac joint
- *Enthesitis* inflammation of tendon insertions eg Achilles
- *Significant family history* and association with HLA-B27

Connective tissue disease

Diseases that affect collagen or elastin structures; often autoimmune (SLE, rheumatoid arthritis, myositis, scleroderma) or inherited (Marfan's)

Vasculitis

Diseases causing blood vessel inflammation eg giant-cell arthritis, polyarteritis, Wegener's granulomatosis, secondary to connective tissue disorder

	History	Examination	Investigations
Rheumatoid arthritis	Symmetrical, hands + wrists, malaise	Inflamed, swollen joints, early deformity	↑ESR, +ve RhF, erosive changes
Osteoarthritis	Chronic onset in hips and knees	Non-inflamed, ↓ROM	Normal blds, distinctive X-ray
Septic arthritis	Fever, single joint, rapid onset	Tender, swollen, hot, red, unable to move	↑WCC/CRP/ESR, +ve culture
Gout	Acute onset, severe single joint pain	Red, tender, swollen, tophi	Urate crystals on joint aspirate
Pseudo-gout	Gradual onset, single joint pain	Red, tender, swollen	CPP crystals on joint aspirate
Polymyalgia rheumatica	Elderly, symmetrical shoulder/pelvic pain	Muscle tenderness, pain on movement	↑↑ESR, ↑ALP
Ankylosing spondylitis	Back pain, stiffness, young male	↓Back flexion and chest expansion	↑ESR, –ve RhF, HLA-B27 +ve
Reactive arthritis (Reiter's)	Lower limb pain, dysuria, eye pain	Inflamed joints, conjunctivitis, keratoderma blennorrhagica	↑ESR, –ve RhF, X-ray normal, +ve chlamydia
Psoriatic arthritis	Psoriasis, variable joint involvement	Psoriasis, nail changes, dactylitis	↑ESR, –ve RhF, erosive changes
SLE	Fever, malaise, weight loss, rash, lethargy	Malar rash, ulcers	ANA, dsDNA +ve, haematuria
Rheumatic fever	Sore throat, migratory joint pain, rash, fever	Murmur, chorea, nodules	↑ESR/CRP, ASOT +ve
IBD	Migratory arthritis, abdo pain, diarrhoea, PR bleeding	Abdo tenderness, erythema nodosum	Distinctive colonoscopy
Endocarditis	Fever, weight loss, oedema	Heart murmur, splinter haemorrhages	Vegetation on echo, ↓Hb, ↑WCC/CRP/ESR
Leukaemia	Weight loss, bruising, weakness	Petechiae, bruises, lymphadenopathy	↑↑WCC, ↓Hb
Sickle cell	Dactylitis in children, septic arthritis all ages	Swollen, hot, tender monoarthritis	Sickle-cell positive, ↓Hb
Haemophilia	Sudden onset, single joint in children	Haemarthrosis, tender, swollen	↑APTTr, ↓factor VIII or IX

Trauma	p352	Leukaemia	p336
Endocarditis	p395	IBD	p259
Sickle cell	p337	Haemophilia	p345

Rheumatoid arthritis

Common joints symmetrical *PIPJs, MCPs,* wrists
Risk factors female sex, family history
Symptoms morning stiffness, malaise, fatigue, mild fever, weight loss
Signs swelling, redness, deformity (see box), nodules (elbows)
Results ↓Hb, normal MCV, ↑ESR, Rh factor +ve (80%), ANA +ve (30%); X-ray shows erosions, cysts, osteopenia, narrow joint space, deformity
Treatment analgesia, NSAIDs, exercise, physiotherapy, corticosteroids, disease-modifying anti-rheumatic drugs (DMARDs) eg sulfasalazine, methotrexate, azathioprine, ciclosporin should be started at diagnosis, biological therapies (anti-TNFα eg infliximab), surgery (reconstructive, synovectomy, joint replacement, fusion)
Flare ups analgesia, splinting, corticosteroids (oral or intra-articular)
Complications joint destruction, episcleritis, pericarditis, pleuritis, hepatitis, vasculitis, neuropathy, septic arthritis

Hand signs in rheumatoid arthritis

Swan neck deformity of fingers	Ulnar deviation of fingers
Z-deformity of the thumb	Dinner-fork deformity of the wrist
Boutonnière's deformity of distal IPJ	Wasting of intrinsic muscles of the hand

Osteoarthritis

Common joints knees, hips, interphalangeal joints
Risk factors age, previous trauma, excess weight
Symptoms pain worse with activity, chronic onset, stiffness on resting
Signs initially none, swelling, deformity, reduced range of movement
Results normal blood tests; X-ray shows loss of joint space, subchondral sclerosis, bone cysts and osteophyte formation
Treatment analgesia (p428), weight loss, walking aids, exercise (especially strengthening of muscles near affected joints), steroid/local anaesthetic joint injections, arthroscopic wash-out, joint replacement/fusion
Complications disability, immobility, chronic pain, joint destruction

Septic arthritis

Common joints single knee or hip
Risk factors joint disease, prosthetic joint, immunosuppression, ↑age, DM, trauma
Symptoms fever, rapid onset painful joint, other joints not involved
Signs held slightly flexed, swollen, warm, tender, red, pain on active and passive movement, reduced range of movement
Results ↑WCC, CRP and ESR, positive blood culture, white cells and positive culture on aspiration, X-ray as baseline
Organisms staph, strep, haemophilus, TB
Treatment analgesia, urgent orthopaedic referral, high-dose IV antibiotics for ≥6wk (eg flucloxacillin 2g/6h IV and benzylpenicillin 2.4g/6h IV) after diagnostic joint aspiration, may need daily aspiration/surgical intervention
Complications joint destruction, secondary osteoarthritis, septicaemia

Gout (urate crystal arthropathy)

Common joints single joint: big toe MTPJ, ankle, wrist, knee
Risk factors family history, ↑age, male sex, thiazide diuretics, red meat, alcohol
Symptoms rapid onset painful joint, other joints not involved, ±fever
Signs swollen, warm, tender, red, shiny skin; ***chronic*** tophi (white/yellow or skin coloured nodules of urate) on Achilles, elbow, knee or ear
Results Exclude septic arthritis, ↑urate, ↑WCC/ESR/CRP, needle-shaped crystals in joint aspirate with negative birefringence, X-ray normal
Treatment NSAIDs (eg diclofenac 50mg/8h PO), rest, high fluid intake, reduce thiazide diuretics, alcohol and red meat, allopurinol is reserved for chronic gout (can trigger attacks therefore start with an NSAID)
Chronic gout recurrent attacks, osteoarthritis, tophi

Pseudo-gout (calcium pyrophosphate crystal arthropathy)

Common joints single joint: knee, wrist, shoulder
Risk factors age, family history, trauma, haemochromatosis
Symptoms gradual onset painful joint, other joints not involved, ±fever
Signs swollen, warm, tender, red, shiny skin
Results exclude septic arthritis, ↑WCC/ESR/CRP, rhomboid-shaped CPP crystals in joint aspirate with positive birefringence, calcification on X-ray
Treatment NSAIDs (eg diclofenac 50mg/8h PO), rest, joint aspiration if severe, there is no prophylactic treatment

Polymyalgia rheumatica

Common joints symmetrical, muscles of neck, shoulder, pelvis
Risk factors >50yr, female sex, giant-cell (temporal) arthritis
Symptoms acute onset of morning pain and stiffness in proximal muscles, weight loss, fatigue, malaise, depression, mild fever
Signs muscle tenderness, reduced range of movement from pain
Results ↑↑ESR, ↑CRP, ↑ALP, ↓Hb, normal MCV, normal CK
Treatment prednisolone 20mg/24h PO, gradually reduced (over years)

Ankylosing spondylitis

Common joints sacroiliac, spine
Risk factors male sex, HLA-B27
Symptoms back pain worst at night, stiffness, (mornings/rest), heel pain
Signs fixed curvature of spine despite bending forwards, restricted chest expansion, heel tenderness (enthesitis), pain on loading sacroiliac joints
Results ↑WCC/ESR/CRP, normal RhF, HLA-B27 (95%), X-rays show spinal and sacroiliac erosions, squared vertebrae, syndesmophytes (ossified edges of vertebral discs), fusion of spine (bamboo spine)
Treatment exercise, NSAIDs, sulfasalazine, biological therapies (anti-TNFα eg infliximab), spinal surgery
Complications anterior uveitis, aortic regurgitation, pulmonary fibrosis, amyloidosis, spinal fusion, restricted ventilation

Reactive arthritis (Reiter's syndrome)

Gastro/venereal disease followed by arthritis, enthesitis and associated symptoms 1–3wk later, symptoms usually resolve within 6mth.

Common joints asymmetrical knee, ankle, foot

Organisms chlamydia, shigella, salmonella, streptococcus, yersinia, HIV

Risk factors HLA-B27

Symptoms recent diarrhoea, stiffness worse with rest, dysuria, urethral discharge, urinary frequency, gritty eye, heel pain, mild fever, malaise

Signs bilateral conjunctivitis, swollen joints, tender tendon insertion points (enthesitis), genital ulceration, nail thickening, vesicles, macules or papules on genitals, palms or sole of foot (keratoderma blennorrhagica)

Results positive chlamydia test or stool culture, ↑WCC/ESR/CRP, normal RhF and ANA, X-rays initially normal

Treatment NSAIDs, rest, intra-articular steroid injections, sulfasalazine or methotrexate if severe, 1% chloramphenicol ointment/6h for eyes, doxycycline 100mg PO/12h for 3mth if caused by chlamydia

Complications recurrent/chronic arthritis, ankylosing spondylitis

Psoriatic arthritis

Common joints five distinct patterns of disease:

(1) Oligoarthritis often fingers/toes

(2) Rheumatoid arthritis pattern

(3) Ankylosing spondylitis pattern

(4) Asymmetric DIP arthropathy with nail changes (most common)

(5) Arthritis mutilans (destruction of hands)

Risk factors psoriasis (skin changes may occur afterwards), family history

Symptoms vary with pattern (common joints), history of psoriasis

Signs nail ridging, pitting and lifting (onycholysis), psoriasis (check scalp, perineum, umbilicus), enthesitis, dactylitis (swollen fingers)

Results ↑WCC/ESR/CRP, normal RhF and ANA, X-ray shows mild erosive changes especially in hands and less osteopenia than rheumatoid

Treatment NSAIDs, sulfasalazine, methotrexate biological therapies (anti-TNFα eg infliximab), rest, splinting, reconstructive surgery

Complications joint destruction, immobility

Systemic lupus erythematosus (SLE)

Common joints symmetrical PIPJ, MCPJ, wrists, knees
Risk factors female sex (90%), African ethnicity
Symptoms malaise, fever, weight loss, lethargy, photosensitive rash (butterfly or discoid), mouth/nose ulcers, chest pain, cough, joint pain, seizures, psychosis, abdo pain, diarrhoea
Signs arthritis (swelling, tender), malar/discoid rash, ulcers
Results ***bld*** ↓Hb/WCC/plts, ↓C4±C3, ↑ESR, ANA +ve (90%), dsDNA +ve (60%), anti-Sm +ve (20%), antiphospholipid +ve; ***urine*** blood, protein, casts; ***x-ray*** non-erosive arthritis
Treatment NSAIDs, corticosteroids, azathioprine, cyclophosphamide, hydroxychloroquine, anti-TNFα eg infliximab, rest, aspirin, anticoagulants
Complications glomerulonephritis, stroke, seizures, psychosis, pericarditis, pleuritis, atherosclerosis, haemolytic anaemia, PE
Drug induced several drugs can cause a lupus-like syndrome these include chlorpromazine, isoniazid, methyldopa, hydralazine

Rheumatic fever

Migratory polyarthritis 2–6wk after a streptococcal infection eg tonsillitis.
Risk factors age <15yr, previous rheumatic fever
Symptoms/signs preceding sore throat, see modified Jones criteria below; diagnosis requires 2 major criteria or 1 major and 2 minor criteria:

Major criteria	Minor criteria
Carditis (enlargement, new murmur, valve lesion, CCF, pericarditis)	Prolonged PR interval on ECG (if carditis not counted)
Migratory polyarthritis (asymmetrical, moves between large joints eg ankle/knee)	Arthralgia (if migratory polyarthritis not counted)
Aschoff bodies (firm, painless nodules on extensor surface of wrist, elbow or knee)	Raised WCC, ESR or CRP
Erythema marginatum (pink rings on the trunk or limbs, non-itchy)	Fever
Sydenham's chorea (face or arms)	Previous rheumatic fever

Results diagnosis requires Group A Strep on throat swab or ↑ASOT
Treatment high-dose aspirin for 2mth (see *Children's BNF*), prednisolone if moderate carditis is present, penicillin V, rest
Complications recurrence, mitral/aortic stenosis, chorea

Burns emergency

Airway	If airway involved – **CALL ANAESTHETIST**
Breathing	If no respiratory effort – **CALL ARREST TEAM**
Circulation	If no palpable pulse – **CALL ARREST TEAM**

Call for **senior help** early if patient deteriorating or >10% burns

Airway/C-spine

- **Apply** collar, sandbags and tape if C-spine injury is possible
- **Look** for burns to the face and neck, singed eyebrows, facial hair or nasal hairs, soot around the nostrils or in the sputum, facial swelling
- **Listen** for snoring noises, stridor, hoarse voice
- **Intubation** if inhalation injury suspected to prevent airway obstruction

Breathing

- **15l/min O_2** in all patients
- **Count** RR; rapid breathing suggests inhalation injury
- **Monitor** O_2 sats and RR
- **Escharotomy** if circumferential chest burns are restricting breathing

Circulation

- **Venous access**, send bloods for
    - FBC, U+E, glucose, clotting, G+S
    - carboxyhaemoglobin (COHb) – try the blood gas machine
- **Give** 0.9% saline 1l stat
- **Give** morphine IV (eg 10mg titrated to pain) and cyclizine 50mg IV
- **Monitor** HR with defibrillator ECG leads and BP for signs of shock

Disability

- **Assess GCS** and check glucose
- **Look/feel** for pupil reflexes, limb tone and plantar reflexes

Exposure

- **Measure** the extent of 2nd/3rd degree burn, see opposite
- **Cover the burn** with cling film as analgesia, avoid creams
- Check **temp**

Further resuscitation

- Obtain **history** and **examine** the patient
- **Calculate** fluid requirements and adjust rate accordingly (opposite)
- **Catheterise** to monitor urine output
- **CXR** for trauma and as a baseline (signs of inhalation injury after 24h)
- **ABG** if respiratory distress
- **Monitor** circulation of all limbs with burns
- Call for **senior help**
- **Reassess**, starting with A, B, C . . .

Serious complications

Hypovolaemia	p212	Coexisting trauma	p352
Carbon monoxide poisoning	p417	Limb ischaemia	p414
Inhalation injury	p417	Restriction of breathing	p219

Measuring the burn

Burn sizes are expressed as a percentage of the skin surface covered by second or third degree burns. First degree burns (erythema only) are not counted. The chart below works for children and adults:

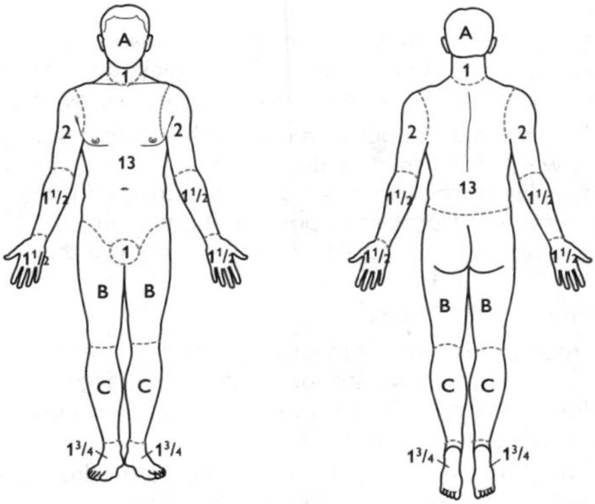

Relative percentage of body surface area affected by growth						
Area	**<1yr**	**1yr**	**5yrs**	**10yrs**	**15yrs**	**Adult**
A (½ of head)	9½	8½	6½	5½	4½	3½
B (½ of one thigh)	2¾	3¼	4	4¼	4½	4¾
C (½ of one leg)	2½	2½	2¾	3	3¼	3½

The palm (not including fingers) of a patient's hand is about 0.75–1% of their body surface area and this can be used for smaller burns. Alternatively the 'rule of nines' can be used for adults:

Head	Each arm	Each leg	Trunk front	Trunk back	Perineum
9%	9%	18%	18%	18%	1%

Burns fluid resuscitation

The burn size is used to calculate fluid requirement for resuscitation using the following formula:

- (4 x weight (kg)) x percentage of burn = volume over 24h (ml)

Give half over the first 8h after injury (ie over 6h if presented at 2h):

- (Volume over 24h (ml) ÷ 2) ÷ 8 = rate per hour (ml)

The other half is given over 16h:

- (Volume over 24h (ml) ÷ 2) ÷ 16 = rate per hour (ml)

So for a 70kg man with 30% burns the rate is 525ml/h for the first 8h then 263ml/h for the next 16h. This is only a guide, monitor the volume status and urine output to maintain volume (p319).

Burns

Worrying features HR>100, systolic BP<100mmHg, RR >30, O_2 sats <92%, signs of inhalation injury, full thickness burn, fires indoors, >10% skin involvement

Think about *life/limb threatening* see box on previous page; ***most likely*** superficial burn, partial thickness burn, full thickness burn, chemical burn, electrical burn, carbon monoxide poisoning, non-accidental injury

Ask about mechanism of burn, time of burn, explosions, smoke, cause of fire, place where fire occurred, duration of exposure, immediate treatment, falls/jumping out of windows, trauma, breathing difficulty, pain; ***PMH*** cardiac or respiratory problems, previous burns/trauma; ***DH*** allergies, tetanus status; ***SH*** smoking (COHb result), housing (do they have somewhere to go?)

Obs temp, RR, BP, HR, O_2 sats

Look for soot around nostrils/mouth, facial burns, swelling, singed facial hair, nostril hair or eyebrows, stridor, hoarse voice, degree of burn (see below), colour, sensation, blistering, extent of burn, location of burn, circumferential burns, other trauma

Depth of burn is assessed by the appearance, blanching, sensation and bleeding when pricked with a needle; it can be difficult to assess especially as different depths may be close together so that a patient may report pain in an area of full thickness burn. If in doubt ask a senior.

Depth	Superficial	Partial dermal	Deep dermal	Full thickness
Degree	1st	2nd		3rd
Colour	Red	Pink, blisters	Bright red, mottled	White, brown, black, leathery
Blanching	Yes	Yes	No	No
Sensation	Yes	Yes	Yes	No
Bleeding	Yes	Yes	Slow	No

Investigations ***blds*** COHb if fire occurred inside; ***consider*** ABG, CXR

Treatment

Major burns (>10% skin surface) resuscitate as per protocol p414
Minor burns cool with running cold water for 10–20min as soon as possible after the injury. Offer analgesia (p428) and cover the burn with cling film until management has been determined. The following should be referred to plastics for assessment (p533):

- All burns to the face, hand or genitalia unless small and first degree
- All deep dermal/full thickness burns larger than a postage stamp

Ask for their advice on dressings (often minimal as some dressings alter the appearance of the burn).
Other burns should be cleaned with water and dressed.

Dressings

If referring straight to plastics just cover the burn in cling film. Otherwise aim to keep the burn covered with a sterile and non-adherent dressing:

Silver sulfadiazine cream (eg Flamazine®) silver has antibiotic effects to reduce the risk of infection; it should be pasted on 3-5mm thick

Paraffin impregnated gauze (eg Jelonet®) this is a non-adherent dressing; it can be applied over silver sulfadiazine cream

Sterile gauze and crepe bandages can be used on top of Jelonet®

Polythene bag/glove this can be placed over a burn to the hand treated with silver sulfadiazine cream

Paraffin wax/Vaseline can be applied frequently for areas which are difficult to dress

The burn should be reviewed and redressed in 2–3d

Tetanus

Burns can cause inoculation with tetanus. They should be managed in the same manner as wounds, see p357.

Inhalation injury

Inhalation of smoke can cause delayed obstruction of the airway.

Symptoms breathlessness, hoarse voice, dysphagia, confusion

Signs singed facial hair or eyebrows, soot around the nostrils or palate, facial/neck burns, stridor, drooling, swelling near the airways, wheeze

Results ↓PEFR; ***blds*** ↑COHb (see below); ***ABG*** acidosis, hypoxia, hypercapnia; ***ECG*** exclude arrhythmia/ischaemia; ***CXR*** ARDS after 24h

Management symptoms or signs of inhalation injury should prompt early intubation, high-flow humidified O_2, salbutamol

Complications pulmonary oedema, ARDS, upper airway obstruction

Carbon monoxide poisoning

This must be considered in all patients involved in a fire indoors.

Symptoms headache, vomiting, malaise, lethargy, arrhythmias

Signs often none, O_2 sats will be falsely high, cherry-red lips are rare

Results COHb >5% suggests moderate inhalation, >15% is serious but it is not a reliable measure of severity; smokers may have a COHb of 8%, ABG may show metabolic acidosis, ECG to exclude arrhythmia/ischaemia

Management 15l/min O_2 by tight fitting mask and reservoir; consider mannitol, ventilation, hyperbaric O_2

Complications cerebral oedema, pulmonary oedema, MI, arrhythmia

Chemical burns

These can be severe, especially if alkalis are involved. They should be washed in running water for at least 20min; larger burns may need fluid replacement as for thermal burns (p414). Toxbase (p305) will give advice on the treatment of specific chemical burns.

Electrical burns

These can cause arrhythmias, cardiac damage and severe muscle damage resulting in renal failure or compartment syndrome. ECG in all patients and FBC, U+E, CK and urine dipstick if severe or high voltage (>1000V).

Weight loss/low appetite

Worrying features ↑HR, arrhythmia, ↑glucose, metabolic acidosis

Think about *emergency* thyrotoxicosis, DKA; ***common*** malignancy, chronic infection (eg TB, HIV), depression, anorexia nervosa, DM, hyperthyroid, malabsorption (eg coeliac, inflammatory bowel disease), chronic disease (eg COPD, heart failure, renal failure, liver failure, neurological conditions, pancreatitis), severe systemic disease, alcoholism, poverty/social isolation, poor diet; ***rare*** Addison's, immunocompromised, vasculitis/connective tissue disease

Ask about amount of weight loss, duration of weight loss, change in clothes' sizes, appetite, dietary intake, thirst, urine output, haematuria, abdo pain, vomiting, dysphagia, change in bowel habit, diarrhoea, steatorrhoea, melaena, rectal bleeding, breathing problems, cough (?bld), chest pain, palpitations, orthopnoea, swelling, fever, night sweats, joint pain, stiffness, rashes, headache, visual disturbance, weakness, mood, suicidal ideation; ***PMH*** heart, lung, kidney, liver problems, malignancy, TB; ***DH*** BCG vaccination, allergies; ***FH*** significant illness or malignancy; ***SH*** foreign travel (where and when), contact with infection, sexual history, drugs of abuse, smoking, alcohol, ability to purchase, prepare and eat food

Obs temp, glucose, RR, HR, BP, postural BP, GCS

Look for needs a thorough examination of all organ systems including neurological and mental state. In particular: clubbing, tremor, muscle wasting, signs of chronic liver failure (p263), lymphadenopathy, goitre, ↑JVP, jaundice, uraemia (lemon colour), downy hair (lanugo), skin lesions (eg erythema nodosum, acanthosis nigrans), pigmented skin folds/gums, displaced apex beat, pleural effusion, creps, wheeze, oedema, organomegally, ascites, PR

Investigations weight, height, BMI (see p640); ***blds*** FBC, U+E, LFT, Ca^{2+}, Mg^{2+}, PO_4^{3-}, amylase, TFT, glucose, CRP, ESR, clotting, G+S, iron, ferritin, TIBC, B_{12}, folate, blood gas; ***urine*** dipstick (ketones). Consider blood cultures, CXR, ECG, coeliac screen and further investigations and imaging as guided by history/examination.

Treatment the key to diagnosing the cause of weight loss is a thorough history and examination. Since there are so many causes it is essential to ask specific questions about each organ system to find likely causes. Aim to localise the cause to a system or category of illness (eg lungs or infection) then focus the investigations on the specific cause.

	History	Examination	Investigations
Diabetes mellitus	Tiredness, polyuria, thirst, abdo pain, vomiting	Ketotic smell, signs of complications	↑Glucose, acidotic, urine ketones
Hyperthyroid	Palpitations, anxiety, heat intolerance, diarrhoea	Tremor, tachycardia, goitre, exophthalmos	↑T_4, ↓or↑TSH
Malignancy	Low appetite, tired, night sweats, specific risk factors	Lymphadenopathy, organomegally, bone pain, masses	Deranged LFT, ↑Ca^{2+}, lesion on imaging
Infection	Fever, night sweats, foreign travel, contact with infection	Focal signs, lymphadenopathy	↑CRP/ESR, ↓PLTS, ↑WCC, positive BLD cultures
Lungs	Cough, pleuritic chest pain, breathlessness, smoker, haemoptysis	Clubbing, hyperinflated, wheeze, creps, effusion, tachypnoea	CXR (hyperexpanded, effusions, focal lesions)
Heart	Chest pain, palpitations, orthopnoea	Arrhythmia, murmurs, displaced apex beat, oedema, basal creps	CXR (big heart, pulmonary oedema), abnormal ECG
Gastro-intestinal and liver	Abdo pain, dysphagia, change in bowel habit, rectal bleeding, alcohol	Organomegally, tenderness, lymphadenopathy, jaundice, ascites, rectal mass	Deranged LFT, faecal occult blood
Renal	Tiredness, small urine output, haematuria	Uraemic, tremor	↑ Urea and Cr, haematuria, proteinuria
Neurological	Weakness, headache, vomiting, visual disturbance, confusion	Abnormal neurological /mental state (p535) exam, papilloedema	Abnormal CT/ MRI brain
Depression	Low mood, poor concentration, suicidal ideation, life events,	Abnormal mental state exam, self-harm	Normal unless organic cause (p309)
Anorexia nervosa	Deranged self-image, unusual diet	Eroded teeth, calluses on back of hand	Normal
Addison's	Vomiting, tiredness, dizziness	Hyperpigmentation (scars, gums), postural BP drop	↑K^+, ↓Na^+, ↓cortisol
Connective tissue	Raynaud's, Sjögren's, joint pain	Joint inflammation	↑CRP/ESR, autoantibodies

Specific Symptoms/Diseases

Abdo pain p235
Breathlessness p219
Confusion p281
Cough p323
Depression p311
DM and DKA p273
Focal neurology p291
Heart failure p226
Hypercalcaemia p330
Jaundice/deranged LFT p268
Joint pain p408
Renal failure p321

Eating disorders

- ***Anorexia nervosa*** BMI ≤17.5 (see p640) with self-induced weight loss and a distorted body image
- ***Bulimia nervosa*** as for anorexia except BMI >17.5 and usually with periods of overeating (binges)

Symptoms distorted body image, weight loss, reduced food consumption, self-induced vomiting, use of diuretics, excessive exercise, depression, obsessions, amenorrhoea, lethargy, social withdrawal

Signs thin, calluses on back of hand, acid erosion of teeth, gaunt face, enlarged salivary glands, lanugo hair (very fine body hair), dry skin, atrophic breasts, scanty pubic hair, peripheral oedema, ↓HR, neuropathy

Investigations ***blds*** electrolytes may be low (especially K^+, Cl^-), may show dehydration otherwise should be relatively normal; ***ABG*** metabolic alkalosis from vomiting; ***ECG*** may show arrhythmias or sinus bradycardia

Treatment combination of antidepressants, counselling (including family therapy) and education; severe cases may need admission for feeding

Complications hypotension, arrhythmias, electrolyte imbalance, constipation, peripheral neuropathy, infertility, osteoporosis

Prognosis anorexia nervosa has a high mortality (15%) with only 33% making a complete recovery; bulimia has a much better prognosis

Hyperthyroid

Excess of thyroxine.

Symptoms weight loss, agitation, anxiety, psychosis, sweating, heat intolerance, diarrhoea, tremor, oligomenorrhoea

Signs thin, ↑temp, ↑HR, irregular pulse, warm hands, tremor, goitre, ±nodules, lid lag

Investigations ↑T_4,↑T_3, ↑↓ or normal TSH (if raised suspect pituitary tumour), positive thyroid autoantibodies, ECG to exclude AF, may need a thyroid scan

Treatment propranolol 40mg/6h for symptoms (unless asthmatic or co-existent heart or vascular problems – see *BNF*), 4wk of oral carbimazole to suppress thyroid. May also be treated by surgery or radioiodine.

Complications AF, ophthalmopathy, osteoporosis

Thyrotoxic storm Caused by infection, severe illness, recent thyroid surgery or radioiodine. Presents with tachycardia, ±AF, agitation, confusion or coma with a ↑T_4 or ↑T_3. Resuscitate as required (p186) and get senior help. Propranolol, carbimazole and hydrocortisone are the main treatments.

Addison's disease

Deficiency of cortisol and aldosterone.

Symptoms tiredness, lethargy, weight loss, weakness, dizziness, depression, abdo pain, diarrhoea or constipation, vomiting, aches and pains

Signs vitiligo, postural hypotension, hyperpigmentation of creases, scars and mouth (buccal)

Investigations ↓Na^+, ↑K^+, ↑urea, may have abnormal FBC and LFT. If suspected perform short Synacthen® test: order 250μg Synacthen® from pharmacy, once this arrives send a blood sample for cortisol levels, give the Synacthen® IM/IV (p564) and repeat cortisol levels in 30min. Addison's is excluded if initial cortisol or 30 min cortisol are >550nmol/l.

Treatment hydrocortisone 20mg PO om and 10mg PO on, may need fludrocortisone 50μg PO alternate days if electrolytes deranged. If unwell, trauma or post-op double all steroid doses for at least 1wk. Replace oral dose with hydrocortisone 100mg IM/IV if vomiting.

Addisonian crisis shock, ↓GCS or hypoglycaemia in a patient with Addison's disease or stopping long-term steroid therapy. Resuscitate according to p208, send bloods for cortisol levels and give hydrocortisone 100mg IV stat followed by cefuroxime 1.5g IV.

Cancer

About 0.4% of the population will be diagnosed with cancer each year. Cancer of the breast, lung, bowel or prostate account for half of these.

Symptoms weight loss, bone pain, lethargy, lumps, abnormal bleeding, bruising, jaundice

Signs lymphadenopathy, cachexia, palpable masses

Investigations deranged LFT, ↑Ca^{2+}, ↑ALP, anaemia, tumour markers

Prognosis about half of all patients diagnosed with cancer will die from it

Pancreatic cancer

Symptoms/signs weight loss, epigastric pain, jaundice, itching, ascites

Management diagnosed by ERCP, CT ±biopsy; surgical resection is occasionally possible, stenting of the bile duct is used for palliative treatment

Prognosis 3% 5yr survival, 10% 1yr survival

Liver cancer

Symptoms/signs jaundice, weight loss, RUQ pain, hepatomegaly, ascites

Management LFT, liver USS, CT and biopsy; treated by localized ablation, surgery (resection or liver transplant) or chemotherapy

Prognosis 75% 5yr survival with liver transplant, 5% 5yr survival overall

Pages where other types of cancer are discussed

Bile duct	p269	Lymphoma	p336	Prostate	p425
Breast	p422	Kidney	p314	Sarcoma	p373
Cervix	p435	Myeloma	p330	Skin	p385
Colorectal	p424	Neck	p374	Stomach	p424
Leukaemia	p336	Oesophagus	p424	Testicle	p378
Lung	p423	Ovary	p435	Uterus	p434

Breast cancer

Epidemiology 45 cases per 100,000 people per year (1% male).
Types vast majority are adenocarcinomas which may be in the duct tissue (ductal, 60–70%) or the lobules (lobular, 10–20%)
Risk factors age, family history, early menarche, late menopause, no children, previous breast cancer
Screening 3-yearly mammogram for women aged 50–70yr
Symptoms finding on screening (mammography), breast lump, change in breast shape or size, nipple inversion or bloody discharge, skin changes bone pain, weight loss, jaundice, breathlessness
Signs palpable lump (often hard, may be firm, poorly defined, tethered, fixed, non-tender,), distorted breast shape, skin dimpling, peau d'orange (prominent pores), eczema around nipple (Paget's), lymphadenopathy
Investigations ***mammogram*** an X-ray of the breast, they are uncomfortable; ***USS*** for women <35yr with dense breasts that give poor mammogram images; ***biopsy/FNA*** for histological evidence of cancer
Staging tests LFT, Ca^{2+}, USS liver, CXR, bone scan
Staging The TNM system by the American Joint Committee on Cancer (AJCC) is usually used; this is a summary of the key points:

Stage	Features
0	Carcinoma-in-situ (DCIS or ICIS depending if it is ductal or lobular)
I	≤2cm with no spread
IIa	≤2cm and spread to axillary lymph nodes **or** 2–5cm with no spread
IIb	2–5cm and spread to axillary lymph nodes **or** >5cm with no spread
IIIa	Fixation of axillary lymph nodes to surrounding structures or each other
IIIb	Invasion of overlying chest wall or skin
IIIc	Spread to lymph nodes beyond the axilla on the same side
IV	Distant metastases

Grading histological appearance of the breast biopsy is also very important; tumours are graded as low, intermediate or high. The presence or absence of oestrogen receptors has a big impact on chemotherapy.
Treatment varies with tumour stage and grade and the patient's wishes:

- *Surgery* the main treatment modality; tumours <4cm may be suitable for breast conservation surgery (lumpectomy or quadrectomy), larger tumours may need mastectomy or rarely radical mastectomy (removal of breast, axillary nodes and pectoralis minor)
- *Radiotherapy* often used after breast surgery to prevent recurrence
- *Chemotherapy* used pre/post-surgery or alone for advanced disease
- *Hormonal therapy* eg tamoxifen given for 5yr after surgery to reduce recurrence in oestrogen receptor-positive tumours
- *Biological therapies* eg Herceptin® monoclonal antibodies that reduce recurrence if the tumour expresses the HER2 growth factor

Prognosis 5yr survival depends on staging and grade and ranges from 99% (carcinoma-in-situ) to 20%. Overall 5yr survival is 80%.
Complications metastases (bones, lung, liver, brain), recurrence, lymphoedema, seroma, cosmetic appearance

Lung cancer

Epidemiology 38 cases per 100,000 people per year
Types non-small-cell (most common, includes adenocarcinoma, squamous- and large-cell), small-cell, mesothelioma
Risk factors smoking (active and passive), age, asbestos, radon gas
Screening none available
Symptoms cough, haemoptysis, breathlessness, chest pain, recurrent pneumonia, anorexia, weight loss, bone pain, incidental shadow on CXR
Signs clubbing, lymphadenopathy, pleural effusion, Horner's syndrome
Investigations ***cytology*** of sputum or pleural aspirate; ***CXR*** with lateral views; ***bronchoscopy*** to visualise and biopsy central lesions, bronchial washings if the lesion is not visible; ***transthoracic*** peripheral lesions can be visualised (thoracoscopy) and biopsied via the chest wall ***CT/MRI/PET*** scan used to identify lung lesions and stage lung cancer
Staging tests LFT, abdo USS, CT, PET scan
Staging of non-small-cell tumours uses a TNM system:

	Tumour	Nodes	Metastases
0	None found	None	None
1	<3cm	Hilar or bronchopulmomary nodes on same side	Present
2	>3cm	Any other nodes on the same side except scalene or supraclavicular	
3	Invasion of surrounding structures **or** <2cm from carina	Any nodes on opposite side or any scalene or supraclavicular nodes	
4	Malignant pleural effusion **or** invasion of carina, vertebral body, heart, oesophagus or great vessels		

The TNM scores give a stage that determines prognosis and treatment:

Stage	TNM	5yr survival	Treatment
Ia	T1N0M0	80%	Surgery, radiotherapy
Ib	T2N0M0	60%	Surgery, radiotherapy
IIa	T1N1M0	50%	Surgery, radiotherapy
IIb	T2N1M0 or T3N0M0	40%	Surgery, radiotherapy
IIIa	T1–3N2M0 or T3N1M0	25%	Surgery, radiotherapy
IIIb	T4N0–3M0 or T1-3N3M0	10%	Radiotherapy, chemotherapy
IV	T1–4N0–3M1	2%	Radiotherapy, chemotherapy

Prognosis 5–10% overall 5yr survival due to advanced disease at diagnosis
Complications metastases (pleura, brain, bones, liver, adrenals), pleural effusion, SVC or airway obstruction (p231), SIADH, Cushing's syndrome, hypercalcaemia, nerve palsies, peripheral neuropathy
Small-cell cancers have a poor prognosis (5yr survival 20%–1%); extremely rapid progression unless treated with chemotherapy

Colorectal cancer

Epidemiology 36 cases per 100,000 people per year
Types almost all are adenocarcinomas; differentiated by location:
- *Right colon* abdominal pain, anaemia, late presentation
- *Left colon* change in bowel habit, bleeding, obstruction
- *Rectum* change in bowel habit, rectal bleeding, tenesmus

Risk factors age, family history, inflammatory bowel disease, polyps, diet (fibre and fish decrease risk, red or processed meat increase risk)
Screening faecal occult blood is offered every 2yr to 60–69yr olds
Symptoms change in bowel habit, PR bleeding, melaena, anaemia, tenesmus (desire to defecate without stool), abdo pain, bowel obstruction, anorexia, weight loss, positive faecal occult blood test (screening)
Signs rectal mass, PR blood, hepatomegaly, ascites, abdominal mass
Investigations ***faecal occult blood*** non-specific screening test; ***sigmoid/colonoscopy*** to visualise and biopsy tumours; ***contrast enema*** can identify tumours not seen on colonoscopy; ***tumour markers*** CEA and CA 19-9
Staging tests LFT, abdo USS, CT, surgery for histology
Staging is via the Dukes' system:

Dukes	Features	5yr survival	Treatment
A	Bowel wall only	>90%	Surgery
B	Through the bowel wall	80%	Surgery ± chemotherapy
C1	Local lymph nodes	60%	Surgery and chemotherapy
C2	Proximal lymph nodes	30%	Surgery and chemotherapy
D	Distant metastases	5%	Chemotherapy

Treatment curative surgical resection is the main treatment; it may involve end-to-end anastomosis or a stoma (temporary or permanent). The usual operation is a right or left hemicolectomy for colon cancer and anterior resection or abdomino-peroneal resection for rectal cancer.
Chemotherapy may be offered as an adjuvant (in addition to surgery) or alone as palliative treatment if surgery is not appropriate. Radiotherapy is rarely used since it is difficult to pinpoint the affected area.
Prognosis overall 5yr survival is 35%
Complications metastases (mainly liver), anaemia, bowel obstruction, bowel perforation

Oesophageal cancer

Symptoms dysphagia, retrosternal pain, weight loss, coughing
Management diagnosed by contrast swallow or endoscopy; distal tumours may be resectable otherwise radiotherapy or stent insertion
Prognosis 20% 5yr survival with surgery, 7% 5yr survival overall

Stomach cancer

Symptoms weight loss, dysphagia, epigastric pain, vomiting
Signs supraclavicular lymph node, palpable epigastric mass
Management endoscopy or contrast meal for diagnosis then gastrectomy
Prognosis 10% 5yr survival overall

Prostate cancer

Epidemiology 35 cases per 100,000 people per year
Types vast majority are adenocarcinomas
Risk factors age, smoking, family history
Screening no formal screening; GP may offer PSA and PR exam if >50yr
Symptoms poor urinary stream, urinary hesitancy, bladder obstruction, haematuria, blood in sperm, pelvic pain, constipation, weight loss, anorexia, ↑Ca^{2+}, bone pain, jaundice, anaemia
Signs mass on PR examination, swelling of legs/scrotum, bony tenderness
Investigations ***transrectal ultrasound*** to assess the prostate, capsule and seminal vesicles for evidence of spread; a biopsy is usually taken to assess grade; prostate ***specific antigen (PSA)*** blood test is usually raised in prostate cancer:

PSA result (ng/ml)	Interpretation
<3	Normal for man aged <60yr
<4	Normal if aged >60yr
<5	Normal if aged >70yr
<10	Probable benign prostatic hypertrophy, monitor
>10	Increasing likelihood of cancer
>40	High chance of cancer with metastases

Staging tests LFT, Ca^{2+}, IVU, lumbar spine X-ray, CXR, bone scan, CT
Staging

1	Small cancer inside a prostate gland that feels normal on PR examination
2	Cancer inside prostate capsule but palpable
3	Cancer outside the prostate capsule
4	Spread to bladder, rectum, pelvic wall, lymph nodes or distant metastases

Grading histological appearance of the prostate biopsy is also very important. Tumours are given a Gleason grade from 1–10 where grade 1 is slow growing whilst 10 is aggressive and likely to metastasise.
Treatment depends on the tumour stage and grade and the patients age:

- Watch and wait monitoring PSA levels for low grade, early stage tumours in elderly patients
- *Radical prostatectomy* offers a cure in younger patients with low stage disease but often causes urinary leakage and erectile dysfunction
- *Radiotherapy* often causes erectile dysfunction
- *Reducing testosterone levels* this can be achieved by removing both testicles or more commonly using medications eg LHRH agonists, oestrogens, androgen antagonists; they can be used palliatively or with radiotherapy
- *Chemotherapy* used for advanced disease with metastases

Prognosis depends on staging and Gleason score and ranges from >95% to 10%. Overall 5yr survival is 70%.
Complications metastases (bladder, rectum, bones, lung, liver, brain), acute urinary retention, hypercalcaemia, anaemia

HIV/AIDS

Transmission mother to child (vertical), sexual contact (oral, penile, vaginal, anal, abroad especially Sub-Saharan Africa), blood contact (IV drug users, needle-stick injuries, blood products), bodily fluid contact (eg splash injuries)
Stages of infection
- *Acute seroconversion* flu-like symptoms 2–6wk after infection eg sore throat, fever, malaise, myalgia, maculopapular rash, lymphadenopathy
- *Asymptomatic* a symptom-free period lasting 10yr on average; may have persistent generalised lymphadenopathy
- *Symptomatic* HIV as the immune system fails the patient becomes more susceptible to common pathogens (eg colds, gastroenteritis, thrush) they may also suffer constitutional symptoms (eg weight loss, low energy)
- *AIDS* diagnosis with an AIDS-defining illness, see box

Symptoms most cases present with PCP (*Pneumocystis jirovecii* pneumonia) or Kaposi's sarcoma: cough, shortness of breath, rashes, weight loss, lethargy, recurrent fever, chronic diarrhoea, confusion, memory loss, headaches, abdominal pain, dysphagia
Signs rashes (Kaposi's sarcoma is a red/purple, slightly raised papule or plaque often on the head, neck, trunk or mucous membranes), wasting, generalised lymphadenopathy, oral/genital candidiasis
Counselling never order an HIV test without consent; the patient should be counselled on the benefits and risks of testing along with the implications of a positive result by a GUM specialist (eg HIV nurse specialist)
Investigations ***HIV antibody*** tests used for diagnosis; it takes up to 3mth to give a positive result after infection; ***HIV PCR*** used to monitor treatment; more sensitive than the antibody tests and gives a viral load to quantify infection; ***CD4 count*** also used to monitor treatment
Label all bodily fluid samples as 'high risk' if HIV is suspected
Treatment combination therapy or HAART (Highly Active Anti-Retroviral Therapy); there are four classes:
- Nucleoside reverse-transcriptase inhibitors (NRTIs)
- Non-nucleoside reverse transcriptase inhibitors (NNRTIs)
- Protease inhibitors (PLS)
- Fusion inhibitors

Treatment is usually led by a GUM or infectious diseases specialist. Co-trimoxazole and isoniazid are sometimes used as prophylaxis against *Pneumocystis jirovecii* and TB respectively. Of note, HIV-positive patients should not have BCG or yellow fever vaccinations.
Prognosis 12% progress to AIDS in 5yr but depends on viral load/CD4

Common AIDS-defining conditions

Kaposi's sarcoma	Progressive multifocal leukoencephalopathy
Pneumocystis jirovecii pneumonia (PCP)	Recurrent non-typhi salmonella septicaemia
CMV retinitis	Cerebral toxoplasmosis
Chronic mucocutaneous herpes	Cryptococcal meningitis
Mycobacterium avium intracellulare	Non-Hodgkin's lymphoma
Miliary or extrapulmonary TB	Primary cerebral lymphoma
Oesophageal candidiasis	HIV-associated wasting
Chronic cryptosporidial diarrhoea	HIV-associated dementia

Tuberculosis (TB)

Transmission airborne, ingested, transcutaneous
Risk factors TB exposure, travel, immunocompromise, non-vaccination
Types of infection

- *Primary TB* initial infection may cause mild cough, breathlessness or be asymptomatic; detectable by Mantoux test and scars on CXR
- *Latent TB* after primary infection most patients become asymptomatic with the TB walled off in a tubercule; it may not progress further
- *Active TB* this is when infection causes disease in a specific organ (see box) or throughout the body (miliary); it is usually a reactivation of latent TB (eg due to immunocompromise) or a continuation of primary TB

Sites of tuberculosis infection

Pulmonary	Most common (80%): cough, breathlessness, effusion
Miliary	Haematological spread to all tissues: liver, spleen, lungs, marrow
Meningeal	Sub-acute meningitic symptoms: fever, headache, photophobia
Genitourinary	Frequency, dysuria, loin pain, haematuria
Bone	Vertebral collapse adjacent to paravertebral abscess
Skin	Jelly-like nodules/ulcers on face and neck (lupus vulgaris)
Heart	Acute/chronic pericarditis, pericardial effusion

Symptoms fever, night sweats, weight loss, anorexia, lethargy, malaise, cough, haemoptysis, pleuritic chest pain, breathlessness, diarrhoea, lumps
Signs lymphadenopathy, erythema nodosum, consolidation, apical bronchial breathing, pleural effusion, masses
Isolation see p119; all sputum-positive TB patients (ie those with positive sputum culture) should be isolated and all visitors/staff should wear a face mask; if the patient is moved through the hospital they should wear a mask. After 2wk of anti-TB treatment they should not be infectious.
Investigations ***CXR*** consolidation (often apical), cavitation, fibrosis, calcification, hilar lymphadenopathy, pleural effusion; ***sputum*** three early morning cultures for Ziehl-Nielsen (ZN) stain looking for acid-fast bacilli (AFB), takes 3-12wk; ***histology*** typically caseating granuloma; ***Mantoux*** tuberculin skin test difficult to interpret if immunocompromised or vaccinated; ***interferon testing*** eg Elispot more sensitive and specific than Mantoux used for borderline cases; ***HIV*** consider testing in all patients
Treatment ***initial phase (8wk)*** rifampicin, isoniazid, pyrazinamide and either ethambutol or streptomycin if resistance suspected; ***continuation phase (4mth)*** rifampicin and isoniazid, add ethambutol if resistance suspected; side-effects are common eg thrombocytopenia (rifampicin), hepatitis (all antibiotics), neuropathy (isoniazid), visual changes (ethambutol). Full compliance is essential, consider Directly Observed Therapy – Short course (DOTS).
Drug resistance multi-drug resistance TB (MDR-TB) is a growing problem; consult with infectious disease specialists early
Contact tracing all individuals who have shared a kitchen or bathroom with someone with active TB should have a CXR and Mantoux test
Vaccination BCG (bacille Calmette-Guérin) is a live vaccine that decreases the risk of developing TB by between 50 and 70%; it used to be given to everyone at 13yr but is now given at birth to at-risk groups only

Pain

Worrying features ↓↑HR, ↓↑BP, ↓↑RR, ↓GCS, sweating, vomiting, chest pain

Think about headache p298, chest pain p177, abdominal pain p234, back pain p296, limb pain p402, infection p392; ***common*** postoperative, musculoskeletal, chronic pain

Ask about (SOCRATES) **S**ite, **O**nset, **C**haracter, **R**adiation, **A**lleviating factors, **T**iming (duration, frequency), **E**xacerbating factors, **S**everity, associated features (sweating, nausea, vomiting); ***PMH*** stomach problems, asthma, cardiac problems; ***DH*** allergies, analgesia already taken and perceived benefit; ***SH*** previous drug abuse

Ward round assess the effectiveness of analgesia daily and ask specifically about drowsiness, nausea, vomiting and constipation

Obs ↑HR and ↑BP suggests pain; RR, pupil size and GCS if on opioids

Look for source of pain

Investigations these should be guided by your history and examination; none are specifically required for pain

Treatment no patient should be left in severe pain, consider titrating an IV opiate after an antiemetic (p252). Use the steps of the WHO pain ladder. Ensure regular analgesia is prescribed, with adequate prn analgesia for break-through pain. If a patient has moderate or severe pain start at step 3 or 4; using paracetamol and NSAIDs reduces opiate requirement and side-effects.

	Step 1	Step 2	Step 3	Step 4
Strong opioids				✓
Weak opioids			✓	
NSAIDs		✓	✓	✓
Paracetamol	✓	✓	✓	✓

Paracetamol ***contraindications*** moderate liver failure; ***side-effects*** rare

- **Paracetamol** 1g/4h, max 4g/24h PO/PR/IV

NSAIDs good for inflammatory pain, renal or biliary colic and bone pain; ***contraindications*** (BARS) **B**leeding (pre-op, coagulopathy), **A**sthma, **R**enal disease, **S**tomach (peptic ulcer or gastritis). 10% of asthmatics are NSAID-sensitive, try a low dose if they have never used them before. Use with caution in the elderly and prescribe with a PPI to protect the stomach; ***side-effects*** GI upset (ulceration and bleeding), worsen renal function.

- ***Ibuprofen*** 400mg/8h, max 2.4g/24h PO, weaker anti-inflammatory action, but less risk of GI ulceration
- ***Diclofenac*** 50mg/8h, max 150mg/24h PO/PR (also IM/IV, see *BNF*)

COX-2 inhibitors are similar to NSAIDs but with less risk of gastroduodenal ulceration. They have been shown to increase the risk of thromboembolic events (eg MI, CVA) and should be used with **caution.**

Weak opioids dependence and tolerance to opioids do not occur with short-term use for acute pain. Consider prescribing regular laxatives and PRN anti-emetics, use with ***caution*** if head injury, ↑ICP, respiratory depression, alcohol intoxication; ***side-effects*** N+V, constipation, drowsiness, hypotension; ***toxicity*** ↓RR, ↓GCS, pinpoint pupils

- ***Codeine*** 30–60mg/4h, max 240mg/24h PO/IM, constipating
- ***Dihydrocodeine (DF118)*** 30mg/4h, max 240mg/24h PO, constipating
- ***Tramadol*** 50–100mg/4h, max 400–600mg/24h PO/IM, stronger than others and less constipating for long-term use

Paracetamol and weak opioid combinations useful for TTO analgesia; it is better to prescribe the components separately in hospital:

- ***Co-codamol*** 30mg codeine and 500mg paracetamol; two tablets/6h PO, nurses must give 8/500 dose if 30/500 not specified
- ***Co-dydramol*** 10mg dihydrocodeine and 500mg paracetamol; two tablets/6h PO
- ***Co-proxamol*** contained dextropropoxyphene and has been withdrawn owing to its potential toxicity and poor analgesic properties. Some patients may still be taking this, but it is not prescribed to new patients.

Weak opiate to oral morphine converter

Drug and dose (oral route)	Equivalent to 1mg oral morphine
Codeine 8mg	1mg oral morphine
Codeine 60mg/6h	30mg oral morphine/24h
Dihydrocodeine 8mg	1mg oral morphine
Dihydrocodeine 60mg/6h	30mg oral morphine/24h
Tramadol 5mg	1mg oral morphine
Tramadol 50mg/6h	40mg oral morphine/24h

Strong opioids morphine is used for severe pain; diamorphine is reserved for rapid action or palliative care. Use regular fast-acting opioids for acute pain with regular laxatives and PRN or regular anti-emetics. See 'weak opioids' for ***cautions, side effects*** and ***toxicity***. Use only one method of administration (ie PO, SC, IM, or IV) to avoid overdose:

- ***Oral*** eg Sevredol® or Oramorph® 10mg/2–4h
- ***SC/IM*** morphine 10mg/2–4h or diamorphine 5mg/2–4h
- ***IV*** titrate to pain; dilute 10mg morphine into 10ml H_2O for injections (1mg/ml), give 2mg initially and wait 2min for response. Give 1mg/2min until pain settled observing RR and responsiveness

Long-acting opioids are used after major surgery or in chronic pain. Use standard opioids initially until morphine requirements known (p122) then prescribe a regular long-acting dose along with PRN fast-acting opioids to cover breakthrough pain (equivalent to 15% or one-sixth of daily requirements). Laxatives will be needed.

- ***Oral*** MST dose = half total daily oral morphine requirement (p122) given every 12h, usually 10–30mg/12h, max 400mg/24h
- ***Topical*** fentanyl patch lasts 72h, available in 25–100μg/h doses

Other analgesic options/adjuncts

Nefopam a non-opioid analgesia that can be given with paracetamol, NSAIDs and opioids; ***contraindications*** epilepsy and convulsions; ***side-effects*** urinary retention, pink urine, dry mouth, light-headedness

- ***Nefopam*** 30–60mg/8h PO or 20mg/6h IM

Hyoscine gives good analgesia in colicky abdo pain; ***contraindications*** paralytic ileus, prostatism, glaucoma, myasthenia gravis, porphyria; ***side-effects*** constipation, dry mouth, confusion, urine retention

- ***Buscopan®*** (hyoscine butylbromide) 20mg/6h PO/IM/IV

Diazepam acts as a muscle relaxant, eg spasm with back pain ***contraindications*** respiratory compromise/failure, sleep apnoea ***side-effects*** drowsiness, confusion, physical dependence (use for short-term only)

- ***Diazepam*** 2mg/8h PO

Quinine used for nocturnal leg cramps; ***contraindications*** haemoglobinuria, optic neuritis, arrhythmias; ***side-effects*** abdo pain, tinnitus, confusion

- ***Quinine*** 200mg/24h PO – at night

Patient-controlled analgesia (PCA) a syringe driver that gives a bolus of IV opiate (usually morphine, but occasionally tramadol or fentanyl) when the patient activates a button. A background infusion rate, bolus dose and maximum bolus frequency can be adjusted to prevent overdose/pain; changes to the PCA are usually undertaken by the pain team (see below). The patient must be alert, cooperative, have IV access and their pain under control before starting. Check hospital protocols.

Epidural are inserted by the anaesthetist in theatre usually prior to surgery. A local anaesthetic infusion (±opiate) anaesthetises the spinal nerves, and usually produces a sensory level below which the patient has little or no feeling; if this level rises too high (higher than T4 (nipples)) there is risk of respiratory failure. The anaesthetist or pain team (see below) usually look after epidurals and their dosing post-op. Complications include local haematoma, abscess (causes cord compression, p297) or local infection which requires epidural removal and treatment with IV antibiotics.

Syringe driver These are used mainly for palliative analgesia and symptom control, see p122

Pain team

Most hospitals have acute and chronic pain teams, comprising nurses and a pain specialist (usually an anaesthetist). The acute pain service is often run by the Outreach Team (p455).

Inpatients with pain issues can be referred to the teams for assessment, though ensure all simple measures have been undertaken to address the patient's pain first, namely identify and treat cause of pain, and ensure the patient is receiving adequate simple analgesia (regular paracetamol, NSAIDs (if not contraindicated) and an opiate (if appropriate)).

Neuropathic and chronic pain

Neuropathic pain is caused by damage to nerves, eg radiculopathy (nerve root pain), peripheral neuropathy, neuralgia and phantom limb pain. The pain tends to be difficult to describe or pinpoint and is often aching, burning, sharp, stabbing or shooting in nature. Chronic conditions can cause significant pain, eg chronic pancreatitis, arthritis, post-traumatic, DM, trigeminal neuralgia; there is frequently a psychogenic component. Standard analgesia is often ineffective and the services of a chronic pain specialist should be sought. Commoner chronic pain therapies include:

Tricyclic antidepressants given at a low dose; ***contraindications*** recent MI, arrhythmias; ***side-effects*** dry mouth, constipation, sedation

- ***Amitriptyline*** 10mg/24h PO – ideally at night

Gabapentin contraindications previous psychosis; ***side-effects*** dizziness, tiredness, cerebellar signs; **NB** do not stop suddenly, taper off the dose

- *Gabapentin* gradually build up, start at 300mg/day PO, see *BNF*

Capsaicin a cream made from extracts of chillies; ***side-effects*** burning sensation

- *Capsaicin* small amount every 6h topical

TENS **T**ranscutaneous **E**lectrical **N**erve **S**timulation is believed to affect the gate mechanism of pain fibres in the spine and/or to stimulate the production of endorphins. Use at a high frequency for acute pain or slow frequency for chronic/neuropathic pain.

Steroids and nerve blocks injections of steroids combined with local anaesthetic into joints or around nerves can reduce pain for long periods. This needs to be done by a specialist.

Sympathectomy and nerve ablation The ablation of sensory and sympathetic nerves by surgery or injection; used as a last resort in some forms of chronic pain.

Acupuncture effective in some trials and with a greater evidence base than most complementary therapies (p64).

Counselling and cognitive–behavioural therapy (CBT) have been looked at widely in chronic pain, but it remains unclear if this helps; there is some suggestion that it might make things worse for some patients.

Some terms in chronic pain

Allodynia	Seemingly harmless stimuli such as light touch can provoke pain
Hyperpathia	A short episode of discomfort causes prolonged, severe pain
Hyperalgesia	Discomfort which would otherwise be mild is felt as severe pain

Vaginal bleeding

Worrying features ↑HR, ↓BP, weight loss, anaemia, abdominal pain, positive pregnancy test

Think about *emergency* massive bleed, ectopic pregnancy, miscarriage; ***common*** menstruation, dysfunctional uterine bleeding, trauma, ectropion, contraceptive-related, infection, cervical or endometrial polyps, malignancy (cervix, uterus, ovaries), foreign body, miscarriage, fibroids, pelvic inflammatory disease; ***rare*** clotting abnormalities, hypothyroid

Causes of vaginal bleeding	
Menorrhagia	Dysfunctional uterine bleeding, fibroids, endometriosis, polyps, pelvic inflammatory disease, endometrial cancer, IUCD/foreign body, clotting disorder, hypothyroid
Postcoital	Ectropion, polyps, infection, cancer (cervix, uterus), trauma
Intermenstrual	Polyps, ectropion, infection, IUCD/foreign body, pregnancy, hormonal contraception, cancer (cervix, uterus)
Postmenopausal	Endometrial cancer until proven otherwise, other cancer (cervix, ovarian), atrophic vaginitis, infection, polyps

Ask about possibility of pregnancy, timing of bleeding (between periods, during periods, after intercourse), duration of bleeding, amount of bleeding (pads, tampons, clots, flooding), menstrual pain, effect on lifestyle, other vaginal discharge, usual cycle and bleeding, weight loss, abdo pain, trauma, pain during intercourse, lumps; ***PMH*** anaemia, clotting problems, thyroid problems; ***DH*** contraceptive pills or injections, IUCDs, aspirin; ***SH*** sexual activity; ***O+GH*** pregnancies, miscarriages, terminations, last smear test and result, STIs, date of last menstrual period (LMP)

Obs HR, BP, postural BP, temp, pregnancy test

Look for abdo tenderness/guarding, pelvic masses, inguinal lymphadenopathy, exclude PR bleeding; *internal examination* (p487) vulval lesions, size of uterus, uterine masses, adnexal tenderness or masses, presence of blood/discharge; *speculum exam* (p487) ulceration, ectropion, bleeding, lumps, prolapse, triple swab if infection is suspected

Investigations A *pregnancy test* is absolutely essential, remember urine β-hCG may give a false-negative after 20wk; consider serum β-hCG, FBC, CRP, clotting, U+E, LFT, TFT, pelvic USS. May need diagnostic laparoscopy or hysteroscopy (looking inside the uterus with fibreoptics).

Treatment

- ***Signs of shock*** resuscitate as for other causes of blood loss (p212), call for senior help
- ***Positive pregnancy*** test and abdominal tenderness assume an ectopic pregnancy (p243); secure two sites of good IV access (grey or bigger) and contact a gynaecologist immediately
- ***Postmenopausal bleeding*** refer to rule out endometrial cancer
- ***Otherwise*** consider likely diagnoses and rule out serious conditions

	History	Examination	Investigations
Ectopic	Abdo pain, last LMP >4wk, PV bleeding	Abdo tenderness ± peritonism, shock	+ve β-hCG, seen on USS, ↓Hb
Miscarriage	PV bleeding, crampy pain	Open/closed os, products of conception	β-hCG +ve, ±fetus on uss
Dysfunctional uterine bleeding	Menorrhagia	Normal	Normal
Fibroids	Menorrhagia	Bulky uterus	Visible on USS
Endometrial cancer	Postmenopausal bleeding, abdo pain	Usually normal	Seen on USS or hysteroscopy
Pelvic inflammatory disease	Abdominal pain, vaginal discharge, dyspareunia	Abdominal tenderness, foul-smelling discharge	Positive cultures
Infection	Vaginal discharge, itching, foul odour	Erythema, swelling, discharge	Positive cultures
Ectropion/erosion	Intermenstrual or postcoital bleeding; on the pill or pregnant	Red ring or flare around external os	Normal
Polyps	Intermenstrual or postcoital bleeding	Polyp may be visible on speculum examination	Polyp on hysteroscopy
Cervical cancer	Postcoital bleeding, dyspareunia, discharge	Mass, ulcer or bleeding cervix	Colposcopy and biopsy
Ovarian cancer	Lower abdo pain, weight loss, ±bleeding	Adnexal mass, abdominal distension	↑CA-125, USS or CT appearance
Hypothyroid	Constipation, cold intolerance, tiredness, menorrhagia	Dry skin, goitre, bradycardia, slow relaxing reflexes	↓T_4, ↑TSH
Clotting abnormality	Family history, bleeding, bruising, joint swelling	Bruises, joint swelling or deformity	Abnormal clotting or bleeding time

Ectopic pregnancy	p243	Miscarriage	p437
Pelvic inflammatory disease	p242	Hypothyroid	p473
Clotting abnormalities	p344		

Dysfunctional uterine bleeding

This is menorrhagia without any detectable abnormality.
Symptoms heavy bleeding during periods only, interfering with daily activities, otherwise well
Signs normal system and gynaecological exam
Investigations may have mild iron deficiency anaemia, otherwise normal
Management tranexamic acid 1g/6h PO or mefenamic acid 500mg/8h PO (both started on the first day of periods and whilst flow is heavy), cyclical progesterone, combined oral contraceptive pill (COC), Mirena® coil, in severe cases endometrial ablation/resection or hysterectomy may be considered.

Fibroids (uterine leiomyoma)

Benign tumours of the smooth muscle in the uterus
Symptoms may be asymptomatic, menorrhagia, prolonged periods, pelvic pain, urinary frequency or incontinence, infertility, abdominal mass
Signs palpable mass on abdominal or vaginal examination, bulky uterus
Investigations visible on pelvic USS, may have anaemia
Treatment symptoms improve after menopause so treatment is often unnecessary; ***medical*** GnRH agonists eg goserelin, leuprorelin cause a temporary menopause to shrink the tumour; ***radiology*** uterine artery ablation; ***surgery*** myomectomy, hysterectomy

Endometrial (uterine) cancer

This is common and presents early, so all postmenopausal or irregular perimenopausal bleeding must be referred to gynaecologists.
Risk factors age, overweight, high fat diet, polycystic ovaries, late menopause, no pregnancies, family history, tamoxifen; COC pill is protective
Symptoms postmenopausal or intermenstrual bleeding, menorrhagia, watery vaginal discharge, lower abdo pain, pain on intercourse
Signs usually normal unless advanced
Investigations transvaginal USS to assess endometrial thickness, biopsy via aspiration sampling, hysteroscopy and dilation and curettage (D+C)
Treatment total abdominal hysterectomy and bilateral salpingo-oophrectomy ±radiotherapy or palliative treatment with radiotherapy
Prognosis overall 5yr survival 80%

Infection (cervicitis, vaginitis)

Infection with candida or STIs; similar symptoms can be caused by a lack oestrogen (atrophic vaginitis), allergy or foreign body
Symptoms itching, vaginal discharge, dysuria, superficial dyspareunia (pain on intercourse), abnormal odour, small amounts of bleeding
Signs vaginal or cervical erythema, swelling, exudates, discharge
Investigation high vaginal, endocervical and chlamydial swabs
Treatment treat the cause eg antibiotics, antifungals, oestrogens

Cervical ectropion/erosion

Temporary extension of the uterine epithelium into the vagina in response to oestrogen eg combined oral contraceptive or pregnancy.
Symptoms often asymptomatic, intermenstrual bleeding, postcoital bleeding, menorrhagia
Signs red flare or ring around the external os on speculum examination
Investigation none required but must have usual smear test screens
Treatment usually none, change of contraceptive, cautery/cryosurgery

Cervical and endometrial polyps

Uterine growths that may pass through the external os into the vagina.
Symptoms often asymptomatic, menorrhagia, intermenstrual, postcoital or postmenopausal bleeding
Signs may be visible on speculum examination
Investigation endometrial polyps may be seen on hysteroscopy; if removed they should be sent for histology, but 99% are benign
Treatment surgical removal with cautery of the base with silver nitrate via speculum or hysteroscopy

Cervical cancer

Risk factors human papillomavirus, early first intercourse, multiple partners, smoking, others STIs, lack of screening
Symptoms usually presents with abnormal smear tests; postcoital, intermenstrual or postmenopausal bleeding, pain on intercourse, abnormal vaginal discharge
Signs ulceration, mass or bleeding on cervix
Investigations colposcopy and biopsy, CT/MRI
Treatment **low stage (1a)** hysterectomy and radiotherapy; ***high stage (>1b)*** chemotherapy and radiotherapy
Prognosis overall 5yr survival 65%

Ovarian cancer

Risk factors family history, age, early menarche, late menopause, no pregnancies, infertility, overweight; COC pill is protective
Symptoms lower abdo pain (similar to ovarian torsion p243), weight loss, bloating, irregular periods, postmenopausal bleeding, urinary frequency, constipation, pain on intercourse
Signs adnexal mass, abdominal distension/mass, ascites, leg oedema, DVT
Investigations raised CA-125, CA-19.9, CEA, α-FP, β-hCG, mass on USS or CT abdomen/pelvis
Treatment surgical removal of all visible tissues (uterus, ovaries, omentum) and chemotherapy
Prognosis usually poor due to late presentation; overall 5yr survival 30%

Early Pregnancy (1st trimester)

Diagnosing pregnancy

Symptoms missed period, urinary frequency, nausea, vomiting, malaise, nipple tingling/itching, breast enlargement, positive pregnancy test
Signs enlarged uterus, cervix looks bluish (venous engorgement)
Investigations
- *Urine β-hCG* positive from the first day of the missed period until about 20/40 gestation
- *Serum β-hCG* only measure if urine β-hCG is +ve; useful for assessing 1st trimester complications as it should double every 2d
- *Transvaginal uss* positive from about 6/40 gestation or if serum β-hCG ≥1500iu/l

Management give the news sensitively, consider who is present (eg relatives), offer congratulations if appropriate, start folic acid 0.4mg/24h PO (more if on anticonvulsants); GP to refer to antenatal clinic
Health promotion exercise, no smoking or alcohol, no vitamin supplements (vitamin A is teratogenic), avoid unpasteurised cheese, shellfish and raw eggs (listeria), avoid cat faeces (toxoplasmosis)
Antenatal care see p514 for schedule of appointments and tests

Prescribing in pregnancy

Check *BNF* Appendix 4
- Make sure the benefits to the mother outweigh the risk to the fetus
- Use the smallest effective dose for the shortest possible time
- Try to avoid all drugs (except folic acid) in the first trimester

Acceptable drugs penicillins, cephalosporins, heparin, ranitidine, paracetamol, codeine
Drugs to avoid tetracyclines, streptomycin, quinolones, warfarin, thiazide diuretics, ACEi, lithium, NSAIDs, vitamin A and retinoids, barbiturates, cytotoxic drugs, phenytoin

Anti-D in rhesus (D)-negative women

<20/40 Anti-D 250iu IM (deltoid) within 72h of the following situations:
- Ectopic pregnancy
- Spontaneous miscarriage <12/40 with instrumentation eg EPRC
- Spontaneous miscarriage >12/40
- Threatened miscarriage >12/40 if bleeding persists this is repeated every 6wk until delivery
- Surgical or medical terminations <20/40
- Amniocentesis/chorionic villus sampling (CVS)
- Abdominal trauma

>20/40 Anti-D 500iu IM (deltoid) within 72h of the following situations:
- Routinely at 28/40 and 34/40 gestation
- Antepartum haemorrhage
- External cephalic version (ECV) attempts
- Abdominal trauma
- Delivery of rhesus-positive baby (none if baby rhesus-negative)

Miscarriage

Loss of pregnancy <24/40 gestation

Differentials ectopic pregnancy (p243), ectropion, infection, polyp

Symptoms positive pregnancy test, vaginal bleeding (may see products of conception), crampy lower abdominal pain, nausea, vomiting, dizziness

Signs may be shocked (HR, BP), abdominal tenderness suggests ectopic; ***vaginal*** check size of uterus, exclude adnexal tenderness; ***speculum*** open/closed cervical os, clots, products of conception

Investigations ***blds*** FBC, G+S, serum β-hCG ***urine*** β-hCG ***USS abdo***

Miscarriage	Description	USS finding
Threatened	Bleeding, closed os	Intrauterine pregnancy with heart beat
Inevitable	Bleeding, open os	Intrauterine pregnancy with heart beat
Missed	None/bleeding	Intrauterine pregnancy, no heart beat
Incomplete	Bleeding, open os	Retained products of conception
Complete	Bleeding settling	Empty uterus

Management if there is marked abdo/cervical tenderness exclude an ectopic (p243) by USS and serial serum β-hCG. If shocked insert a grey cannula, fluid resuscitate (p212) and remove products of conception from the os (can cause vasovagal); ergometrine 0.5mg IM is given for severe bleeding. Offer all patients analgesia (p428).

- ***Threatened*** no treatment has demonstrated any benefit; bed rest is often suggested but does not affect outcome; 25–50% will abort
- ***Inevitable/incomplete*** the products of conception usually pass without intervention or with mifepristone; surgical removal by ERPC may be considered for pain, bleeding or large quantities of tissue in the uterus
- ***Missed*** evacuation of products of conception medically eg mifepristone or surgically by EPRC

ERPC Evacuation of Retained Products of Conception is performed under spinal or general anaesthetic; the products of conception should be sent for karotyping and histology

Counselling Offer couples a chance to ask questions and provide written material for them to take away. Up to 40% of pregnancies end in miscarriage and of these 80% are due to a fetal abnormality eg chromosomal and it is almost never due to the actions of the mother.

Recurrence ≥3 miscarriages should prompt investigation eg parental karyotypes, karotype of the products of conception, maternal antiphospholipid antibodies, maternal pelvic USS

Termination of pregnancy (TOP)

Patients are referred by GPs or family planning centres. Future contraception should be discussed.

Methods medical (<9wk) mifepristone 600mg PO, then 1mg gemeprost PV 36–48h later; ***surgical*** dilatation and evacuation or vacuum aspiration

Complications haemorrhage, infection, retained products of conception, uterine perforation, feelings of guilt, depression

Later pregnancy (2nd/3rd trimester)

Normal ranges in pregnancy

Feature	Range	Feature	Range
Haematocrit	No change	Albumin	28–40mmol/l
Haemoglobin	11–15g/dl	Urea	1.6–6μmol/l
WCC	5–16 x 10^9/l	Creatinine	70–150μmol/l
Platelets	150–400 x 10^9/l	PaO_2	10.0–13.3kPa
ESR	44–114mm/h	$PaCO_2$	3.6–4.2kPa
Fibrinogen	400–600mg/dl	HCO_3^-	18–23mmol/l

Pregnancy-induced hypertension (PIH)/Pre-eclampsia

- Pregnancy-induced hypertension (PIH) BP >140/90mmHg
- Pre-eclampsia PIH with proteinuria (>0.3g/24h), ≥20/40 gestation
- Eclampsia seizures in a patient with pre-eclampsia

Risk factors <20yr or >35yr, first pregnancy, multiple pregnancies, BMI >34, ↑BP, DM, previous of family pre-eclampsia
Symptoms usually asymptomatic, headache, vomiting, visual disturbance
Signs RUQ tenderness, oedema, papilloedema, hyperreflexia, clonus
Investigations ***urine*** M,C+S, 24h collection; ***blds*** FBC, U+E, urate, LFT, clotting, G+S
Assess the fetus USS (fetal growth, size, presentation, liquor volume, fetal movements), umbilical artery Doppler, CTG
Management refer to antenatal medical clinic for monitoring ±antihypertensive therapy, if severe admit ±treat as for eclampsia below

HELLP (Haemolysis, Elevated Liver enzymes , Low Platelets)

A variant of pre-eclampsia.
Symptoms upper abdominal pain, headache, malaise, vomiting
Signs RUQ tenderness, oedema, ↑BP
Results ↓Hb, ↑bilirubin, ↑ALT, ↓plts
Management resuscitate, FFP/plts/blood transfusion, urgent delivery
Complications DIC, haemorrhage (brain, liver), eclampsia

Eclampsia

Seizures or pre-eclampsia with ↑reflexes or clonus.
Crash call obstetrician and anaesthetist, move into left lateral position
Airway manoeuvres/adjuncts
Breathing 15l/min O_2
Circulation check BP, IV access (FBC, U+E, LFT, clotting, G+S)
Disability check glucose, 4g $MgSO_4$ IV/IM over 20min then at maintenance dose of 2g/h IV; if diastolic >105mmHg give hydralazine or labetalol IV (p201)
Urgent delivery use oxytocin instead of Syntometrine® for third stage
After delivery treat BP >160/110mmHg (p201), strict fluid balance, monitor FBC, U+E, LFT, observe for ≥5d, medical review

Anaemia in pregnancy

Screening FBC is checked at 12, 28 and 36wk, treat if Hb <11g/dl
Treatment ferrous sulphate 200mg/24h PO and folic acid 0.4mg/24h PO

Gestational diabetes mellitus

Fasting glucose >7.0mmol/l, GTT glucose of ≥7.8mmol/l at 2h.
Screening GTT offered at 28wk if: previous gestational DM, large baby, polyhydramnios, BMI >27, 1st degree relative with DM, previous stillbirth
Symptoms often asymptomatic, glucose on urine dipstick
Signs large for dates, polyhydramnios
Investigations if persistent glycosuria then check fasting glucose, oral glucose tolerance test (GTT p277) if >5.5mmol/l; regular USS to assess fetal growth
Treatment diet changes, exercise, 15% require insulin, oral hypoglycaemics contraindicated in pregnancy, stop insulin after birth and repeat GTT (p277) in 6wk
Complications large babies, congenital abnormalities, stillbirths, pre-eclampsia, polyhydramnios, malpresentation, cord prolapse

Antepartum haemorrhage

Vaginal bleeding after 24/40 gestation.
Causes placenta praevia, placental abruption, gynae causes see p432
Severe bleeding call help, 15l/min O_2, elevate legs, large bore IV access x 2 (take blood for FBC, clotting, G+S), give 0.9% saline until able to give blood (O –ve blood or crossmatched), urgent delivery
Mild bleeding admit, IV access (FBC, clotting, G+S), monitor HR and BP, vaginal examination only if placental site known, USS, consider anti-D

Breech presentation

Should be noted from antenatal examination and scans. External cephalic version can be attempted at 37/40 gestation (Rhesus –ve mothers will need anti-D p436). Elective Caesarean section is often performed.

Gestation >41/40

The risk of stillbirth increases after 42/40 gestation. If the baby has not been delivered by 41/40 then the mother is seen in antenatal clinic to discuss induction. Induction methods include:

- Prostaglandin vaginal gel to 'ripen' the cervix
- Artificial rupture of membranes (AROM, amniotomy)
- Oxytocin infusion

Delivery

See p594 for the procedure for normal vaginal delivery

Prematurity

Birth between before 37/40 gestation can have serious effects on the baby's survival and risk of disability, especially <32/40. The key components of management include: informing neonate/paediatric dept giving two doses of steroids (beclometasone 12mg/12h IM) if 24–34/40, considering tocolysis, considering transfer to a hospital with neonatal intensive care.

Premature rupture of membranes (PROM)

Delivery should occur within 24h of the membranes rupturing to reduce the risk of maternal/fetal infection. If labour does not start spontaneously the delivery may be induced; monitor maternal temp. If gestation is <37/40 then antibiotics may be given instead of induction.

Fetal monitoring

- *Doppler probe* listen for decelerations at the end of a contraction
- *CTG* see box for interpretation
- *Fetal blood* samples can be taken to check for acidosis (representing hypoxia) the normal value is pH >7.25

If there is fetal distress (worrying CTG, abnormal fetal blood sample) call a senior immediately; the baby may need to be delivered urgently.

Reading the Cardiotocograph (CTG)

CTGs measure fetal HR and uterine tone (contractions). They are usually printed with a scale of 1cm/min. There are four features to note:

- **Baseline** fetal HR (should be 110–160bpm)
- **Variability** (spikes and dips, should be ≥5bpm)
- **Acceleration** (transient increase in HR of >15bpm for >15s)
- **Decelerations** (transient decrease in HR of >15bpm for >15s)

There are three types of deceleration:

- **Early** occur with contractions; the lowest HR is when uterine tone is highest – physiological (compression of the fetal head)
- **Late** occur after the contraction; the lowest fetal HR is 20–30s after the maximal uterine tone – pathological (fetal hypoxia)
- **Variable** the relation to uterine tone and the degree of deceleration vary between contractions – pathological (compression of the cord)

Worrying features baseline outside of normal, reduced variability, early decelerations of >40bpm, late decelerations, persistent variable decelerations, prolonged decelerations

Difficult deliveries

Failure to progress if the baby is not coming out get senior help and consider: maternal position, maternal technique, episiotomy, instrumental delivery (forceps/ventouse), emergency LSCS

Shoulder dystocia 'HELPERR': call **H**elp, **E**pisiotomy, hyperextend the mother's **L**egs onto the abdomen, suprapubic **P**ressure, **E**nter (turn the shoulder with fingers), **R**emove the posterior arm, **R**oll onto all fours

After delivery (post-partum)

Post-partum haemorrhage

Loss of >500ml blood during the first 24h after delivery.

Causes failure of uterus to contract, tears, retained placenta, clotting disorders

Severe bleeding call help, 15l/min O_2, large-bore IV access x 2 (take blood for FBC, U+E, clotting, G+S), give Gelofusine® until able to give blood (O–ve blood or crossmatched), compress the uterus bimanually, give Syntocinon® 10units/h in 500ml 0.9% saline, deliver/check placenta, remove any retained placental tissue and repair tears, may need evacuation under anaesthetic or emergency hysterectomy

Mild bleeding IV access (FBC, clotting, G+S), 0.9% saline, monitor HR and BP, vaginal examination

Pyrexia

Causes endometritis, wound infection, mastitis, UTI, URTI, DVT

Ask about mode of delivery, premature ruptured membranes, pyrexia in labour, pain, cough/SOB, PV bleeding/discharge, dysuria, breast pain

Look for abdo/loin tenderness; ***PV*** uterine/adnexal tenderness, lochia (period-like discharge), breast tenderness, leg swelling

Investigations urine M,C+S; ***blds*** FBC, CRP, G+S, bld cultures; ***culture*** high vaginal swab, sputum, wound swab

Management according to the cause:

- *Wound infection* of tear, episiotomy, flucloxacillin 250–500mg/6h PO, metronidazole 400mg/8h PO
- *Endometritis* tender uterus, offensive lochia (vaginal discharge), treat with cefuroxime 750mg/8h IV, metronidazole 500mg/8h IV
- *Mastitis* tender, red breast, flucloxacillin 250mg/6h PO, continue breast. feeding (to prevent milk stagnation), ibuprofen

Breast problems

Cracked nipples nipple shields or Kamillosan® cream

Mastitis flucloxacillin 250mg/6h PO, continue breast-feeding, ibuprofen

Breast abscess refer to surgical team for incision and drainage

Psychiatric problems

- ***Baby blues*** many women feel 'down' 1–10d after delivery; it rarely requires specific treatment.
- ***Postnatal depression*** affects 10–15% of women 6–16wk after delivery; may necessitate antidepressants, counselling or psychiatric referral
- ***Puerperal psychosis*** affects 0.2% of women 3–7d after delivery; presents with acute psychosis (p308); refer to psychiatry

Prescribing in breast-feeding

Check *BNF* Appendix 5

- ***Safe drugs*** warfarin, aminoglycosides, NSAIDs, penicillins, cephalosporins, antihypertensive drugs, salbutamol, anticonvulsants
- ***Drugs to avoid*** benzodiazepines, barbiturates, amiodarone, COC, cytotoxics, aspirin

Chapter 10
Specialities

Anaesthetics

Role The anaesthetist has many roles: providing anaesthesia and analgesia for surgical procedures and obstetrics, caring for patients on ITU and in other high-dependency areas, part of the trauma, cardiac- and paediatric-arrest teams, inpatient and outpatient pain management and in the teaching of medical and nursing staff.

Anaesthetic history

Alongside taking a standard history (p98) the following are important:

Previous anaesthetics ask about previous general or local anaesthetics and any problems the patient was aware of such as post-operative N+V (PONV). Check the notes for previous anaesthetic records.

Past medical history asthma/COPD, IHD, DM, rheumatoid arthritis; are these well controlled?

Indigestion/reflux are they being treated for this or do they suffer with acid regurgitation or reflux after meals or lying flat?

General health exercise tolerance; can they climb a flight of stairs?

Current health do they have a cold or a chest infection?

Drug history anticoagulants, antiplatelet agents, cardiac medications

Allergy document allergies and reaction encountered

Family history have other family members had problems with either general or local anaesthetics?

Social history smoking, alcohol and recreational drugs

Teeth document site of caps, crowns, false or loose teeth (p493)

Fasting status when was their last meal and last drink, see p445

Consent see p69

ASA classification (American Society of Anesthesiologists)

ASA 1	Healthy, no comorbidities
ASA 2	Mild systemic disease, but with no limitation on activity eg hypertension, stable asthma
ASA 3	Severe systemic disease that limits activity; not incapacitating eg exertional angina, mild COPD
ASA 4	Incapacitating systemic disease which poses a threat to life eg unstable angina, severe pneumonia
ASA 5	Moribund. Not expected to survive 24h even with operation.
ASA 6	Brain-dead patient whose organs are being removed for donor purposes

Anaesthetic examination

All patients should have a CVS and RS examination before going to theatre (p100). Identification of heart failure, murmurs, wheeze, pleural effusions, pneumothorax or focal chest infections pre-operatively can allow treatment to be commenced or alternative anaesthetic techniques to be used.

Airway assessment reduced mouth opening, a short and fat neck, limited neck movement, prominent upper teeth, limited protrusion of the mandible and a small chin (micrognathia) are indicators that airway maintenance and intubation may be difficult.

Weight and BMI assessment documenting a child's weight is important as most anaesthetic drugs are given on a dose/kg basis. In adults, a ↑BMI is associated with potential difficulties with the airway and with patient positioning and theatre equipment.

Pre-operative investigations

Most hospitals will have specific guidelines which usually follow the 2003 NICE guidelines (www.guidance.nice.org.uk/cg3/guidance/pdf/English) Common tests and indications are shown below:

- ***FBC*** age >60yr, anaemia suspected or transfusion anticipated
- ***Sickle-cell trait*** African, Caribbean, Middle Eastern or Mediterranean
- ***Group and save/crossmatch*** depends on type of surgery, see p128
- ***U+E*** age >60yr, DM or other chronic disease, diuretic therapy
- ***Clotting*** anticoagulation therapy, liver disease or bleeding tendency
- ***ECG*** age >60yr, suspected or known IHD, DM, obesity
- ***Echocardiogram*** history suggests cardiac failure, new murmur
- ***CXR*** unexplained breathlessness or abnormal physical findings
- ***Respiratory function tests*** severe asthma, severe COPD/emphysema

Fasting times

Oral ingestion of clear fluids should be encouraged up to 2h before theatre. Clear fluids are those **without** particular matter and in some trusts this includes tea or coffee with a small amount of semi-skimmed milk; **check your local guidelines.** Tablets should be taken as normal[1].

Adults	2h pre-op	Nil by mouth[1]
	2–6h pre-op	Clear fluids
	>6h pre-op	Solids (food, drinks with particulate matter)
Babies and children	2h pre-op	Nil by mouth[1]
	2–4h pre-op	Clear fluids
	4–6h pre-op	Breast milk
	>6h pre-op	Formula milk/solids

[1] Tablets can be taken with a sip of water, even if 0–2h before theatre.

Anaesthetic referrals

Checklist

Name, hospital number, age, gender, location, relevant comorbidity/ current health

Planned operation, urgency, operating surgeon/consultant

Fasting status, bloods, ECG, if a crossmatch/G+S has been done

If post-op: surgery undertaken, pain relief given, fluid balance

Referrals for cases to be added to emergency lists are usually made to the on-call anaesthetist. To discuss an elective case, identify from the anaesthetic office who will be anaesthetising that list and speak to them directly or, if they are unavailable, speak to the on-call anaesthetist.

- *Add case to emergency list* most non-elective cases will need to be reviewed on the ward by an anaesthetist prior to theatre
- *Ward review* if the patient has post-operative pain, there is a problem with an epidural or PCA or if there is an airway problem
- *Discuss an elective patient* if a patient seen in pre-assessment has a complex medical/drug history that could interfere with the anaesthetic or post-operative recovery period (see p128)
- *Central lines* if the patient needs central venous access and your team, including the consultant, is unable to perform this, the patient may be added to the emergency list for the line to be sited in theatre

Urgency of surgery

The National Confidential Enquiry into Perioperative Deaths (NCEPOD) have devised a system which encourages the need for surgery to be categorised according to urgency. Various modifications of this are used, but the original categories are as follows:

CEPOD 1 Immediate life-, limb- or organ-saving intervention – resuscitation simultaneous with intervention. Normally within **minutes** of decision to operate, eg ruptured AAA.

CEPOD 2 Acute onset or deterioration of conditions that threaten life, limb or organ survival; fixation of fractures; relief of distressing symptoms. Normally within **hours** of decision to operate, eg laparotomy for perforation, debridement plus fixation of fracture.

CEPOD 3 Stable patient requiring early intervention for a condition that is not an immediate threat to life, limb or organ survival. Normally within **days** of decision to operate, eg repair of tendon and nerve injuries.

CEPOD 4 Surgical procedure planned or booked in advance of routine admission to hospital. Planned surgery, eg varicose vein surgery, joint replacement, elective AAA repair.

Anaesthetics as an F1/F2

This is becoming a more common FP job in both the F1 and F2 years. Anaesthetic problems are also encountered in EDs and on the wards.

Structure anaesthetics has four main components:

- ***Anaesthesia*** providing anaesthesia for surgical procedures
- ***Pain*** acute and chronic pain management
- ***Intensive care*** traditionally this was run by anaesthetists, but intensive care is now a speciality in its own right (p452)
- ***Resuscitation*** in trauma, cardiac and paediatric emergency calls

The job you will be expected to perform the following roles:

- Pre-operatively assess patients for theatre
- Learn to give a general anaesthetic and a spinal anaesthetic
- Manage acute pain issues in theatre recovery and on the wards
- Carry the crash bleep for adult cardiac arrests

Aims try to do the following during your placement:

- Become familiar with assessing patients for theatre
- Learn to plan an anaesthetic in advance; have plans B and C in reserve
- Become confident in giving a general and spinal anaesthetic
- Become more confident with cannulation (p558)
- Learn how to site central venous (p574) and arterial lines
- Learn how to manage acute severe pain safely (p428)
- Learn/practise emergency airway management during arrests (p162)

Common cases

Acute appendicitis (p239) usually young adults who have no other comorbidity but usually require a rapid sequence intubation (RSI) as gastric emptying is likely to be delayed which poses a risk of aspiration

Evacuation of retained products following miscarriage (p437) usually fit, young, fasted women who can often be managed on a facemask

Emergency laparotomy often an older patient with coexisting disease and an acute abdomen. Will require senior anaesthetic support, likely invasive BP monitoring ±central venous access, and careful post-operative care/monitoring (often ITU/HDU).

Varicose vein surgery often a day case procedure. Can be undertaken under a spinal anaesthetic or general anaesthetic. Sometimes patient needs to go prone if short saphenous vein is to be stripped.

Post-operative problems following surgery (p138) pain and N+V are the commonest problems in the recovery room and also on the ward. Careful assessment is needed and treating symptoms with several agents may be effective, but increases the risk of drug complications.

Training

Initial route CT1 in anaesthetics or CT1 in Acute Care Common Stem (ACCS) though this second route takes an extra year (p28)

Further training competitive application for ST3 anaesthetics

Exams Primary FRCA required for ST3; Final FRCA to progress to ST5

Breast surgery

Role Breast surgeons look after patients with breast cancer but can also specialise in cosmetic or reconstructive surgery. Dealing mostly with cancer patients can be a difficult job and the speciality relies heavily on associated specialists such as breast care nurses both for practical and psychological support for patients.

Breast surgery history

Alongside taking a standard history (p98), when clerking patients with breast disease the following areas must be covered:

Lump size, duration, mobility, pain, nipple discharge/bleeding/inversion, skin changes, previous breast lumps

Past obs/gynae history parity, age of first pregnancy, breast-feeding, menarche, menopause

Past medical history DM, asthma, ↑BP, IHD, clotting problems, liver disease, anaemia, previous malignancy, epilepsy

FH breast cancer, gynae cancer

DH HRT, COC

Breast surgery examination

Examine both breasts (normal side first): ***inspection*** asymmetry, scars, skin changes, nipple discharge/inversion, skin tethering, erythema, oedema; ***palpation*** ask the patient to show you where the lump is, palpate all four quadrants (see below), axillary tail, assess any palpable masses; ***lymphadenopathy*** axilla, cervical, supraclavicular; ***other*** liver, spine

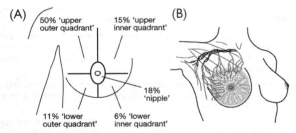

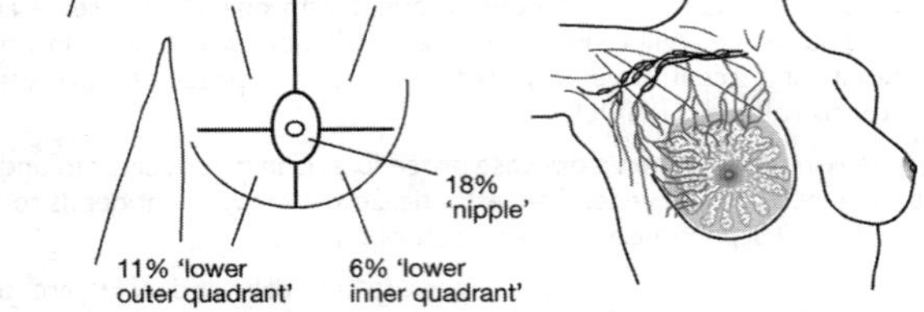

(A) Quadrants of the breast showing proportion of breast cancer by location.
(B) Glands and lymphatics of the right breast.

Breast surgery referrals

Checklist

Name, hospital number, age, gender, location

Breast pain, breast lumps, changes with menstrual cycles, family history

Examination findings (lumps, mobility, skin changes, nipple changes, lymph nodes)

What the patient has been told about their diagnosis

Referrals are usually made to the breast surgery registrar on-call. Try to give an impression of the urgency of the problem and which of the following would be appropriate:

- *Ward review* if the patient has a breast problem which requires review but is immobile or bed-bound
- *Urgent clinic review* if the patient is stable and mobile but with a condition requiring urgent review (eg suspected breast cancer), they could be seen in clinic
- *Routine outpatient clinic* if the patient is stable and has a non-urgent breast problem

Breast surgery as an F1/F2

Breast surgery may be part of F1 general surgery or a specialist attachment. The job is often combined with another surgical speciality eg managing both breast surgery and general surgery patients. If you have any free time you can attend clinics and theatre.

The job you will be expected to perform the following roles:

- Assess patients pre-operatively
- Assist in theatre
- Perform daily ward round and completing ensuing jobs
- Manage post-op problems (p138)
- Attend outpatient clinics

Aims try to do the following during your placement:

- Develop history and examination skills for breast surgery patients
- Learn the different surgical options of how to manage breast cancer and spend time in theatre assisting with procedures
- Learn basic surgical skills including suturing (p600)
- Spend time in outpatient clinics
- Spend time with breast care specialist nurses

Training

Initial route CT1 in 'surgery in general' general surgery (p28)

Further training competitive application for ST3 general surgery then subspecialise during training; a separate breast surgery ST3 may develop

Exams MRCS required to apply for ST3 general surgery

Cardiology

Cardiology history

Alongside taking a standard history (p98) the following are important:

Major symptoms chest pain or heaviness, dyspnoea (exertional, orthopnoea, paroxysmal nocturnal), ankle swelling, palpitations, syncope, intermittent claudication, fatigue

Past medical history rheumatic fever, recent dental work, thyroid disease, cardiac surgery, previous palpitations/pain

Drug history cardiac medications (and compliance), allergies

Social history tobacco, alcohol and caffeine consumption, occupation, exercise tolerance on the flat and ability to climb stairs

Family history IHD, ↑lipids, cardiomyopathy, congenital heart disease

Coronary artery disease risk factors previous IHD, smoking, ↑BP, ↑lipids, family history of IHD, DM, obesity and physical inactivity, male sex

Functional status of established heart disease

Class I – disease present but no symptoms during ordinary activity
Class II – angina or dyspnoea during ordinary activity
Class III – angina or dyspnoea during minimal activity
Class IV – angina or dyspnoea at rest

Cardiology examination

Lying at 45°

General inspection Marfan's, Turner's, Down's syndromes, rheumatological disorders, acromegaly, dyspnoea at rest, cyanosis

Hands radial pulses (right and left, collapsing pulse), clubbing, splinter haemorrhages, Osler's nodes, peripheral cyanosis, xanthomata

Face eyes (pallor, jaundice, xanthelasma), malar flush, mouth (cyanosis, high arched palate, dentition)

Neck JVP, carotids (pulse character)

Precordium inspection (scars, deformity, apex beat), palpate (apex beat, thrills, heave), auscultate (heart sounds, murmurs (also auscultate with the patient in both left lateral and sitting forward positions))

Back scars, sacral oedema, pleural effusions, pulmonary oedema

Abdomen palpate liver, spleen, aorta, ballot kidneys, percuss for ascites, femoral and renal artery bruits, radiofemoral delay

Legs peripheral pulses, cold limbs, ulceration, oedema, calf tenderness, pigmentation

Blood pressure left and right arms, lying and standing

Other urine analysis, fundoscopy, temperature chart

Cardiology referrals

Checklist

Name, hospital number, age, gender, location

Presenting complaint, cardiac risk factors (opposite)

Initial clinical findings, observations, ECG and management

Subsequent events and response to treatment; cardiac markers if appropriate

Latest clinical findings and ECG/exercise ECG/echo/angiogram results

Cardiology referrals are usually made to the cardiology registrar on-call; for new patients (ED or acute admissions) the general medical team is usually the first port of call:

- ***Request cardiology review*** some inpatients may be initially cared for by a non-cardiology team (endocrine, general surgery etc) but have a new cardiac problem or a longstanding history of cardiac disease for which discussion with a cardiologist is necessary. This is often prior to surgery or before discharge, regarding follow-up and investigations.
- ***Request echocardiogram/24h ECG*** urgent out-of-hours echocardiograms must be discussed with a cardiologist; in some hospitals requesting echos and 24h ECGs at any time requires cardiologist approval
- ***Urgent cardiology advice*** for complex, seriously ill, cardiology patients

Cardiology as an F1/F2

A cardiology placement may be part of general medicine as an F1 or as a specialist attachment. These patients can deteriorate extremely fast necessitating urgent life-saving treatment.

The job you will be expected to perform the following roles:

- Clerk new admissions and initiate treatment plans
- Perform daily ward round and ensuing jobs
- Provide medical cover for exercise tolerance testing
- Provide on-call cover for cardiology ±general medicine

Aims try to do the following during your placement:

- Become familiar with history and examination in cardiology patients
- Become confident at interpreting ECGs (p610)
- Learn about the acute and chronic treatment of heart failure (p226)
- Learn to manage acute chest pain (p176) and arrhythmias (p184/192)
- Observe echocardiography and learn to interpret the images
- Observe cardiac catheterisation and pacemaker placement
- Spend time in outpatient clinics

Training

Initial route CT1 in core medical training (p28)

Further training competitive application for ST3 cardiology

Exams MRCP part 1 required to apply for ST3 cardiology

Critical care (ITU/HDU)

Critical care is the term generally used to refer to ITU and HDU.

Role Intensivists were traditionally anaesthetists, but this has now changed and individuals with medical, surgical and emergency medicine backgrounds are also running critical care areas. Critically ill patients who are presenting acutely to the hospital via ED or GP admissions, as well as inpatients who are deteriorating, form the basis of emergency admissions; the critical care team spend a significant amount of time assessing and managing these patients. Elective admissions are usually admitted from theatre post-operatively.

Critical care history

There is no standardised history for patients being admitted to critical care areas as the range of presentations is so vast (respiratory, obstetric, trauma, burns, paediatrics etc). A relevant, thorough history from the patient (if possible) or referring team should be obtained. The following are important aspects which should be clearly documented:

General health exercise tolerance (on flat, climbing stairs, ability to leave the house); independence with ADLs (eg fully self-caring, help getting dressed, eating etc)

Drug history usual medications; agents affecting coagulation (antiplatelets, warfarin), antihypertensives, agents for airway disease, agents which are potentially nephrotoxic (NSAIDs) and drugs affecting protein binding (antiepileptics, the OCP). It is essential to know if a patient takes regular oral steroids (p118).

Allergy document all allergies and note what reaction is encountered

Social history smoking, alcohol consumption and recreational drugs

Levels of critical illness	
Level 0	Patients whose needs can be met through normal ward care in an acute hospital
Level 1	Patients at risk of their condition deteriorating, or those recently relocated from higher levels of care, whose needs can be met on an acute ward with additional advice and support from the critical care team
Level 2	Patients requiring more detailed observations or interventions including support for a single failing organ system or post-operative care and those 'stepping down' from higher levels of care
Level 3	Patients requiring advanced respiratory support alone or basic respiratory support together with the support of at least two organs systems; this level includes all complex patients requiring support for multi-organ failure

Critical care examination

The assessment of an **unstable** critically ill patient should begin with a logical **A**irway, **B**reathing and **C**irculation approach, followed by a methodical and thorough systems-based examination.

Clinical assessment of a **stable** critical care patient is a continuous process throughout the day and night, though formal examination and documentation of this is undertaken at least once a day in most centres; below is one method for approaching this:

Airway Is the patient protecting their own airway or are they intubated or have a tracheostomy? How long have these been in place, do they need changing or will the patient cope without them? Are there problems with the airway which need addressing (moving ETT, cuff leak)?

Breathing Is the patient breathing unaided or are they requiring ventilatory support (note mode of ventilation)? Has the level of support or inspired O_2 requirement altered since the last review? How do the latest set of blood gases compare to previous results? Are there any new clinical chest signs or change in secretions/chest drain activity? When was the last CXR or other imaging undertaken; is another required?

Circulation HR, BP, CVP, ECG. Does the patient feel warm and vasodilated or cool and shut down? Are there new clinical signs (murmurs, splinter haemorrhages, oedema)? What are the other haemodynamic parameters (cardiac output, wedge pressure); if not already being measured should these be? Has the need for inotropes or vasopressors changed since the last review? What is the urine output and overall fluid balance? Is the patient getting DVT prophylaxis?

Disability What is the patient's GCS or their degree of consciousness if being pharmacologically sedated? What sedating agents are being used, has there been a sedation holiday? Are there any new abnormal neurological signs (limbs, pupils, seizure activity)? Has there been a change in ICP or volume draining from EVD if present?

Everything else

- Fluid balance, choice of fluids, renal function (U+E), renal support
- Gut and nutrition, ulcer protection, absorbing feed, constipation prevention, position of feeding tubes, need for TPN, trace elements
- Lines, when put in, infection at site, are they still necessary?
- Microbiology, temperature, WCC, latest results, antibiotics, antibiotic plasma levels, side-effects
- Other teams, input from other teams and allied healthcare workers
- Results, blood, urine, stool, CSF, radiology, ECG
- Skin, pressure areas

Critical care referrals

Checklist

Name, hospital number, age, gender, location

Presenting complaint, clinical findings, observations, relevant investigation results

Presumed diagnosis, management commenced, response to treatment

Pre-morbid health, exercise tolerance, reversibility of condition

Referrals to the critical care team usually involve patients with one or more organ systems failure. Acute deterioration of a chronic process is commonly seen, as is acute presentation of critical illness in a previously healthy individual. Elective admission from theatre is the other common route of referral.

Acute on chronic deterioration it is not uncommon for chronic disease processes to fluctuate, and acute deteriorations can be life-threatening and require organ support (eg asthma, DM, epilepsy etc). It is important to recognise the difference between acute reversible deterioration and irreversible progression of a disease process.

Previously healthy patients most of these patients present via the ED, and the commoner causes are polytrauma (RTAs), burns and infectious diseases (meningitis, septicaemia etc)

Elective admissions patients undergoing major surgery (usually major neuro, thoracic or abdominal surgery), or patients who have significant comorbidity (such as obstructive sleep apnoea) and require surgery may be considered for a critical care bed for immediate postoperative recovery to allow closer monitoring and earlier detection of post-operative complications

Critical care transfers

Movement of any patient from a critical care area (including resus) constitutes a patient transfer; this includes taking a patient to theatre, to the radiology department, to other ward areas or between hospitals. The potential for problems to arise during any transfer is great, even when there has been adequate preparation of staff and equipment.

The risks of **every** transfer should be assessed by a senior member of the team on an individual basis, and from that the skill mix and seniority of the transfer team should be decided.

For patients who are intubated at least one member of the transfer team should be airway-trained and be capable of re-intubating the patient should the original airway become dislodged or fail in another way.

Critical care as an F1/F2

This is a specialist FP job available in both the F1 and F2 years. Critically ill patients are encountered in all aspects of medicine, so this will give you valuable skills for later in your career.

Structure

- *ITU* the hub of critical care with the most unwell patients; many patients have multiple organ failure and require continuous assessment and changes to their management
- *HDU* usually level 1 or level 2 patients (p452), may physically be part of ITU or another ward within the hospital. Surgical and medical HDU may be in different locations and cater for different critical illnesses.
- *Outreach* critical care nurses who support ward nursing staff with problem patients to prevent patients from deteriorating and identify the sickest patients who need critical care beds
- *Resuscitation* critical care nurses and doctors form a crucial part of the resuscitation team

The job you will be expected to perform the following roles:

- Participate in critical care ward rounds
- Assess acute critical care referrals, under supervision
- Admit patients to critical care areas
- Site invasive monitoring lines (arterial, central venous etc)
- Carry the crash bleep for adult cardiac arrests

Aims try to do the following during your placement:

- Learn how to recognise the critically ill patient
- Learn how to manage critically ill patients
- Learn how to site central venous and arterial lines
- Learn/practise emergency airway management during cardiac arrests

Common cases

Polytrauma (p168) Often otherwise healthy patients who have multiple fractures and soft tissue injury, including lung contusion. May need several trips to theatre. Development of ARDS (p227) is common.

Exacerbation of asthma (p223) Often young, brittle asthmatics. Severe bronchospasm can be very difficult to treat and intubation does not cure bronchospasm; ventilation of bronchospastic lungs is difficult and barotrauma and pneumothoracies in these patients are common.

Post-elective AAA repair after major surgery these patients are slowly warmed up; electrolyte and acid/base disturbance needs correcting prior to extubation, maximising the patient's potential for recovery

Training

Initial route critical care does not have a single clear point of entry; you need to finish core training in anaesthetics, ACCS, medicine or surgery

Further training after core training you need to secure a run-through post in one of these specialities; training in critical care should be possible within these posts, but check before you commit to run-through training

Exams membership exams will be required to start run-through training

Dermatology

Role Dermatology is largely an outpatient speciality, though some patients do require admission to either general wards or dedicated dermatology wards. Identification of new skin lesions and rashes, management of established dermatological disease and minor surgical procedures forms the bulk of the dermatologist's workload. Unlike most other medical specialities, dermatology remains largely a clinical one, with little reliance on imaging or laboratory investigation.

Dermatology history

Alongside taking a standard history (p98) the following are important:

Presenting skin complaint timing how long present for, sudden or gradual onset, getting better or worse; ***location*** original site and subsequent sites affected; ***symptoms*** itch (localised or generalised), pain, burning, bleeding, weeping; ***exacerbating factors*** dietary components, drugs, sunlight (seasonal variability), pet dander, night-time, water; ***relieving factors*** emollient cream, topical steroids

Past skin history previous skin disease(s), sensitivity of skin to sun exposure, lifelong history of sun exposure, measures taken to prevent sunburn (eg suncream), use of sun beds

Current health anorexia, diarrhoea, fever, headache, fatigue, weight loss, depression, sore throat, joint pain

Past medical history DM, sarcoid, IBD, porphyria, SLE, malignancy, endocrine disease, asthma/atopy

Drug history dermatological agents being used at present and their effects, previous drugs used and their effects, other drugs being taken, drug allergies

Allergy hayfever, pet dander, dust mite etc

Occupational history current and previous jobs and effect of work upon skin, exposure to chemicals; hobbies and recreational activities

Family history anyone else in the family affected; need to differentiate inherited pathology versus infectious pathology

Travel history recent foreign travel and relationship of any travel to skin disease – vaccinations/prophylaxis taken for foreign travel

Changes to pigmented lesion changes to size, shape, colour, outline, surface (raised, rough); new symptoms (eg bleeding, itching), family history of multiple pigmented lesions or skin cancers

Dermatology examination

After a thorough history, it will often be clear what the possible diagnoses are likely to be. Some dermatological conditions have a typical distribution or classical appearance and this can aid in making a quick diagnosis. The whole body should be examined in good natural light; patients complaining of a rash on their arm may well have other tell-tale signs elsewhere on the body. Examination of hair and nails is also often useful as these are commonly involved in many conditions.

Distribution solitary lesion, flexor aspects of limbs/trunk, extensor aspects of limbs/trunk, scalp/eyebrows/gutters of nose, sun-exposed sites, tip of nose, helix of ear, in webspaces of hands or feet, periumbilical

Morphology noting or describing the appearance of the rash using the terms on p458 refines the list of differential diagnoses

Hair alopecia (hair loss) may be generalised or localised, hirsuitism (hair in the distribution typically seen in the male), hypertrichosis (excessive hair growth)

Nails pitting, ridging, onycholysis, nail loss, thinning of nail plate, yellow nail syndrome

Dermatology referrals

Checklist

Name, hospital number, age, gender, location, mobility of patient

Presenting complaint, working diagnosis, infection, foreign travel, allergens

Previous dermatological problems including treatments

Description of rash (see definitions on next page)

Inpatient referrals are usually made to the dermatology registrar on-call. Dermatologists spend a lot of time in clinics and are often keen for the patients to be transferred to clinic rather than coming to the ward. Think about the patient's mobility and what action you require:

- *Inpatient review* dermatology review may be required for two reasons: (1) a new rash that complicates the patient's management either as part of their underlying diagnosis or as a result of treatment eg drug rash (2) pre-existing skin disease that requires treatment eg eczema or psoriasis
- *Urgent clinic review* incidental finding of unusual moles (p456) or ulcers requires a two-week clinic review to exclude skin cancer
- *Outpatient review* for incidental findings of rashes that do not need urgent diagnosis or management

Dermatology definitions

Non-palpable	
Ecchymosis	Bruising; discolouration from blood leaking into the skin
Macule	Flat well-defined area of altered skin pigmentation
Petechia	Non-blanching pinpoint-sized purple macule
Purpura	Purple lesion resulting from free red blood cells in the skin non-blanching
Telangiectasia	Abnormal visible dilatation of blood vessels (spider naevi)

Palpable	
Nodule	Solid, mostly subcutaneous lesion (>0.5cm diameter)
Papule	Raised well-defined lesion (<0.5cm diameter)
Plaque	Raised flat-topped lesion, usually >2cm diameter
Weal	Transient raised lesion with pink margin
Urticaria	Weals with pale centres and well-defined pink margins

Blisters	
Abscess	Fluctuant swelling containing pus beneath the epidermis
Bulla	Fluid-filled blister larger than a vesicle (>0.5cm diameter)
Pustule	Well-defined pus-filled lesion
Vesicle	Fluid-filled blister (<0.5cm diameter)

Skin defects	
Excoriation	Linear break in the skin surface (a scratch)
Atrophy	Thinning and loss of skin substance
Crust	Dried brownish/yellow exudates
Erosion	Superficial break in the continuity of the epidermis
Abrasion	Scraping off superficial layers of the skin (a graze)
Fissure	Crack, often through keratin
Incisional wound	Break to the skin by sharp object
Laceration	Break to the skin caused by blunt trauma/tearing injury
Lichenification	Skin thickening with exaggerated skin markings
Scale	Fragment of dry skin
Ulcer	Loss of epidermis and dermis resulting in scar

Dermatology as an F1/F2

Dermatology may be part of general medicine as an F1 or a specialist attachment. Sometimes this role is paired with another medical speciality such as rheumatology.

Structure dermatology has three main components:

- *Outpatients* the vast majority of the patients under the care of a dermatologist will be in the community and seen regularly in clinic
- *Inpatients* if a patient's disease flares up and they are unable to cope at home or need intensive treatment, admission may be necessary
- *Surgery* most dermatologists spend at least half a day a week performing minor surgical procedures

The job you will be expected to perform the following roles:

- Manage inpatients (investigations, referrals, prescriptions etc)
- Assist in outpatient clinics
- Take and review referrals from other teams, under supervision
- Attend and participate in minor surgical procedures, under supervision
- Contribute at meetings and to the educational programme

Aims try to do the following during your placement:

- Learn to manage a ward of inpatients and their care
- Refine clerking skills and knowledge of skin diseases
- Participate in outpatient clinics
- Acquire minor surgical skills and the use of local anaesthetics
- Contribute to departmental audit or research

Common cases and treatments

Mole that has changed appearance (p456) this is a common referral from GPs to the dermatologist in clinic. By taking a note of the symptoms the patient describes and by examining the mole closely most experienced dermatologists will be able to assess the risk of the mole being malignant and surgically remove it if appropriate.

Basal cell carcinoma (p385) this is another common referral from GPs, especially in the elderly population. Most are excised surgically or treated with cryotherapy.

Cryotherapy liquid nitrogen is sprayed in a fine jet at a small area of skin. Freezing of the superficial layers of the skin results in cell lysis and eventual necrosis of the area. Used to treat warts, moles, skin tags and solar keratoses. Also used by some GPs.

Eczema and psoriasis (p369) these two diseases occupy much of the dermatologists time and pose difficulties in therapeutic management. They often cause considerable emotional and psychological upset to the patient.

Training

Initial route CT1 in core medical training

Further training competitive application for ST3 dermatology

Exams MRCP part 1 required to apply for ST3 dermatology

Ear, nose and throat (ENT)

Role ENT is a separate surgical speciality which covers a wide range of common conditions seen in the ED and by the GP.

ENT history

As well as a good general history, specific symptoms to note include:

- *Ears* pain, blocked ears, wax, discharge, tinnitus, deafness, unilateral/bilateral features, vertigo, trauma, itching, foreign bodies (FB), noise exposure, occupation
- *Nose* blocked nose, watery discharge, sneezing, itching, coughing, change in voice, altered sensation of smell/taste, external deformity/recent trauma, epistaxis, sinusitis; ask about daytime variation in symptom severity, pattern of obstruction, effects on speech and sleep
- *Throat* dysphagia, pain on swallowing, hoarseness, difficulty opening jaw (trismus), stridor, sleep apnoea/snoring; ask about neck lumps, vomiting, heartburn, waterbrash (acid regurgitation or filling or mouth with saliva)

ENT examination

- *Ears* ***inspect*** the pinna, auditory meatus, tenderness over pinna or mastoid; ***otoscopy*** examine all four quadrants of the eardrum (colour, bulging/retraction, perforation, exudate); ***test hearing*** (see below)
- *Nose* ***look*** for obvious scars, deviations/deformities, tilt the head back and look down each nostril; ***rhinoscopy*** (administer lidocaine spray first), look for polyps, inflamed turbinates, pus
- *Throat* ***inspect*** the lips, around and inside the mouth; ***examine*** the tongue and tonsils using a torch and tongue depressor, check palate movements by asking the patient to say 'ah'
- *Neck* ***look*** for swellings, asymmetry, scars; ***ask*** the patient to swallow, protrude the tongue; ***palpate*** the neck from behind and ask the patient to take a sip of water; ***feel*** for tracheal deviation, lymphadenopathy, tenderness; ***auscultate*** for a bruit; ***examine*** any lumps (see p374)

Hearing tests (*OHCS*7 p540)

- *Whisper* a different number into each ear, standing 30cm away whilst blocking the other ear. Ask the patient to repeat it in turn.
- *Tuning fork tests*
    - ***Rinne's test*** place the tuning fork on the patient's mastoid bone until it is no longer heard; then place the fork near the external auditory meatus where it is still heard in a normal ear, but not in an ear with conductive deafness
    - ***Weber's test*** place the tuning fork in the middle of the forehead and ask which side the sound is loudest; in nerve deafness the sound is loudest in the normal ear, in conductive deafness the sound is loudest in the abnormal ear

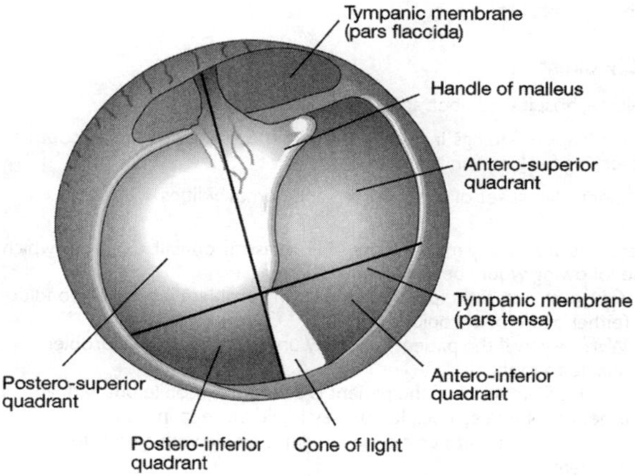

Structures and quadrants of the right tympanic membrane (eardrum) as seen on otoscopy

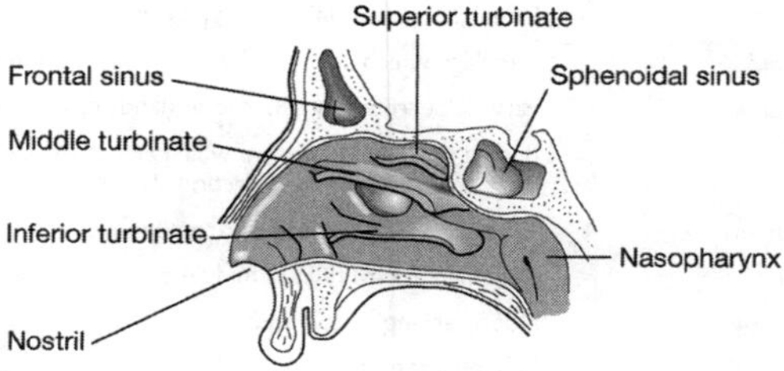

Anatomy of the nose

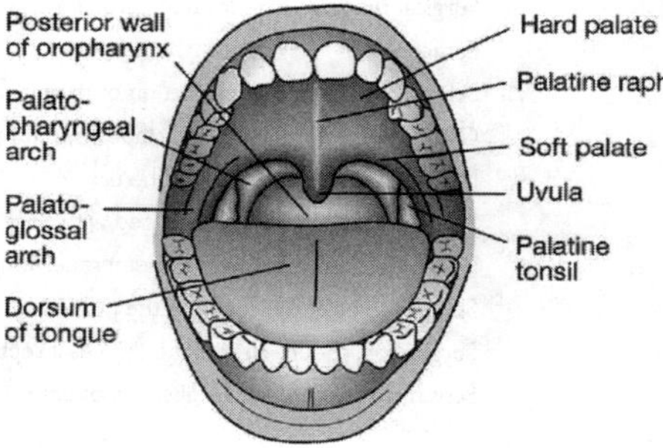

Mouth and oropharynx

ENT referrals

Checklist

Name, hospital number, age, gender, location

Examination findings including looking in the ear, nose and mouth and checking for lumps in the neck

Patient's latest set of observations and comorbidities

Referrals are usually made to the ENT registrar on-call. Consider which of the following would be most appropriate:

- *Take over care* if the patient's underlying problem is an ENT condition (either acute or chronic)
- *Ward review* if the patient is acutely unwell with an ENT problem or unable to mobilise
- *Urgent clinic review* if the patient is stable and mobile but with an urgent problem eg neck lump, they could be seen in clinic
- *Routine outpatient clinic* if the patient is stable with a non-urgent problem

ENT definitions

Adenoid	Lymphatic tissues in the nasopharynx
Arytenoid	Cartilage which support the vocal cords in the larynx
Cerumen	Earwax, secreted by sebaceous glands of ear canal
Cholesteatoma	Benign growth of eardrum which can cause local invasion and introduce infection into the CNS
Eustachian tube	Tube connecting middle ear to pharynx
Glue ear	Accumulation of fluid in middle ear causing deafness
Laryngomalacia	Floppy ary-epiglottic folds
Mastoiditis	Inflammation of the mastoid
Mastoid process	Bony prominence of the temporal bone behind ear
Myringoplasty	Surgical repair of a perforated eardrum
Otalgia	Earache
Otoplasty	Surgical repair or reconstruction of the pinna
Otosclerosis	Overgrowth of bone around stapes causing deafness
Pinna	Fleshy (cartilaginous) part of the ear
Presbyacusis	Sensorineural deafness associated with ↑age
Rhinitis	Inflammation of the mucous membranes of the nose
Rhinoplasty	Surgery to alter the shape of the nose
Septoplasty	Surgical procedure to reshape the nasal septum
Tinnitus	Sensation of sound in the absence of external stimulus
Tracheostomy	Surgical opening (hole) in the neck into the trachea

ENT as an F1/F2

ENT is usually an F2 specialist attachment though rarely may be part of general surgery as an F1. It is a varied job with medical and surgical components so you will meet a wide range of patients; often you will be covering the on-call general surgical rota too.

Structure ENT specialists work closely with the following:

- *Audiologist* assess hearing and balance, fit hearing aids
- *Audiovestibular medicine* doctors who deal with hearing and balance
- *Speech therapist* assess and treat defects in speech
- *Maxillofacial surgery* surgeons specialising in the face, teeth or jaw
- *Plastic surgery* experts at cosmetic repair

The job you will be expected to perform the following roles:

- Clerk new admissions and initiate treatment plans
- Perform daily ward round and job lists
- Pre-op assessment of patients (including children)
- Attend ENT clinics
- Assist in theatre
- Manage post-op complications

Aims try to do the following during your placement:

- Become familiar with history and examination in ENT patients
- Learn how to pack a nose post-operatively or following epistaxis
- Learn how to perform cautery (nasal and pharyngeal)
- Learn how to remove foreign bodies
- Learn to use a flexible endoscope to examine the pharynx
- Gain experience in simple surgical procedures eg grommet insertion

Common referrals/cases

Adenotonsillectomy this is a common operation usually performed on children with recurrent tonsillitis

Grommet insertion an operation used to treat glue ear (secretory otitis media) if the child is having difficulty with hearing or speech

Epistaxis (p357) this is a common problem, especially in elderly patients. Simple nosebleeds are treated in the ED but recurrent or severe bleeds may require nasal packing or cautery.

Foreign bodies a variety of interesting objects find their way into children's ears and noses; most of these are relatively simple to treat but inhaled objects require emergency endoscopic removal to prevent respiratory compromise and potentially death

Tumour excision this is the opposite extreme of ENT; tumours can require long and complicated operations for removal often with input from other surgical specialists (see structure above)

Training

Initial route CT1 in 'surgery in general' otolaryngology (p28)

Further training competitive application for ST3 otolaryngology

Exams completion of MRCS required for ST3 application

Emergency medicine (EM)

Starting in the emergency department (ED, formerly A+E) can be a daunting experience due to the wide variety of presentations (eg sick children, foreign bodies in eyes) and severity of illness (paper cuts to cardiac arrests). Like any speciality you should ask a senior if you are at all unsure; remember that in your F1 year you should not discharge any patients from the ED without a senior review.

Main areas in an emergency department

Triage ('sorting' in French) This is where experienced nurses take a full set of obs and assess how urgently patients need to be seen; relevant investigations may also be ordered (eg X-rays, bloods). Patients are often scored on a 1–5 scale with 1 being an emergency (eg cardiac arrest) and 5 being inappropriate attendance.

'See and treat' This is when a senior doctor (usually middle grade or consultant) sees minor injuries. Many can be treated and discharged at once without the need for investigations.

Minors or ambulatory This is where minor injuries and the 'walking wounded' go, it often includes minor head injuries, cuts, fractures and sprains. This area can be especially scary when you start since it is so different from the conditions seen in other departments. The term 'minor' can be a misnomer since the injuries can be significant (eg multiple rib fractures with pneumothorax) and medically 'minor' injuries can be highly disabling if treated badly, eg finger/hand injuries.

Majors or trolleys The medically unwell, seriously injured and those unable to walk tend to be seen in majors. These patients often require investigations and about 25% are admitted under specialist teams.

Resuscitation The sickest patients who need close monitoring and more individual nursing care are brought into 'resus'. Includes acute resuscitations and ambulance patients that have been phoned ahead.

Paediatrics Most departments have a separate children's area with paediatric medical equipment and a separate toy-filled waiting room.

Staff

Many ED nurses are able to do practical procedures including cannulas and taking bloods. Highly qualified nurses may be trained as Emergency Nurse Practitioners (ENPs) who see and treat patients with specific conditions (according to their training). They are often excellent at practical procedures (including suturing), very experienced and a good source of advice.

Four-hour target

Emergency departments are expected to discharge or admit 98% of patients within four hours of their arrival. While it is important not to let this target compromise your care, try to be efficient to avoid delays. Refer patients early if they clearly need admission regardless of investigation results and keep other staff informed of your management plan so that beds or transport can be arranged in advance.

Emergency medicine as an F1/F2

A common FP job in both the F1 and F2 years. Management of minor injuries is useful in all aspects of medicine, as is the skill of recognising the critically ill patient and initiating immediate resuscitation/treatment.

The job you will be expected to perform the following roles:
- See all groups of patients (minors, majors, paediatrics, resus patients)
- Diagnose and treat simple injuries and minor medical ailments
- Decide which patients should be admitted and which should be discharged, following discussion with a senior, as appropriate
- Be a part of the trauma team for major injuries

Aims try to become familiar with the following during your placement:
- Assessment and management of major trauma
- Assessment and management of minor trauma
- Identification, assessment and management of the critically ill
- Assessment and management of children
- Analgesic options in the emergency department
- Simple surgical skills (suturing, shoulder relocation, ring block etc)
- Taking a focused history and appropriate use of investigations

Five tips for emergency medicine

AMPLE history **A**llergies, **M**edicines, **P**ast history (medical, surgical, drugs), **L**ast meal, **E**vents or description of the injury. A useful approach in taking a history in all types of injury/trauma.

Minor injuries (p352) A good history alone allows the probable diagnosis to be established in many cases; examination either confirms or refutes this, demonstrates the severity of the injury and identifies any other injuries/problems.

Uncertainty It is not uncommon for patients to present with symptoms and signs which do not fit with any specific diagnosis. Ensure a senior has been consulted ±seen the patient, and do not be afraid to tell the patient you cannot give them a diagnosis, but reassure them that you haven't found anything worrying (as long as you haven't). Advise them to seek medical advice again (GP or ED) if things change or get worse.

Investigations X-rays are the commonest form of investigations undertaken in EDs. Document clearly the mechanism of injury, the clinical findings and your suspicion or the potential diagnoses – this will help the radiographer taking the image and the person formally reporting the film.

Documentation The need for clear, concise and thorough documentation is paramount in the ED. Noting some negative findings can be just as important as some positive findings (eg no proximal fibular tenderness in a patient with a severe ankle 'sprain' or an ankle fracture).

Training

Initial route CT1 in Acute Care Common Stem (ACCS, p28)

Further training competitive application for ST4 emergency medicine

Exams completion of MCEM required for ST4 application

Endocrinology

Role Endocrinologists look after patients with hormonal disorders. This can range from common conditions such as DM and thyroid disease which are encountered in daily practice, to very specialised conditions such as pituitary tumours and their associated conditions. Patients range from newborns to the elderly and endocrinologists often work in conjunction with other specialities such as gynaecology, paediatrics and surgery.

Endocrinology history

Alongside taking a standard history (p98) the following are important:

Systemic features weight loss, weight gain, appetite, sweating, heat/cold intolerance, tremor, weakness, tiredness, dizziness, hirsuitism, joint pain/swelling, change in appearance (skin, hair, nails, face, eyes), change in clothes/shoe/hat size

Cardiorespiratory features chest pain, breathlessness, palpitations, sleep apnoea

GI/urinary features diarrhoea, constipation, nausea, vomiting, abdominal pain, thirst, polyuria

Reproductive features menstrual irregularities, infertility, galactorrhoea, impotence

Psychiatric features anxiety, mood changes, memory problems

Eye features blurred vision, visual field defects, bulging eyes

Past medical history thyroid surgery, stroke, heart failure, liver failure, renal artery stenosis, adrenal surgery, brain surgery

Drug history steroids, diuretics, OCP, HRT, levothyroxine, insulin

Family history DM, thyroid disease, pituitary tumours

Endocrinology examination

General inspection body habitus, 'buffalo hump', facial appearance ('moon face'), striae, bruising, muscle wasting, hyperpigmentation, coarse skin, prominent jaw and brow ridge, goitre

Hands temperature, sweating, size, tremor

Eyes lid lag, proptosis, exophthalmos, bitemporal hemianopia, cranial nerve III, IV or VI palsy, fundoscopy

Neck goitre, thyroid lumps

Cardiorespiratory ↑↓HR, ↑↓BP, postural hypotension, irregular pulse, peripheral oedema, bibasal crackles (LVF)

Neurological cranial nerve III/IV/VI palsy, peripheral neuropathy, slow relaxing reflexes

Other joints, skin, genitalia, fundoscopy, urine analysis, U+E, early morning cortisol, TFTs, short Synacthen® test, GTT – more specialist tests on advice from an endocrinologist

Endocrinology referrals

Checklist

Name, hospital number, age, gender, location

Usual insulin/oral hypoglycaemic regime, last dose, time of last dose, last meal

Latest blood glucose and pH; urine ketones and glucose

Referrals are usually made to the endocrinology registrar on-call. Try to give an impression of the urgency of the problem and which of the following would be appropriate:
- *Take over care* if the patient's underlying problem is suspected to be or is a newly diagnosed endocrinological condition, or poorly controlled previous problem (eg uncontrollable blood sugars in diabetics)
- *Ward review* if the patient is acutely unwell with a endocrinological problem or unable to mobilise
- *Urgent clinic review* if the patient is stable and mobile but with a condition requiring urgent review, they could be seen in clinic
- *Routine outpatient* clinic if the patient is stable and has a non-urgent endocrinological problem

Endocrinology as an F1/F2

Endocrinology may be part of general medicine as an F1 or a specialist attachment. However, common endocrinological conditions such as DM and thyroid disease will be encountered in any medical or surgical job, so it is important to learn how to manage these conditions.

The job you will be expected to perform the following roles:
- Clerk new admissions and initiate treatment plans
- Manage patients with both acute and chronic illnesses on the ward
- Perform functional endocrine tests such as:
  - oral glucose tolerance tests (p277)
  - short Synacthen® tests (p609)
  - anterior pituitary function testing
  - water deprivation tests
- Attend clinics and learn how to manage chronic disease

Aims try to do the following during your placement:
- Become familiar with taking a history and examining patients with a range of endocrinological conditions
- Learn to perform endocrine tests and interpret their results (p609)
- Learn how to initiate insulin therapy and adjust regimes accordingly
- Spend time in outpatient clinics
- Learn how chronic disease can impact on a patient's life

Training

Initial route CT1 in core medical training
Further training competitive application for ST3 endocrinology
Exams MRCP part 1 required to apply for ST3 endocrinology

Gastroenterology

Role care of patients with gastrointestinal or liver dysfunction; liver failure and GI bleeds make up a large proportion of the ward-based work.

Gastroenterology history

Along with a standard clerking (p98) ask about the following:

General abdo pain, association with eating, vomiting or opening bowels, weight loss, appetite, bruising, bleeding, nausea, vomiting (appearance), dysphagia, dysuria, urinary frequency and urgency, possibility of pregnancy; **stool** change in bowel habit, frequency, consistency, colour, pain on passing, recurrent urge, blood (bowl or paper), offensive smell, mucus

Past medical history GI bleeds, GORD, varices, gallstones, liver problems, jaundice, IBD, haemorrhoids, polyps

Drug history NSAIDs, warfarin, hepatotoxic drugs (p148)

Alcohol intake per day (in units, p116), CAGE questions (p116)

Family history IBD, liver disease, cancer

Gastroenterology examination

General inspection oedema, wasting, jaundice, orientation, nail colour, clubbing, anaemia, palm colour, flap, jaundice, lymphadenopathy, breath, mouth ulcers, gynaecomastia, spider naevi, bruises

Abdomen distension (fat, faeces, flatus, fluid, fetus), prominent veins, tenderness (guarding, rebound), masses, organomegaly (see tables), ascites, hernial orifices (inguinal, femoral, incisional), bowel sounds

PR visible haemorrhoids, fissures and skin tags, anal tone, prostate, rectal masses, appearance of faeces ±blood

Common abdominal masses – if in doubt check with USS	
Liver	RUQ, extends to RLQ, unable to get above, dull to percussion
Spleen	LUQ extends to RLQ, unable to get above, notch
Kidney	RUQ and/or LUQ, ballotable, able to get above it, smooth outline
Faeces	Indentable mass away from umbilicus

Common causes of enlarged liver and spleen

Hepatomegaly alcohol, hepatitis, EBV, CMV, thin patient, autoimmune hepatitis, toxins, liver metastases, lymphoma, leukaemia, haemochromatosis, amyloidosis, hyperexpanded chest eg COPD, heart failure

Splenomegaly chronic liver disease, autoimmune disease, thrombocytopenia, EBV, CMV, hepatitis, HIV, haemolytic anaemia, leukaemia, lymphoma, endocarditis, thalassaemia, sickle cell, myelofibrosis, sarcoid, amyloidosis, malaria, leishmaniasis

Hepatosplenomegaly hepatitis, EBV, CMV, chronic liver disease, leukaemia, lymphoma, myelofibrosis, amyloidosis

Gastroenterology referrals

Checklist

Name, hospital number, age, gender, location

Alcohol consumption, need for withdrawal medication (p116)

Examination findings of hernial orifices and PR

Latest observations including haemodynamic status (HR and BP) and GCS

Results of urine dipstick (and β-hCG if female), FBC, LFT, clotting

Referrals are usually made to the gastroenterology registrar on-call. Try to give an impression of the urgency of the problem and which of the following would be appropriate:

- *Emergency review* for severe GI bleeds requiring urgent management
- *Take over care* if the patient's underlying problem is with the bowel or liver; they might not accept uncomplicated alcohol withdrawal. Note that pancreatitis is conventionally managed by surgeons.
- *Ward review* if the patient has a gastroenterological problem that is complicating their care on another ward
- *Urgent clinic review* for undiagnosed lower GI bleeding in a well patient as a two-week (cancer) referral
- *Routine outpatient clinic* if the patient is stable and has a non-urgent gastroenterological problem

Gastroenterology as an F1/F2

Gastroenterology may be part of general medicine as an F1 or a specialist attachment. The ward-based patients can rapidly become unwell (eg massive upper GI bleed); there is a high proportion of alcohol dependence which can lead to challenging behaviour.

The job you will be expected to perform the following roles:

- Clerk new admissions and initiate treatment plans
- Perform daily ward round and ensuing jobs
- Prepare patients for GI investigations eg bowel prep for colonoscopy
- Manage liver failure and GI bleed emergencies

Aims try to do the following during your placement:

- Become familiar with GI history taking and examination
- Become familiar with taking a detailed alcohol history (p116)
- Learn how to perform ascitic taps and drains (p590)
- Learn to manage upper and lower GI bleeds (p245/248) including resuscitation of massive GI bleeds (p244)
- Spend time in outpatient clinics
- Observe upper and lower GI endoscopy

Training

Initial route CT1 in core medical training
Further training competitive application for ST3 gastroenterology
Exams MRCP part 1 required to apply for ST3 gastroenterology

General practice – cardiology/diabetes

Avoid the following cardiac drug contraindications:
- β-blockers in patients with asthma
- β-blockers with Ca^{2+} channel blockers (verapamil and diltiazem)
- Aspirin with warfarin

Cardiac risk factors (*OHGP*2 p314)

Many causes of coronary heart disease are reversible. The OHGP2 and the back of *BNF* have Framingham charts to estimate a well patient's 10yr risk. All patients should be encouraged to exercise, stop smoking and improve their diet (↓salt/fat). As risk increases the reversible risk factors should be targeted (cholesterol, smoking, BP, DM control, weight).

Hypertension (p199, *OHGP*2 p316)

Red flags BP ≥200/110, headache, ↓GCS, visual problems, pregnancy

Causes essential/idiopathic (95%), DM, steroids, renal disease, alcohol, Conn's, phaeochromocytoma, acromegaly, pregnancy, aortic coarctation

Symptoms usually asymptomatic, eye, kidney, heart or renal problems

Signs BP>140/90mmHg, displaced apex, heart failure, retinopathy

GP monitoring hypertension should be recorded on ≥3 occasions before starting treatment unless red flags are present. Checks can be done by the practice nurse and should take place over weeks if BP is 199/109 to 160/100 or months if 159/99 to 140/90. Consider 24h ambulatory monitoring if patient is anxious or there is diagnostic doubt.

Investigations FBC, U+E, fasting glucose, lipids, urine dipstick, ECG, consider echo if LVH/LVF suspected (p226), echo if murmur or new SOB

Management education, exercise, stop smoking, reduce alcohol, restrict salt, diet, relaxation. Aspirin 75–150mg/24h PO if ≥50yr. Antihypertensive medications include thiazides, ACEi (see starting ACEi p203), β-blockers, Ca^{2+} blockers. ACEi, thiazides and Ca^{2+} blockers are common 1st line treatments (p203). Warn patients about side-effects (eg cold hands, erectile dysfunction).

Safety net seek advice if visual problems; regular monitoring

Ischaemic heart disease (IHD) (chest pain p177, *OHGP*2 p328)

Red flags pain at rest or mild exertion, increasing frequency/severity

Symptoms central/left chest pain or tightness, radiating to left arm or jaw, brought on by exertion/cold/emotion, improved with rest/GTN

Signs often normal, may have displaced apex, exclude arrhythmias

Investigations FBC, ESR, TFT, fasting glucose, lipids, ECG (p568)

Acute see p176, sit up, O_2, GTN, aspirin, dial 999

Management if new onset or worsening, refer to rapid access chest pain clinic/cardiology. Control risk factors (see above), start aspirin 75–150mg/24h PO and prescribe a GTN spray. Medications to improve symptoms: nitrates (eg ISMN), β-blockers, Ca^{2+} channel blockers.

Safety net seek advice if frequent attacks, ED if SOB/chest pain >20min

Post MI (*OHGP*2 p332)

Educate regarding need to continue meds, check U+E (ACEi and statin), enforce need to stop smoking, exercise, eat healthily, tight DM control

Heart failure (*OHGP*2 p334)

Red flags chest pain, arrhythmia, tachypnoea, oedema above ankles

LVF symptoms short of breath, reduced exercise tolerance, tiredness, orthopnoea, cough worse at night, pink/frothy sputum

RVF symptoms swollen ankles, tiredness, nausea

Signs ↑JVP, 3rd heart sound, displaced apex, symmetrical basal creps, wheeze, pleural effusions, ascites, tender hepatomegaly, pitting oedema

Investigations FBC, U+E, LFT, TFT, glucose, cholesterol and lipids, ECG (p568), CXR (enlarged heart, p620), echo

Acute see p225, sit up, 15l/min O_2, dial 999

Management stop smoking, exercise, adequate diet (↓salt), control BP. Drugs with a life-prolonging effect: β-blockers, ACEi (see starting an ACEi, p203), spironolactone, nitrates; other drugs with only symptomatic improvement: diuretics and digoxin. Regular review and involve chronic/long-term conditions nursing team.

Safety net seek advice if swelling or SOB worsen, attend the ED if acutely SOB or new onset chest pain

High cholesterol (*OHGP*2 p324)

Management low cholesterol diet (fish, vegetables, margarine) can lower cholesterol by 10%. Statins improve prognosis if total cholesterol is ≥5mmol/l; control is especially important if Framingham risk ≥30%, ischaemic heart disease (IHD), post MI/CVA or DM.

Aspirin (*OHGP*2 p314)

Prescribed to patients with ↑BP and age ≥50yr, previous angina, MI, stroke, intermittent claudication, atrial fibrillation (unless on warfarin)

Diabetes (DM) (p276, *OHGP*2 p404)

Red flags weight loss, polyuria, thirst, vomiting, ketones

Acute management refer all new type 1 DM to acute admissions or dial 999 if DKA suspected. Start treatment and monitoring in type 2 (p277).

Chronic management regular reviews often with the practice nurse:

- Education
- Dietary modification
- Lifestyle modification (exercise and smoking)
- Self-monitoring (usually urine; finger-prick if on insulin or poor control)
- Pneumovax® and yearly flu vaccines
- Control cardiac risk factors (BP, cholesterol, smoking, weight) ie keep BP <140/80, ACEi to reduce nephropathy, statin if ↑cholesterol
- Strict glucose control, aim for HbA_{1C} of ≤7.4% to reduce complications; hard to achieve as type-2 DM progresses
- Early detection and treatment of complications including regular ophthalmology ±laser photocoagulation and chiropody

Monitoring urine dipsticks, finger-prick glucose, HbA_{1C}, BP, cholesterol

Safety net seek advice if feeling acutely unwell or losing weight

Diabetic review

Check for chest pain, leg pain, numbness/tingling, erectile problems; review foot care and problems, inspect feet and pulses; check visual acuity and retina; check urine dipstick; discuss cardiac risk factors and their treatment/prevention, check BP; discuss other reviews and appointments

General practice – respiratory

Coughs and colds (SOB p219)

Red flags very unwell, unable to swallow, drooling, stridor, night sweats, weight loss, haemoptysis, SOB, chest pain

Acute causes URTI, croup, pneumonia, asthma, COPD, postnasal drip

Chronic causes (>2WK) ***serious*** lung cancer, TB; ***common*** postviral, post-nasal drip, asthma, smoker's cough, COPD, bronchiectasis. oesophageal reflux, heart failure, ACE inhibitors, restrictive lung disease

Ask about duration, time of day, sputum quantity and colour (?bld), shortness of breath, chest pain, malaise, runny nose, ability to eat and drink, night sweats, weight loss, calf pain, parental anxiety (children)

Look for pyrexia, RR, tonsils, lymphadenopathy, air entry, creps, bronchial breathing, ↑JVP, heart murmur, swollen calves or ankles

Management most coughs and colds require minimal treatment; offer advice on self-management (eg paracetamol, decongestants) and follow up in anxious. Consider PEFR. Specific treatments include:

- ***Postnasal drip*** beclometasone 2puffs/12h intranasal or antihistamines
- ***Asthma*** and ***COPD*** see below
- ***Pneumonia*** amoxicillin 500mg/8h PO, refer if unwell (p224)

Persistent consider FBC, U+E, CRP, CXR and respiratory function tests. Advice about reducing smoking.

Safety net seek advice if no better in 1wk, ED if severely SOB

Asthma (p223 and *OHGP*2 p376)

Red flags ↓O_2 sats, PEFR <50%, incomplete sentences, recession, ↑RR/HR

Symptoms chronic cough, night/morning cough, poor exercise tolerance, short of breath, tight chest, atopy (allergies, hayfever, eczema), family history of atopy, diurnal variation

Signs ↓PEFR, wheeze, recession, tracheal tug

Diagnosis symptom diary, PEFR diary (pre and post-inhaler), spirometry

Exacerbation regular salbutamol inhalers, ±oral steroids, ±amoxicillin

Chronic use the treatment steps p223, the aim is for no symptoms with minimal treatment. Practice nurses can monitor symptoms, check inhaler technique, encourage smoking cessation and recommend therapy.

Safety net seek urgent advice if symptoms worsen, ED if SOB

COPD (p221 and *OHGP*2 p382)

Red flags ↓GCS, cyanosis, ↑RR, haemoptysis, night sweats, weight loss

Symptoms chronic cough, ±productive (?colour/bld), breathless, recurrent resp infection, wheeze, reduced exercise tolerance, weight loss

Signs ↑RR, ↓O_2 sats, ↓PEFR, wheeze, creps, pursed lips

Diagnosis CXR, spirometry, trial of steroids

Exacerbation regular inhalers, ±oral steroids, ±amoxicillin, consider involving COPD home service to prevent unnecessary admission

Management smoking cessation advice and encourage exercise (p222), refer to a specialist for diagnosis and treatment. Long term may require home nebulisers or home O_2, as advised by specialist.

Safety net seek urgent advice if symptoms worsen, ED if severely SOB

General practice

Fatigue and tiredness (*OHGP*2 p582)

Red flags weight loss, polyuria, bone pain, haemoptysis, melaena, suicidal *Causes* **serious** DM, cancer; ***common*** depression, anxiety, alcohol, recreational drugs, anaemia, hypothyroid, infections (EBV, CMV), menopause, insomnia, heart/renal failure, antihistamines, sedatives, chronic fatigue

Ask about duration, onset, exacerbating factors (exertion suggests physical illness), change through day, sleep quality and hygiene, early morning waking, snoring, weight loss, urinary frequency, thirst, swelling, recent colds or sore throat, SOB, cough, worries, anorexia, anhedonia

Look for pyrexia, lymphadenopathy, tonsils, CVS, resp, abdo and neuro for physical disease, consider depression scoring (p307)

Management investigate physical illnesses suggested by history/examination; consider FBC, U+E, ESR, TFT, fasting glucose, EBV serology and urine dipstick; further investigations rarely help. Reassurance, regular review and sleep hygiene advice p153.

Chronic fatigue acute onset, often following a viral infection, fatigue is worse after exertion and accompanied by muscle/joint pain, headaches, sore throat or poor concentration. Treat with reassurance, cognitive behavioural therapy and antidepressants. See OHGP2 p583.

Safety net seek advice if feeling acutely unwell or losing weight

Hypothyroid

Symptoms tiredness, lethargy, weight gain, depression, confusion, dementia, cold intolerance, constipation, menorrhagia, infertility

Signs obese, bradycardia, ↓temp, cold/dry hands, non-pitting oedema, goitre, peripheral neuropathy, slow relaxing reflexes

Investigations ↓T_4, ↑TSH, positive thyroid autoantibodies

Treatment refer to specialist to start levothyroxine (usually 100µg/24h PO, less if elderly/heart problems) the dose is then increased over months until symptoms resolve and TSH is normal. Yearly TFT once stable. Consider propranolol 40mg/6h PO if ischaemic heart disease present.

Complications angina from treatment, myxoedema coma

Health promotion

Smoking (*OHGP*2 p234) repeated advice will help 5% people give up per year. Encourage picking a day to throw all the cigarettes and lighters away. Nicotine gum, patches and sprays are prescribable. Repeated reviews and support groups help to prevent and limit relapses.

Alcohol (p116 and *OHGP*2 p236) targets are: <21units/wk for men (>50units is high intake) and <14units for women (>35units is high intake). Monitor FBC (↑MCV) and LFT (↑γGT). Strategies include drink diaries, Alcoholics Anonymous, community alcohol teams.

Exercise (*OHGP*2 p232) Aim for ≥30min of exercise twice a week at a level that induces slight breathlessness. Walking, cycling and swimming are all good low-impact sports.

Diet and obesity (*OHGP*2 p226) Encourage patients to eat fresh vegetables and fruit with less fat, sugar and salt. Exercise, low-calorie healthy diets and encouragement all help weight loss.

General practice – psychiatry

See p534 for psychiatric history and mental state examination; see p309 for mood disturbance and psychosis.

Depression (p311 or *OHGP*2 p968)

Common and under-diagnosed, especially in the elderly and adolescents.
Red flags anhedonia, suicidal intent and plans, psychosis

Symptoms low mood, lack of pleasure (anhedonia), suicidal, early morning waking, insomnia, tiredness, lack of energy, poor concentration, agitated, feeling worthless/guilty, anorexia, weight change, stressful events

Signs self-neglect, poor eye contact, objectively low mood

Treatment acute psychiatric review/crisis team if suicidal or psychotic. Treatment options include: education, problem-solving strategies, self-help groups, exercise, counselling, cognitive behavioural therapy (CBT), other psychological therapies, regular GP review. Consider referral if not improving despite ≥2 attempts at treatment.

Antidepressants can be prescribed for persistent or moderate/severe depression, eg tricyclics (dangerous in overdose) and SSRIs. Tell the patient that they take 2–6wk to have an effect, are usually continued for 6mth after symptoms resolved then weaned off because stopping them suddenly can cause withdrawal. Monitor regularly.

Safety net monitor new diagnoses every 1–2wk

Anxiety (p313 of *OHGP*2 p960)

Red flags recurrent sudden headaches, weight loss, severe chest pain
Anxiety can be psychological (fearful, restless, poor concentration, obsessions) or physical (tingling, chest discomfort, fluttering heart). There are several types of anxiety disorder:

- Simple phobias (eg jellyfish)
- Social phobias (eg agoraphobia)
- Post-traumatic stress disorder
- Obsessive–compulsive disorder
- Panic
- Somatisation ('hypochondria')

Differentials physical illness can cause anxiety: hyperthyroid, hypoglycaemia, phaechromocytoma, Cushing's, stroke/TIAs, chronic fatigue

Physical illness be open to the possibility of new physical illness, eg MI

Treatment explore beliefs, reassurance, education, avoid phobias, ↓caffeine, counselling, self-help groups, CBT, antidepressants, refer if diagnostic doubt or uncontrollable anxiety, try to avoid benzodiazepines

Safety net monitor regularly (1–2wk), seek advice if acutely unwell

Dementia (p282 or *OHGP*2 p978)

Red flags acute onset, weakness, headache, confusion, slurred speech

Symptoms forgetful, neglect, unable to cope, altered personality

Signs self-neglect, falls, check mini-mental state (p283)

Investigations FBC, U+E, LFT, Ca^{2+}, TFT, glucose, ESR, B_{12}, folate, CXR, MSU, consider VDRL (syphilis) and HIV. Consider depression.

Treatment refer to a psychogeriatrican to confirm diagnosis, social services, benefits, check vision, hearing, exclude UTI and offer treatment (eg anticholinesterase inhibitors)

Safety net seek advice if acute deterioration/new symptoms

General practice – orthopaedics

Back pain (p296 or *OHGP*2 p550)

Red flags bilateral leg pain, bladder/bowel changes, progressive/night pain, weight loss, age <20yr or >55yr, steroids, thoracic or non-mechanical pain, previous cancer

Causes serious cauda equina, cancer (eg myeloma, bone mets); ***common*** mechanical pain, Paget's, ankylosing spondylitis, vertebral collapse (osteoporosis/cancer)

Ask about trauma, onset, duration, leg pain, numbness, weakness, location, bladder and bowel changes, weight loss, worse at night, work

Look for back movements whilst standing, tenderness, leg power, sensation and reflexes, straight leg raise (mechanical if pain at <45°)

Investigations if red flag symptoms FBC, ESR, Ca^{2+}, PO_4^{3-}, ALP, lumbar spine and pelvic X-rays, MRI

Management prescribe adequate analgesia:
- ***Mechanical*** reassure and educate regarding posture, weight, lifting; offer analgesia. Suggest physiotherapy and back exercises. Consider orthopaedic referral for persistent or severe sciatica.
- *Red flag symptoms* refer and perform investigations above
- *Cauda equina* p297, admit urgently to orthopaedics/neurosurgeons

Safety net seek advice if not improving, ED if bladder/bowel problems or bilateral neurology

Osteoarthritis (p410 or *OHGP*2 p570)

Red flags pyrexia, hot and swollen joint

Symptoms joint pain and stiffness, clicking, deformity

Signs effusion, pain on moving, reduced movement, crepitus

Investigations X-rays show ↓joint space, cysts, osteophytes and sclerosis

Management exercise and muscle strengthening, weight reduction, walking aids, hot/cold pads may help. Pain relief (p428), creams eg capsaicin and Deep Heat®, steroid injections. Refer if diagnosis in doubt or symptoms uncontrolled (wash out, joint replacement).

Safety net seek advice if symptoms worse or unable to cope at home

Osteoporosis (*OHGP*2 p568)

Aim to prevent prior to a fracture or treat aggressively afterwards. Risk factors include early menopause, age, female, ↓BMI (especially previous eating disorder), family history, dairy intolerance, steroids, alcohol. Screen those at risk by DXA scan to check bone mineral density (BMD).

Management stop smoking, regular weight-bearing exercise, reducing falls, Ca^{2+} and vitamin D supplements, bisphosphonates (especially if on steroids), Protelos® (strontium ranelate). HRT should only be used for short-term relief of menopausal symptoms (<5yr).

General practice – ENT

See p460 for examination and treatment of common ENT conditions.

Earache and deafness (*OHGP2* p922/924)

Red flags unwell, unilateral hearing loss/tinnitus, mastoid pain

Acute causes serious mastoiditis, foreign body; ***common*** URTI, otitis media, otitis externa, earwax

Chronic causes serious cholesteatoma, acoustic neuroma; ***common*** glue ear, chronic suppurative otitis media (CSOM), earwax, presbyacusis

Ask about onset, duration, discharge, itching, hearing loss, speech problems, runny nose, sore throat, trauma, malaise

Look for pyrexia, appearance of eardrum (?perforated), effusion, colour of canal, discharge, tonsils, lymphadenopathy, sinus pain, teeth, mastoid

Management most earache simply requires analgesia, consider:
- ***Otitis media*** pus/bloody discharge if drum perforated, red, bulging drum, ±effusion; analgesia, amoxicillin if ≥3d, perforated or unilateral
- ***Otitis externa*** itching, tender, discharge, ±pus; clean canal and keep dry (may need aural toilet by ENT), give gentamicin + steroid ear drops

Persistent consider hearing tests:
- ***Ear wax*** olive oil, ±syringing so long as drum not perforated
- ***Presbyacusis*** bilateral hearing loss with age, consider hearing aid
- ***Glue ear*** persistent middle ear effusion with deafness usually lasts 3–6mth; a 2–6wk course of amoxicillin may help. ENT referral for grommets is only required if persistent and falling behind at school.
- ***CSOM*** central perforation of drum, treat as for otitis externa

Peripheral perforations, cholesteatoma and ***unilateral deafness*** (acoustic neuroma) require ENT referral

Safety net seek advice if persistent discharge or hearing/speech problems

Sore throats (*OHGP2* p914)

Red flags unilateral tonsillar enlargement, unable to swallow, tonsils meeting in midline, stridor, very unwell, night sweats, weight loss

Causes serious quinsy (peritonsillar abscess – seen in adults), retropharyngeal abscess (children), leukaemia; ***common*** viral, tonsillitis, glandular fever

Ask about duration, cough, malaise, runny nose, ability to eat and drink, night sweats, weight loss

Look for pyrexia, enlarged tonsils, red throat, pus, lymphadenopathy

Management reassurance, gargle with salt water or dissolvable aspirin, regular analgesia (paracetamol and ibuprofen), hot drinks, over-the-counter medications (Difflam®, Lemsip®, Strepsils®, see *BNF*). Consider antibiotics (penicillin V 500mg/6h PO or erythromycin 500mg/6h PO) if persistent or pus seen.

Persistent consider alternative diagnosis including FBC and EBV serology. May need referral to ENT for tonsillectomy if:
- ≥5 sore throats needing time off each year for two years
- ≥3mth sore throat
- Sleep apnoea or unilateral enlargement

Safety net seek advice if no improvement in 3–5d or feeling unwell

General practice – gynaecology

See p486 for gynaecology history and examination.

Smear test (*OHGP*2 p716)

Screening for cervical cancer should be offered every 3yr to all women aged 25–64yr (or younger if sexually active for >3yr). It is often performed by a practice nurse; follow up in colposcopy clinic if abnormal.

Menopause and HRT (*OHGP*2 p732)

HRT should only be prescribed for 5yr to treat acute symptoms unless menopause/ovarian failure is premature (eg age 35–40yr).

Pill checks (*OHGP*2 p750)

Women on the COC or POP need reviews every 3–6mth:
- ***Problems*** headaches, weight gain, bloating, breakthrough bleeding, depression, acne, breast tenderness
- Check ***BP***
- ***Education*** stop smoking, DVT risks, missed pill rules (see box)

Safety net reattend in 6mth, immediately if painful ±swollen leg

Missed pill or vomiting/diarrhoea

COC if **<12h** since missed dose, take the pill immediately then at the usual time; no extra precautions. If **>12h** take next pill at normal time; alternative contraception for next 7d, start another pack without a break if due to finish pack within 7d.

POP if >3h since missed dose, take pill immediately and then take the next dose at the normal time; alternative contraception for 7d.

Contraception (*OHGP*2 p766)

Ideally, this should be discussed with both partners; options include:
- ***Barrier methods*** condoms, caps, diaphragm, femidoms, sponges; reduce transmission of STIs (no other contraceptives have this effect)
- ***IUCD*** local progesterone-releasing (Mirena®) or copper-containing plastic device; ***side-effects*** bleeding, pain, pelvic infection, ectopic pregnancies, expulsion
- ***Oral contraceptive pill*** either oestrogen and progesterone (combined, COC) or progesterone only (POP); ***side-effects*** acne, bleeding, breast tenderness, bloating, weight gain, mood changes, nausea, DVT/PE
- ***Hormones by other routes*** eg implants (3yr) and injections (3mth)
- ***Sterilisation*** for couples who have completed families; NB male sterilisation is 10 times more effective than female sterilisation
- ***Effectiveness*** Male sterilisation >99.9%, female sterilisation 99.7%, Mirena® 99.9%, COC 99.7%, POP 99.5%, Depo 99.5%, Implants 99.9%, IUCD 99%, barrier methods 85–98%, coitus interruptus 70%

Emergency contraception

Discuss timings, LMP, PE/focal migraine, future contraception, STI testing
- ***Levonorgestrel*** available over the counter as a single 1500μg tablet within 72h then barrier contraception until next period
- ***Copper IUCD*** inserted within 5d; more effective but infection is a risk so needs STI screen (p484) and consider prophylactic antibiotics

General practice – paediatrics

See p524 for vaccinations, history, examination and development.

Child health (*OHGP2* p814)

Children are usually seen by the GP 6wk after birth; further child health check-ups are conducted by the health visiting team. Child vaccination is important, the current schedule can be seen on p524; these are usually given by the practice nurse.

Rashes (p363 and *OHGP2* p876)

Red flags unwell, headache, not acting normal self, non-blanching

Causes serious septicaemia, HSP, ITP; ***common*** viral, eczema, nappy rash

Ask about onset, location, spread, itching, painful, trauma, malaise, urine output, eating and drinking

Look for location, distribution, character (p457), red ears/throat

Management

- ***Non-blanching*** dial 999 if unwell; consider benzylpenicillin IM
- ***Nappy rash*** caused by contact with urine/faeces, use absorbent nappies, regular changing and time without nappies; zinc barrier creams and aqueous cream instead of soap; antifungal cream if not clearing
- ***Eczema*** aqueous cream, bath emollients, topical steroids, antibiotics if signs of infection, antihistamines if itching is a problem
- ***Viral rash*** try to identify the source (eyes, ears, urine), if well discharge with safety netting, if unwell consider referring

Safety net reattend if rash not improving or becomes unwell

Acne (*OHGP2* p644)

Red flags ↑BP, DM, weight gain, vasculitis

Symptoms spots over head, neck and back, otherwise well

Signs whiteheads, blackheads, pustules, scars and sinuses

Treatment ask if bothered by spots (may be embarrassed), reassurance, wash twice daily with soap, moisturisers, topical benzoyl peroxide, retinoids (topical or oral – Roaccutane® requires dermatology referral), antibiotics (topical or oral). Note, if prescribing females tetracycline then give contraception as well (teratogenic), Dianette® may also help the acne.

Safety net reattend if not improving – there are other treatments

Epiglottitis

This is an *emergency*; infection of the epiglottis (rare since HiB vaccine).

Red flags stridor at rest, ↓O_2 sats, severe recession, septic

Symptoms/signs <3yr, stridor, fever, sepsis, drooling, respiratory distress

Management do not look in the mouth or upset the child, dial 999, and contact the ED so that an anaesthetist and ENT surgeon are ready for urgent intubation/tracheostomy

Croup

Viral inflammation of the upper airway (laryngotracheobronchitis).

Red flags stridor at rest, ↓O_2 sats, recession, not eating

Symptoms/signs <4yr, gradual onset stridor, barking cough, resp distress

Management one-off oral dexamethasone dose (150μg/kg) in all children; if severe dial 999; if mild review/refer if stridor at rest persists

Bronchiolitis

Common respiratory infection in <2yr olds causing respiratory distress.

Red flags ↑RR, ↓O_2 sats, severe recession, not eating
Symptoms coryza, cough, fever, apnoea, poor feeding
Signs wheeze, creps, resp distress, exclude cardiac abnormality
Diagnosis usually clinical, CXR if pneumonia suspected
Management no specific treatment; symptoms usually last about 10d with the peak at day 3. If recessing, has ↓O_2 sats or not feeding consider referral to paediatrics for O_2 or NG feeding. If severe may need ITU.

Hayfever and atopy (*OHGP*2 p920)

Red flags ↑HR, ↓BP, stridor, ↑RR, perioral oedema
Symptoms runny nose, recurrent blocked nose, cough, headaches, itchy and watering eyes, sneezing, rash, allergens (pollen, animals, nuts)
Signs clear nasal discharge, red/swollen nostrils
Management allergen avoidance and encourage self-medication with over-the-counter medications including antihistamines (eg loratadine, cetirizine) and sodium cromoglicate eye drops. Intranasal steroid sprays or drops may be required if these do not help.
Safety net ED if swelling, itching or SOB

Neonatal jaundice

Red flags fever, poor feeding, vomiting, tired
Types early <24h, common 2–5d, prolonged >14d
Causes neonatal sepsis, haemolysis (rhesus, ABO), polycythaemia, bruising, prematurity, metabolic; ***prolonged*** breast milk, sepsis, UTI, biliary atresia, haemolysis, hypothyroid, genetic
Management refer unwell babies or early jaundice immediately; prolonged jaundice should be referred to prolonged jaundice clinic
Safety net reattend if jaundice does not resolve

Fever

Red flags no focus, fever >39°C, non-blanching rash, irritable
Symptoms runny nose, cough, miserable, sore throat, off food, pulling ears, vomiting, diarrhoea
Signs coryza, resp distress, rash, lymphadenopathy, red ears, red throat, abdo pain, meningism, impetigo
Management fever may be the only sign of sepsis in young children; refer all babies <6mth with fever to paediatrics. >6mth look carefully for a source (eg URTI, UTI), refer if no source is evident.
Safety net reattend if not resolving, ED if unwell, non-blanching rash

Urinary tract infection

Red flags recurrent, male, ↑BP, haematuria
Symptoms/signs vomiting, fever, abdo pain, offensive nappy
Management UTI in children <2yr requires investigation to exclude vesicoureteric reflux; obtain two clean catch urines prior to treating and refer to paediatrics for investigation
Safety net reattend for repeat urine dipstick after UTI resolved

Referring/writing to GPs

Checklist

Name, hospital number, age, gender, date of birth

Diagnosis, key investigation, management

Follow-up, future management, what you hope the GP will do

Make it clear if the referral is for information or for action

A referral to a GP is the most common referral that F1/F2s will make in the form of a TTO (p106). It is essential that these are done well so that the patient and GP can understand future management.

There are also situations where you may wish to write specifically to the GP for example:

- *To make a referral* some departments will only accept referrals from GPs. If you think your patient needs to be seen by a specialist write a letter to their GP clearly stating why they need referral, how urgently this is needed and who the referral will be to.
- *Complicated management* if a patient's future management is complicated or you feel their understanding is poor then write a letter to their GP explaining it and send a copy to the patient
- *Sensitive issues* this can cover a wide range of topics eg unusual family dynamics, GUM problems, concerns about relatives; consider phoning or writing to the GP – they may well have similar concerns

Referrals by GPs

Referrals

GPs are the gatekeepers to the NHS, accordingly there are many referral and review options available. Hospital admission can often be avoided by considering alternative routes of referral. Options include:

Some referral options	
Emergency department (dial 999)	Midwife
GP admission (ambulance, taxi, own car)	Health visitor
Acute psychiatry team	School nurse
Acute social services	Practice nurse
Hospital speciality 2wk wait (cancer)	Asthma nurse
Hospital speciality normal referral	Diabetic nurse
Yourself eg review in a week	Community nurse
Another member of your practice	Counsellor
Family planning clinic	Occupational health
GUM clinic	Complementary therapy
COPD home service	Social services

General practice as an F1/F2

80% of junior doctors will do a GP placement as part of their F2 year. It gives an opportunity to experience the acute and chronic management of a wide range of conditions in an environment away from instant investigations. The following pages cover some common GP consultations; however you should consider buying the excellent *Oxford Handbook of General Practice 2e.*

The job you will be expected to perform the following roles:
- See patients, initially alongside a GP, but then on your own
- Make management plans for the patients that you see
- Perform home visits
- Participate in practice meetings and audit

Aims try to become familiar with the following during your placement:
- Taking a focused history and relevant examination
- Assessment and management of common medical problems
- Learn about time management
- Learn about sources of out-of-hours care
- Understand the role of referral to the different sources (opposite)
- Performing home visits including nursing homes
- Addressing GP targets eg hypertension, vaccination, screening
- Learn about the management and organisation of general practice
- Awareness of social and occupational aspects of illness

You should not:
- Discharge patients home who you are unsure about
- Prescribe outside the practice or local formulary

Investigations GPs have immediate access to far fewer investigations than in a hospital. The following are usually available:
- *Home visit* HR, BP, RR, urine dipstick, glucose, PEFR, ±O_2 sats
- *GP consultation* HR, BP, RR, urine dipstick, glucose, PEFR, ±O_2 sats, cervical swabs, ±ECG, phlebotomy (1–10d for results), spirometry
- *Hospital* X-rays, USS, ±CT, ±MRI, microbiology, histology, ABG, respiratory function, echo, ECG, phlebotomy

Patient education A patient who understands their condition is much more likely to comply with treatment and take appropriate steps if their condition changes. Taking 15min to explain what hypertension is and why it needs treating can have a life-saving effect.

Leaflets and further information Patients will remember only a fraction of what you have said. Writing down important points and giving leaflets will improve compliance and recall. The internet is a useful resource – suggest some of the better sites (see p637).

Training
Initial route ST1 in general practice (p28)
Further training no more competitive applications are essential for CCT; two years are spent in hospital specialities and one as a GP registrar
Exams nMRCGP must be completed during ST3

General surgery

Role General surgeons look after patients with gastrointestinal disease, performing elective and emergency surgery. In larger centres, general surgeons tend to be divided into either upper GI or lower GI surgeons and may be even further specialised eg hepatobiliary surgeons. General surgeons often have joint care of patients with other specialities, including gynaecology, medicine and paediatrics.

General surgery history

Alongside taking a standard history (p98), when clerking surgical patients the following areas must be covered thoroughly:

Abdominal pain site (localised, general), onset (gradual, rapid, sudden, constant, intermittent) character (burning, stabbing, aching, dull, sharp), radiation (to back, groin, shoulder tip, loin), associations (nausea, vomiting, urinary symptoms, jaundice), timing, exacerbating/relieving factors

Change in bowel habit diarrhoea, mucus, constipation, duration of symptoms, stool colour, PR bleeding (whether mixed with stool, streaking the outside or on toilet paper), usual bowel habit, how many motions per day, when last opened bowels, passing flatus, pain on defecation, haemorrhoids, tenesmus, urgency of defecation, faecal incontinence

Dysphagia duration of symptoms, constant or worsening, solids/liquids, aggravating/relieving factors, positional, pain, sensation of food 'getting stuck', what level, regurgitation, vomiting, coughing, appetite, weight loss

Past surgical history previous operations, malignancy

Past medical history DM, asthma, ↑BP, IHD, clotting problems, liver disease, jaundice, thyroid problems, anaemia, malignancy, epilepsy

Family history DM, malignancy, IBD

Drug history NSAIDs, warfarin, steroids, insulin

Social history smoking, alcohol

General surgery examination

Alongside performing a standard examination (p100) include the following:

General jaundice, wasting, anaemia, lymphadenopathy

Abdominal tenderness, guarding, rebound tenderness, percussion tenderness, masses, ascites

PR pain, masses, stool colour, blood, melaena, prostate size

Hernial orifices inguinal, femoral or incisional hernias

General surgery referrals

Checklist

Name, hospital number, age, gender, location

Time of last food/drink, pre-morbid state, are they peritonitic?

FBC, U+E, LFT, amylase, CRP, clotting, G+S, erect CXR, AXR

Haemodynamic status/shock, why you feel it is a surgical problem

Referrals are usually made to the surgical registrar on-call. Try to give an impression of the urgency of the problem and which of the following would be appropriate:

- *Take over care* if the patient's underlying problem is surgical and requires urgent intervention
- *Joint care* if the patient has a non-urgent surgical problem but would ideally be reviewed during their inpatient stay (eg prolapsed haemorrhoids during late pregnancy)
- *Urgent clinic review* if the patient is stable and mobile but with a condition requiring urgent review (eg suspected GI malignancy), they could be seen in clinic
- *Routine outpatient clinic* if the patient is stable and has a non-urgent surgical problem

General surgery as an F1/F2

General surgery is an F1 placement but can also be a specialist attachment in F2. Patients range from children to the elderly and you may share care of a patient with another team. Much of the work involves preparing patients for theatre and monitoring them carefully post-op.

The job you will be expected to perform the following roles:

- Assess patients pre-operatively (p128)
- Clerk acute admissions in the ED and initiate management plans
- Assist in theatre
- Perform daily ward round and completing ensuing jobs
- Manage post-op problems (p139)
- Attend outpatient clinics

Aims try to do the following during your placement:

- Develop history and examination skills for surgery patients
- Learn some basic surgical skills eg suturing (p600)
- Learn the ward and theatre-based management of surgical conditions
- Attend endoscopy lists
- Spend time with associated professionals eg stoma specialist nurses

Training

Initial route CT1 in 'surgery in general' general surgery (p28)
Further training competitive application for ST3 general surgery
Exams MRCS required to apply for ST3 general surgery

Genitourinary medicine (GUM)

Role Diagnosis and treatment of sexually transmitted infections; this often includes HIV though this may be managed by infectious disease doctors

GUM/sexual history

Alongside taking a standard history (p98) the following are important:

Major symptoms dysuria, haematuria, penile/vaginal discharge, genital/perineal lesion, scrotal pain, itch, dyspareunia, foreign body (vaginal, urethral, anal), anal/perianal problems, sore throat

Past medical history previous STIs, immunosuppression (steroids, HIV), last cervical smear and result

Drug history oral contraception used, vaccinations, allergies

Sexual history:

- Last sexual intercourse (LSI) – gender of partner, type of intercourse (vaginal, anal, oral), barrier contraception used, relationship of partner (casual, long-term), problems or symptoms in partner, date of LSI
- Repeat the above for all partners in the last 3mth
- All men should also be asked if they have ever had sex with another man in the past

Social history foreign travel, sex abroad, illicit drug use (smoke, oral, IV)

Examining male genitalia	p545
Examining female genitalia	p487

GUM investigations

The following is a guide. Investigations should be requested as per local policy or as indicated following a thorough history and examination:

Men urine for ***chlamydia***, urethra swab for gonorrhoea, urethra swab for M,C+S and venous blood for syphilis serology. All patients are usually offered counselling and HIV testing.

Women the following swabs are frequently performed in GUM and gynaecology; there are often referred to as 'triple swabs':

- *High vaginal swab* use a charcoal swab to sweep the posterior fornix (vagina, posterior to the cervix); this is sent for M,C+S
- *Endocervical swab* insert a second charcoal swab into the cervical os and rotate 360°; this is tested for gonorrhoea
- *Endocervical swab* insert a ***chlamydial*** swab into the cervical os and rotate 360°; this is tested for ***chlamydia***

Women may also be offered blood testing for syphilis serology and HIV testing (with counselling).

GUM referrals

Checklist

Name, hospital number, age, gender, location

Presenting complaint, initial findings and investigations, presumed diagnosis

Initial management and response to treatment

Inpatient referrals to the GUM team are usually for advice on HIV-related issues, and in some hospitals GUM provide advice for needlestick injuries.

- *Counselling for HIV testing* the GUM team (medical and nursing staff) are often requested to talk to patients about HIV screening, as they are trained in counselling and in the testing process itself and in HIV treatment and care (p426)
- *Admitted HIV patients* as the prevalence of HIV increases, these patients often present with unrelated pathology. Specialist advice about HIV treatments, drugs interactions etc should be discussed with an HIV/GUM specialist.
- *Needlestick injuries* in some hospitals, 24h advice on needlestick injuries is coordinated by the GUM team – check local policy, p127
- *Outpatient review* for non-urgent GUM problems the patient can be referred to a GUM clinic; they often have a walk-in service

Sexually transmitted infections (STIs)

Chlamydia Symptoms usually appear 1–3wk after exposure though infection can go unnoticed (especially in women). Watery/white discharge ±dysuria in both sexes. Usually sensitive to tetracyclines or macrolides.

Genital herpes Symptoms usually appear 2–7d after exposure, causing itching, tingling or small fluid-filled vesicles in genital area. Episodes can be treated with antivirals (eg aciclovir), but this does not 'cure' the disease.

Genital warts Small fleshy tags or larger cauliflower-shaped lesions. Treated with topical keratolytic or cryotherapy or surgically removed. Likely to recur.

Gonorrhoea Symptoms usually appear 1–14d after exposure. Yellow/green discharge with dysuria in both sexes. Usually sensitive to cephalosporins, as increasingly resistant to fluoroquinolones (ciprofloxacin, levofloxacin).

Syphilis Symptoms can take up to 3mth to appear. Primary disease causes a painless genital ulcer. Secondary disease causes perianal plaques, a non-itchy rash and flu-like symptoms. Diagnosed by either microscopy of tissue from an ulcer or serologically. Treat with IM benzylpenicillin.

Pubic lice Symptoms take 1–14d after exposure. Itch in hairy infected areas in both sexes. Treat with parasiticidal topical preparation which should be repeated at 7d to kill lice emerging from surviving eggs.

Gynaecology

Role Gynaecologists deal with disorders of the female reproductive tract and also look after acute problems in pregnancy up to 20wk gestation (eg threatened miscarriage and ectopic pregnancies). The speciality is surgical but with a strong medical and outpatient component.

Gynaecology history

Alongside taking a standard history (p98) the following are important:

Menstrual history date of last period, length of menstrual cycle (regular or irregular), length of period, associated pain/symptoms, age when periods started/stopped; **bleeding/discharge** severity of periods (number of pads/tampons, clots, flooding), bleeding between periods, after intercourse or after menopause, rectal/urinary bleeding, effect on lifestyle, other vaginal discharge (colour, consistency and smell)

Sexual history pain on superficial or deep penetration (dyspareunia), type of intercourse, use of contraception, intercourse in foreign countries, previous sexually transmitted infections; **contraception** current and previous types, problems/benefits

Cervical smear date of last test and result, previous results and any treatment (repeat smears, colposcopy clinic, laser ablation)

Past gynae history previous problems and/or operations (where and name of surgeon), breast or thyroid problems, use of HRT, prolapse

Past obstetric history number of pregnancies, number of births, type of delivery, complications, fertility problems (see p514 for full obstetric history)

Past medical history clotting problems, thyroid problems, anaemia, malignancy

Urinary problems incontinence (on laughing/coughing/exercising or spontaneous), dysuria, urgency, frequency, haematuria, if symptomatic ask about fluid intake, leg weakness, faecal incontinence, back pain and previous spinal problems/surgery, effect on lifestyle

Other vaginal lumps, weight loss, other concerns

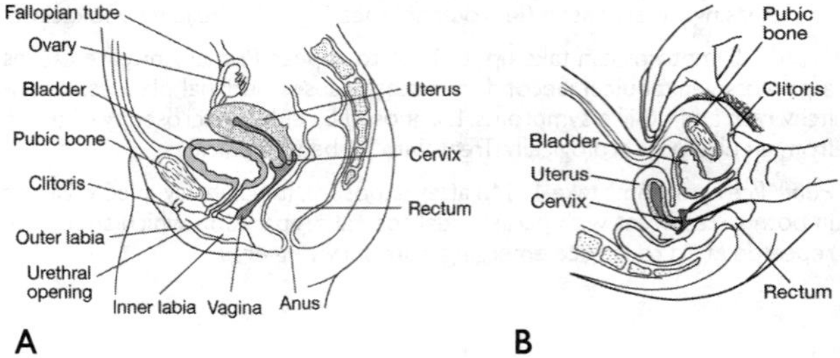

Gynaecology examination

Always have a chaperone who can also watch the door. Ask friends and family members to leave, unless the patient wants them to stay (this also provides an opportunity to ask questions which the patient may not have answered fully with others present). As with any examination it is essential to keep the patient informed about what you are going to do. Start with the patient lying flat on their back with arms by their sides.

Abdominal Assess for scars, striae, hernias, body hair distribution, everted umbilicus, distension, tenderness including loins (±guarding, rebound), masses, organomegaly, percuss (masses, shifting dullness)

Ask the patient to move her feet apart, bend her knees and let her legs flop outwards. Have a strong light source directed at the vulva and gloves on both hands.

Vaginal Look carefully for rashes, ulcers, warts, lumps or other lesions. Spread the labia majora using your dominant thumb and index finger and look for lesions, lumps, discharge (urethral/vaginal), bleeding. Ask the patient to push down (look for prolapse) and cough (make sure you are not in the firing line and look for incontinence).

Insert a well-lubricated index and middle finger (dominant hand) into the vagina and feel for the cervix, noting the size, shape, consistency and whether it is mobile or tender. Feel above, below and to the sides (adnexae) for masses or tenderness. Finally palpate the uterus by placing your other hand above the pubic symphysis and press down with the fingers at the cervix; pressing up feel for uterine position (anteverted/retroverted), size, shape, consistency, mobility and tenderness. Inspect the finger afterwards for blood or discharge.

Cuscoe's speculum Whilst the patient is in the same position insert a well lubricated and warmed speculum into the vagina. Look at the cervix for ulceration, bleeding, cysts or other lesions and the cervical os. If required take swabs and/or a cervical smear.

Consider Sim's speculum (for examining prolapses), rectal examination

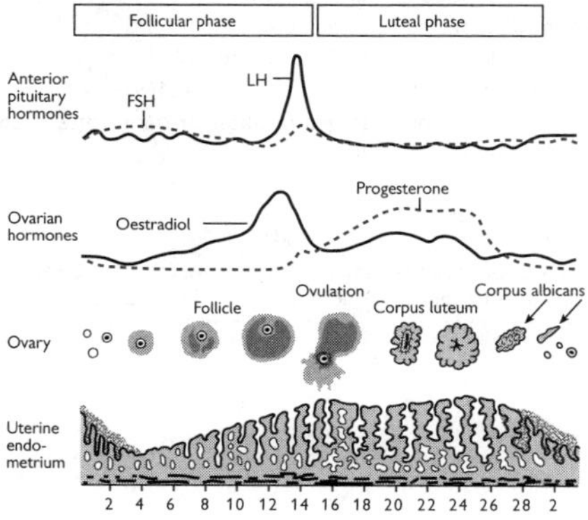

Gynaecology referrals

Checklist

Name, hospital number, age, location

Menstrual history, last menstrual period, urine dipstick, urine β-hCG result

Why you suspect a gynaecological, rather than abdominal/surgical problem

Latest set of observations including HR and BP

Referrals are usually made to the gynaecology registrar on-call. Try to give an impression of the urgency of the problem and which of the following would be appropriate:

- *Take over care* if the patient's underlying problem is gynaecological
- *Ward review* if the patient is acutely unwell with a gynaecological problem or unable to mobilise
- *Urgent clinic* review if the patient is stable and mobile they could be seen in gynae clinic where all the correct equipment and USS will be available
- *Routine outpatient clinic* if the patient is stable and has a non-urgent gynaecological problem

Gynaecology definitions

Anatomy

Introitus the entrance to the vagina

Adnexae the areas lateral to the cervix where the ovaries are located

Abnormal bleeding

Climacteric phase of irregular periods and associated symptoms prior to menopause

Intermenstrual bleeding between periods

Oligomenorrhoea infrequent periods, >42d cycle

Menopause the end of menstruation

Menorrhagia excessive blood loss during periods, >80ml/period

Postcoital bleeding after sexual intercourse

Postmenopausal bleeding >6mth after the menopause

Primary amenorrhoea failure to start menstruating by 16yr

Secondary amenorrhoea absence of menstruation for >6mth after menstruation has started and not due to pregnancy

Pain

Dysmenorrhoea pain associated with periods

Dyspareunia pain associated with sexual intercourse, can be superficial (eg vulval or entrance to vagina) or deep (only on deep penetration)

Gynaecology as an F1/F2

This may form part of a gynaecology and obstetrics placement in the F1 or F2 year. Gynaecological problems are also encountered in the ED and on the wards.

Structure most gynaecologists are also obstetricians though they may specialise more in one area. They may also have a special interest or specialise in a specific area:

- *Gynaeoncology* managing gynaecological cancers
- *Urogynaecology* managing urinary problems eg incontinence
- *Reproductive medicine* helping couples with fertility problems
- *Sexual and reproductive health* contraceptive advice and screening
- *Fetomaternal medicine* care of complicated pregnancies and fetal abnormality

The job you will be expected to perform the following roles:

- Provide medical care for the patients on the gynaecology ward
- Clerk new admissions from ED or GPs and initiate treatment plans
- See patients in gynaecology clinics
- Assist in theatre
- See also job list under obstetrics p517

Aims try to do the following during your placement:

- Become familiar with gynaecology history and examination (p486)
- Learn how to take triple swabs (p484)
- Become familiar with the management of vaginal bleeding (p432)
- Learn to manage bleeding or pain in early pregnancy (p436)
- Become familiar with common gynaecological operations
- Learn to advise on different types of contraception (p477)
- Learn how to insert an intrauterine contraceptive device (IUCD)
- Attend specialist clinics (eg oncology, urogynaecology)

Common cases

Bleeding/pain in early pregnancy (p434) this could be an ectopic pregnancy or an early miscarriage; they may need fluid resuscitation or emergency surgery along with sympathy and counselling

Postmenopausal bleeding (p432) this can be a sign of serious pathology, particularly endometrial cancer

Menorrhagia (p432) heavy periods can have a dramatic impact on a patient's quality of life; there are many treatment options but it is important to choose one appropriate to the patient

Incontinence (p322) this is a common problem in older women; there are a wide range of interventions to help depending on the cause

Training

Initial route ST1 in obstetrics and gynaecology

Further training no more competitive applications are essential for CCT

Exams MRCOG part 1 required for ST3

Haematology

Role Haematology services are provided 24h a day allowing urgent laboratory investigations to be undertaken, blood products to be on hand and specialist medical advice to be available. Haematologists oversee all the laboratory investigations undertaken providing advice where appropriate on further tests or clinical management, as well as providing care for their own inpatients and outpatients.

Haematology history

Alongside taking a standard history (p98) the following are important:

Presenting symptoms ***anaemia*** weakness, lethargy, shortness of breath on exertion, fatigue, postural dizziness; ***platelet dysfunction/clotting disorder*** easy bruising, recurrent epistaxis, haemarthrosis, heavy menstrual loss, recurrent miscarriage; ***other*** recurrent infections, weight loss, swellings (lymphadenopathy), fevers, focal neurology, recurrent thrombosis

Past history previous gastric or small bowel surgery, malabsorption, chronic disease (eg RA), previous blood transfusions, splenectomy

Drug history iron, B_{12}/folate, aspirin, warfarin, vaccinations post-splenectomy, long-term antibiotics, OCP

Social history racial origin, diet (vegan, vegetarian), recreational drug use

Family history thalassaemia, sickle-cell anaemia, haemophilia, von Willebrand's disease, pernicious anaemia, spherocytosis, thrombophilia

Haematology examination

The patient should have a thorough examination, looking especially for:

General inspection bruising, pigmentation, rashes and nodules, ulceration, cyanosis, plethora, jaundice, excoriations, racial origin

Hands nails (koilonychias, pallor), palmar crease pallor, arthropathy

Face eyes (jaundice, pallor), mouth (gum hypertrophy or bleeding, ulceration, candida, atrophic glossitis, angular stomatitis)

Lymph nodes cervical, axillary, epitrochlear (elbow), inguinal

Bones bony pain in sternum, spine, clavicles, scapulae

Abdomen hepatomegaly, splenomegaly, para-aortic nodes, ascites

Legs vasculitis, bruising, pigmentation, ulceration, neurological signs

Other fundi (haemorrhages, engorged veins, papilloedema), temperature chart, urinalysis

Haematology referrals

Checklist

Name, hospital number, age, gender, location

Presenting complaint, family history, previous transfusions, evidence of infection

Bleeding, bruising, organomegaly, lymphadenopathy

Hb, MCV, WCC, plts, clotting, blood film

Haematology referrals are usually centred around abnormal laboratory results, advice about management of complex patients or to discuss a potential blood product transfusion.

- ***Abnormal laboratory results*** discussion with a haematologist about this will aid in deciding which further investigations are necessary
- ***Complex patients*** with existing haematological conditions (such as sickle-cell anaemia) often present with unrelated pathology and it can be useful to discuss these patients with a haematologist to plan their care and prevent potentially avoidable complications
- ***Blood product transfusions*** where massive transfusions are required or correction of complex bleeding disorders; it is often useful to discuss this with the haematologist first

Haematology as an F1/F2

There are not many F1/F2 jobs in haematology, but those who do undertake it often find it very useful; sometimes haematology forms part of a 'clinical laboratory' rotation job.

The job you will be expected to perform the following roles:

- Participate in laboratory handling and analysis of all clinical samples
- Take enquiries about specimens and results
- Telephone urgent results to doctors (under supervision)
- Attend outpatient clinics and inpatient ward rounds

Aims try to do the following during your placement:

- Learn the microscopic morphology of normal and abnormal cells (p333)
- Learn how to manage abnormal coagulation (p344)
- Learn about transfusion medicine (p338)
- Attend and participate in ward rounds with your seniors
- Attend and participate in outpatients, under supervision
- Observe and learn practical procedures (venesections, bone marrow aspirations and trephines)

Training

Initial route CT1 in core medical training
Further training competitive application for ST3 haematology
Exams MRCP part 1 required to apply for ST3 haematology; completion of MRCP and MRCPath (Haem) will be required during training

Maxillofacial surgery

Role Maxillofacial surgeons manage surgical problems of the face, jaws, mouth and neck. They cover a wide range of diseases from trauma to cancer; they work closely with ENT and plastic surgeons amongst others.

Maxillofacial history

These pages will focus on the acute aspects of maxillofacial surgery; there is considerable elective work too. Alongside taking a standard history (p98) the following are important:

*Major symptoms/signs **trauma*** pain, swelling, deformity, double vision/loss of vision, inability to open/close mouth, lacerations, bleeding, inability to swallow, loose teeth, steps in teeth, numbness in lip/face; ***infection*** pain (jaw pain or toothache), swelling, fever, anorexia

Past medical/dental history previous dental problems, name and address of dentist, interval since last visit; cardiac disease, respiratory disease, neurological disease, DM

Drug history analgesics taken and their effects, antibiotics (date started and compliance), other medications; allergies; tetanus

Social history alcohol/drug intoxication, ability to cope if discharged

Maxillofacial examination

*Face **inspect*** symmetry, lacerations, bruising, bleeding, CSF leak, swelling/deformity, steps in teeth, swelling of gums, dental hygiene; ***palpate*** for bony tenderness from TMJ along mandible, maxilla, zygomas, orbital ring, nose, forehead and temples, feel for loose/tender teeth or for steps in the teeth; ***move*** get patient to open and close mouth whilst feeling over the TMJs

Eyes always check visual acuity in trauma and note any diplopia which may suggest orbital floor fracture

Neck always examine the C-spine in head/face trauma (p360)

GCS ↓GCS may be due to intracranial trauma; consult NICE guidelines (p358) on head injury management

Other perform top to toe examination to identify other injuries

Maxillofacial investigations

*Radiology **trauma*** as with fractures at other sites of the body, it is important to try and get two views; writing the site of the potential fracture on the request card helps the radiographer select the best views ***infection*** if the patient is to be referred to the maxillofacial team, discuss X-rays with them first as acute imaging of dental infections is rarely necessary

Maxillofacial referrals

Checklist

Name, hospital number, age, gender, location

Presenting complaint, mechanism of injury or duration of symptoms

Clinical findings, teeth affected, observations, results of investigations

Last food or drink, fitness for theatre

Referrals to the maxillofacial team are usually from ED, but sometimes from the wards and often related to facial trauma or dental problems.

- *Facial trauma* most hospitals have guidelines on the management of facial lacerations, though the on-call maxillofacial surgeon often sutures lacerations crossing the vermillion border of the lips. Facial fractures should all be referred for consideration of surgery/admission.
- *Dental problems* most dental problems can be referred back to the patient's own dentist or the community emergency dentist (switchboard should have the contact details) with oral analgesia ±antibiotics. Dental abscesses with gross swelling should be referred for consideration of drainage.

Teeth nomenclature

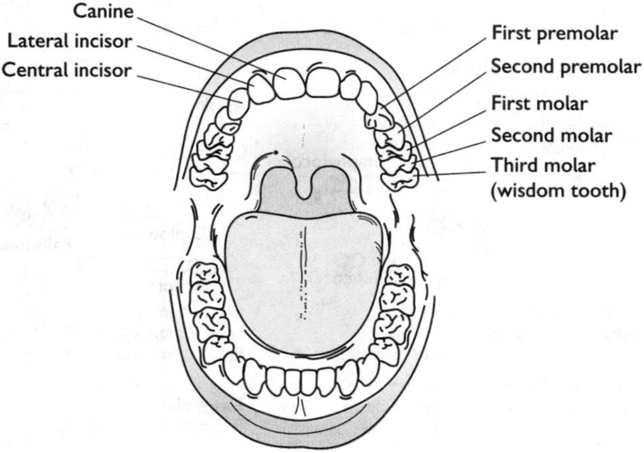

Microbiology

Role Microbiologists manage the microbiology labs, provide advice on complex patients and often attend ITU and haematology ward rounds.

Microbiology history

Alongside taking a standard history (p98) the following are important:

Presenting symptoms timing and order symptoms appeared, any prodromal illness, pattern of fever, systems affected (eg RS, joints, neuro)

Past history previous episodes, factors predisposing to infections including: splenectomy, immunosuppression (steroids, HIV), mechanical heart valves, other indwelling foreign materials (prosthetic hips, stents, mesh); malignancy, haemoglobinopathy, dental surgery/problems, renal problems

Drug history long-term steroids, long-term antibiotics, previous antibiotics and effect/tolerability, allergies, vaccination history

Social history occupation, pets/animal exposure, symptoms in family members/colleagues, foreign travel (vaccinations and prophylaxis taken and compliance with this), intravenous drug use, sexual history (p484)

Microbiology examination

Repeated clinical examination is essential in all unwell patients whether the focus is believed to be known or not. Consider a septic screen (p393) if the focus is unknown or the patient is systemically unwell.

Observations cyclical changes in HR and temp suggest abscesses

Serial clinical examination to aid in identifying the focus/source of infection; this includes a thorough examination of all the skin

Bacterial classification

	Cocci	Bacilli
Morphology	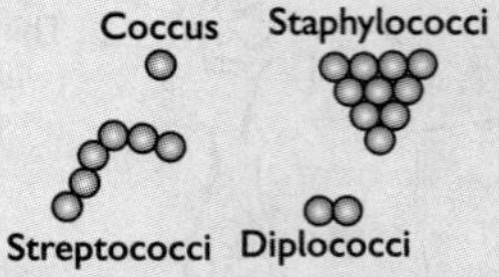	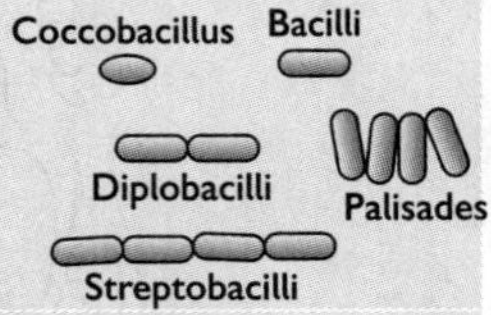
Gram-positive (stain blue)	Enterococcus spp. Staphylococcus aureus Streptococcus pneumoniae	Clostridium spp. Listeria monocytogenes Propionibacterium acnes
Gram-negative (stain pink)	Neisseria gonorrhoeae Neisseria meningitides Moraxella catarrhalis	Haemophilus ducreyi Escherichia coli Pseudomonas aeruginosa

Microbiology referrals

Checklist

Name, hospital number, age, gender, location, weight, latest U+E (or GFR)

Clinical symptoms and signs (including observations) and any investigation results

Management commenced (previous and present antibiotics including doses)

Response to treatment and latest clinical observations and blood results

Microbiology advice is often sought when a patient is failing to respond to treatment, when the patient has complex and multiple pathology or when specific advice is needed about investigations, antibiotics or probable microbial sensitivities.

- *Failing to respond to treatment* persistent symptoms and signs of infection even after commencement of antibiotics may suggest that treatment has been too short, the dose is ineffective, the most appropriate agents are not being used or that the diagnosis is wrong
- *Complex patients* many patients in ITU have multiple potential sources of infection and so choice of antibiotic agent is complex. Antibiotics are chosen by taking samples from the patient for culture and sensitivity, checking previous culture results for the organism and sensitivity, noting the patient's prior antibiotic history and the likely source of infection; often broad-spectrum antibiotics are commenced at the onset.
- *Specific questions* the microbiologist will be able to advise on the most appropriate laboratory investigations for complex patients, and their knowledge of the pharmacology of antimicrobials allows them to offer immediate advice in most situations

Microbiology as an F1/F2

Microbiology is an uncommon specialist FP job, usually in F2. Those who do undertake it often find it very useful.

The job you will be expected to perform the following roles:

- Participate in laboratory handling of clinical samples
- Take enquiries about specimens and results
- Telephone urgent results to doctors (under supervision)
- Attend and contribute to ward rounds
- Participate in on going research and teaching activities

Aims try to do the following during your placement:

- Learn practical laboratory skills and how samples are processed
- Broaden knowledge about antimicrobial agents and their use
- Attend and participate in ward rounds with your seniors
- Contribute to departmental research projects and audits

Training

Initial route ST1 in medical microbiology/virology
Further training no more competitive applications are essential for CCT
Exams MRCPath required during training along with yearly assessments

Musculoskeletal

Role Musculoskeletal specialities include trauma and orthopaedics, sports medicine, musculoskeletal medicine and rheumatology. There are varying degrees of overlap between these, but generally trauma is concerned with injury (fractures, sprains etc), orthopaedics with congenital and acquired bone and joint disease (congenital hip dislocation, osteoarthritis of the hip etc) and rheumatology with inflammatory joint and soft tissue disease (rheumatoid arthritis, fibromyalgia etc).

Musculoskeletal history

Alongside taking a standard history (p98) the following are important:

Major symptoms joint pain, swelling, deformity, morning stiffness, instability, sensory changes, back pain, limb pain, muscle/soft tissue aches, cold fingers and toes, dry eyes and mouth, red eyes, systemic symptoms (fatigue, weight loss, tight skin, fever, rash, diarrhoea), injury/trauma (mechanism, timing, change in symptoms since), bleeding tendency

Past medical history previous trauma/surgery, recent infections (streptococcal, gonorrhoeal, tuberculosis etc), insect/tick bites, inflammatory bowel disease, skin disease (psoriasis), childhood arthritis, haemophilia

Drug history previous anti-arthritic agents (NSAIDs, steroids (oral/intraarticular), DMARDs) with beneficial effects and tolerability/side effects, long-standing steroids, Ca^{2+} supplements, vitamin D analogues, bisphosphonates, other concurrent medications (antihypertensives etc), allergies

Activities of daily living ability to: bathe, dress (and undress), eat, transfer from bed or chair and back, use of the toilet. Effect presenting symptom(s) has upon ADLs, and coping strategies.

Social history domestic arrangements (who else is at home, location of bathroom in relation to bed), smoking history, drug and alcohol use

Family history rheumatoid, gout, osteoarthritis, haemochromatosis, inflammatory bowel disease, haemophilia

Musculoskeletal examination

There are well-established ways of examining all the specific joints, though the underlying principles for each are very similar:

General inspection gross appearance of the patient and their gait

Look close inspection of the joint, comparing left to right

Feel assessment of warmth, tenderness, crepitus, effusions etc

Move active and passive movements; stressing joint where appropriate

Measure range of movements (in degrees) and degree of joint laxity

Hip examination (*OHCS*7 p680)

Inspection Look for leg shortening or internal rotation (hip dislocation) or external rotation (fractured neck of femur). Examine skin over joint for signs of surgical scars, sinuses, cellulitis or bruising.

Palpation feel for bony landmarks (greater trochanter, anterior superior iliac crest), are these at a similar level on either side? Palpate joint for warmth and as it is moved to feel for crepitus, clicks etc.

Supine Active (allow patient to demonstrate their ROM) and passive movements (ask the patient to relax and move the joint yourself); flexion (straight leg flexion 0–90°, flexion with knee bent 0–135°), abduction (0–50°) and adduction, internal (0–45°) and external (0–45°) rotation. Check for fixed flexion deformity by placing hand in lumbar lordosis and checking the hips can extend to allow the popliteal fossa to touch the couch.

Prone Active and passive movement to check hip extension (0–20°)

Stressing is not generally undertaken for the hip

Gait Trendelenburg gait, uses stick on side opposite to diseased hip

Other joints Examine the knee and lower spine/sacroiliac joints

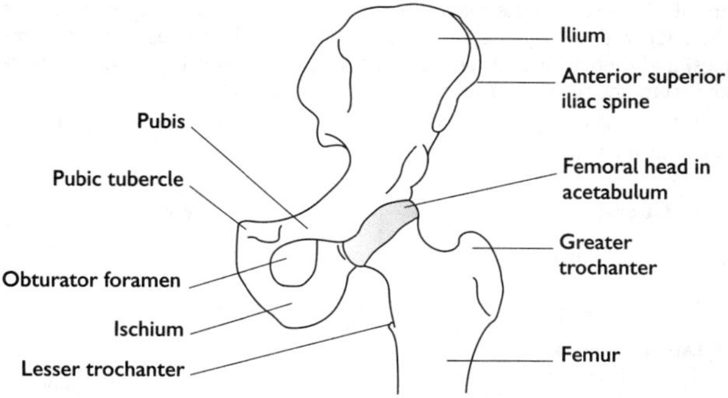

Knee examination (*OHCS7* p686)

Inspection Look for swelling, erythema and the position that the knee is held in by the patient. Is there any varus (bow-legs) or valgus (knock-knees) deformity? Examine the skin over the joint for signs of surgical scars, sinuses or cellulitis. Is there any wasting of the thigh muscles compared to the other side (especially vastus medialis)?

Palpation Feel for temperature, bony landmarks (head of fibula, medial and lateral joint lines, patella). Is there an effusion (if large infra-patella sulci will be bulging outwards with a positive patella tap, if small try milking fluid down from thigh and stroking fluid from one side to the other)? Palpate joint as it is moved to feel for crepitus, clicks. Palpate patella for position, tenderness and mobility (stability).

Supine Active (allow patient to demonstrate their ROM) and passive movements (ask the patient to relax and move the joint yourself); flexion (0–135°), extension (0°).

Prone Examine the popliteal fossa for cysts and popliteal aneurysms.

Stressing Flex knee to 90°, sit on the patient's foot so the foot is immobilised and perform anterior and posterior draw tests to check for anterior and posterior cruciate ligament integrity, respectively. Holding the knee at about 30° flexed, fix the thigh with your left hand on inner aspect and stress the knee with a valgus strain (force applied over lower leg to mimic bow-legs) and then a varus strain (force applied over lower leg to mimic knock-knees) to check for medial and lateral collateral integrity.

Gait Limp or using walking aids. Gives way on mobilising or patient cautious or in pain.

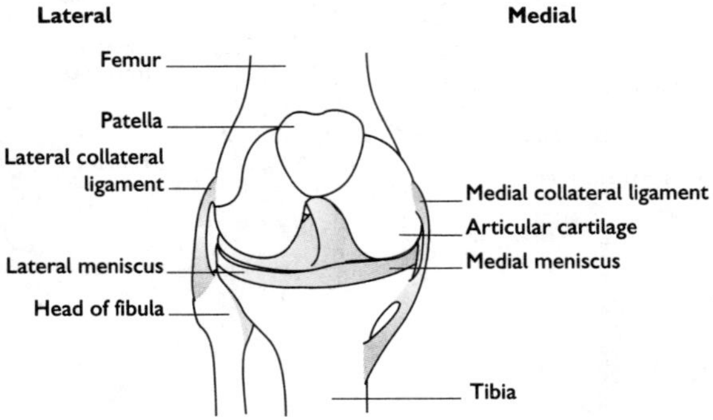

Ankle examination (*OHCS7* p692)

Inspection Look for swelling, erythema and the position that the foot is held in by the patient, if there is marked deviation of the foot in trauma consider fracture–dislocation and summon senior help immediately as it requires immediate reduction before undertaking X-rays due to risk of neurovascular compromise to the foot (p355).

Palpation Feel for temperature, bony landmarks (medial and lateral malleolus, tibiotalar joint) for crepitus or pain; always feel the proximal fibula head in ankle injury to exclude its fracture (Maisonneuve fracture). For Ottawa ankle rules see p355. Is there any swelling, if so is it soft tissue or an effusion in the joint? Palpate joint as it is moved to feel for crepitus, clicks etc. Check for foot pulses, cap-refill and sensation.

Movement Active (allow patient to demonstrate their ROM) and passive movements (ask the patient to relax and move the joints yourself); flexion (plantarflexion (normally 0–50°)) extension (dorsiflexion (0–15°)) across the tibiotalar joint (tibiotaler joint), inversion (0–30°) and eversion (0–15°) across the subtalar joint (talocalcaneal joint).

Stressing is not generally undertaken for the ankle

Gait Is the patient able to weight-bear (able to walk two paces unaided)?

Other joints Examine the knee and foot

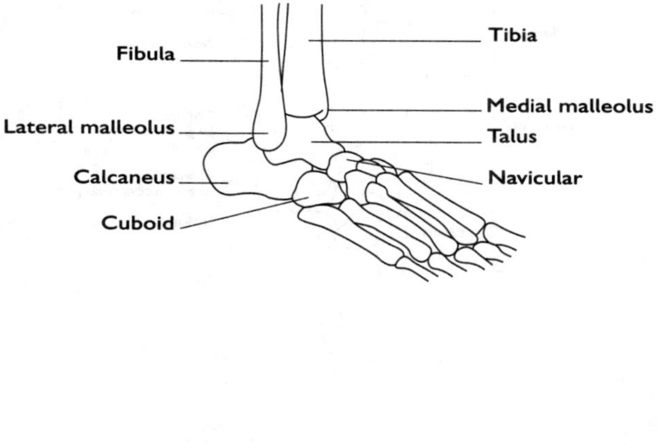

Foot examination

Inspection Look for swelling, erythema, high-arch, bunions and the position that the foot is held in by the patient; are the toes all in a normal alignment?

Palpation Feel for temperature and along each metatarsal and adjacent phalanx, assessing for pain or crepitus. Palpate forefoot bones (navicular, cuboid and medial, intermediate and lateral cuneiform bones). Check for foot pulses, cap-refill and sensation.

Movement Active (allow patient to demonstrate their ROM) and passive movements (ask the patient to relax and move the joints yourself); flexion (plantarflexion (normally 0–50°)), extension (dorsiflexion (0–15°)) across the tibiotalar joint (tibiotaler joint), inversion (0–30°) and eversion (0–15°) across the subtalar joint (talocalcaneal joint) and adduction and abduction across the talonavicular and calcaneocuboid joints.

Stressing is not generally undertaken for the foot

Gait Is the patient able to weight-bear (able to walk two paces unaided)?

Other joints Examine the ankle

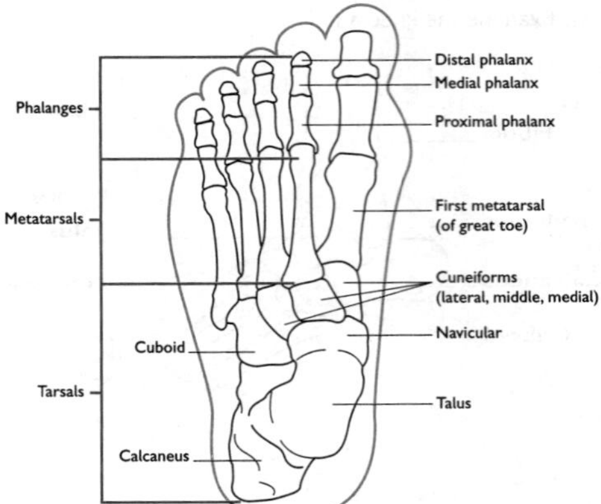

Shoulder examination (glenohumeral joint, *OHCS7* p662)

Inspection Look for swelling, erythema, abnormal bony prominences and the position that the arm and shoulder are held in by the patient; look at the joint from the front, side and back. Examine the skin over the joint and clavicle for signs of surgical scars, sinuses, cellulitis, swelling or deformity (loss of angle of the deltoid). Is there any wasting of the muscles around the shoulder girdle compared to the other side (deltoid, supraspinatus, infraspinatus)?

Palpation Feel for temp and bony landmarks (acromioclavicular joint, clavicle and spine of scapula). Check the cervical and upper thoracic vertebrae for tenderness. Feel the joint as it is moved for crepitus, clicks and instability.

Movement Active (allow patient to demonstrate their ROM) and passive movements (ask the patient to relax and move the joint yourself); abduction (0–90° with elbow flexed, 0–180° with elbow extended), adduction, internal (0–90°) and external (0–65°) rotation, flexion (0–180°) and extension (0–65°). Easing the arm through a painful arc (on abduction) should be undertaken carefully and passively.

Stressing ***Impingement test***: arm held at 90° abduction and internally rotated, if pain detected it is a positive test. ***Scarf test:*** left hand placed over right shoulder and vice versa, if pain detected it is a positive test (acromioclavicular joint pathology).

Other joints Examine the neck and scapulae

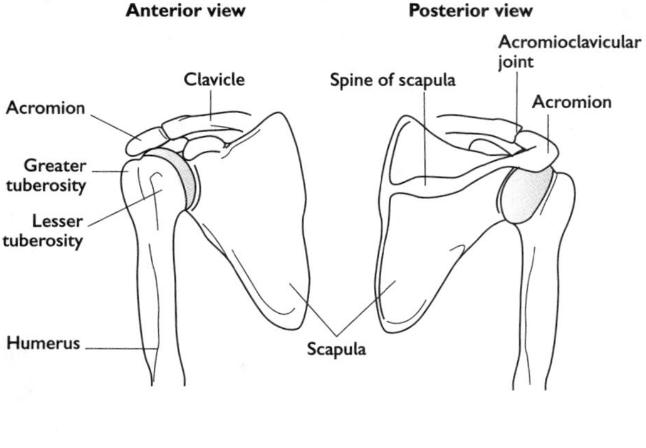

Elbow examination (*OHCS7* p666)

Inspection Look for swelling, erythema.

Palpation Feel for temperature and bony landmarks (medial and lateral epicondyles, olecranon). Pain over lateral epicondyle suggests 'tennis elbow' and over the medial epicondyle 'golfer's elbow'. Feel the joint as it is moved for crepitus, clicks and instability. Examine for rheumatoid nodules or psoriatic plaques over the olecranon.

Movement Active (allow patient to demonstrate their ROM) and passive movements (ask the patient to relax and move the joint yourself); flexion (0–150°) and extension (0°); pronation and supination.

Stressing is not generally undertaken for the elbow

Other joints Examine the shoulder and wrist

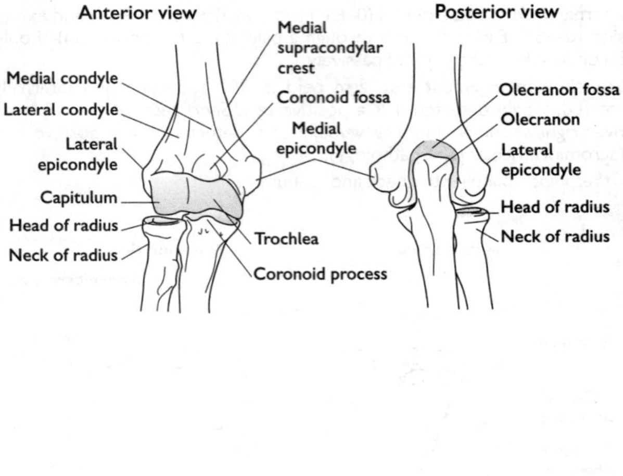

Wrist examination (*OHCS7* p668)

Inspection Look for deformity (eg Colles' fracture), break to the skin (open fracture) or features of rheumatoid disease (p410), scars over carpel tunnel

Palpation Feel for temperature, bony landmarks (styloid process of radius, head and styloid process of ulna) and for scaphoid in the base of the anatomical snuff-box

Movement Active (allow patient to demonstrate their ROM) and passive movements (ask the patient to relax and move the joint yourself); flexion (0–75°), extension (0–75°), radial (0–20°) and ulna deviation (0–20°), circumduction of the wrist relies on all four movements; pronation and supination

Stressing To see if painful

Other joints Examine the forearm and elbow

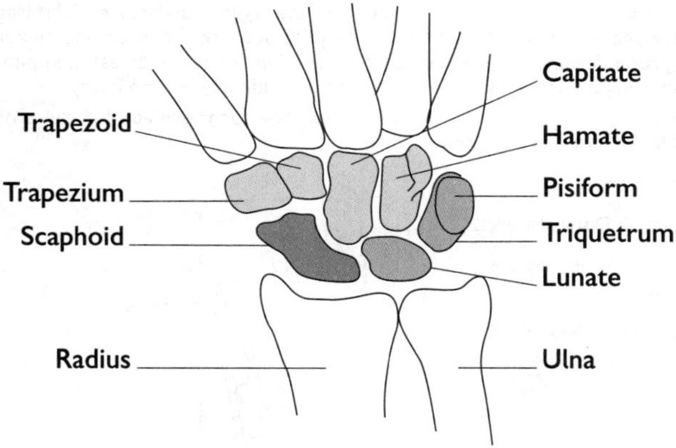

Hand examination (*OHCS7* p668)

Inspection Look for erythema, swelling, breaks to the skin, features of rheumatoid disease (p410) or osteoarthritis (p410), deformity or dislocation, muscle wasting, pitting of the nails.

Palpation Feel for temperature and along each metacarpal and adjacent phalanx, assessing for pain or crepitus. Check for cap-refill and cutaneous sensation.

Movement Active (allow patient to demonstrate their ROM by making a fist and opening hand fully) and passive movements (ask the patient to relax and move the joints yourself); flexion and extension of all MTPJ, PIPJ and DIPJ, abduction and adduction of all MTPJ and opposition and circumduction of the thumb MTPJ. Ask the patient to hold a pencil and write, pick up a mug, undo a button on a shirt or blouse, demonstrate pincer grip and then ask them to oppose their thumb and little finger and assess strength of this union.

Stressing Of the collateral ligaments of the digits is undertaken following trauma and dislocation to establish joint stability. Extensor and flexor (profundus and superficialis) tendon function should be assessed in penetrating or lacerating trauma to the hand to identify tendon injury.

Other joints Examine the wrist and examine for rheumatoid nodules or psoriatic rash at the elbows.

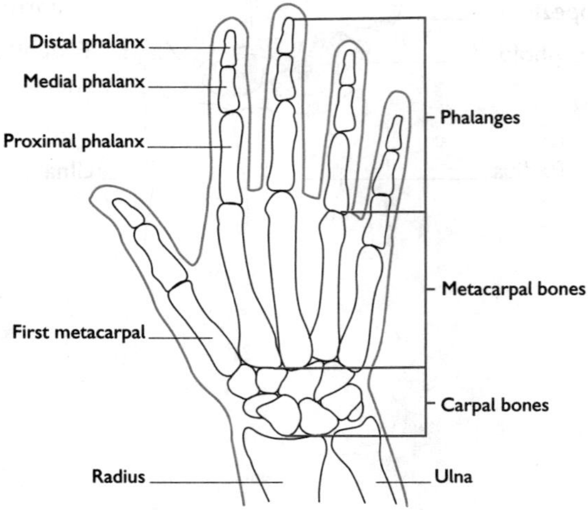

Back examination (thoracolumbar spine, *OHCS7* p670)

Inspection Look for deformity, especially loss of thoracic kyphosis or lumbar lordosis and lateral deviation from the midline (scoliosis).

Palpation Feel each vertebra for pain and with the patient prone palpate below the dimples of Venus on each side for sacroiliac tenderness.

Movement Active (allow patient to demonstrate flexion (touching of the toes with knees locked in extension) most people can touch their shins, if not their toes), extension (leaning backwards), lateral bending (lateral flexion) and rotation (best assessed with patient seated so pelvis is fixed). Passive – with patient supine, perform straight leg raise by elevating each leg in turn with the knee in extension (0–85°).

Measure Lumbar flexion can be measured using Schober's test (mark the level of the posterior iliac spine in the midline; make a further two marks, one 5cm below this and one 10cm above this; the distance between these two new marks measured when the patient is standing and then in full flexion – an increase of <5cm suggests limited lumbar flexion).

Other joints Examine the wrist and examine for rheumatoid nodules or psoriatic rash at the elbows.

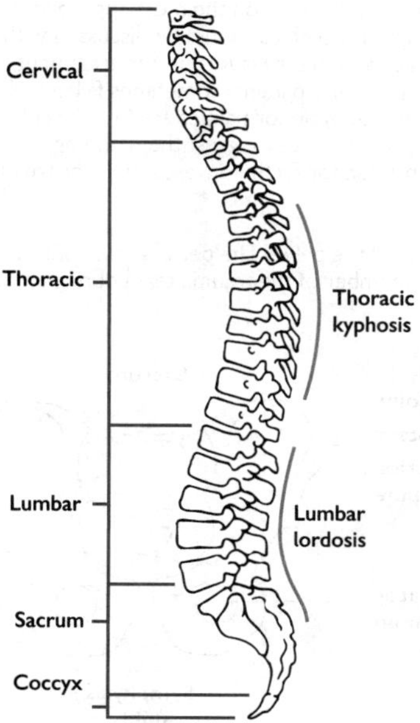

Musculoskeletal referrals

Checklist

Name, hospital number, age, gender, location

Presenting complaint, mechanism of injury, range of movement, rash, observations

X-ray results, inflammatory markers

Last food or drink, fitness for theatre

Inpatient referrals about musculoskeletal issues are usually about a hot swollen joint, to help manage an undiagnosed polyarthropathy or worsening of an existing polyarthropathy or to review a patient following an abnormal X-ray:

- *A hot swollen joint* this should always raise the question of whether this is a septic arthritis (p410). Early communication with an orthopaedic surgeon is essential to confirm or refute diagnosis and commence treatment as appropriate.
- *Managing polyarthropathy* most patients with an existing polyarthropathy are known to the rheumatology service and they will be happy to review the patient and advise on the most appropriate management. New-onset polyarthropathies should be discussed with a rheumatologist to ensure appropriate investigation and treatment.
- *Abnormal X-rays* elderly patients sometimes fall in hospital and sustain fractures or other bony abnormalities are found incidentally on X-ray. A radiology report will often suggest the pathology, but a surgeon may need to be consulted for further investigations or treatment.

Pelvis

Bony components of the pelvis. The pelvis should only be tested for instability by a senior member of the trauma team during a trauma emergency.

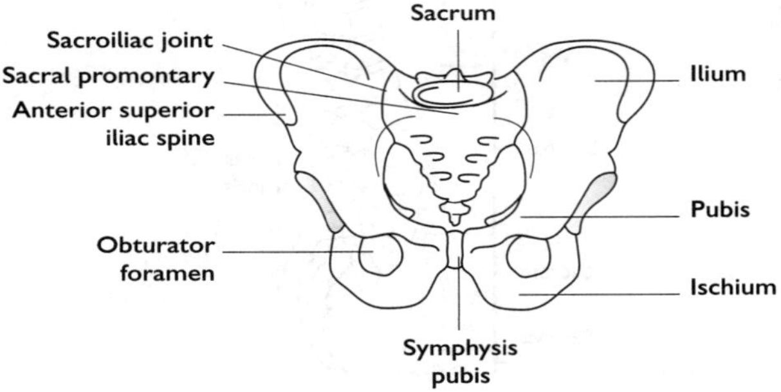

Musculoskeletal specialities as an F1/F2

Musculoskeletal jobs may be part of general surgery as an F1 (orthopaedics), general medicine as an F1 (rheumatology) or a specialist attachment.

Structure

- *Orthopaedics* elective surgery in patients of all age groups
- *Trauma* bone and soft tissue injury often requiring surgery
- *Rheumatology* mostly inflammatory conditions of joints and soft tissues, with a predominantly outpatient population

The job you will be expected to perform the following roles:

- Manage inpatients (investigations, referrals, theatre lists, prescriptions)
- Pre-operatively assess elective patients for theatre
- Clerk emergency admissions and instigate initial management
- Coordinate multidisciplinary post-operative rehabilitation
- Assist seniors in theatre
- Attend outpatient clinics, including fracture clinic

Aims try to do the following during your placement:

- Refine clerking skills and knowledge of the immediate and subsequent management of the more common emergency presentations
- Appreciate the roles of allied healthcare professionals in the assessment and rehabilitation of patients following illness/surgery
- Gain exposure to practical procedures in the ED/theatre/clinic
- Participate in outpatient clinics

Common cases

Fractured neck of femur (p355) often an elderly patient with coexisting pathology (eg renal impairment, dementia, COPD). Needs thorough medical work-up prior to surgery. Surgery should be undertaken within 24–48h to minimise complications of being bed-bound.

Elective hip replacement usually in their 60s and 70s, often with a good quality of life and usually with well-controlled comorbidity if any comorbidity at all; ideally very motivated and compliant with rehabilitation

Fractured long bones often young patients following sporting trauma or road traffic accidents; usually no pre-existing comorbidities, but may have other injuries (pneumothorax, facial injuries)

Septic arthritis (p410) this is a medical emergency and should be seen early by a senior member of the team

Rheumatology training

Initial route CT1 in core medical training
Further training competitive application for ST3 rheumatology
Exams MRCP part 1 required to apply for ST3 rheumatology

Trauma and orthopaedics training

Initial route CT1 in 'surgery in general' trauma and orthopaedics (p28)
Further training competitive application for ST3 trauma and orthopaedics
Exams MRCS required to apply for ST3 trauma and orthopaedics

Neurology

Role Neurologists look after the medical care of patients with organic brain disease or diseases affecting the nerves. They work closely with neurosurgeons and have some contact with psychiatrists. Much of the work is clinic-based, though there is a significant ward-based component.

Neurology history

Alongside taking a standard history (p98) the following are important:

Presenting complaint onset, duration, course (improving, worsening, relapsing–remitting), aggravating or alleviating factors, change with time of day, trauma

Neurological symptoms headache, pain, numbness, tingling, weakness, tremor, twitching, abnormal movements, loss of consciousness, seizures, abnormal smells, vision (loss, diplopia, flashing lights), hearing, swallowing, speech, balance, vertigo, nausea, vomiting, coordination, urinary incontinence or retention, impotence, faecal incontinence, constipation, personality, memory, language, visuospatial skills, change in intellect

Corroborating history in many neurological conditions the patient may not be able to describe all the symptoms eg seizure; try to get a history from a witness (acute) or family member (chronic)

Past medical history similar episodes, meningitis, migraines, strokes, seizures, heart problems, hypertension, psychiatric problems

Family history draw a family tree with all four grandparents and all their children and grandchildren, ask specifically about learning difficulties, disability, epilepsy, dementia, CVAs, psychiatric problems

Social history alcohol, smoking, illicit drugs, occupation, travel abroad, dominant hand

General examination

Alongside a standard examination (p100) the following are important:

Obs GCS, BP, HR, RR, glucose

General appearance posture, neglect, nutrition, mobility aids

Cognition tested using the Mini-Mental State Exam (p283) or 10-point Abbreviated Mental State Exam (p281)

Meningism photophobia, neck stiffness, Brudzinski's sign (flexion of both knees on testing neck stiffness), Kernig's sign (hamstring spasm on attempting to straighten the knee with hip and knee flexed), straight leg raise (hamstring spasm on passively flexing the hip)

Skin birthmarks, vitiligo, café-au-lait spots, lumps, tufts of hair/dimples at the base of the spine

Cranial nerve examination

Nerve		Function	Tests
Olfactory	I	Smell	Rarely tested
Optic	II	Vision	Visual acuity, visual fields, pupil reflexes, fundoscopy
Oculomotor	III	Eye movements, lift the eyelid, pupil construction	Eye movements, pupil reflexes
Trochlear	IV	Superior oblique	Move eye down and out
Trigeminal	V	Sensation to face, movement of jaw muscles	Facial sensation, jaw power, corneal reflex
Abducens	VI	Lateral rectus muscle	Move eye laterally
Facial	VII	Facial muscle movement, taste (anterior 2/3rd), salivary and lacrimal glands, stapedius muscle	Facial power
Vestibulo-cochlear	VIII	Hearing and balance	Whispering numbers, Weber's (forehead), Rinne's (behind ear)
Glosso-pharyngeal	IX	Taste (posterior 1/3rd), parotid gland, sensation of pharynx, nasopharynx, middle ear	Saying 'Ahh', swallow, gag reflex
Vagus	X	Sensation of pharynx and larynx, movement of palette, pharynx, larynx	Saying 'Ahh' (deviates away from defect), cough, swallow, speech, gag reflex
Accessory	XI	Movement of sternomastoid and trapezius	Shrug shoulders, turn head
Hypoglossal	XII	Movement of tongue	Stick tongue out (deviates towards defect), speech

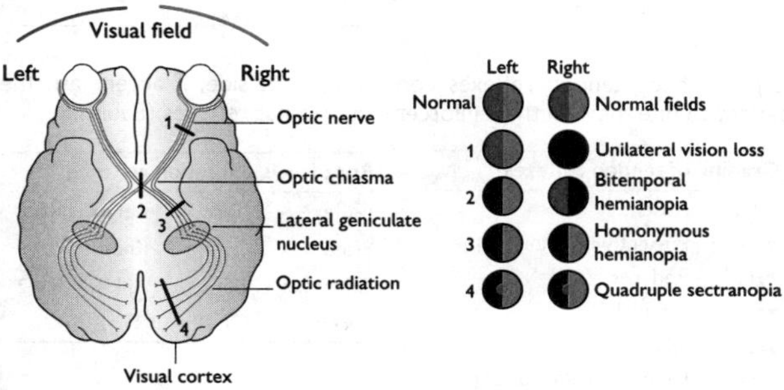

Optic pathways and effect of a lesion on the visual fields at various locations.

Peripheral nerve examination

Appearance posture, tremor, muscle wasting, fasciculation, abnormal movements, facial expression and symmetry, neglect

Hold out hands with palms up and eyes closed; look for drift (pyramidal defect), tremor or involuntary finger movement (loss of position sense)

Tone tone at wrist, elbow, knee and ankle (increased, decreased, clasp knife, cog-wheeling), clonus at the ankle (≥5 beats is abnormal)

Power isolate each joint with one hand so that only the muscle group you are testing can be used for the movement; compare each side:

Medical Research Council (MRC) grading of muscle power

Grade 0	No movement
Grade 1	Flicker of movement
Grade 2	Movement but not against gravity
Grade 3	Weakness but movement against gravity
Grade 4	Weakness but movement against resistance
Grade 5	Normal power

Root levels of main limb movements

Joint	Movement	Root	Joint	Movement	Root
Shoulder	Abduction	C5	Hip	Flexion	L1–2
	Adduction	C5–7		Adduction	L2–3
Elbow	Flexion	C5–6	Knee	Extension	L5–S1
	Extension	C7		Flexion	L5–S1
Wrist	Flexion	C7–8	Ankle	Extension	L3–4
	Extension	C7		Dorsiflexion	L4
Fingers	Flexion	C8	Big toe	Plantarflexion	S1–2
	Extension	C7		Extension	L5
	Abduction	T1			

Reflexes deep tendon reflexes comparing each side, if absent ask the patient to bite their teeth (reinforcement); plantar reflexes (Babinski)

Grading of tendon reflexes

0	Absent
±	Present with reinforcement
+	Reduced
++	Normal
+++	Increased
++++	Increased with clonus

Root levels of tendon reflexes

Reflex	Root	Reflex	Root
Bicep	C5–6	Knee	L3–4
Supinator	C5–6	Ankle	S1–2
Tricep	C7–8		

Coordination finger–nose, dysdiadochokinesia, tapping, heel–shin

Romberg's tested with patient standing with eyes open then closed, positive if more unbalanced with eyes closed; suggests sensory ataxia

Sensation pinprick, light touch, vibration, joint position; the spinal dermatomes of the front and back are shown below and spinal tracts on p512

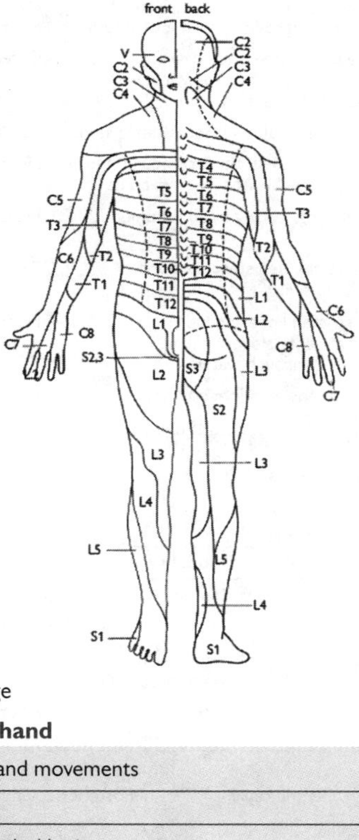

Gait see next page

Nerves of the hand

Innervation of hand movements

Movement	Nerve
Finger abduction and adduction	Ulnar
Thumb opposition and abduction	Median
Finger extension	Radial

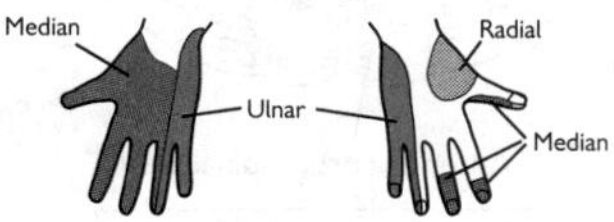

Gait

Gait	Description	Cause
Antalgic	Painful gait, limping, short weight-bearing on painful side	Mechanical injury, sciatica
Apraxic	Unable to lift legs despite normal power, magnetic steps/stuck to floor	Hydrocephalus, frontal lesions
Ataxic	Uncoordinated, wide-based, unsteady (as if drunk), worse with eyes shut if sensory	Cerebellar, sensory
Festinating	A shuffling gait with accelerating steps	Parkinson's
Hemiparetic	Knee extended, hip circumducts and drags leg; elbow may be flexed up	Hemiplegia eg CVA
Myopathic	Waddling, leaning back, abdomen sticking out	Proximal myopathy
Shuffling	Short, shuffled steps, stooped, no arm swing	Parkinson's
Spastic	Restricted knee and hip movements, slow, shuffling, 'wading through water'	Pyramidal tract lesion eg MS
Steppage	High steps with foot slapping, 'foot drop'	Peripheral neuropathy

Spinal tracts

Spinal tracts and anatomy

Tract	Modality	Crosses (decussates) at
Lateral corticospinal (pyramidal)	Motor	Medulla
Anterior corticospinal	Motor	Level of exit of the cord
Posterior columns (dorsal)	Light touch, vibration, position	Medulla
Spinothalamic	Hard touch, pain, temperature	Level of entry to the cord

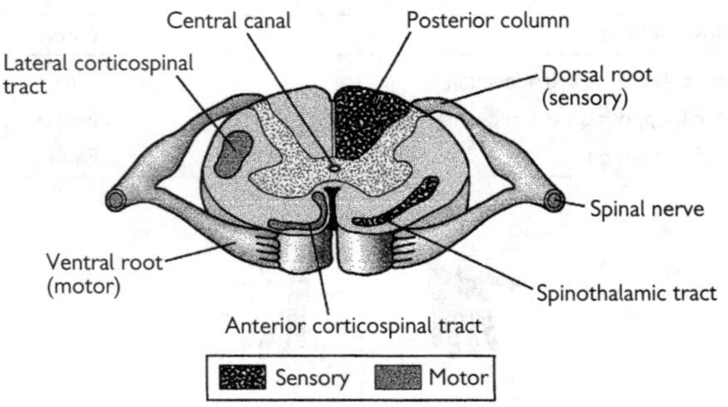

Neurology referrals

Checklist

Name, hospital number, age, gender, location

Description of neurology including plantar reflex, ±PR sensation/tone if appropriate

Latest set of observations including GCS, HR and BP

Referrals are usually made to the neurology registrar on-call. Try to give an impression of the urgency of the problem and which of the following would be appropriate:

- *Take over care* if the patient's underlying problem is neurological other than a cerebrovascular accident (CVA)
- *Ward review* if the patient has a neurological condition that is interfering with their care eg multiple sclerosis, poor epileptic control
- *Urgent clinic review* for urgent neurological conditions that do not need to be seen immediately eg suspected brain tumour
- *Routine outpatient clinic* for non-urgent neurological problems eg migraine

Neurology as an F1/F2

Neurology may be part of general medicine as an F1 or a specialist attachment. It can be a challenging speciality since many of the patients will have conditions that are extremely rare and may not have been even mentioned at medical school. The patients tend to have complex chronic problems often with minimal treatment available. An attachment in neurology is an excellent opportunity to become familiar with an area of medicine that many doctors find difficult.

The job you will be expected to perform the following roles:

- Clerk new admissions and initiate treatment plans
- Perform daily ward round and ensuing jobs
- Organising complicated blood tests
- Perform elective lumbar punctures for diagnosis and treatment

Aims try to do the following during your placement:

- Become familiar with neurological history taking and examination
- Learn to locate neurological lesions from examination findings (p508)
- Learn to interpret neurological imaging eg CT and MRI
- Learn how to perform lumbar punctures (p592)
- Learn about the social support and welfare available for chronic neurological conditions
- Spend time in neurological outpatient clinics
- Attend radiological and academic meetings

Training

Initial route CT1 in core medical training
Further training competitive application for ST3 neurology
Exams MRCP part 1 required to apply for ST3 neurology

Obstetrics

Role Obstetricians look after complex pregnancies from 12wk gestation to 6wk after birth; for uncomplicated pregnancies this is from 20wk gestation. The obstetrician should be informed about all women of ≥20wk gestation who present to hospital.

Obstetric history

Alongside taking a standard history (p98) the following are important:

Current pregnancy expected due date (EDD), gestation, last menstrual period (LMP), method of conception, scan results, site of placenta, rhesus status, concerns, attitude to pregnancy; ***current symptoms*** bleeding, other vaginal discharge, headache, visual disturbance, dysuria, urinary frequency or urgency, constipation, vomiting, GORD

Previous pregnancies number of pregnancies (gravida), number of deliveries ≥24/40wks (parity), miscarriages, terminations (reason, gestation, method), stillbirths, complications: vomiting, anaemia, bleeding, group B strep, BP, proteinuria, gestational DM, poor fetal growth, admission

Delivery history method of delivery and reason (vaginal, ventouse, forceps, elective/emergency Caesarean), gestation, birthweight, sex, complications (fever, prolonged rupture of membranes, CTG trace), postnatal baby problems (feeding, infection, jaundice), admission to SCBU/NNU, outcome (how is the child now), postnatal maternal problems (pain, fever, bleeding, depression)

Past gynae history previous problems, operations, STIs, see p484/486

Past medical history DVT, PE, DM, admissions, psychiatric problems

Family history DM, ↑BP, pre-eclampsia, congenital abnormalities, DVT, PE, multiple pregnancies

Social history support from family/partner, type of housing, employment, financial problems, smoking, alcohol, substance abuse

Gestation (wk)	Standard antenatal care: purpose of each visit
Booking	FBC, G+S, red cell antibodies, rubella, syphilis, hepatitis B, HIV serology, sickle-cell disease, BMI, BP, urine dipstick and culture
11–14	USS for gestational assessment and nuchal screening
16	Urine, BP, serum screening (for Down's and neural tube defects)
20	USS for anomalies
28	Fundal height, BP, urine, FBC, red cell antibodies, anti-D if rhesus –ve
25*, 31*	Fundal height, BP, urine
34	Fundal height, BP, urine, anti-D if rhesus –ve
36, 38, 40*	Fetal position, fundal height, BP, urine
41	Discuss induction, fetal position, fundal height, BP, urine

* For the first pregnancy only.

Obstetric examination

Fetal heart audible from 12wk using a Doppler ultrasound and 24wk using a Pinard stethoscope; it is faster than the mothers (110–160bpm)

Weight plot mother's weight and BMI (p640) at the booking visit only

Inspection striae, linea nigra (line of pigmentation from the pubic symphysis to the navel that darkens during the 1st trimester), venous distension, scars, oedema

Fundal height the fundus (top of the uterus) is palpable from about 12wk gestation; it should be measured from the top of the pubic symphysis to the top of the fundus with a tape measure. Between 16 and 36wk the fundal height in centimetres should be the same as the gestation ±2cm eg 23–27cm at 25wk. Fundal height is unreliable after 36wk.

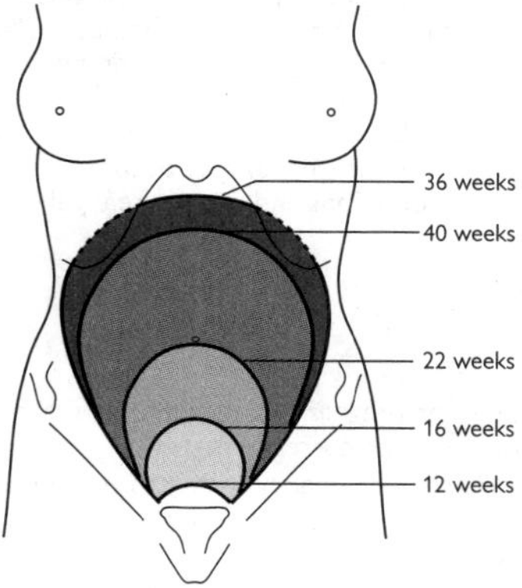

Fetal lie after 32wk it is possible to assess the position of the fetus by palpating across the abdomen for the fetal head:
- *Longitudinal* head palpable in midline
- *Oblique* head palpable in iliac fossa
- *Transverse* head palpable in lateral abdomen

Presentation palpation after 32wk can also assess the presentation though this is liable to change until about 36wk. By palpating both ends of the fetus the position of the head can be determined:
- *Cephalic* head is at the bottom
- *Breech* head is at the top

Engagement this is assessed by palpating the base of the uterus above the pubic symphysis between two hands to assess how much of the presenting part is palpable. If only the top 1/5th of the presenting part is palpable the fetus has 'engaged'

Blood pressure must be monitored regularly to assess for pregnancy induced ↑BP; consider urine dipstick and fundoscopy too

Urine dipstick for protein (pre-eclampsia) and glucose (DM)

USS lie, presentation and engagement can be confirmed on USS

Obstetric referrals

Checklist

Name, hospital number, age, location

EDD, gestation, LMP, gravida, parity

BP, urine dipstick result, latest set of observations

It is uncommon to make a referral to obstetricians except from the ED. If the women is <20/40 the referral should be made to gynaecology. Referrals should be made to the obstetric registrar on-call.

- *Joint care* acute medical or surgical problems in late pregnancy can be extremely challenging and need joint care from obstetricians and relevant specialists; admission may be to an antenatal, labour or non-obstetric ward depending on gestation and condition
- *Labour* women in other parts of the hospital may enter labour and need urgent transfer to obstetrics
- *Undisclosed pregnancy* late pregnancy may become apparent during investigation for other conditions and require referral for assessment and antenatal care

Obstetric definitions

General

Gravida total number of pregnancies including miscarriages, terminations, stillbirths, live births and current pregnancy

Miscarriage delivery/loss of pregnancy with no signs of life <24/40

Parity total number of live or stillbirths ≥24/40

Pre-term labour labour at <37/40

Puerperium the 6wk after delivery, often called the postnatal period

Stillbirth delivery of a fetus showing no signs of life ≥24/40

Termination medical/surgical removal of an unwanted pregnancy <24/40

Trimester pregnancy is described in three trimesters: first ≤14/40, second 15–28/40 and third 28-birth/40

Bleeding

Antepartum haemorrhage bleeding from the genital tract ≥20/40

Placental abruption early placental separation causing bleeding and pain

Placenta praevia part or all of the placenta in lower uterine segment

Postpartum haemorrhage blood loss >500ml in first 24h post-delivery (primary) or excessive blood loss between 24h and 6wk (secondary)

Delivery

1st stage of labour from regular contractions and 3cm cervical dilation to full dilation of the cervix

2nd stage of labour from full dilation of the cervix until birth of the baby

3rd stage of labour from after the birth of the baby until delivery of the placenta

Obstetrics as an F1/F2

May be part of a gynaecology and obstetrics placement in the F2 year. It is unusual to encounter women >20wk gestation in other specialities.

Structure most obstetricians are also gynaecologists though they may specialise more in one area. They have contact with two main specialities:

- ***Feto-maternal medicine*** obstetric specialists who look after high-risk pregnancies due to maternal medical conditions or fetal abnormality
- ***Neonatal medicine*** paediatricians run the neonatal intensive care unit and special care baby unit (SCBU); they will be present to resuscitate the baby at all births that are abnormal

The job you will be expected to perform the following roles:

- Carry the labour ward bleep for difficult deliveries and emergencies
- Clerk new admissions to labour ward or antenatal ward
- Perform daily ward round of antenatal, labour and postnatal ward
- Assist with instrumental deliveries and Caesarean sections
- Assist with other labour theatre operations eg repairing perineal tears
- See also job list under gynaecology p489

Aims try to do the following during your placement:

- Become familiar with obstetric history and examination
- Manage common problems in pregnancy eg ↑BP and pre-eclampsia
- Learn to help deliver babies by normal vaginal delivery (p594)
- Learn to interpret a cardiotocograph (CTG, p440)
- Observe/perform ventouse and forcep deliveries
- Assist with and perform Caesarean sections
- Become familiar with the management of postnatal problems
- Learn obstetric (p174) and neonatal (p172) resuscitation

Common cases

Pre-eclampsia (p438) ↑BP with proteinuria must be detected and treated to prevent life-threatening eclamptic seizures

Suboptimal CTG (p440) this suggests fetal distress so the fetus needs to be delivered urgently; this may require an emergency Caesarean

Antepartum haemorrhage (p439) this poses a serious risk to the mother and fetus; resuscitation and emergency Caesarean often offer the best chance of survival for both

Postpartum haemorrhage (p441) excess bleeding after delivery is an emergency that requires resuscitation and surgical treatment

Postpartum pyrexia (p441) along with the usual causes of pyrexia (p392) women can develop reproductive tract or breast infections after delivery, especially if the birth was difficult or prolonged

Training

Initial route ST1 in obstetrics and gynaecology

Further training no more competitive applications are essential for CCT

Exams MRCOG part 1 required for ST3

Oncology

Role Oncology is a speciality concerned with the diagnosis and management of patients with cancer. Oncologists treat cancers in every body system and there is usually ample opportunity for research and teaching.

Oncology history

Alongside taking a standard history (p98), the following areas should be covered:

Symptoms from the tumour lumps, swelling, pain (SOCRATES questions, see p428), cough, SOB, haemoptysis, secretions, infection, nausea, vomiting, anorexia, diarrhoea, constipation, PR bleeding, ascites, fractures, bone pain, polyuria, prostatism

General features of malignancy weight loss, fatigue, myopathy, weakness, mood disturbance

Effect on activities of daily living washing, dressing, personal hygiene needs, shopping, cooking, driving

Symptoms of treatment nausea, vomiting, oral/skin ulcers, stomatitis, gingivitis, diarrhoea, constipation, pain, anorexia

Past medical history DM, asthma, ↑BP, IHD, liver disease, jaundice, thyroid problems, anaemia, malignancy (and radiotherapy), epilepsy

Drug history chemotherapy regime, date of last dose, allergies

Family history malignancy

Social history smoking, alcohol, family support, living circumstances, home help, occupation, previous exposure to dyes/asbestos/coal tar

Oncology examination

The specific focus of the examination depends on the location of the tumour eg a patient with breast cancer should have a thorough breast exam (both sides), with attention also being paid to axillary lymph nodes, liver and spine. A thorough clinical examination is essential in all patients with cancer in order to recognise any comorbidities which may affect the treatment plan and also to identify any metastatic disease.

General examination	p100
Abdominal examination	p482
Respiratory examination	p542
Breast examination	p448
PR examination	p482

Oncology referrals

Checklist

Name, hospital number, age, gender, location

Type of cancer, stage/staging investigations, date of last chemotherapy

What the patient has been told about their diagnosis

Referrals are usually made in writing directly to a consultant oncologist. It is important to include the patient's pre-morbid condition and reports of staging scans in your referral letter so the oncologist is able to judge the best route of treatment for the patient. There are three subspecialities of oncology, so check with your consultant which would be the most appropriate to refer to:

- *Medical oncologists* specialise in chemotherapy
- *Clinical oncologists* provide chemotherapy and radiotherapy
- *Surgical oncologists* specialise in the operative removal of tumours

Chemotherapy definitions	
Neoadjuvant	Shrinks the tumour prior to surgery
Primary therapy	Curative treatment (eg leukaemia)
Adjuvant	Reduce the chance of relapse
Palliative	Aids symptom relief

Oncology as an F1/F2

Oncology is usually an F2 specialist attachment; it may rarely be part of general medicine as an F1.

The job you will be expected to perform the following roles:

- Clerk new admissions and initiate treatment plans
- Perform daily ward round and ensuing jobs
- Explain management plans with patients and relatives
- Provide on-call cover for oncology ±haematology/general medicine

Aims try to do the following during your placement:

- Develop the skills of history taking, physical examination, appropriate investigation and rational prescribing in patients with cancer
- Learn how to manage common oncological emergencies
- Become familiar with common chemotherapy regimens as well as their indications and side-effects; you should **never** prescribe or administer chemotherapy
- Gain experience in procedures eg pleural taps (p578)
- Learn the principles of good pain control (p428) and palliative care
- Develop communication skills (p52) with patients and relatives
- Learn about breaking bad news by observing seniors (p57)

Training

Initial route CT1 in core medical training

Further training competitive application for ST3 oncology

Exams MRCP part 1 required to apply for ST3 oncology

Ophthalmology

Role Ophthalmology is a large speciality, often with inpatients and a large outpatient population. Many cities now have 'eye hospitals' and/or 'eye casualty' departments which are dedicated to caring for acute and chronic eye disease. Assessment of ophthalmic disease is often undertaken on an outpatient basis and many of the surgical procedures can be done as day-case operations, allowing the patient to return home the same day.

Ophthalmic history

Alongside taking a standard history (p98) the following are important:

Major symptoms reduced/impaired vision or visual loss, red eye, discomfort (gritty or FB sensation), pain of the eye or soft tissues around the eye, dry eyes or excessive watering, itch, swelling, photophobia or haloes around lights, floaters or flashing lights, diplopia, discharge

Past ophthalmic history glaucoma, myopia, cataracts, previous surgery, glasses/contact lens prescription and last optometry check-up

Past medical history numerous systemic diseases can affect the eye, including DM, ↑BP, vascular disease, RA, SLE, thyroid disease, MS

Drug history ophthalmic medications, steroids, medications for co-existing disease; allergies

Family history glaucoma, retinoblastoma

Social history ability to self-care, impact eye disease has upon ADLs and home support received/needed

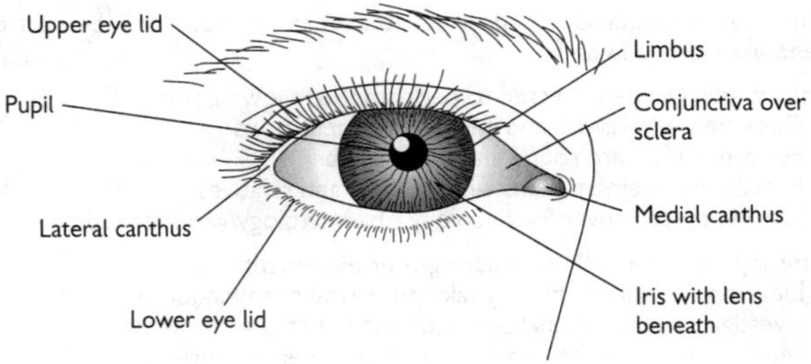

Surface anatomy of the right eye.

Ophthalmic examination

Inspection exophthalmos, proptosis, jaundice, pallor, xanthelasma, eyelids (cysts, inflammation), red eye, corneal arcus, periorbital cellulitis

Visual acuity this ***must*** be tested in ***all*** patients
- Use a Snellen chart at 6m to test visual acuity
- Make sure the patient is using the correct glasses for the test (reading vs. distance) if in doubt use a pin-hole in a piece of card
- If visual acuity is very bad assess ability to ***count fingers, awareness of movement*** (waving hand) or ***perception of light*** (pen torch)

Pupillary response and reflexes check the pupils are equal, reacting to light and accommodation (PERLA) and for a relative afferent papillary defect. Look for the red reflex (absent in dense cataracts).

Visual fields confrontation testing to identify any visual field loss and to establish if the defect is unilateral or bilateral (p509)

Ocular movements look for loss of conjugate gaze or nystagmus

Ophthalmoscopy allows examination of anterior structures and retina:
- With the ophthalmoscope set on +10 the cornea and anterior chambers can be examined. 1 or 2 drops of fluorescein highlights corneal ulcers, abrasions and foreign bodies, especially under the blue light
- With the ophthalmoscope set on 0 the user can visualise the retina. It is important to dilate the pupil with 1 or 2 drops of a weak mydriatic (eg 0.5% or 1% tropicamide) to allow full visualisation of the retina. The risk of causing acute glaucoma with mydriatics is small.

Slit lamp examination requires specialist training before use

Ophthalmology referrals

Checklist

Name, hospital number, age, gender, location, pre-existing ophthalmic disease

Presenting complaint, clinical findings and current management

Visual acuity, pupil reflexes, visual fields, appearance of cornea and retina

Inpatient referrals to ophthalmology are usually because of ophthalmic complications of systemic disease or for advice on pre-existing ophthalmic disease.
- *Ophthalmic complications* The eyes are involved in several systemic processes (shingles, RA) or iatrogenically in the treatment of them (ethambutol, amiodarone). Consultation with an ophthalmologist is often necessary to ensure the patient is receiving the most appropriate management or for advice in dealing with complications.
- *Pre-existing ophthalmic disease* It is not uncommon for patients with pre-existing ophthalmic disease to present to hospital with another pathology. Consultation with an ophthalmologist is sometimes necessary to check the patient's ophthalmic medication regimen.

Ophthalmology definitions

Accommodation	Alteration in lens (and pupil) to focus on near objects
Acuity	Ability of the eye to discriminate fine detail
Anterior chamber	Chamber anterior to the lens, containing aqueous
Aqueous	Fluid-like jelly in the anterior chamber of the eye
Blepharitis	Inflammation/infection of eyelids
Canthus	Medial or lateral junction of the upper and lower eyelids
Chemosis	Conjunctival oedema
Choroid	Layer sandwiched between retina and sclera
Ciliary body	Structure posterior to iris, containing ciliary muscle
Conjunctiva	Mucous membrane covering sclera and cornea anteriorly
Cycloplegia	Ciliary muscle paralysis preventing accommodation
Dacryocystitis	Inflammation of the lacrimal sac
Ectropion	Eyelids evert outwards (away from the cornea)
Entropion	Eyelids invert towards the cornea (lashes irritate cornea)
Fornix	Junction of sclera and lid conjunctiva
Fovea	Highly cone-rich area of the macula (yellow-spot)
Fundus	Area of the retina visible with the ophthalmoscope
Hyphaema	Blood in the anterior chamber seen as a red fluid level
Hypopyon	Pus in the anterior chamber seen as a white fluid level
Limbus	Border between cornea and sclera
Macula	Rim around the fovea, rich in cone cells
Miotic	Agent resulting in pupillary constriction (eg pilocarpine)
Mydriatic	Agents resulting in pupillary dilatation (eg tropicamide)
Papillitis	Inflammation of the optic nerve head (optic disc)
Optic cup	Depression in the centre of the optic disc
Optic disc	Optic nerve head seen as white opacity on fundoscopy
Posterior chamber	Chamber behind the lens, containing vitreous
Presbyopia	Age-related reduction in near acuity (long-sightedness)
Ptosis	Drooping eyelid(s)
Sclera	The visible white fibrous layer of the eye
Scotoma	Defect resulting in loss of a specific area of vision
Strabismus	Squint, loss of conjugate gaze
Tonometer	Apparatus for indirectly measuring intraocular pressure
Uvea	Iris, ciliary body and choroids
Vitrectomy	Surgical removal of the vitreous
Vitreous	Jelly-like matter which occupies the globe behind the lens

Ophthalmology as an F1/F2

Ophthalmology is largely an outpatient speciality, with patients managed medically and surgically (or both). Ophthalmic emergencies often present to the ED (or eye casualty) or via GPs. Preservation of sight in acute and chronic disease is paramount; early senior input should always be sought.

Structure

- *Outpatients* the vast majority of the patients under the care of a ophthalmologist will be in the community and intermittently in clinic
- *Inpatients* ophthalmic inpatients tend to have complex disease/ treatments or comorbidity which prevents their discharge
- *Theatre* most procedures are undertaken as day-case operations and often under local anaesthesia rather than general anaesthesia
- *Eye casualty* acute ophthalmic problems often presents here first. Many can be treated and discharged home ±follow-up.

The job you will be expected to perform the following roles:

- Manage inpatients (investigations, referrals, prescriptions etc)
- Assist in outpatients clinic
- Assess and manage eye casualty patients, under supervision
- Attend and participate in surgical procedures, under supervision
- Contribute at meetings and to the educational programme

Aims try to do the following during your placement:

- Learn to manage a ward of inpatients and their care
- Refine clerking skills and knowledge of eye diseases
- Become competent in basic ophthalmic clinical skills
- Assist in theatre and gain surgical experience
- Contribute to departmental audit or research

Common cases

Foreign body (FB) This is a common presentation to eye casualty and removal of the FB by a direct method or by irrigation is usually successful. Ensure the cornea is intact as corneal abrasions may have developed and should be followed up.

Ophthalmic shingles Herpes zoster reactivation results in shingles and the ophthalmic branch of the trigeminal nerve is often affected; 50% of those with ophthalmic shingles will have globe involvement, so specialist assessment and advice should always be sought.

Cataract surgery These patients are often elderly and may have co-existing disease. Most cataract operations are conducted under local anaesthesia, but this does not mean the patients do not need a good pre-operative assessment.

Training

Initial route ST1 in ophthalmology
Further training no more competitive applications are essential for CCT
Exams FRCOphth is required for ST3

Paediatrics

Role Paediatricians look after all children with medical problems from birth to when they finish year 11 at school (ie after GCSEs). They also provide advice for children admitted under other specialities eg surgeons, orthopaedics and plastics. Paediatricians often share care with these specialities for anything which is not routine.

Paediatric history

Basics age in days (until 1mth), weeks (until 2mth), months (until 2yr) or years, gender, who gave the history, who was present

Current state feeding and drinking, weight gain, wetting nappies/passing urine, fever, bowels, crying, runny nose (coryza), cough, breathing problems, pulling ears, drawing up legs, rash

Birth pregnancy problems and medications, gestation at birth (37–42/40 is normal), type of delivery (NVD, induced, ventouse, forceps, if LSCS ask why), resuscitation, special care, birthweight, premature rupture of membranes (PROM), group B strep (GBS), meconium, maternal pyrexia during labour, vitamin K (IM or oral), feeding (breast, bottle, type of milk)

Development see opposite and ask about school performance

Immunisations check the child is up to date with vaccinations; jabs will be postponed if the child is unwell or febrile beforehand and children often get a slight fever for <24h afterwards

Birth	May get tuberculosis (BCG) and/or hepatitis B
2mth	Diphtheria, tetanus, pertussis, *Haemophilus influenzae* type B (DTwP-Hib), polio, pneumococcal
3mth	Diphtheria, tetanus, pertussis, *Haemophilus influenzae* type B (DTwP-Hib), polio, meningitis C (MCC)
4mth	Diphtheria, tetanus, pertussis, *Haemophilus influenzae* type B (DTwP-Hib), polio, pneumococcal, meningitis C (MCC)
12–18mth	Measles, mumps, rubella (MMR)
4–5yr	Diphtheria, tetanus, pertussis (DTaP), polio, MMR
15–18yr	Diphtheria, tetanus, polio

Social history who the child lives with, who has parental responsibility, parental jobs, smoking, nursery/school attendance, type of school (mainstream, special needs), academic ability, sporting ability, friends at school, enjoyment of school, foreign travel

Family history family tree with parents and siblings, ask diplomatically about consanguinity if relevant, any illnesses in the family, how are their parents and siblings at the moment, asthma, eczema, hayfever, DM, epilepsy, other diseases specific to presenting complaint

Paediatric examination

Much of the examination can be performed by simply observing the child; this usually has the advantage of limiting tears. Approach younger children gently whilst they are sitting on a parent's knee and feeling secure. Examination is much the same as for adult patients, but include the following:

If unwell ABC and resuscitate, see p170

Chaperone ask a nurse to accompany you if a child of either sex is over 10yr, there is a child protection issue or you feel it is necessary

Hydration fontanelle, capillary-refill (≤2s), warm peripheries, mucous membranes, tears if crying, skin turgor, sunken eyes, tachycardia, lethargy

Respiratory grunting, head bobbing, nasal flaring, tracheal tug, cervical lymphadenopathy, recession (sternal, subcostal, intercostal)

Cardiovascular cyanosis (check mouth), clubbing, mottled skin, murmurs may radiate to the back, femoral pulses (coarctation), radiofemoral delay, dextrocardia, hepatomegaly (heart failure)

Abdominal check the external genitalia if young, relevant or boys with abdominal pain (torsion), never do a PR (though seniors might)

Neurological AVPU (**A**lert, responds to **V**oice, responds to **P**ain, **U**nresponsive), fontanelles, tone, reflexes (including Moro and grasp reflex if young), head circumference (growth chart), development:

Age	Gross motor	Fine motor	Speech	Social
6wk	Holds head in line	Eyes follow 90°	Startles to sound	Smiles
3mth	Lifts head up	Eyes follow 180°	Coos	Laughs
6mth	Sits unsupported	Transfers objects	Babbles	Objects to mouth
9mth	Pulls to stand	Finger–thumb grip	'Mama, dada'	Waves goodbye
12mth	Walks unsupported	Points	First words	Finger foods
18mth	Running	Scribbles	Asks for 'wants'	Feeds alone
2yr	Jumps	Copies line	2–3word sentences	Uses fork
3yr	Uses tricycle	Copies circle	Name and age	Dry by day
4yr	Hops	Copies cross	Counts to 10	Dry by night

ENT always check the ears and throat if there is a suspicion of infection; describe the colour, appearance and if an effusion or pus is present

Weight, height should be plotted on a sex-specific growth chart (p641–5)

Head circumference this is especially important in infants and those with neurological disease; the measurement should be plotted on a sex-specific chart

Neonatal examination

The baby check is a key component of life in paediatrics. Every baby should be examined prior to discharge from the hospital with the aim of:

- Identifying unwell babies (tone and respiratory rate are very important)
- Identifying abnormalities (especially reversible ones)

Preparation prior to the examination you should check the maternal notes for: significant maternal illness, gestation at birth, birthweight, type of delivery, problems at delivery (meconium, premature rupture of membranes (PROM), group B strep, low apgar scores)

Introduction introduce yourself to the mother/parents, offer congratulations and explain that you've come to examine their baby. Ask if the baby has passed **faeces** and **urine**, is **feeding** well and if there are any concerns; ask them to undress the baby to the nappy while you wash your hands.

Settled baby consider doing the following first as they are difficult if the baby is crying: listening to the heart and feeling the apex beat, counting the respiratory rate, feeling the femoral pulse and looking in the eyes

Crying baby try getting the baby to suck (pacifier, breast, bottle, parents little finger, your little finger), if this fails swaddle the baby and ask the parents to give the baby a feed then return in 30min

Overall take a few moments just to look, ask yourself is the baby: jaundiced, blue, dysmorphic, moving normally, breathing normally?

Neuro **tone** (degree of head support, spontaneous symmetrical limb movements), Moro reflex is not routinely performed

Head anterior and posterior **fontanelle** (bulging, sunken), **head circumference**, eyes **red reflex** (paler in pigmented babies), **face** (dysmorphic?), **ear** shape and position (tags, pits, top of insertion of pinna should be at the level of the eyes), **palate** (with your little finger), **suck reflex**

Hands/arms **fingers** (number, shape, colour), **palms** (single crease in 60% of Down's and 1% of non-Down's), symmetrical arm movement

Chest **respiratory rate** (RR >60 is abnormal), listen to the **heart**, apex beat, gently feel the clavicles for fractures

Abdo **palpate** (to exclude hepatomegaly, splenomegaly, masses), descended **testes**, patent **anus**, enlarged clitoris, **femoral pulses**

Hips/feet anterior hip creases (symmetrical?), **Barlow** test (flex hip to 90°, press posteriorly, feel for a click/clunk if the hip dislocates), **Ortolani** test (after Barlow's abduct the hips one at a time whilst pressing on the greater trochanter with your middle finger, feel for a click/clunk as the hip relocates), note repetition of these tests can cause hip instability, **ankles** (talipes, correctable or not), **toes** (number, shape, colour)

Turn baby over **spine** (straight), **sacrum** (lumps, dimples, hair tufts, skin defects), **buttocks** (blue spots – make a note), posterior hip creases

Plot in the red book: weight, head circumference, examination

Child protection

As a doctor you get a unique view of how a family works under pressure. Often this is inspiring and uplifting. Sadly it sometimes causes concern for the child's welfare and this must be acted upon. Most paediatric departments organise seminars to raise awareness of child protection.

Non-accidental injury (NAI) the following injuries should raise suspicion:

Injuries hand-shaped bruises (slaps), ring-shaped bruises (bites), bruises in unusual places, femur fractures <12mth, cigarette burns, subdural haematoma (shaking injuries)

History parents unable to account for injuries, mechanism inappropriate to age or injury, vague description of mechanism, inappropriate reaction from parent, recurrent injuries

There are four patterns of child abuse, they can occur together:
- *Physical* injuring a child eg shaking, hitting, burning; see NAI above
- *Emotional* this can be verbal abuse, unfair punishments or degrading behaviour; presentations include: domestic violence, child rapidly forms attachment with strangers, urinary or faecal incontinence in older children, resistance to leaving the ward
- *Neglect* the failure to provide the physical or emotional care that a child needs, presentations include: late disease presentation, dirty child, ±clothing, bad nappy rash, failure to thrive
- *Sexual* any sexual behaviour inappropriate to the child's age including verbal, images or contact; presentations include: allegation from child, trauma to genitalia, vaginal discharge or bleeding, sexually transmitted infection, fear of male staff, sexually inappropriate play/speech

If you suspect child abuse talk to your seniors immediately:
- Fully document any history and examination findings including who was present, ages of other children, where they are, bone or clotting problems in the family and who chaperoned you during the examination
- Do not accuse parents of child abuse at this stage
- If the parents attempt to leave do not stop them, inform social services who will contact the police

A registrar or consultant will take a full history and examination then:
- Treat the medical problems and injuries first
- Alert social services immediately
- Leave examination of the genitalia for a consultant paediatrician and police surgeon if sexual abuse is suspected

Further action may include:
- Checking old notes and X-rays, discussion with health visitor and GP
- Checking the Child Protection Register
- Skeletal survey (X-rays of whole body), FBC, clotting, CT head or cranial USS

Paediatric referrals

Checklist

Name, hospital number, age, gender, location

Weight in kg (p639 for conversion) and growth chart centile (p641–5)

Gestation, birth details, birthweight, pregnancy details

Who will stay with them (must be a parent/legal guardian)

Referrals are usually made to the paediatric registrar on-call. They need to know about every child admitted to paediatric wards and will give permission for the child to take a paediatric bed. Children might be admitted for the following reasons:

- *Medical care* give a full history and management plan
- *Injury* give full details of mechanism of injury and social history with the view to excluding child abuse
- *Surgery* a full history and management plan is often expected since paediatricians often review cases which are not clearcut or routine
- *Social care* rarely a child will be admitted if there is no alternative safe accommodation (eg unwell parent and no support). This is a last resort and the intended duration of admission will need to be stated.

A referral to the paediatricians may also be made to advise on the management of complex children under other specialities eg surgery. Paediatricians resent being used as a phlebotomy/cannulation service, but may be sympathetic for young children or if the referrer has tried (p560).

Paediatrics definitions

Capillary/cap-refill time for the skin to return to its normal colour after being pressed for 5s, <2s is considered normal, prolonged in shock

EBM expressed breast milk, either maternal (MEBM) or donor (DEBM)

Gillick competent describes children who have the capacity to give consent see p68

Infant a baby from birth to 1yr of age

Health visitor a nurse/midwife in the community who may be involved with child protection or development issues

Neonate a newborn baby from birth to 28d of age

NICU neonatal intensive care unit, a ward for the intensive care of newborn babies

NPA nasopharyngeal aspirate, a test for RSV that causes bronchiolitis

Play therapist a member of staff who uses play to inform children about unpleasant procedures (eg MRI), devices (eg central lines) or offers distraction for procedures (eg taking blood)

Postnates the ward that women and babies are admitted to after birth

SCBU special care baby unit, a ward for unwell newborn babies

Paediatrics as an F1/F2

Paediatric placements can form specialist placements of the F1 or F2 year. Many specialities have contact with children and this is a common source of anxiety; even 4mth experience helps to demystify paediatrics.

Structure paediatrics is divided into three main subspecialities:
- *General paediatrics* acute admissions, wards and hospital clinics
- *Community paediatrics* community clinics
- *Neonates* newborn babies until discharged from hospital; intensive care, high-dependency and special care baby units (SCBU)

The job you will be expected to perform the following roles:
- Carry the crash bleep for resuscitations and problematic births
- Clerk new admissions and initiate treatment plans
- Present children on the ward round
- Order and chase investigations
- Baby checks

Aims try to do the following during your placement
- Become familiar with taking a history and examining children
- Learn to examine newborn babies
- Learn to take blood samples from children using heel/finger pricks, winged needles, butterflys and cannulas (p560)
- Learn to cannulate children of all age groups
- Spend time on neonatal intensive care
- Spend time with community paediatricians
- Attend paediatric clinics (general and speciality)
- Attend a seminar on child protection
- Learn paediatric (p170) and neonatal (p172) resuscitation

Common cases

Fever without focus fever is taken very seriously in infants and young children in whom it can be the only sign of sepsis/occult bacteraemia. There is a very low threshold for a full septic screen (blood, urine, CSF and CXR) and admission for IV antibiotics.

Bronchiolitis a viral winter outbreak that makes infants have breathing and feeding difficulties

Viral-induced wheeze children below 3yr often wheeze when they have viral infections, this is different from asthma but treated the same way

Gastroenteritis children are very prone to vomiting and diarrhoea which can be highly infective for family and staff

Neonatal feeding problems neonates are often discharged before breast feeding is established and may present a few days later with dehydration, weight loss, jaundice and ↑Na^+

Training

Initial route ST1 in paediatrics
Further training no more competitive applications are essential for CCT
Exams the MRCPCH exam is required for ST4

Palliative care

Role Palliative care is a speciality concerned with symptom control. Traditionally this is mainly patients with cancer, but any chronic condition with difficult to manage symptoms can benefit from input from a palliative care physician. These doctors usually work closely with specialist nurses including Macmillan, lung, breast and colorectal nurses.

Palliative care history

By the time a patient is referred to a palliative care physician, the diagnosis should already be clear and a management plan formed. However, palliation is based on a holistic approach to patients, so alongside taking a standard history (p98), the following areas should be covered:

Current symptoms pain (SOCRATES questions, see p428), cough, SOB, haemoptysis, secretions, nausea, vomiting, anorexia, diarrhoea, constipation, abdominal swelling (ascites), bone pain, polyuria, pain due to urinary retention, prostatism

Psychological symptoms depression, anxiety, agitation, fears and worries about death and dying

Nutritional status and requirements ability to eat and drink, need for fortified drink supplements/high protein drinks (for comfort rather than treatment), fluid requirements

Family history malignancy, terminal illnesses

Social history smoking, alcohol, family support, children/dependants, living circumstances, home help, previous occupation, religious views, cultural/ethnic beliefs, financial concerns

Palliative care examination

A careful and thorough examination is essential when assessing a patient's palliative care needs. Terminally ill patients can suffer from a wide range of complaints and it is important that the physician picks up on these in order to best manage the symptoms.

General obvious pain at rest, cachexia, bruising, breathlessness, anxiety, restlessness, temp, feeding tubes, venous access

CVS/respiratory bibasal crackles, ↑JVP, wheeze, cough, stridor

Abdomen hepatomegaly, splenomegaly, ascites, palpable faecal loading, bladder

Other oedema (check back and sacrum), pressure sores, ulcers, oral hygiene

Palliative care referrals

Checklist

Name, hospital number, age, gender, location

Diagnosis, prognosis, main symptoms, current analgesia and pain control

Social support, specialist nurse involvement

What the patient and family have been told, resuscitation status

Referrals are usually made to a palliative care consultant in writing, however if the request is urgent you can usually telephone or bleep the palliative care team (physicians or specialist nurses) directly. Try to determine which of the following is appropriate:

- *Urgent ward review* if the patient is in distress from their symptoms despite starting appropriate treatment (p122)
- *Urgent advice* if you simply need to discuss a complex case
- *Ward review* if the patient would benefit from palliative care input but does not require this immediately

Palliative care as an F1/F2

Palliative care is a specialist FP rotation usually in the F2 year. It is an excellent opportunity to work in a unique medical speciality. The skills learnt will be extremely useful throughout medicine.

The job you will be expected to perform the following roles:

- Clerk new admissions and initiate treatment plans
- Daily patient round and ensuing jobs
- Review patients who are in pain
- Explain/discuss management plans with patients and relatives
- Provide on-call cover for palliative care and/or general medicine

Aims try to do the following during your placement:

- Learn to assess a patient from a palliative medicine perspective
- Understand the role of the palliative care team and its members
- Gain experience in pain and symptom control (p122) including pharmacological, psychological and physical interventions for pain
- Develop communication skills (p51) with patients, relatives, carers and multidisciplinary teams
- Improve your awareness of legal and ethical issues in palliative care
- Learn about breaking bad news by observing seniors (p57)
- Learn about bereavement (p124) and caring for dying patients
- Spend time working at a hospice

Training

Initial route CT1 in core medical training

Further training competitive application for ST3 palliative care

Exams MRCP part 1 required to apply for ST3 palliative care

Plastic surgery

Role care of patients with complex wounds (in cosmetically/functionally important locations or missing tissue) and reconstructive surgery (for functional and cosmetic improvement). They also manage severe burns after the initial resuscitation in the ED. In some hospitals plastics manage acute hand injuries, alternatively this may be the realm of orthopaedics.

Plastic surgery history

Along with a standard clerking (p98) ask about the following:

Wound/burn time of injury, mechanism of injury, contaminants (broken glass, gravel), immediate management, management in hospital, pain, other injuries, time of last meal, fluid resuscitation

Ulcers/pressure sores onset, trauma, duration, pain, cause, treatments, types of dressing, quantity of exudate, odour

Function restricted actions, effect on life, mobility

Past medical history DM, varicose veins, peripheral arterial disease, cardiac problems, neurological problems, previous ulcers, trauma

Past plastic history previous wound management or surgery, grafts, flaps, donor site, complications, infections, surgeon, hospital, previous ulcers (location, duration, treatment)

Drug history allergies, reactions to dressings, steroids, tetanus status (p357)

Social history occupation, dominant hand, hobbies/sports, smoking, social support

Plastic surgery examination

General HR, BP, signs of shock (p210), evidence of arterial or venous disease

Wound location, size (measure), shape, surface area (if irregular trace onto transparent sheets with grids), type (eg laceration, ulcer p384), shape of edges, sensation, depth, involvement of deep structures (blood vessels, tendons, bone, muscle), foreign bodies, wound bed (colour, granulation tissue), necrotic tissue, slough, exudate, sinuses, fistulae, odour

Skin by wound colour, temp, swelling, eczema, maceration, tenderness, capillary-refill, damage to skin surrounding the wound

Burns (p414) surface area affected, depth, sensation, evidence of inhalation injury (eg singed facial hair)

Away from wound limb pulses, distal capillary-refill, distal sensation, movement and power of distal structures

Plastic surgery referrals

Checklist

Name, hospital number, age, gender, location

Wound: size, depth, mechanism, location, involvement of deep structures, distal circulation and sensation, distal function (tendon injury)

Burn: surface area, depth/degree, mechanism, resuscitation details

Referrals are usually made to the plastics registrar on-call for:
- *Assessment/treatment* of wounds to cosmetically/functionally sensitive areas (eg hand, face, perineum), wounds with tissue loss or partial/full thickness burns
- *Outpatient clinic* for review of chronic problems eg severe ulcers, reconstructive surgery

Plastic surgery definitions

Langer's lines these correspond to the lines of collagen fibres in the skin; surgeons aim to cut along these lines to give the best cosmetic result

Epidermis the thin top layer of skin; it has no blood vessels

Dermis the layer beneath the epidermis that contains blood vessels, nerve endings and sweat glands

Skin graft skin (epidermis and partial dermis) transferred to another site

Tissue expander an inflatable device that is placed under the skin and inflated over weeks causing skin to expand; the excess is used in surgery

Granulation tissue connective tissue that replaces clots in wounds; it is pale pink, moist and soft to touch

Slough yellow exudate that often covers wound

Flaps

Flaps are when a section of tissue (skin, muscle, bone) is moved to a new site. There are different types depending on the blood supply:
- *Random pattern flap* blood supply from unnamed native vessels
- *Pedicled flap* remains connected to a named blood vessel
- *Free flap* named blood vessel reattached in a new location

There is a high risk of the blood supply failing post-operative so it is essential that the flaps are monitored up to every 15min and a surgeon contacted immediately if the blood supply is in doubt.

Monitoring flaps – if there is any change call for help immediately

	Normal	Arterial problem	Venous problem
Colour	Normal	Pale	Purple
Feel	Soft	Very soft	Hard
Temp	Warm	Cold	Cold
Cap-refill	<3s	>6s	<3s

Psychiatry

Role Psychiatrists diagnose and manage mental illness in patients of all ages. The majority of the work is in outpatient clinics or outside of hospitals, however there is a significant inpatient component.

Psychiatric history

Are you safe sit so the patient is not between you and the door, remove all potential weapons, be familiar with the panic alarm, check notes/ask staff about previous violence, low threshold for a chaperone

Set the scene make sure you are both comfortable, ensure privacy and that you will not be disturbed eg give the bleep to someone else, have tissues available, emphasise confidentiality

A psychiatric history requires all the components of a standard history (p98) along with the following specific features.

Basics full name, age, marital status, occupation, who were they referred by, current status under Mental Health Act

Past psychiatric history previous psychiatric diagnoses, inpatient/day patient/outpatient care, do they have a community psychiatric nurse (CPN), previous deliberate self-harm (DSH), previous treatments and effects, ever been admitted under the Mental Health Act

Medication history current and previous medications, effects, have they/did they take it, allergies/reactions, alternative/herbal remedies

Personal history

- *Childhood* pregnancy, birth, development (p525), associated memories, names of schools attended, reason if changed schools, types of school (mainstream/specialist), age of leaving school, qualifications
- *Employment* loss of jobs, which did they enjoy, why did they change, ask about unemployment and why
- *Relationships* current relationship(s) and sexual orientation, list of major relationships and reasons for ending, any children and who they live with and relationship to patient

Forensic contact with police, convictions or charges, sentences, outstanding charges

Personality how would they describe their personality now and before the illness? How would others describe it?

Social history occupation and duration of employment/unemployment, where they live, concerns over money, friends and relationships, hobbies

Drug and alcohol smoking, alcohol, illicit drugs

Family history family tree with parents and siblings, ages, occupations, relationships, illnesses

Mental state examination

Psychiatrists examine the mind through talking to the patient. Much of the information is gleaned whilst taking the history and should be organised under the following headings:

Appearance racial origin, age, dress, make-up, hairstyle, jewellery, tattoos, cleanliness, neglect, physical condition

Behaviour appropriateness, posture, movement (excessive, slow, exaggerated), gestures, tics, facial expression, eye contact, anxiety, suspiciousness, rapport, abnormal movements, aggression, distraction, concentration

Mood the patient's subjective assessment of their mood

Affect interviewer's objective assessment of mood and appropriateness of patient's response eg flat, reactive, blunted

Speech ***form*** accent, volume, rate, tone, quantity, hesitations, stuttering; ***content*** associations (derailment, changing between subjects), puns

Thought ***form*** rate, flow (eg blocked), connection (eg flight of ideas, derailment); ***content*** beliefs about self, beliefs about others, thought insertion/withdrawal/control/broadcast, beliefs about the world/future, delusions, overvalued ideas, obsessions, compulsions, ruminations, rituals, phobias

Perception illusions, hallucinations (visual, auditory, tactile, olfactory), unusual experiences, depersonalisation, derealisation

Cognition this can be tested formally using the Mini-Mental State Examination (MMSE) on p281, often the Abbreviated Mental Test Score (AMTS) is used instead (p279)

Risk thoughts of deliberate self-harm, suicide, harming others, plans, acquiring equipment, writing notes, previous suicide attempts

Insight awareness of illness and need for treatment

The Mental Health Act 1983

This table gives a brief summary of the commonly used sections for formally admitting patients under the Mental Health Act:

Section	Length	Applicant	Doctors	Comments
2	28d	Nearest relative or approved social worker	Two (one approved)	Assessment only
3	6m	Nearest relative or approved social worker	Two (one approved)	Allows treatment, can be extended
4	72h	Nearest relative or approved social worker	One	Allows emergency treatment
5(2)	72h	The doctor running the ward or a representative eg F2	One	Prevents inpatients from leaving ward
5(4)	6h	A nurse on the ward	None	Prevents inpatients from leaving

Psychiatric referrals

Checklist

Name, hospital number, age, gender, location

Previous psychiatric problems including current and previous status under Mental Health Act (p535) and psychiatric consultant

Current mental state including suicidal ideation and risk (p307)

Referrals are usually made to the psychiatry registrar on-call. Try to be clear about the urgency of assessment (inpatient vs. outpatient). The majority of referrals made during the foundation years will be:

- *Assessment of an inpatient* give details of why a mental health problem is being considered for this patient, current medical problems and the extent to which an alternative cause has been ruled out
- *Deliberate self-harm* the patient should be 'medically stable' before they are referred to psychiatry, this means that all injuries should be suitably treated and observation periods completed so that the patient is ready for discharge except for their mental state
- *Acute psychosis* the patient may need to be held under the Mental Health Act so psychiatric input is required early on

Psychiatry definitions

Approved doctor a doctor entitled to recommend admission under Section 2 or 3 Mental Health Act; they are approved under Section 12(2)

Cognition the process of thinking, reasoning and remembering

Compulsion repetitive behaviours in response to obsessions; often to relieve the distress caused by them eg washing hands

Delirium acute onset of severe confusion may be associated with hallucinations; caused by an organic process eg sepsis

Delusion a fixed, false belief that goes against available evidence and is not explained by the person's religious or cultural background

Dementia deterioration of cognition that affects daily life

Derailment rapid switching of topics without an obvious common thread

Derealisation altered sense of reality as if detached from surroundings

Depersonalisation altered sense of self as if detached or outside the body

Flight of ideas rapid switching of topics where the thread of connection can be determined (eg sound, content), cf derailment

Formal admission admission under a section of the Mental Health Act

Hallucination a false sensory perception eg hearing voices

Illusion misinterpreting a sensory perception eg seeing a shadow and thinking it is a person

Informal admission voluntary admission as a psychiatric inpatient

Obsession recurrent unwanted thoughts or images eg my hands are dirty

Ruminations a compulsion to consider an idea or phrase

Psychosis disordered thinking and perception manifesting as delusions and/or hallucinations

Psychiatry as an F1/F2

Psychiatry may be a specialist placement in F1 or F2. The approach is very different from other specialities which may be disconcerting, however psychiatric problems are common at all ages so the experience will be useful.

Structure you may have contact with the following sub-specialities:
- *Liaison* psychiatrists who see patients on non-psychiatric wards with mental health problems eg depression, anxiety, delirium
- *Adult* the main speciality seeing inpatients and outpatients
- *Old age* specialise in the mental health problems of the elderly
- *Child and adolescent* specialise in the mental health problems of the young (cut-off is the same as for paediatrics ~16y see p525)
- Other specialities include learning disability, rehabilitation, substance misuse, psychotherapy and forensics

The job you will be expected to perform the following roles:
- Carry the bleep for urgent psychiatric problems
- Clerk new admissions and initiate management plans
- Manage any coexisting medical problems of the psychiatric inpatients
- Attend outpatient clinics
- Attend multidisciplinary meetings

Aims try to do the following during your placement:
- Become familiar with psychiatric history and mental state examination
- Gain experience in diagnosing and treating acute psychiatric illness
- Learn about treatment modalities in psychiatry including medications and psychotherapy
- Spend time in other psychiatric subspecialities
- Learn about the Mental Health Act and how it is applied to patients

Common cases

Depression (p311) psychiatrists encounter a complete range of low mood from single mild episodes to severe recurrent episodes associated with psychosis

Deliberate self-harm (p305) this may be a medication overdose or superficial cutting; a risk assessment is a vital part of the management

Schizophrenia (p312) a chronic psychotic disorder that often presents acutely requiring inpatient assessment and treatment

Bipolar disorder (p310) Severe fluctuations in mood from depression to mania

Obsessive-compulsive disorder anxiety disorder presenting with repetitive and intrusive thoughts, images or sounds; often associated with compulsive behaviours which are an attempt to reduce the distress

Training

Initial route CT1 in psychiatry
Further training competitive application for ST4 in psychiatry specialities
Exams parts 1 and 2 of MRCPsych required for ST4 application

Radiology

Role The radiology department is a crucial lynchpin at the centre of most hospitals, with most other specialities now heavily dependent upon radiological imaging for all aspects of patient care (screening, diagnosis and treatment). With advances in diagnostic radiology and the birth of interventional radiology this has become a high-tech and dynamic speciality in which to work.

Radiology history

Radiologists don't often fully clerk their patients, but there are some salient features in the patient's history it is useful to ascertain:

Allergy it is crucial to know if the patient has ever had an allergic reaction to contrast media or iodine

Drugs it is important to know if a patient is taking anticoagulants or antiplatelet agents prior to performing some interventional procedures

Metal implants or metal fragments MRI relies on the creation of strong magnetic fields which attract ferromagnetic metals. There are strict guidelines on what implantable metals can be exposed to MRI scans, and local guidelines should be checked.

Ability to lay flat some investigations require the patient to lay flat (such as CT and MRI scans). If the patient has severe orthopnoea then alternative imaging modalities may have to be considered.

Ability to lay still some investigations require the patient to lay still for potentially long periods (eg CT and MRI imaging). This is often hardest for small children and for patients with learning difficulties. It is sometimes necessary for an anaesthetist to attend and administer a general anaesthetic.

Claustrophobia some patients are highly claustrophobic and would be unable to tolerate having an MRI scan. Sedation or even a general anaesthetic may be necessary.

Radiology preparation

Blood tests radiological contrast is nephrotoxic in susceptible patients, and so the radiologist may want to know the latest set of U+Es. When performing procedures which have the potential to bleed, it is often normal to check the patient's clotting and platelets beforehand.

Contrast oral contrast is usually given on the ward, whereas intravenous contrast is usually given during the procedure itself

Ultrasound for abdominal ultrasound, it is common to ask the patient to be fasted and for them to have a full bladder

Radiology referrals

Checklist

Name, hospital number, age, gender, location

Possible diagnoses and diagnoses which need to be excluded

Specific question(s) which can be answered by imaging

Renal failure (contrast), urine β-hCG (radiation), metal objects (MRI)

The radiology request form is essentially a referral from one team to another and as such it should contain as much information about the patient as would be given in any other situation; it just has to be very condensed. As well as your name and signature, it must include:

- *Patient details* name, address, DoB, location within the hospital
- *Examination required* the specific examination required
- *Clinical details* a very brief summary of the history, clinical findings, results of relevant investigations and presumed diagnosis
- *Questions to be answered* every diagnostic investigation should be undertaken to answer specific questions, even if these are negative findings – does the patient have: pneumonia, pneumothorax, PE?
- *Urgency* how quickly does this investigation need to be undertaken?

Talking to a radiologist prior to submitting a more complex radiology request will ensure the most appropriate investigation is undertaken to answer the specific questions your team has raised.

Radiology as an F1/F2

Radiology may be undertaken as an F2 specialist placement, or rarely F1. It is a chance to learn some extremely valuable skills that will be of use in almost all specialities.

The job you will be expected to perform the following roles:

- Work alongside various members of the radiology team
- Learn how radiological images are obtained
- Attend and participate in radiology reporting sessions
- Attend and participate in radiology lists
- Participate in educational programmes (learning and teaching)

Aims try to do the following during your placement:

- Be able to report CXR, AXR and contrast studies
- Become confident in interpreting limb X-rays
- Be able to perform basic ultrasound techniques
- Gain basic understanding of CT and MRI image interpretation
- Spend time working with an interventional radiologist
- Observe less familiar radiological techniques eg radio-isotope imaging

Training

Initial route ST1 in clinical radiology
Further training no more competitive applications are essential for CCT
Exams the FRCR exam should be completed by the end of ST3

Renal medicine

Role Renal physicians manage patients with renal failure (including dialysis and post-transplant) and renal disease (eg glomerulonephritis)

Renal medicine history

Alongside taking a standard history (p98) the following are important:

Major symptoms polyuria, anuria, prostatism (urgency, hesitancy, poor stream, terminal dribble), haematuria, oedema, renal colic, incontinence, malaise, lethargy, N+V, anorexia, weight loss, itching

Past medical history DM, ↑BP, recurrent UTIs, renal/ureteric stones, myeloma, known renal impairment/failure, previous vesicoureteric reflux

Drug history nephrotoxics (including NSAIDs, ACEi, aminoglycosides)

Social history foreign travel

Occupational history past and present jobs, exposure to dyes

Family history polycystic kidney disease, DM, ↑BP

Renal medicine examination

Lying flat, supine

General inspection mental state, RR (?Kussmaul breathing), hiccups, comlexion (?sallow), hydration (***dehydrated***: sunken eyes, dry lips/tongue; ***fluid-overload:*** peripheral oedema, pulmonary oedema)

Hands leuconychia, brown nails

Arms bruising (purpura), pigmentation, scratch marks, fistula, BP (lying and standing)

Face eyes (anaemia, jaundice), mouth (dehydration, ulcers, fetor), rash

Neck JVP

Abdomen inspect (scars, transplanted kidney, dialysis port), palpate (ballot kidneys, bladder, liver, spleen, lymph nodes), percuss (ascites), auscultate (renal artery bruits), PR for prostate

Back oedema, loin tenderness on percussion

Chest CVS and RS examination (pericarditis, heart failure, fluid overload)

Legs oedema, bruising, pigmentation, scratch marks, neuropathy, proximal weakness (myopathy)

Urinalysis glucose, blood, protein, nitrites

Other fundoscopy (DM and ↑BP changes), blood glucose, weight

Renal medicine referrals

Checklist

Name, hospital number, age, gender, location

Presenting complaint, hydration status, observations, initial U+E and blood gas

Previous history including renal biopsy, dialysis, transplant

Response to treatment, urine output, current U+E and GFR (if known, p321)

Referrals to the renal team are usually for advice on the management of acute or chronic renal impairment/failure, or to discuss the possibility of urgent dialysis for established or newly diagnosed renal failure.

- *Acute renal failure advice* some inpatients may be initially cared for by a non-renal team (endocrine, general surgery etc) but develop a new renal problem or have existing renal disease for which discussion with a renal physician may be necessary to ensure appropriate steps are being taken to prevent further renal damage and maximise the potential to restore renal function.
- *Consideration of urgent dialysis* it's not uncommon for patients who are established on dialysis to present acutely to hospital and subsequently need transferring to a dialysis centre for urgent dialysis to offload fluid or correct an electrolyte imbalance. Occasionally a patient who has not had dialysis before will need this, and the decision between ITU dialysis (often haemofiltration) and transferring to a dialysis unit will be decided by senior team members. Hyperkalaemia (p326) should usually be addressed prior to interhospital transfers.

Renal replacement therapy

Haemodialysis The patient's blood is pumped past a semi-permeable membrane on the other side of which is a dialysis solution (dialysate). Small molecules (ions, urea etc) and water cross from the blood to the dialysate due to concentration gradients. This form of renal replacement can leave the patient intravascularly depleted, so postural hypotension immediately following is relatively common. Typically patients need 3–4 sessions per week, each lasting 3–4h. This commonly relies on a fistula.

Haemofiltration The patient's blood is pumped past a semi-permeable membrane, and increased hydrostatic force causes molecules and water to be filtered out and form the haemofiltrate, which is discarded. Water and electrolytes are added back to the filtered blood before it is returned to the patient. Haemofiltration is a slow process and often runs for 12–24h at a time, and is usually used mainly in critical care areas.

CAPD **C**ontinuous **A**mbulatory **P**eritoneal **D**ialysis is when the peritoneum is filled with a hyperosmolar fluid and left for about 8h. Water, ions and waste products are drawn into the fluid which is then drained off and discarded. The whole cycle can then be repeated. This relies on a CAPD catheter being in situ, usually on the lower anterior abdominal wall.

Respiratory medicine

Role Respiratory physicians manage patients with chest disease. A large proportion of this is asthma, COPD, lung cancer and pneumonia.

Respiratory medicine history

Alongside taking a standard history (p98) the following are important:

Major symptoms cough, sputum, shortness of breath, wheeze, chest pain, fevers and sweats, weight loss, hoarseness, snoring, day sleepiness

Past medical history chest infections/pneumonias (as child or adult), tuberculosis, HIV status and risk factors, allergy, rheumatoid disease

Drug history respiratory drugs (inhalers, steroids etc), vaccination history (especially BCG, Hib, pneumococcus), drugs known to cause respiratory problems (bleomycin, methotrexate, amiodarone etc), allergies

Social history tobacco use (expressed in pack years (ie 20 cigarettes a day for 1year = 1pack year)) and social exposure to tobacco smoke if non-smoker, pets, exposure to other family members with respiratory problems (TB etc), illicit drug use (cannabis)

Occupational history past and present jobs, asking specifically about dust exposure, asbestos, animal dander

Family history asthma/atopy, cystic fibrosis, emphysema

Functional status of breathlessness (NYHA classification)
Class I – disease present but no dyspnoea during ordinary activity
Class II – dyspnoea during ordinary activities (eg walking to the shops)
Class III – dyspnoea during minimal activities (eg making a cup of tea)
Class IV – dyspnoea at rest

Respiratory medicine examination

Lying at 45°

General inspection O_2 requirements, cough, audible wheeze or stridor, rate and depth of respiration, use of accessory muscles, body habitus

Hands clubbing, peripheral cyanosis, tar staining, wasting/weakness of intrinsic muscles, HR, fine tremor of β-agonists, flapping tremor of CO_2 retention

Face eyes (Horner's syndrome, anaemia), mouth (central cyanosis), voice

Neck trachea position (±scars), JVP

Chest anteriorly inspect (shape, scars, radiotherapy marks), palpate (supraclavicular nodes, axillary nodes, expansion, vocal fremitus, apex beat, parasternal heave), percuss, auscultate

Chest posteriorly inspect, palpate (including cervical nodes), percuss, auscultate

Other peripheral oedema, calf erythema/tenderness, temperature chart, breast examination, abdominal examination, PEFR, sputum pot

Respiratory medicine referrals

Checklist

Name, hospital number, age, gender, location

Probable diagnosis, severity and previous (home) and current treatments

Observations, PEFR O_2 saturations and ABG on air unless very O_2 dependant

Usual exercise tolerance. Serial CXR findings/inflammatory markers.

Referrals to the respiratory team are usually about management of chronic disease, though urgent referrals for advice or intervention are sometimes necessary.

- *Request respiratory review* some inpatients may be initially cared for by a non-respiratory team (endocrine, general surgery etc) but have an acute or chronic respiratory problem requiring discussion with a respiratory physician
- *Urgent respiratory advice* the on-call general medical team are usually the first port of call for medical problems in the ED and inpatients, but sometimes a respiratory opinion is still needed for advice (eg open TB) or for an interventional procedure (eg urgent bronchoscopy)

Respiratory medicine as an F1/F2

Respiratory medicine may be part of general medicine as an F1 or a specialist attachment. Respiratory disease is common throughout medicine so it is important to learn how to manage these conditions well.

The job you will be expected to perform the following roles:

- Clerk new admissions and initiate treatment plans
- Perform daily ward round and ensuing jobs
- Manage acute respiratory deteriorations on the ward
- Explain the diagnosis and treatment plan to the patient and relatives

Aims try to do the following during your placement:

- Become familiar with history taking and examining respiratory patients
- Become confident at interpreting CXRs (p620)
- Learn to interpret respiratory function tests (p624)
- Learn to perform pleural taps (p578) and insert chest drains (p580)
- Learn to manage COPD (p221) and asthma (p223)
- Spend time in outpatient clinics
- Learn the role of non-invasive ventilation (NIV, p221)
- Learn about breaking bad news by observing seniors (p57)
- Observe bronchoscopy ±thoracoscopy
- Gain exposure to patients on medical HDU (if possible)

Training

Initial route CT1 in core medical training
Further training competitive application for ST3 respiratory medicine
Exams MRCP part 1 required to apply for ST3 respiratory medicine

Urology

Role Urology is a big surgical speciality, often with inpatients (planned and unplanned admissions) and a large outpatient population. The speciality is concerned with the urogenital tract in both males and females and there is some overlap with gynaecology, plastic surgery, nephrology and paediatric surgery.

Urology history

Alongside taking a standard history (p98) the following are important:

Major symptoms prostatism (urgency, hesitancy, terminal dribble, poor stream, nocturia), haematuria, renal colic, passing stones in the urine, incontinence, malaise, N+V, anorexia, weight loss, itching, impotence, infertility, problem with long-term urinary catheter (urethral or suprapubic), bone pain, tight foreskin, recurrent balanitis, testicular pain/swelling

Past medical history DM, ↑BP, recurrent UTIs, renal/ureteric stones, known renal impairment/failure, gout, neurological disease

Obstetric history number of children, mode of delivery and any complications

Drug history nephrotoxics (including NSAIDs, ACEi, aminoglycosides), bladder neck relaxants, infertility or impotence drugs, antiandrogens; allergies

Social history foreign travel, ability to cope with ADLs

Occupational history past and present jobs, exposure to dyes

Family history polycystic kidney disease, DM

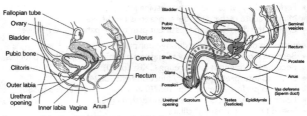

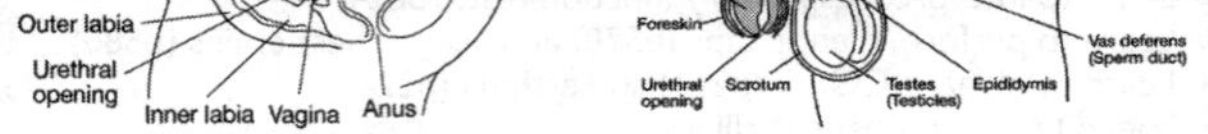

Anatomy of the female (left) and male (right) urogenital systems.

Urology examination

General inspection pain or discomfort, hydration

Hands leuconychia, brown nails, pale nail beds, HR

Arms BP

Face eyes (anaemia, jaundice), mouth (dehydration)

Neck JVP

Abdomen inspect (distended bladder, scars, transplanted kidney, dialysis port), palpate (ballot kidneys, bladder, liver, spleen, lymph nodes), percuss (enlarged bladed, ascites), auscultate (renal artery bruits)

Back oedema, loin tenderness on percussion

Genitalia see below

Rectum palpate nature of the prostate in the male, feeling for size, surface, consistency and symmetry. Rectal examination may also be useful in the female who has lower urinary tract symptoms.

Neurology check for neurological signs in the legs (tone, power, sensation, reflexes)

Examining male genitalia

General inspection look for any ulceration (including retracting foreskin and checking the glans), warts, scars or sinuses, urethral discharge, tight foreskin (phimosis) or retracted foreskin which is stuck leaving the glans exposed (paraphimosis). Observe the scrotum for skin changes or oedema and, whilst the patient is standing, the lie of the testes (the left testis usually hangs lower than the right and both testes lie longitudinally – a high testis with a transverse lie may indicate torsion, though a torted testis may also appear normal).

Palpate each testis in turn between the fingers and the thumb feeling for texture, tenderness, nodules and to compare left to right. An absent testis may be maldescended and trapped in the inguinal canal. Examine epididymis and follow it up superiorly to the spermatic cord and up into the inguinal ring. Palpate inguinal lymph nodes or maldescended testis.

Examining female genitalia

See p487

Urology referrals

Checklist

Name, hospital number, age, gender, location

Presenting complaint, symptoms of prostatism, trauma, renal/urological disease, weight loss

Observations, PR findings, palpable bladder, hydration status (p319)

Urine dipstick, urine microscopy, PSA, if catherised volume of urine drained

Inpatient referrals to a urologist are often related to acute on chronic retention of urine, problems with catheters or interspeciality referrals during surgery or following radiological examinations.

- *Urinary retention* acute on chronic retention is common in middle-aged men and often related to an enlarged prostate. The acute episode is usually resolved by urethral catheterisation, though follow-up is necessary to perform a trial without catheter (TWOC) and to fully investigate the patient.
- *Catheterisation* this is usually achieved through the urethra with ease, though there are occasions where it can be difficult or where a suprapubic catheter is indicated. A urologist is usually the most skilled person at catheterisation, though they will not take kindly to being bleeped at 3am to perform a routine catheter change.
- *Abdominal malignancy* intra-abdominal malignancy often involves the urogenital tract and urologists are often consulted by general surgeons during a surgical procedure or when planning surgery to avoid causing unnecessary damage.

Urodynamic investigations

Investigations of the lower urinary tract	
Urinary flow rate	Flow rate during micturition is recorded. Peak flow rate of <12ml/s suggests bladder outflow obstruction (BOO) or detrusor failure.
Urodynamics	A specialised catheter is sited into the bladder and another into the rectum. Pressure in both the bladder and rectum (a reflection of intra-abdominal pressure) is recorded during bladder filling and during micturition. Subtraction of one from the other allows true intravesicular (bladder) pressure to be determined to establish detrusor function.

Urology as an F1/F2

Urology may be part of general surgery as an F1 or a specialist attachment. The job has a good mix of inpatients, outpatients and theatre time; you will often be part of the general surgery on-call rota.

Structure urologists work very closely with the following specialities:
- ***Radiologists*** urology often requires imaging
- ***Oncologists*** a very high proportion of the work load is diagnosing and treating prostate cancer; oncologists manage the chemotherapy side
- ***Gynaecologists*** both specialities deal with incontinence; there is also surgical cooperation since the ureters are closely related to the uterus

The job you will be expected to perform the following roles:
- Manage inpatients (investigations, referrals, prescriptions etc)
- Assist in outpatient clinic.
- Clerk and initiate management of emergency admissions
- Attend and participate in theatre
- Contribute at meetings and to the educational programme

Aims try to do the following during your placement:
- Learn to manage a ward of inpatients and their care
- Refine clerking skills and knowledge of urological diseases
- Participate in outpatient clinics
- Acquire minor surgical skills including suturing (p600)
- Contribute to departmental audit or research

Common cases

Acute on chronic retention p320 a common presentation in middle-aged men, who often have previously undiagnosed prostatism. The pain of acute retention is rapidly relieved with catheterisation; highly rewarding for patient and junior doctor. An overnight stay in hospital often allows renal function and BP to be monitored following catheterisation.

Haematuria p314 frank haematuria is seen from time to time and has many causes. Bladder irrigation is often needed to prevent blood clots from causing urethral obstruction. Often a 3-way catheter is used which is like a normal urethral catheter, but has a wider diameter and an extra lumen to allow irrigation of the bladder with sterile fluid.

Post-TURP transurethral resection of the prostate is a common operation and patients often stay in hospital for a few days following surgery. Common post-operative problems include haematuria, electrolyte abnormalities (TURP syndrome) and sepsis.

Pre-ops elderly patients undergoing major surgery are often admitted the day before surgery, allowing final investigations to be undertaken and giving the anaesthetist an opportunity to assess them thoroughly.

Training

Initial route CT1 in 'surgery in general' urology (p28)
Further training competitive application for ST3 urology
Exams MRCS required to apply for ST3 urology

Vascular surgery

Role Vascular surgeons look after patients with a range of blood vessel conditions. It is a challenging speciality which requires technical skill and dexterity.

Vascular surgery history

Alongside taking a standard history (p98), when clerking vascular patients the following areas must be covered specifically:

General pain in muscles when walking, pain at rest, temperature of hands and feet, impotence in men, poor healing of injuries to the lower limb, ulcers, numbness, limb swelling, itching, varicose veins

Risk factors ↑age, male sex, smoking, ↑BP, DM, ↑lipids, family history

Past medical/surgical history asthma, IHD, MI, clotting problems, liver disease, jaundice, anaemia, malignancy, epilepsy, previous operations

Vascular surgery examination

As well as performing a thorough cardiovascular exam, you should also:

Look for pallor and cyanosis of limbs, temperature, loss of pulses (see below), venous guttering, arterial bruits, thin shiny skin, loss of hair, gangrene, varicose veins, eczema, haemosiderin pigmentation of the skin (particularly above the medial malleolus), lipodermatosclerosis ('inverted champagne bottle leg'), venous ulcers (see p384)

Examine pulses

Arms

- ***Radial*** two fingers pressed on the radial aspect of the inner wrist
- ***Ulnar*** two fingers pressed on the ulnar aspect of the inner wrist
- ***Brachial*** two fingers pressed into the antecubital fossa, just medial to the biceps tendon (ask patient to flex arm against resistance to find the tendon)

Legs

- ***Femoral*** two fingers pressed firmly into the middle of the crease in the groin, halfway between the symphysis pubis and the anterior superior iliac spine
- ***Popliteal*** ask patient to flex their knee, put both your thumbs either side of the patella and press firmly with your fingertips into the popliteal fossa
- ***Posterior tibial*** two fingers pressed 1cm posterior to the medial malleolus
- ***Dorsalis pedis*** two fingers pressed between the 1st and 2nd metatarsals

Central

- ***Carotid*** two fingers, medial to the sternocleidomastoid muscle and lateral to the thyroid cartilage (do not palpate both sides together)
- ***Abdominal aorta*** both fingertips, halfway between umbilicus and xiphisternum

Vascular surgery referrals

Checklist

Name, hospital number, age, gender, location

Cardiac risk factors (p450), comorbidities, exercise tolerance, anticoagulation

Pulses, limb capillary-refill, heart rhythm

Last food or drink, fitness for surgery

Referrals are usually made to the vascular registrar on-call. Try to give an impression of the urgency of the problem and which of the following would be appropriate:

- *Take over care* if the patient's underlying problem is vascular and requires urgent surgical intervention
- *Ward review* if the patient has a vascular problem which requires review but is immobile or bed-ridden
- *Urgent clinic* review if the patient is stable and mobile but with a condition requiring review, they could be seen in clinic
- *Routine outpatient* clinic if the patient is stable and has a non-urgent vascular problem

Vascular surgery as an F1/F2

Vascular surgery may be part of general surgery as an F1 or a specialist attachment. It is an exciting job as a junior. Patients admitted under a vascular team are often extremely unwell and can deteriorate suddenly, so management decisions often have to be made quickly.

The job you will be expected to perform the following roles:

- Assess patients pre-operatively (p128)
- Clerk acute admissions in the ED and initiate management plans
- Assist in theatre
- Perform daily ward round and complete ensuing jobs
- Manage post-op problems (p139)
- Attend outpatient clinics

Aims try to do the following during your placement:

- Develop history and examination skills for vascular surgery patients
- Learn some basic surgical skills eg suturing (p600)
- Learn about different arterial bypasses (eg fem–fem and fem–pop) and spend time in theatre assisting with these procedures
- Gain some exposure to amputation operations
- Spend time in outpatient clinics

Training

Initial route CT1 in 'surgery in general' general surgery (p28)
Further training competitive application for ST3 general surgery then subspecialise during training; a separate vascular surgery ST3 may start
Exams MRCS required to apply for ST3 general surgery

Chapter 11

Procedures

Practical procedures

In experienced hands procedures seem easy and highly rewarding, but it takes practice. Learning new procedures can make you feel frustrated, embarrassed and guilty about inflicting pain. When you are learning a new procedure, especially if it is your first time, ask one of your seniors to take you through it and supervise you. Try to get as much practical experience as you can so that you can work more efficiently and eventually teach others.

Before starting always introduce yourself and obtain informed consent (verbal or written, p69) before carrying out the procedure. Explain what the procedure involves, how it will feel and why it is necessary in clear, simple language and ask if they have any questions. Mentally prepare yourself by thinking through each step of the procedure.

The procedure as you perform the procedure take your time, plan ahead and be confident in your actions. Make sure you and the patient are comfortable and in the right position. Ask for an assistant – useful if you have forgotten anything.

If things go well at the end of the procedure always clean up and always dispose of your own sharps. Check the patient is alert, comfortable and well.

If things go wrong ask for help early. Stay calm and reassure the patient while you wait. See p74 if there is a serious problem.

Writing in the notes write your name, date and time of the procedure. Document that you obtained informed consent, why the procedure was undertaken, if there were any problems during it, who supervised and/or assisted you, and what your management plan is eg sending CSF sample for M,C+S. You should also document the details of any equipment used, such as putting the reference sticker from a urinary catheter wrapping in the notes. Always write that the patient is comfortable afterwards, assuming this is true.

Improving make sure you get feedback and hints from supervisors so that next time you can do it better. Reflect on your efforts, think about what you did well, what you could do differently and how you would teach someone else doing the procedure.

Things to remember to put on a procedures trolley

- Gloves ±sterile
- Needles (various sizes)
- 0.9% saline
- Antiseptic solution
- Syringes
- Local anaesthetic
- Plenty of swabs – you can never have too many
- Dressings and tape
- Specimen pots/bottles
- Kidney dishes/galipots
- Sharps bin

Laboratories

There are six main laboratories associated with a hospital:
- Biochemistry
- Haematology and blood bank
- Microbiology
- Histopathology (including cytology)
- Immunology
- Genetics

Biochemistry this department deals with the processing of blood samples for salt and mineral levels eg U+E, LFT and hormone levels such as cortisol, TFT etc. It also deals with monitoring drug levels eg sodium valproate and ABG samples if there is not a blood gas machine in the clinical areas. In general 'glucose separating gel' bottles (p557) are used for biochemistry samples but check with your lab if you are unsure or taking blood for an unusual test (see p557).

Haematology this lab processes samples for FBC, ESR, clotting studies, G+S and crossmatching. It also examines blood films if there is clinical suspicion of haematological disease eg haemolytic anaemia, leukaemia or malaria.

Microbiology this speciality is concerned with growing bugs in samples of various bodily fluids from patients. It examines specimens under the microscope to look for cells, it cultures them in an incubator to try and grow pathogens and if any bugs grow, it investigates which antibiotics can be used to kill them. It deals with specimens such as blood, urine, faeces, CSF and swabs taken from any site on the body. Microbiologists also assay antibiotic levels and are a useful source of advice when prescribing antibiotics. They usually produce the hospital antibiotic guideline policy in combination with the pharmacists. As well as bacteria, the lab also deals with samples looking for viruses, fungi and other pathogens.

Histopathology this speciality deals with tissue samples eg biopsies and specimens removed during operations or post-mortems. Pathologists examine these samples both macro- and microscopically to determine the nature of the tissue and the underlying disease process. They use different slicing and staining techniques to examine specimens under the microscope to obtain an accurate representation of disease activity.

Immunology performs tests to assess the immune system for underactivity (immunosupression) or overactivity (autoimmune disease); many of these involve measuring antibody levels eg ANA. Samples for antibody analysis usually go in the plain tubes (p557).

Genetics this lab has two subdivisions:
- Cytogenetics that look for chromosomal abnormalities by microscopy eg assessing an amniocentesis sample for trisomy 21 (Down's)
- Molecular genetics that look for mutations in DNA eg cystic fibrosis

The blood tube used for these tests varies between centres; the sample quality (fresh, free-flowing) is especially important for cytogenetics.

Taking blood (venepuncture)

Indications diagnosis, monitoring physiological state, therapeutic drug monitoring

Contraindications ***absolute*** patient refusal, AV fistula

Consent verbal; explain why a blood sample is required

Site usually antecubital fossa but can use any vein (eg hands, arms, feet and groin (femoral stab p556)); never use a limb with an AV fistula (dialysis) or an IV infusion distal to the venepuncture site

Equipment non-sterile gloves, tourniquet, alcohol swab, vacutainer hub and needle, gauze, tape, sharps bin, blood bottles (see p557)

Checks patient comfortable, vein exposed, accessible and not pulsing, cotton wool to hand, no IV fluids going into the limb of selected vein

Patient position ***upper limb*** sit the patient upright, with arm extended and below the heart; ***lower limb*** lay patient flat on their back

Procedure wash hands and wear non-sterile gloves. Assess both arms and select an appropriate vein. Tighten the tourniquet proximally and palpate along the course of the vein to assess its direction and depth. Swab the skin and hold the vein steady with your non-dominant hand. Warn the patient and advance the needle into the vein at 20° to the skin; feel for the slight 'give' as you enter the vein and hold your position as you insert the blood bottle into the hub. Unclip the tourniquet and apply pressure to the puncture site with cotton wool as you withdraw the needle. Press (or ask the patient to press) on the cotton wool for 2min (longer if bleeding) then tape it in place. Dispose of the needle and hub into the sharps bin. Fill the blood tubes at the patient's bedside, label them and complete the accompanying request forms.

Confirmation blood flows freely into the bottle

Complications pain, bleeding, haematoma, infection, failure

Safety steady the patient's arm on a pillow to reduce movement and risk of needle-stick injury, dispose of needles into a sharps bin immediately, do not resheath them

Alternatives

- Blood samples can be taken from cannulas when they are first inserted. It is sometimes possible to take blood at a later date; dispose of the first 5ml and interpret results with caution
- Needle and syringes can be used for smaller veins which may collapse from the suction from vacutainers
- For fine veins use a small needle (eg blue, 23G) or 'butterfly' (p555) but beware of haemolysis causing artificially ↑K^+ and ↑LDH
- If you are unable to obtain blood from the upper limb look at the veins in the leg/foot; if you still cannot find veins ask your senior to try before considering a femoral stab

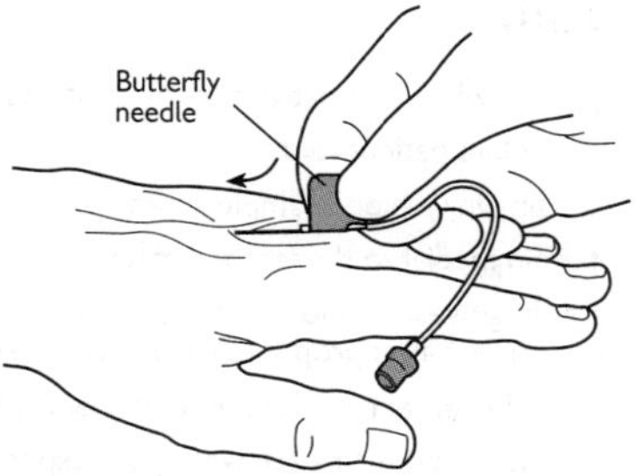

Taking blood using a butterfly needle.

Hints and tips

- In patients with poor veins spend a long time finding a suitable vein rather than stabbing blindly
- In children use topical local anaesthetic, see p561
- In adults choose veins by palpation with the tourniquet on rather than their appearance; a bouncy vein is usually easy to take blood from
- Tie the tourniquet tightly and ask the patient to clench their fist repeatedly with their arm below their heart; tap the vein to make it more prominent
- It is best to use a green (21G) vacutainer needle for U+E samples to prevent haemolysis and ↑K^+; if using a needle and syringe, extract blood slowly and gently with blue (23G) needles
- Pull the skin and vein taut to prevent movement away from the needle, especially in older patients
- Going through the skin is the most painful bit, once under the skin you can take several attempts to manoeuvre the needle into the vein
- If you can only obtain a small sample consider using paediatric tubes; see the minimum blood requirements on p557
- If you decide to use a needle and syringe, never force blood into blood tubes; the results are spectacular, messy and embarrassing. Consider pulling the top off or withdrawing air.

Procedure for taking blood cultures

Indicated by a repeated/persistent temp >37°C or one-off ≥38°C

Taking antibiotics is a relative contraindication

If bacterial endocarditis is suspected take 3 sets (6 bottles) from 3 separate veins

Procedure as for normal blood-taking with needle and syringe except:

- Wear sterile gloves (strict aseptic technique for deep veins)
- A set of blood cultures is two bottles (one aerobic and one anaerobic)
- After using the alcohol swab do not touch the vein again
- Once the blood has been obtained replace the used needle with a fresh one
- Flip off the culture bottle lids, swab the top with a clean alcohol wipe, insert the needle and fill each bottle with 5–10ml

Femoral stab

Indications taking blood when alternative sites are not possible

Contraindications ***absolute*** patient refusal

Consent verbal; explain why a blood sample is required

Site either side of groin medial to the femoral artery

Equipment non-sterile gloves, alcohol swab, 10–20ml syringe, 21G green needle, gauze, tape, sharps bin, appropriate blood bottles (see p557)

Checks patient comfortable, vein exposed, cotton wool to hand

Patient position patient flat on their back with groin exposed

Procedure wash hands and wear non-sterile gloves. Feel for the femoral pulse and choose the side where it is most prominent. Swab the skin thoroughly then place your fingers over the artery; warn the patient and insert the needle vertically 1cm medial to your fingers. Pull back on the syringe as you advance and stop moving as soon as you get flashback. Fill the syringe then withdraw. Exert pressure over the area with cotton wool for at least 2min and dress it with a plaster once bleeding has subsided. Fill the blood tubes, dispose of the needle and syringe in a sharps bin, label the tubes and complete the accompanying request forms

Confirmation blood flows freely into the syringe

Complications pain, bleeding, haematoma, infection, failure; bright red, pulsatile flashback suggests you hit the artery; aspirate the required amount of blood (arterial blood can be used for all routine tests) but press firmly for ≥5min after withdrawing the needle

Hints and tips to remember the anatomy of the femoral region, work in a lateral to medial direction and think 'NAVY':
- **N**erve (femoral nerve, most lateral)
- **A**rtery (femoral artery)
- **V**ein (femoral vein)
- **Y**-fronts (vital undergarment, best removed prior to procedure)

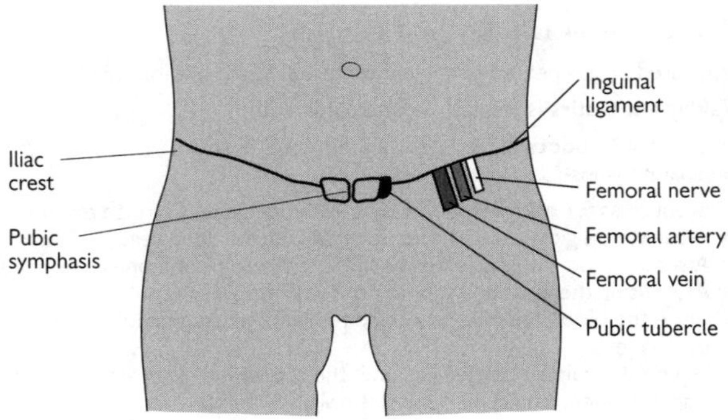

Anatomy of the femoral region.

Blood tubes

The colours and roles of the various blood bottles vary between hospitals. Use this page as a guide to which bottle is used for each test and to make sure the sample is suitable. Fill in the colour of blood bottles and specific blood tests used in your hospital. We have left space at the bottom for other blood tubes.

Colour	Contents	Tests	Special instructions
	EDTA	FBC, reticulocytes, HbA_{1C}, sickle screen, Hb electrophoresis, malaria screen	1ml minimum but aim to fill; gently mix to prevent clotting
	EDTA	ESR	Always fill to the line and gently mix to prevent clotting
	EDTA	Blood transfusion (G+S, crossmatch)	4ml minimum; always handwrite ≥3 forms of patient identification
	Sodium citrate	D-dimer, APTTr, INR, thrombophilia screen, fibrinogen	**Always** fill to the line and gently mix to prevent clotting
	Glucose separating gel	U+E, LFT, amylase, TFT, CRP, Cl^-, Mg^{2+}, Ca^{2+}, PO_4^{3-}, HCO_3^-, urate, LDH, total protein, digoxin, paracetamol and salicylate, lithium, other drug levels, tumour markers, β-hCG, protein electrophoresis, cardiac markers	1.5ml minimum but aim to fill; try to use a green vacutainer needle to prevent haemolysis and inaccurate K^+ result
	Plain	Some endocrine tests, drug levels, serology	1.5ml minimum but aim to fill
	Fluoride oxalate	***Blood*** glucose, lactate, alcohol; ***CSF*** glucose, protein, oligoclonal bands	***Blood*** fill to the line, mix gently; ***CSF*** 6 drops; mix gently
	Heparin	Some endocrine tests	Mix gently, may need to be transported on ice

IV cannulation

Indications unwell patients, shock, IV fluids/drugs, blood product transfusions, other routes of drug administration not tolerated

Contraindications ***absolute*** patient refusal, AV fistula

Consent verbal; explain why a cannula is required

Site the forearm and back of the hand on the non-dominant arm are best, but any vein can be used (eg hands, arms, feet, legs), antecubital fossa in an emergency, never use a limb with an AV fistula (dialysis)

Equipment tourniquet, non-sterile gloves, alcohol swab, cannulas (appropriate size, see opposite), cannula dressing, 5ml syringe with saline flush, cotton wool, 5–20ml syringe if blood sample required, sharps bin

Checks patient comfortable, skin is clean and free of infection, vein exposed, accessible and not pulsing, cotton wool ±syringe to hand

Patient position ***upper limb*** sit the patient upright, with arm extended and below the heart; ***lower limb*** lie patient flat on their back

Procedure wash hands and wear non-sterile gloves. Assess both arms and select an appropriate vein. Tighten the tourniquet proximally and palpate along the course of the vein to assess its direction and depth. Swab the skin and hold the vein steady with your non-dominant hand. Warn the patient and advance the cannula through the skin at 20° with the bevel facing upwards and proximally. Look for flashback, then advance the cannula and needle a little further before withdrawing the metal needle whilst firmly advancing the plastic cannula. Press with your thumb over the tip of the cannula in the vein.

- *Taking blood* if blood leaks out try lifting the arm, if still leaking remove the tourniquet. Attach the syringe, take the blood (easier with gentle pressure) and remove the tourniquet then the syringe.
- *Not taking blood* remove the tourniquet

Place the cap on the end of the cannula, secure with the adhesive dressing and flush with 2–5ml 0.9% saline through the flip-top cap. Dispose of the needle into a sharps bin.

Confirmation flashback seen, saline flush requires minimal pressure and does not form a proximal subcutaneous 'bleb' or hurt

Complications ***early*** haematoma, tissuing (fluid/drugs enter subcutaneous tissues), local damage, air embolism; ***late*** thrombophlebitis, cellulitis

Safety never reinsert the metal needle into the plastic cannula once you have fully removed it as this increases the risk of needle-stick injuries and bits of the plastic cannula may shear off and embolise, steady the patient's arm on a pillow to reduce movement and the risk of needle-stick injury, dispose of needles into a sharps bin immediately

Alternatives central venous cannulation (p574), alternative route of drug administration (PO/IM/SC/PR)

Hints and tips

- See comments under 'Taking blood'
- Start distally in a limb and work your way proximally if you fail to cannulate initially
- Veins are easier to cannulate at the junction of two veins
- Try to avoid cannulas over a joint as these are uncomfortable and more likely to tissue
- If you go through the wall of the vein, withdraw a small distance until flashback recurs and try to advance the plastic cannula
- In confused patients and children, always cover the cannula with a crêpe bandage and tape the IV line to their skin to minimise auto-extraction and further cannulation practice

Size and function of different cannulae

Colour	Size	Flow rate (ml/min)	Use
Blue	22G	31	Small fragile veins
Pink	20G	55	IV drugs and fluids ±blood
Green	18G	90	Blood, fluids, drugs
White	17G	135	Blood, fluids, drugs
Grey	16G	170	Rapid blood, fluids, drugs
Brown	14G	265	Emergency situations

Cannula care

- Inspect cannula daily, looking for inflammation and replace it every 72h
- If asked to replace it, check cannula is still necessary
- If blocked, try flushing the line gently with 0.9% saline and check it isn't kinked
- Remove the cannula if the surrounding skin is red, swollen or tender

Taking blood in children

Never use a needle and syringe, ***never*** use a snapped off needle/broken needle

Indications diagnosis, monitoring physiological state
Contraindications ***absolute*** parental refusal; ***relative*** preserving veins
Consent verbal from parent ±child; explain why it is required
Planning before you take the blood get all the equipment ready, think about the amount of blood and which bottles you need, work out where the child, parent and staff will go, think about distraction
Choosing a vein the appearance of the vein is more important than the feel (they are often too small to palpate); common sites include hands, feet and forearms. Antecubital fossa and saphenous veins should only be used if there is no chance of a long line being inserted.

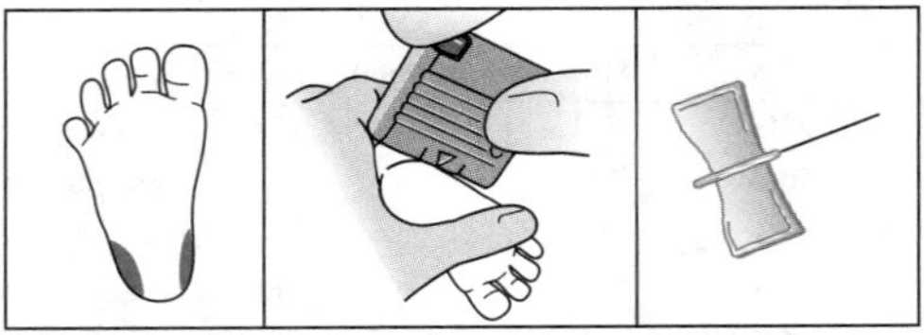

(A) Site for heel prick (B) Heel prick (Tenderfoot) (C) Winged needle

Heel prick

Age range babies <10d; though works on fingers at all ages if desperate
Samples <1ml of blood ie 2 bottles, not K^+, clotting or blood cultures
Analgesia pacifier dipped in 20% dextrose, swaddling
Staff can be performed alone in babies
Technique grip the heel tightly between index finger and thumb. Choose a site on the outside of the heel (Fig. (A)) and wipe with a Steret® then apply a small amount of Vaseline®. Hold the lancet (Fig. (B)) firmly against the skin and squeeze the heel as you release the lancet. Catch the blood as it drips out; you may need to gently squeeze the foot. Apply cotton wool.
Advantages easy, usually quick, does not use up a site for cannulation
Disadvantages small quantities, can take a long time, messy

Winged needle/cut-off butterfly (Fig. C)

Age range <1yr (but works at any age)
Samples not blood cultures
Analgesia pacifier dipped in 20% dextrose, swaddling, Ametop®/EMLA®
Staff two extra – one to hold the child, one to act as tourniquet
Technique locate suitable vein (between the knuckles can be surprisingly good if no others are visible). Ask a colleague to act as a tourniquet. Stretch the skin to fix the vein; a baby's fist fits well between the thumb and index finger if their wrist is flexed. Insert the needle slowly until blood drips out of the needle; catch sufficient blood then remove the needle and apply cotton wool.
Advantages relatively easy to hit the vein, can get large quantities
Disadvantages very messy, can clot if flowing slowly

Butterfly

Age range >1yr
Samples not blood cultures
Analgesia Ametop®/EMLA®, cold spray, distraction (play therapist)
Staff two extra – one to hold the child, one as tourniquet and distraction
Technique locate suitable vein. Ask a colleague to act as a tourniquet. Stretch the skin to fix the vein; insert the needle slowly until there is flash back. Hold the butterfly in place whilst gently filling the syringe until there is sufficient blood; remove the butterfly and apply cotton wool.
Advantages clean, can get large quantities
Disadvantages hard to hold butterfly whilst drawing on syringe

Keeping it 'fun' it is essential to make the experience as pleasant as possible – not least of all to make it easier the next time. Use a special treatment room, involve the play therapist, keep their parents with them, smile, offer distraction and, most importantly, give out stickers.

Cannula

Age range any
Samples any including blood cultures
Analgesia pacifier dipped in 20% dextrose, swaddling, Ametop®/EMLA®, cold spray, distraction (play therapist)
Staff two extra – one to hold the child, one as tourniquet and distraction
Technique locate a suitable vein, it needs to be straight. Ask a colleague to act as a tourniquet. Stretch the skin to fix the vein; insert the needle slowly until there is flash back. Advance the cannula whilst withdrawing the stylet. Blood can be obtained by three methods:

- Dripping into bottles (non-sterile)
- Sucking from the cannula with a needle and syringe (risk of needle-stick and partially sterile, but main method in babies)
- Attaching sterile extender and syringe (sterile)

If blood does not come, gently withdraw the cannula until blood flows. Once blood has been obtained either fix the cannula in place or remove and apply cotton wool.
Advantages sterile, easy to obtain large samples, clean
Disadvantages makes future cannulation harder, can be difficult

Topical local anaesthetic ('magic cream') is used for taking blood or cannulation. It is applied directly to the skin (often to multiple sites) and covered with Tegaderm® until it has 'cooked'. There are two types:

- **Ametop®** (>1mth) takes 30–40min
- **EMLA®** (>1yr) takes 1h

Cold spray (ethyl chloride) as this evaporates it numbs the skin and provides distraction. The effects last about 5s

Pacifier (dummy) the sucking reflex has an analgesic effect in babies and this can be augmented by dipping the pacifier in 20% dextrose solution

Swaddling tightly wrapping an infant in a sheet has an analgesic effect and also helps to keep them still

Arterial blood gas (ABG)

Indications assessment of hypoxia, CO_2 retention, acutely ill patients

Contraindications ***absolute*** patient refusal; ***radial*** AV fistula, poor/absent collateral circulation, bony fractures; ***femoral*** femoral artery graft; ***relative*** abnormal blood coagulation

Consent verbal; explain why the test is required

Site radial artery (usual), femoral artery, ulnar artery, brachial artery (last resort)

Equipment non-sterile gloves, alcohol swab, heparin-filled syringe and cap, needle (blue for radial, green for femoral), gauze/cotton ball, tape, sharps bin

Checks note the concentration of O_2 the patient is on and their temperature. Locate the nearest ABG analysis machine. ***Radial ABG*** check ulnar circulation adequacy by squeezing the hand into a fist, occluding the radial and ulnar arteries in the wrist, holding for 10s then opening the hand and releasing the pressure on the ulnar artery only; looking for reperfusion of the whole hand (Allen's test)

Patient position ***upper limb*** sit the patient upright, arm and wrist extended, put a pillow under the wrist to hold the position; ***femoral ABG*** lie patient flat on their back with their groin exposed and curtains shut

Procedure wash hands and wear non-sterile gloves. Attach needle to syringe and expel excess heparin (if present). Palpate both radial pulses and select the better side. Roll your finger back and forth over the artery to assess its width and course. Do not use a tourniquet. Place a finger on the radial pulse, hold the syringe like a pen with the bevel facing upwards and proximally. Warn the patient and insert the syringe at 30° to the skin, aiming for the centre of the artery against the direction of blood flow. Once you hit the artery the blood should pulse into the syringe (best method of assessing whether arterial or venous). If not reassess the positions of the pulse and needle by feeling for the needle tip as you gently press the syringe upwards. Once you have about 1ml of blood apply gentle pressure to the puncture site with cotton wool and withdraw the needle. Press firmly for at least 3min (do not let the patient do this). Remove the needle using a sharps bin and put the cap on the syringe. Label the syringe at the bedside with the patient's details, O_2 concentration and temp and take it to the ABG machine.

Confirmations ***during procedure*** pulsatile, bright-red blood fills the syringe automatically; ***post-procedure*** blood O_2 saturation is the same as that measured with a sats probe

Complications bleeding, haematoma, arterial damage and peripheral ischaemia, pain, infection, local tendon/nerve damage

Safety steady the patient's arm on a pillow to reduce movement and risk of needle-stick injury, dispose of needles into a sharps container immediately, do not resheath them

Alternatives

- ***Femoral blood gas*** similar to femoral stab (p556) but aim for the femoral pulse (usually 2 fingers width below the inguinal ligament), with the patient lying flat on their back. Insert the green (21G) needle at 90° to the skin.
- ***Brachial artery gas*** (if unable to get radial or femoral) extend the patient's arm and insert needle at 45° into the brachial artery (medial to the biceps tendon, on the inner aspect of the upper forearm)
- ***Arterial cannula*** used for repeated arterial samples or direct BP measurement (seek senior/specialist advice)

Hints and tips

- Consider applying topical (p561) or infiltrated local anaesthetic (bleb of 1% lidocaine over the artery using an orange needle)
- If no blood is seen reposition the needle without withdrawing it completely from the skin; ask the patient to dorsiflex the wrist fully
- You may miss the artery and hit the bone (painful); if this happens gently withdraw the needle to just under the skin, reposition the needle in line with the pulse and try again, taking your time
- The ED, ITU, HDU, neonatal and labour wards often have ABG machines; if you cannot process the ABG immediately put it in a fridge or on ice
- Expel air bubbles from the syringe before presenting the sample to the analysis machine

Interpretation see p622

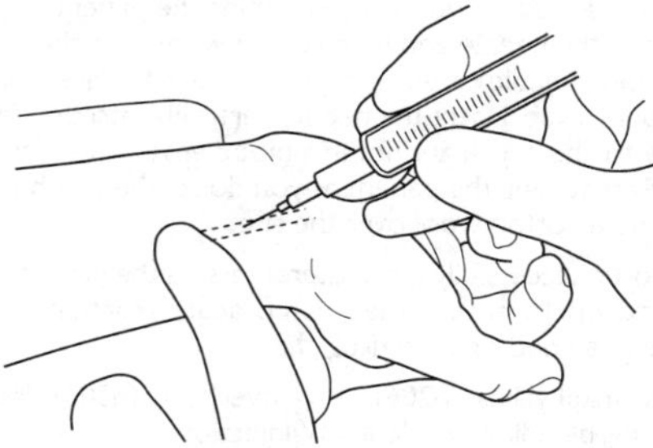

Obtaining an arterial blood sample from the right radial artery.

SC/IM injections

Indications only route of administration available or tolerated

Contraindications ***absolute*** patient refusal, drug allergy, bleeding disorder, ↓platelets, ↑INR, ↑APTTr

Consent verbal; explain why you are giving the drug

Site
- *SC* upper arm (tricep/deltoid), anterior abdominal wall, anterior thigh
- *IM* shoulder (deltoid), lateral thigh, superior lateral quadrant of the buttocks (to avoid the sciatic nerve)

Equipment non-sterile gloves, alcohol swab, drug, syringe, green (21G) and blue (23G) or orange (25G) needle, cotton wool

Checks patient's name and DoB (ask patient or check ID band), dose and strength prescribed, batch number and expiry date, allergies (ask patient, check allergy bands or drug chart)

Patient position so that target site is exposed and accessible

Procedure wash hands and wear non-sterile gloves. Draw up the medication into a syringe using a green needle and expel any air bubbles:
- *SC* attach an orange needle to the syringe and clean the area for injection with an alcohol swab. Raise the skin and subcutaneous tissue between your fingers by pinching it and insert the needle at 45° into the skin. Pull the syringe back slightly to check you are not in a blood vessel. Inject the medication slowly, watching the patient as you do so, then withdraw the needle and hold cotton wool over the site.
- *IM* attach a blue needle to the syringe and clean the area for injection with an alcohol swab. Insert the needle vertically into the skin and pull back slightly to check you are not in a blood vessel. Inject the medication slowly, watching the patient as you do so, then withdraw the needle and hold cotton wool over the site.

Confirmation drug successfully administered, assess the patient and monitor the HR, BP and RR to ensure there is no acute reaction, remember to write the time given and sign the drug chart

Complications anaphylaxis (p206), drug overdose (p304), local swelling, pain and bruising, bleeding, accidental IV injection

Safety stay on the ward for at least 5min after giving drugs in case of an acute reaction. Dispose of sharps in a sharps bin.

Alternatives consider other routes (PO/IV/PR/SL/IN) or other drugs

Hints and tips
- Use a larger needle in obese patients
- If blood is aspirated, withdraw and repeat the procedure in a different area with a clean needle
- Rotate injection sites to limit local reactions
- Most nurses can give IM/SC injections and are more experienced at it
- Try to avoid IM injections as much as possible as they are fairly painful

Drugs commonly given via SC and IM routes

Subcutaneous	Intramuscular
• Insulin	• Metoclopramide
• LMWH	• Cyclizine
• Diamorphine	• Tramadol/pethidine
	• Chlorphenamine
	• Haloperidol

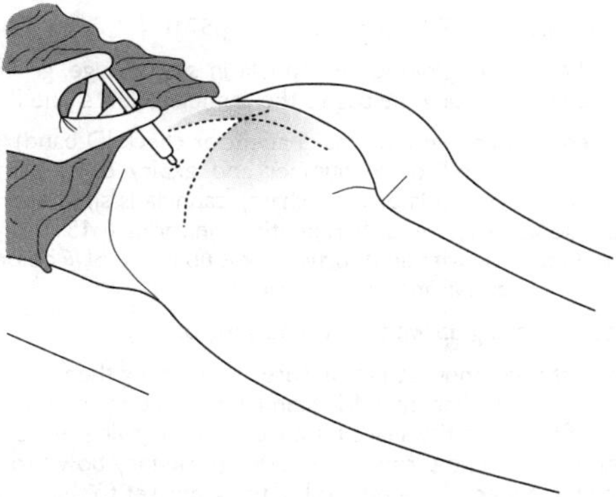

Safe area for IM injection in the buttock.

IV injections (intravenous)

Blood transfusions	p388	Heparin infusion	p347
Insulin sliding scale	p275	GTN infusion	p201
IV fluids	p323	Morphine injection	p429

Indications rapid or direct drug administration, steady plasma concentration from infusion, only route of administration available or tolerated
Contraindications ***absolute*** patient refusal, drug allergy

Consent verbal; explain what fluid/drug/blood you are injecting and why

Site via a cannula (see p558) or central line (p574)

Equipment IV fluid/drug/blood, IV cannula *in situ*, syringe, green needle, giving set (tube connecting the bag to the cannula), 0.9% saline flush

Checks patient's name and DoB (ask patient or check ID band), dose and infusion rate prescribed, batch number and expiry date, allergies (ask patient, check allergy bands or drug chart), cannula is sited appropriately and flushing, some drugs need therapeutic monitoring (p151)
- If you are unfamiliar with an IV drug look it up in the *BNF* before giving
- Always follow the *BNF* and drug instructions

Patient position sitting up with the cannula exposed

Procedure flush the cannula to make sure it is working then:
- *IV infusion* hang the bag on a drip stand and puncture the port on the bag of fluids with the sharp plastic end of the giving set. Open the valve and run the fluid through into a sink (or kidney bowl) to remove air bubbles. Connect the other end of the giving set to the horizontal cannula porthole (not the coloured top). Alter the drip speed and tape a loop of the tubing to the patient's arm to limit traction on the cannula.
- *Drawing up IV drugs* if the drug is in powder form reconstitute with solvent as directed (often 0.9% saline/water; Appendix 6 of *BNF*). Draw solvent into a syringe and inject it into the drug vial with a green 21G needle. Shake well then draw the solution back into the syringe. If the drug is already in liquid form in a glass ampoule, use a filter needle to draw up the drug to prevent aspiration of tiny shards of glass.
- *Giving IV drugs* tap the syringe to bring air bubbles to the top then expel any air and remove the needle. Attach the syringe to the coloured cannula port and slowly administer the medication according to the drug manufacturer's instructions or the *BNF*. Flush with 5ml 0.9% saline.

Confirmation infusion running/IV drug successfully administered, assess the patient and monitor the HR, BP and RR to ensure there is no acute reaction, remember to write the time given and sign the drug chart

Complications anaphylaxis (p206), drug overdose (p304), local irritation/thrombophlebitis, leakage of drug from tissued cannula, haematoma

Safety if multiple infusions are set up check they can be given through the same cannula. If not, insert a second cannula or give the drugs at different times. Stay on the ward for at least 5min after giving IV drugs in case of an acute adverse reaction.

Alternatives consider other routes of administration (PO, IM, SC, PR, SL, IN). As a last resort IV fluids (0.9% saline or dextrose saline without KCl) can be given very slowly SC (no faster than 1l over 12h). Never give 5% dextrose SC due to infection risk. Blood transfusions (p388) can only be given IV. You may need a central line (p574) for some IV infusions/drugs.

Hints and tips
- Flush the cannula, especially after giving irritant drugs
- If you are unsure of infusion rates, consult the *BNF*
- Some medications must be given at a constant rate using a syringe driver (eg heparin, magnesium, GTN, opiates)
- Keep IV infusions above the level of the patient's heart to prevent blood loss
- Keep syringe drivers below the level of the patient's heart to prevent drug siphoning
- Most nurses can administer IV infusions or drugs though some IV injections must be given by a doctor; there is usually good reason for this – find out what it is before giving the injection

ECGs and cardiac monitors

Indications

- *ECG* chest/back/abdo pain or suspicion of cardiac ischaemia, unexplained SOB, ↓GCS, ↑K^+, arrhythmias, pre-op
- *Cardiac monitoring* peri- and post-cardiorespiratory arrest, peri- and post-MI, ↑K^+, arrhythmias, cardioversion, administration of certain drugs, administration of anaesthesia

Contraindications ***absolute*** patient refusal; ***relative*** patient contaminated with toxic substance or other risk to operator

Consent verbal; explain why the ECG/monitoring is required

Site anterior chest wall and limbs

Equipment ECG/cardiac monitor, adhesive electrodes

Checks sufficient ECG paper, paper moving at 25mm/s

Patient position sitting at 45° for ECG

Procedure

- *ECG* apply adhesive electrodes and connect as shown in the box below then turn the ECG machine on. Ask the patient to sit back and stay still. Press 'record' (often an ECG picture or '12'). The ECG should print once the machine has collected enough data.

Limb leads **red** right shoulder; **yellow** left shoulder; **green** left foot; black right foot

Chest leads **V1** (red) right sternal edge, 4th intercostal space; **V2** (yellow) left sternal edge, 4th intercostal space; **V3** (green) between V2 and V4; **V4** (brown) mid-clavicular line, 5th intercostal space; **V5** (black) anterior-axillary line, horizontal with V4; **V6** (purple) mid-axillary line horizontal with V4 (see Fig. (A) opposite)

- *Cardiac monitoring* apply the leads as follows: ***red*** right shoulder; ***yellow*** left shoulder and ***green/black*** over the apex beat or spleen; see Fig. (B). The machine will show the trace of lead 'II' on a standard 12-lead ECG. Other views can also be obtained with three leads.

Confirmation adequate ECG printout or trace on cardiac monitor

Complications skin reaction to adhesive electrodes (rare)

Safety caution with electricity and wet/bloody environments

Alternatives for posterior MIs the ECG is set up with posterior leads; the leads are attached three places further on ie V1 is connected to V4, V2 to V5, etc. Leads V4–6 are attached round the posterior chest at the same horizontal level as V6 to become V7–9, see Fig. (C). Ensure you document this on the ECG trace.

Hints and tips adhesive electrodes do not stick to hairy skin so you may need to shave a small patch. If the patient is sweaty, clean the skin with an alcohol wipe first. In desperation use a pen to hold single leads in place. The limb leads can be placed on the ankles and wrists or over the hips and shoulders, however comparing ECGs taken by different methods can be hard. Consider a chaperone for female patients.

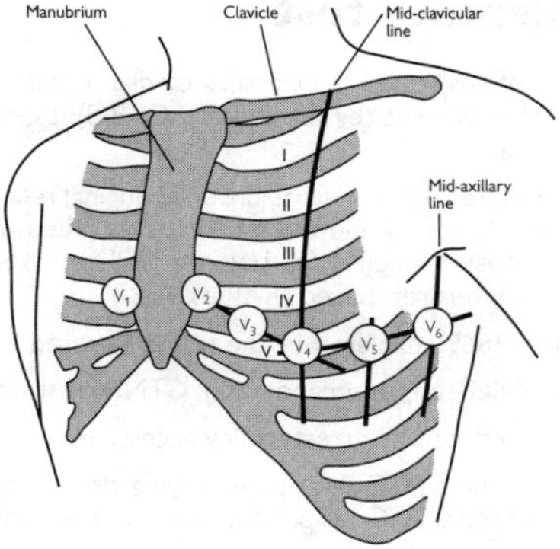

(A) Position of the chest leads for 12-lead ECG.

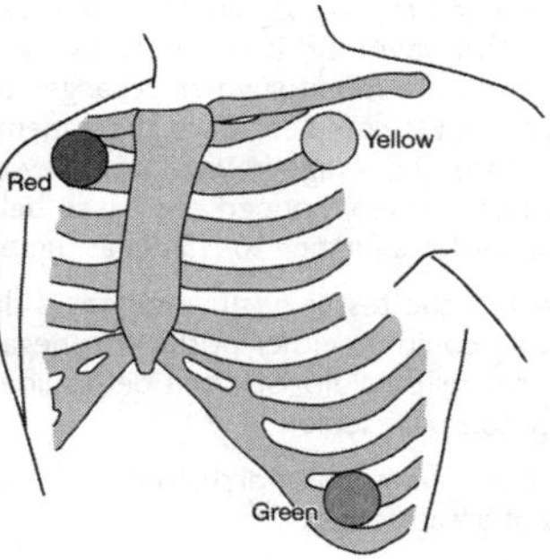

(B) Position of the three leads for cardiac monitoring.

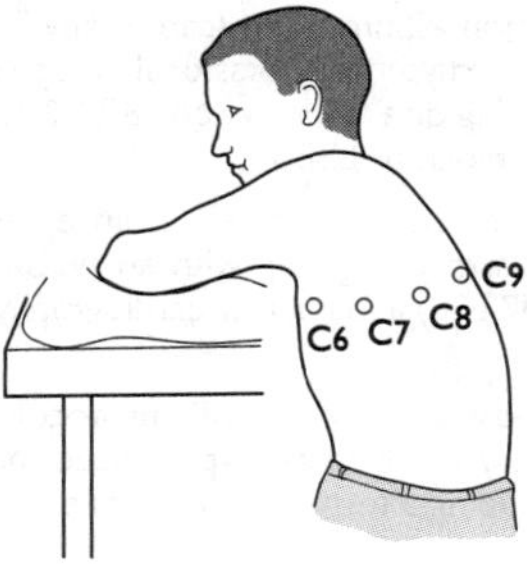

(C) Position of the posterior chest leads; V7–9.

Exercise tolerance test

Indications diagnosis of suspected IHD, assess cardiac fitness, prognosis post-MI, evaluation of treatment (eg angioplasty, CABG), assessing exercise-induced arrhythmias

Contraindications absolute patient refusal, unstable angina; ***relative*** severe aortic stenosis, recent (<5d) ST elevation MI, uncontrolled arrhythmia, ↑BP or heart failure, physical inability (eg severe COPD, stroke, arthritis), β-blockade, inability to interpret (paced rhythms, LBBB)

Consent verbal/written (p69); explain why the test is required

Equipment treadmill, ECG, sphygmomanometer, GTN, arrest trolley

Checks exclude contraindications, arrest trolley accessible

Patient position record first ECG with patient lying down, second with patient standing up and serial ECGs as patient walks on the treadmill

Procedure the technician connects the BP cuff and ECG leads to the patient with a specialised harness; a baseline BP is recorded. The test commences with the treadmill moving slowly then gradually speeding up whilst increasing the gradient; this is pre-programmed and most hospitals use the Bruce protocol (OHCM7 p94). BP is recorded every 3–5min. Real-time ECGs are often shown on a monitor where changes to the ST segment can be observed. The test is complete once the patient reaches ≥90% of their maximal heart rate (220 – age in years) or they complete the protocol (30min). The test is often stopped early (see below). BP and ECG measurement continues for a further 10–15min as the patient rests.

Confirmation deciding if the test is positive or not is difficult, since stopping early (see below) could be either positive or negative depending on the ECG tracing. A senior cardiologist often determines the result. If the test is stopped early consult a senior.

Complications atrial and ventricular arrhythmias (including VF and VT), syncope, shortness of breath, angina, MI

Safety stop the test if:

- Patient has chest pain or shortness of breath
- Patient is exhausted, feeling faint or at risk of falling
- ST segment depression >2mm in any lead or any ST elevation
- Atrial or ventricular arrhythmia (occasional ectopics do not count)
- Systolic BP ≥230mmHg or a fall in systolic BP ≥20mmHg
- Development of AV block or LBBB

Alternatives the test can be performed on an exercise bicycle, an arm bicycle or induced pharmacologically with an IV β-agonist. Stress echocardiography (OHCM7 p98) and nuclear cardiography can also be used to assess cardiac disease.

Hints and tips most hospitals have specific protocols for exercise testing. The technician is usually much more experienced than the junior doctor and if they suggest stopping a test it is worthwhile doing so.

Chemical cardioversion (adenosine)

Indications regular narrow complex tachycardia, known SVT with bundle branch block

Contraindications ***absolute*** serious adverse event with adenosine in past; ***relative*** cardiovascular instability (↓GCS, systolic BP <90mmHg, chest pain, heart failure), second-or third-degree heart block, asthma, accessory-pathways (eg WPW), sick-sinus syndrome, bradycardia

Things to try first vagal manoeuvres: 10s of carotid sinus massage (**never** both sides together); straining down as if passing a stool; trying to blow the plunger out of a clean 10ml syringe from the narrow end; immersing the face in icy cold water (often difficult to perform on the ward)

Consent usually verbal (p69). Explain procedure and possible symptoms patient may experience (see below).

Equipment defibrillator with monitoring strip recorder and paper, BP monitoring, pulse oximetry, large-bore venous access (≥green cannulae in antecubital fossa), O_2 supplementation, arrest trolley (equipment and drugs), adenosine, saline flushes and drawing-up needles and syringes

Patient position allow the patient to get themselves into a position where they are comfortable, either laying flat or at 45° in bed

Patient explanation tell the patient about the procedure including the common symptoms such as facial flushing, lightheadedness, chest tightness and nausea; most symptoms last less than 60s after administration

Pre-procedural checks ensure a 12-lead ECG has been undertaken. Check the patient still has a tachycardia. Give the patient supplemental O_2, ensure O_2 sats and BP monitoring are attached to the patient (on the opposite arm to the venous access) and that observations are being noted every few minutes. Attach leads of defibrillator to monitor heart rhythm (select 'leads' on the defibrillator). Have at least one assistant and at least one member present should be ALS trained. Draw up 6mg of adenosine and a 10ml 0.9% saline flush. Check the cannula is patent and flushing painlessly.

Procedure commence rhythm strip recording/printing on the defibrillator (usually press 'record'). Warn the patient you are going to give the drug. Inject 6mg adenosine rapidly, followed immediately by the 10ml flush and lift the arm to aid venous return. Observe the rhythm strip and patient.

Possible outcomes and further management

- *No effect* on HR or rhythm within 60s; repeat procedure using 12mg of adenosine; if still no response seek senior/specialist advice
- *Transient slowing* of HR, but restoration of original tachycardia; observe underlying rhythm on rhythm strip during slowing; if AF then treat for fast AF (p188), otherwise treat according to ALS (p164)
- *Conversion* of tachycardia into sinus rhythm; success
- *Evolution* of pathological rhythm eg VF/VT; follow appropriate ALS algorithm (p164)

Complications see patient explanation above

Safety never perform this procedure for the first time on your own

Cardioversion and defibrillation

Indications ***emergency*** VF, VT, fast AF (new onset or haemodynamically unstable), SVT if other treatments have failed (p184–5) or patient haemodynamically unstable; ***elective*** AF

Contraindications ***absolute*** patient refusal; ***relative*** wet or bloody environment (moisture and electricity don't mix)

Consent verbal/common law in an emergency, otherwise verbal/written

Site one electrode to the right of the upper sternum below the clavicle and the other electrode level with the 5th left intercostal space in the anterior axillary line (see Figs. (A), (B) opposite). In refractory VF/VT consider shocking in the anterior/posterior position (Fig. (C)).

Equipment defibrillator with paddles and gel-pads or hands-free electrodes, arrest trolley, ECG machine

Checks defibrillator working and battery charged; gel-pads and resuscitation drugs available, at least one assistant, patient's cardiac rhythm requires cardioversion, nobody touching the patient/bed, O_2 removed. In elective cases check the patient is starved and adequately anticoagulated with good IV access.

Patient position supine; left lateral position for AP cardioversion

Procedure

- *Emergency* follow BLS (p162) and ALS (p164)/APLS algorithms. Attach gel-pads or hands-free electrodes. Set defibrillator to required energy, make sure no one is in contact with the patient or bed and the O_2 is removed. **Give a clear verbal warning to stand clear.** Shock. Replace electrodes into defibrillator and continue CPR in accordance with ALS/APLS algorithm.
- *Elective* ensure the anaesthetist is available and inform the nursing staff. Apply gel-pads or hands-free electrodes before the patient is anaesthetised. Once asleep set the defibrillator to 'synchronised shock' and shock in accordance with ALS/APLS algorithms, checking that no one is in contact with the patient/bed and that O_2 is removed. **Give a clear verbal warning to stand clear**. Shock.

Defibrillation energies

Cardiac arrest	Haemodynamically unstable patients
• *Monophasic* 360J, 360J, 360J	***Broad-complex tachycardia and AF***
• *Biphasic* 200J, 360J, 360J	• *Monophasic* 200J, 360J, 360J
	• *Biphasic* 150J, 200J, 360J
	Atrial flutter and narrow-complex tachycardia
	• *Monophasic* 100J, 200J, 360J
	• *Biphasic* 100J, 200J, 360J

Confirmation restoration of sinus rhythm for elective cases or a cardiac output in the emergency situation; perform 12-lead ECG

Complications life-threatening arrhythmias, thromboembolism, aspiration, local burning to skin, risks to user and bystanders

Safety users of the manual defibrillator must have passed an ALS or ILS course; caution with electricity and wet/bloody environments

Alternatives automated external defibrillators (AEDs) are becoming widespread and require no rhythm recognition by the user. Two hands-free electrodes are applied to the patient and the AED determines if a shock is advisable or not; if a shock is advisable the operator just presses the 'shock' button when the AED tells them to. AEDs should not be used for elective cardioversions.

Hints and tips always defibrillate safely; if in doubt contact your resuscitation officer for some extra training

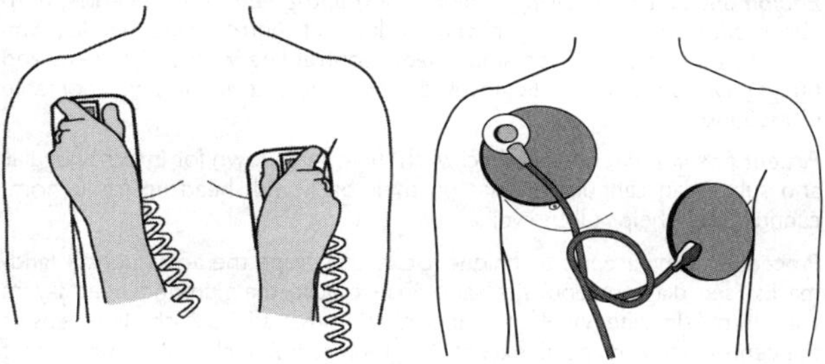

(A) (B)

(A) *Position of manual defibrillator paddles* make sure gel-pads are placed on the skin underneath the paddles as these reduce the impedance and limit skin burns. **(B) *Position of hands-free adhesive defibrillation electrodes*** the electrodes for most hands-free systems indicate where they should be placed: over the right shoulder and over the left side of the chest.

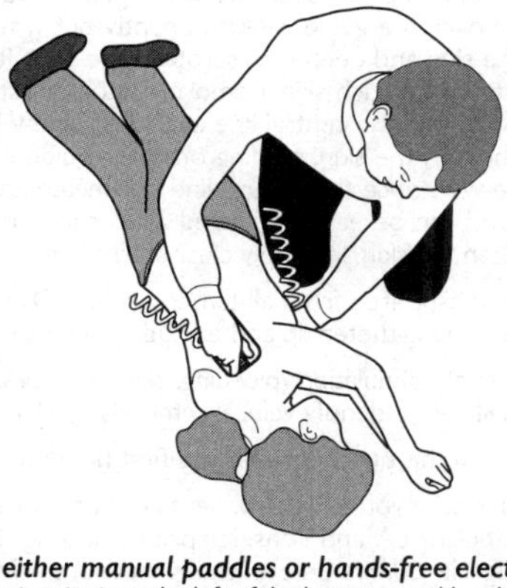

(C) *Position of either manual paddles or hands-free electrodes in the AP position* the anterior site is to the left of the lower sternal border and the posterior position is just inferior to the left scapula.

Central lines

Indications monitoring fluid balance, pulmonary artery catheterisation (Swann-Ganz catheters), temporary pacing wires, drug administration, parenteral feeding, permits blood sampling

Contraindications ***absolute*** patient refusal; ***relative*** infection at site, bleeding diathesis/anticoagulation, shock

Consent verbal/written (p69); explain why the central line is required

Site internal jugular, subclavian or femoral vein

Equipment 5ml/10ml syringes, blue (23G) and green (21G) needles, non-absorbable suture, Seldinger central line kit (introducing needle, 5ml syringe, guide-wire, dilator, small blade, central line with 2–5 lumens and bungs), 1% lidocaine, sterile gloves, dressing pack, sterile drapes, ±portable ultrasound

Patient position flat on their back with their head down for internal jugular and subclavian cannulation; flat on their back with head up for femoral cannulation – helps fill the vein

Procedure using aseptic technique, clean and drape the area. Identify landmarks (see diagram opposite) and anaesthetise the skin and deep layers with 10ml lidocaine. Whilst the anaesthetic takes effect, flush all lumens of the central line and cap all except the green one. Attach 5ml syringe, insert the introducer needle through the skin and towards the vein, aspirating whilst advancing. Once dark red blood is aspirated freely into the syringe, stop advancing. Remove the syringe whilst holding the needle firmly in place. If blood spurts out in a pulsatile fashion it is likely to be an arterial cannulation (see opposite). Advance the guide-wire through the lumen of the needle (should occur without resistance). Once most of the guide-wire is inserted, remove the needle, but always holding onto the guide-wire. Make a small incision in the skin adjacent to the guide-wire with the blade; thread the dilator over the guide-wire and gently but firmly advance the dilator through the skin and deep layers, rotating to ease its passage. Stop once half the dilator is through skin. Remove dilator, whilst always holding on to the guide-wire. Pass the central line over the guide-wire and advance the central line through the skin, holding onto the guide-wire at all times. Remove the guide-wire once the central line is inserted and cap the open lumen. Check blood can be easily aspirated from each lumen. Suture the line to the skin, clean the skin and apply clear sterile dressing.

Confirmation blood aspirated from all lumens, blood O_2 sats < finger O_2 sats, CXR to locate the catheter tip and exclude pneumothorax

Complications arterial cannulation, bleeding, pneumothorax (subclavian > internal jugular), failure to identify vein, air embolism, infection

Safety never perform this procedure for the first time on your own

Hints and tips make sure you and the patient are both comfortable before you start. Use sufficient LA and consider premedicating the patient with good PO/IV analgesia 30min before the procedure. Ultrasound often shows the vascular anatomy very clearly and can aid line placement.

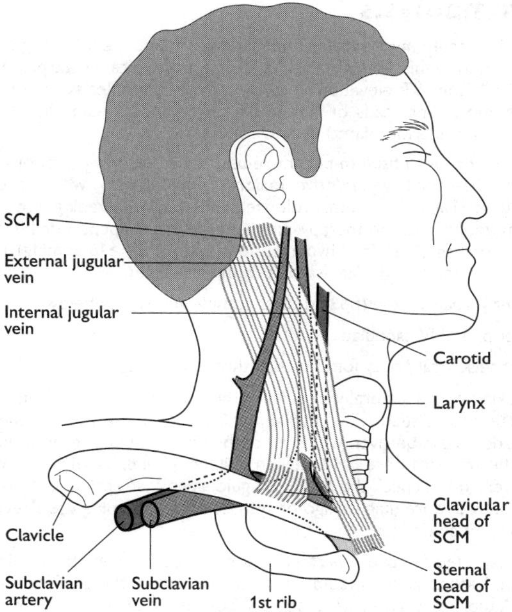

Anatomy of the major vessels in the neck the internal jugular is the commonest site and has fewer complications than subclavian cannulation; femoral cannulation carries a higher rate of infection. The internal jugular lies deep to sternocleidomastoid muscle (SCM). The needle should puncture the skin midway between the mastoid process and the sternoclavicular joint, lateral to the carotid pulse. The needle should then be directed towards the nipple on the same side to hit the vein.

Accidental arterial cannulation

Signs of arterial cannulation

- Bright-red blood, rather than dark-red
- Pulsatile blood, rather than constant low flow
- ↑O_2 sats (>95%) of blood compared with finger O_2 sats
- If the right carotid artery is cannulated the central line will cross the midline on the CXR

What to do if the artery is cannulated

- Identify arterial cannulation
- Remove all lines and press firmly over site for 10min
- Seek senior help

You can reattempt on the same side or the other side; if you don't feel confident, ask your seniors for assistance.

Thrombolysis

Indications acute myocardial infarction which meets the following criteria: presentation within 12h of onset of symptoms; typical chest pain lasting >30min; >2mm ST elevation in two or more chest leads or >1mm in two or more limb leads or >1mm ST segment depression in V1 to V3 (suggesting posterior infarct) or new LBBB

Contraindications ***absolute*** patient refusal, active bleeding, previous intracerebral haemorrhage; ***relative*** major trauma/surgery within previous 4wk, stroke/TIA in last 3mth, prolonged CPR, known bleeding disorder or current anticoagulation therapy, pregnancy, active dyspepsia or history of GI haemorrhage, sustained hypertension (systolic BP >180mmHg), recent head injury, pericarditis. Age is not a contraindication.

Consent verbal/written (p69); discuss complications (see below)

Site peripheral IV cannulae

Agent check local policy for choice of thrombolytic agent

Streptokinase is a naturally occurring thrombolytic derived from streptococcus and as such will cause an antibody response in the patient so repeat doses can be given within 4d of the first dose but never again after that. The standard dose is 1.5 million units in 50ml 0.9% saline by IV infusion over 1h but check the *BNF*/local guidelines. If streptokinase has been administered more than 4d ago or systolic BP <110mmHg use a recombinant thrombolytic agent.

Alteplase, reteplase and *tenecteplase* are all recombinant tissue plasminogen activators; doses should be determined from the *BNF*/local guidelines. Alteplase is given as a bolus followed by an infusion. Reteplase is given as two boluses. Tenecteplase is given as a single bolus. Heparin is commenced following administration of all the recombinant thrombolytics (see p347).

Monitoring during treatment monitor cardiac rhythm continuously and BP every 5min. Reperfusion arrhythmias (including VT) are common and usually self-limiting. Use ALS algorithm if persistent or cause compromise.

Desired outcome eventual normalisation of ST segments and improvement in chest pain. If symptoms and/or ST segment changes persist seek senior cardiology help; a second thrombolysis dose may sometimes be given.

Complications bleeding (intracranial (1%), other major bleed (5%)), reperfusion arrhythmias, hypotension, anaphylaxis. If hypotension occurs during treatment with streptokinase, slow the infusion down.

Safety never perform this procedure for the first time on your own

Alternatives primary coronary angioplasty (PCA) (see *OHCM*7 p102)

Hints and tips only undertake in a well-monitored environment (ED resus, CCU, HDU). Bleeding from cannula sites is common and patients should be warned not to worry about this. In the event of massive life-threatening haemorrhage, antifibrinolytics and FFP can be used to reverse the process.

Pleural tap

Indications diagnosis of effusion, symptomatic relief

Contraindications absolute patient refusal; ***relative*** local infection, contralateral pneumothorax/effusion, anticoagulation

Consent verbal; explain why the pleural tap is required

Site simplest and safest sites are shown opposite (Fig. (A)), directly below the inferior angle of the scapula or in the posterior-axillary line; choose an intercostal space two or three spaces below the top of the effusion; if in doubt request an ultrasound and ask for a site to be marked

Equipment 5, 10, 20, 50ml syringes, orange (25G) and green (21G) needles, ±intravenous cannula (14–16G), 3-way tap, 3 specimen containers and fluoride oxalate blood tube (p557), sterile jug/bowel, 1% lidocaine, sterile gloves, dressing pack, antiseptic cleaning solution

Checks confirm side of the effusion clinically and on CXR; lay equipment out on clean treatment trolley; recruit an assistant

Patient position see Fig. (A) opposite

Procedure wash hands and wear sterile gloves. Clean area thoroughly with Betadine® or chlorhexidine. Infiltrate 2–5ml of LA with orange needle into subcutaneous and then deeper layers towards pleura, avoiding neurovascular bundles (Fig. (C) opposite). Allow 2min to take effect. Using either a green needle on a 20ml syringe or a cannula, gently advance the needle through the anaesthetised area directly towards the pleura. Once in the pleural space, fluid is easily drawn into the syringe or a flashback will be seen in the cannula; if using the cannula then remove the needle, leaving the plastic component in place, and attach a syringe. Aspirate volume required and divide into specimen containers. If performing a therapeutic procedure use the cannula and attach a 3-way tap with a 50ml syringe; withdraw and dispose of fluid into a jug. Once complete withdraw needle/cannula and apply plaster to skin.

Confirmation pleural fluid aspirated, always get a CXR (pneumothorax and reassess the level of the effusion if a therapeutic procedure)

Complications pneumothorax, haemothorax, pain, bleeding, damage to intercostal nerve, local or intrapleural infection, visceral puncture

Safety never perform this procedure for the first time on your own; take care not to allow air into the pleural space

Alternatives retry in a different rib space; radiology might perform a diagnostic tap under ultrasound guidance; chest drain for large effusions

Hints and tips make sure you and the patient are comfortable before you start; try to anaesthetise the skin fully and insert the local anaesthetic needle at right angles to the skin when infiltrating down to the pleura

Aspiration of pneumothorax tension pneumothorax is a medical emergency and requires immediate treatment (p227). Aspiration of 'simple' pneumothoraces can also be performed (p228).

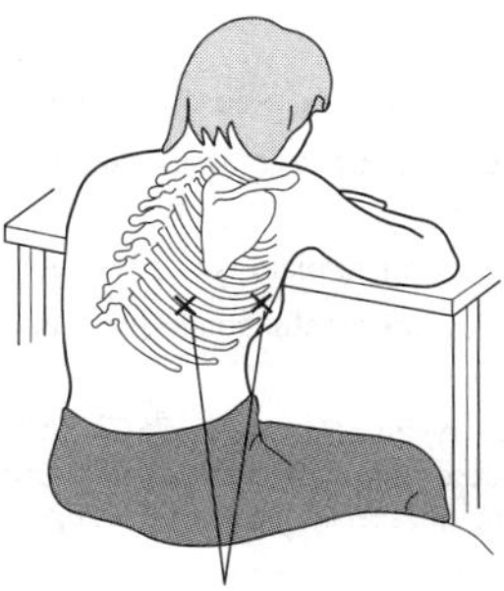

(A) ***Position of the patient for aspiration of pleural fluid*** get the patient to lean forwards over a table or the back of a chair to open up the rib spaces and prevent excessive movement.

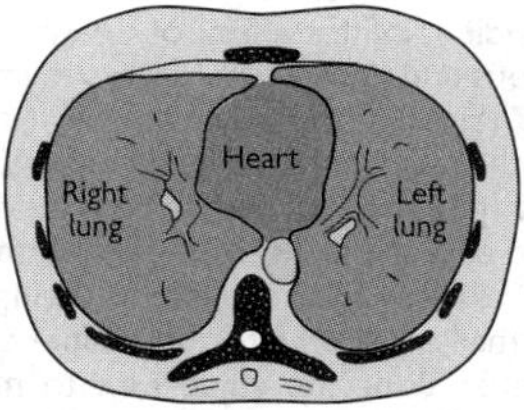

(B) ***Position of the normal heart within the thorax at level of T6/T7 vertebra*** the diaphragm lies between T8/T12. Posterior and lateral approaches for pleural aspiration with standard green (21G) needle or IV cannula are highly unlikely to puncture the heart, even on the left side of the chest.

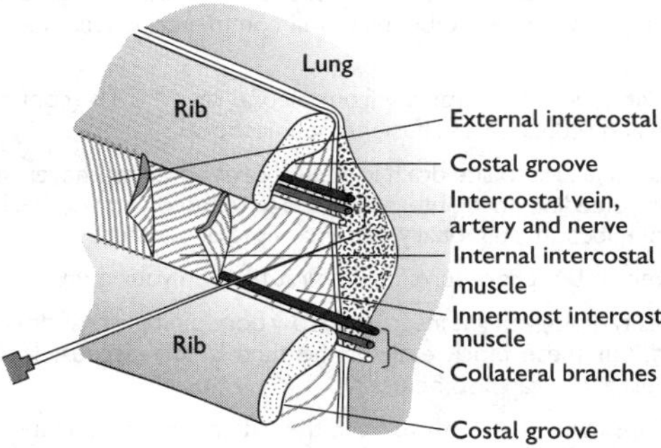

(C) ***Safe pleural aspiration to avoid neurovascular bundles*** the main bundle sits just posterior to the inferior rib edge, though collateral branches are located adjacent to the superior border. The safe approach is to advance the needle above a rib, but not right against its superior edge.

Chest drain

Indications pneumo/haemothorax, pleural effusion, empyema

Contraindications ***absolute*** patient refusal; ***relative*** local infection, bleeding diathesis/anticoagulation

Consent verbal/written (p69); explain why procedure is required

Site mid-axillary line, 5th intercostal space for a pneumothorax or below fluid level in an effusion

Equipment 5, 10, 20ml syringes, orange (25G) and green (21G) needles, suture, Seldinger chest drain pack, bottle with underwater seal (400ml sterile water), 1% lidocaine, sterile gloves, dressing pack, antiseptic cleaning solution

Checks confirm side of the effusion clinically and on CXR; lay equipment out on clean treatment trolley; recruit an assistant

Patient position hunched forwards over a table (Fig. (A)) or reclining back with their arm behind the head (Fig. (B)); choose according to comfort

Procedure wash hands and wear sterile gloves. Clean area thoroughly with Betadine® or chlorhexidine. Infiltrate 5ml of LA with orange then green needle into subcutaneous and then deeper layers towards pleura, avoiding neurovascular bundles (Fig. C, p579). Allow 2min to take effect. Attach Seldinger needle onto the syringe and advance through the area of infiltration as for a pleural tap (p578). Once needle tip is inside the pleural space, remove the syringe and pass the guide-wire through the needle. Never let go of the guide-wire. Withdraw the needle fully leaving half the guide-wire in the chest. Make a small incision with the scalpel alongside the guide-wire and pass the dilator along the guide-wire to make a track to the pleural space. Withdraw dilator, but leave the guide-wire in situ. Pass the chest drain over the guide-wire to the required depth then remove the guide-wire. Attach the 3-way tap to the end of the chest drain and turn 'off to chest'. Suture the chest drain to the chest wall using more LA if needed. Connect the 3-way tap to the tubing of the chest drain bottle and open the 3-way tap. Fluid drainage/bubbling will commence. Cover wound with clear dressings.

Confirmation fluid or air draining from pleural cavity, CXR (confirmation of position and reduction of effusion/pneumothorax)

Complications failure to site drain in pleural cavity, pneumothorax, haemothorax, pain, bleeding (local/internal), damage to intercostal nerve, local or intrapleural infection, pulmonary oedema, visceral puncture

Safety never do this procedure for the first time on your own

Alternatives radiology might insert a narrow bore pig-tail chest drain under ultrasound, but these block easily if the fluid is too viscous. Traditional trochar chest tubes can also be used.

Hints and tips make sure both you and the patient are comfortable before you start; use sufficient LA and consider premedicating the patient with good PO/IV analgesia 30min before the procedure

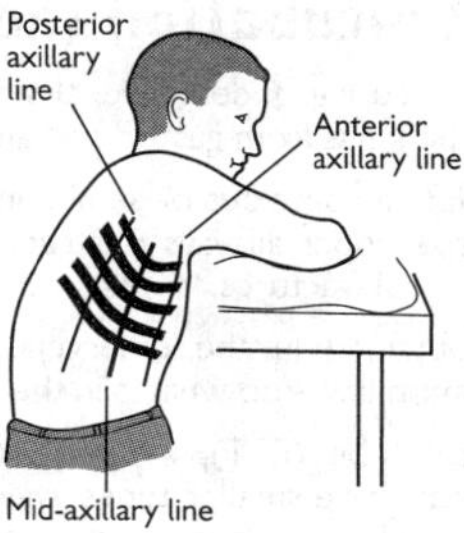

(A) ***Position of the patient for chest drain insertion*** ask the patient to lean forwards over a table or the back of a chair, since this opens up the rib spaces and prevents them from moving too much.

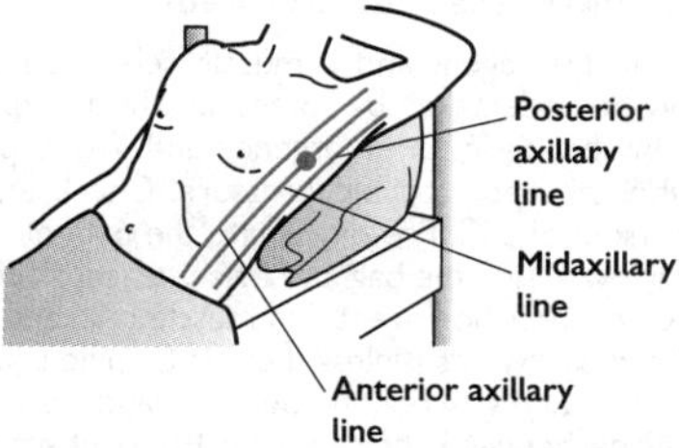

(B) ***Alternative position of the patient for chest drain insertion*** position the patient at about 45° with their arm above and behind the head, exposing the axilla.

Removing a chest drain

- Leave the drain unclamped
- Remove dressings from skin
- Clean skin with Betadine® or chlorhexidine
- Remove all sutures
- Gently but firmly remove drain as patient exhales; occlude wound
- Re-suture mattress sutures around drain site (p600)
- Apply sterile dressing. Sutures should stay in for 5d.
- CXR to ensure no pneumothorax has developed during removal of the drain

Endotracheal intubation (adult)

Emergency indications securing a definitive airway in the unconscious patient and protecting the lungs from gastric contaminants

Contraindications ***absolute*** a conscious or semi-conscious patient, inexperienced operator; ***relative*** upper airways obstruction from foreign body, known or suspected cervical fractures, laryngeal oedema/trauma

Consent not usually obtained in the emergency situation as patient unconscious; apply common law – do what is in the patient's best interests

Equipment endotracheal tube (ETT), 7–8mm internal diameter for a woman, 8–9mm for a man; have smaller tubes available. 10ml syringe and water-based lubricant. Working laryngoscope (commonly size 3 and size 4 Mackintosh) and spare laryngoscope in case batteries fail. Bougie and Magill forceps. Stethoscope. Guedel and nasopharyngeal airways. LMA sizes 3, 4 and 5. Bag and mask for pre-oxygenation. Tape to secure ETT and suction with yanker attached. CO_2 monitor is advised. Gloves.

Patient position laying flat, with single pillow under neck to achieve 'sniffing morning air' position (neck flexed, head extended)

Procedure an IV induction agent and a muscle relaxant must be given, but this should only be undertaken by someone who is experienced and well rehearsed in intubating in an emergency and in the presence of a skilled assistant who can apply cricoid pressure. Check equipment and slightly lubricate outside of ETT. Pre-oxygenate the patient for 3min with 15l/min O_2 if time allows using the bag and mask, assisting their ventilation if it is inadequate. Once induction agent and muscle relaxant have worked, remove mask, tilt head backwards (unless there is C-spine injury) and open the mouth. Holding the laryngoscope in your left hand, advance the tip of the laryngoscope blade between the teeth on the right-hand side of the patient's mouth over the top of the tongue. Sweep the tongue to the left of the patient's mouth. Advance the laryngoscope in the midline until the uvula can be seen, then advance further until the epiglottis is visualised. Lift the laryngoscope away from you, do not lever as this will break the patient's teeth. As you lift the laryngoscope, the epiglottis should also be lifted and the vocal cords and the opening into the trachea (the glottis) visualised. Take the ETT in your right hand and pass it through the mouth and observe it passing between the vocal cords. When the ETT is at about 22cm at the lips the assistant should inflate the cuff; gently remove the laryngoscope, holding the ETT securely in place. Attach the CO_2 monitor and re-inflating bag to the ETT and gently squeeze. Once satisfied with the position of the ETT allow assistant to release cricoid pressure and secure ETT in place with tape and continue to ventilate, giving sedatives/hypnotics as required.

Confirmation the chest should rise and fall, the ETT should mist up and the CO_2 monitor should detect CO_2 as the chest falls (expiration). Auscultate in both axilla to listen for breath sounds and over the epigastrium to exclude air entering the stomach. Obtain a CXR to check the ETT is not in too far, as it is often past the carina in the right main bronchus.

Complications ***failure to visualize the vocal cords*** – revert to bag and mask ventilation ±Guedel/nasopharyngeal airway, or attempt to put in an LMA until expert help arrives. ***Oesophageal intubation*** – no air entering chest, no CO_2, gurgling in stomach; remove ETT immediately and revert to bag and mask ventilation ±Guedel/nasopharyngeal airway, or attempt to put in an LMA until expert help arrives. ***Endobronchial intubation*** – difficulty in ventilating the patient, only one side of the chest wall moves and breath sounds only audible on that side; withdraw the ETT a centimetre at a time and re-check.

Safety never undertake this procedure on your own. If in doubt bag and mask ventilate a patient until expert help arrives or insert an LMA if appropriately trained to do so (see below). You will never be criticised for supporting an obtunded patient's breathing with bag and mask ventilation alone, but you will be if you unsuccessfully undertake a procedure you are unfamiliar with and untrained to perform.

Hints and tips speak to a friendly anaesthetist and ask to go to theatre to watch and help at intubations and other airway skills. Consult Chapter 6 of the *Advanced Life Support Providers' Manual* (5th edition 2006).

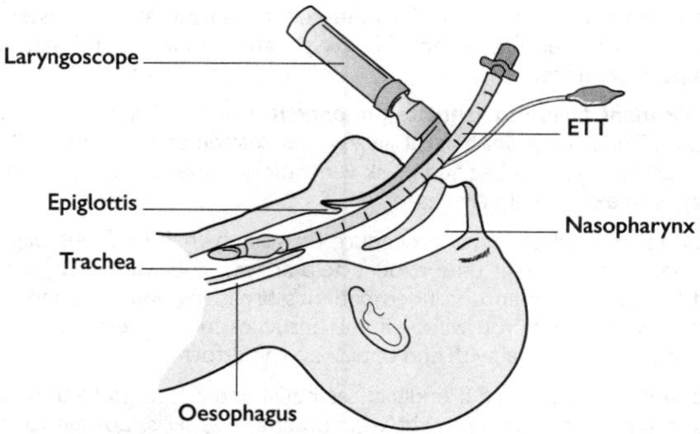

(A) Position of the laryngoscope and ETT once inserted.

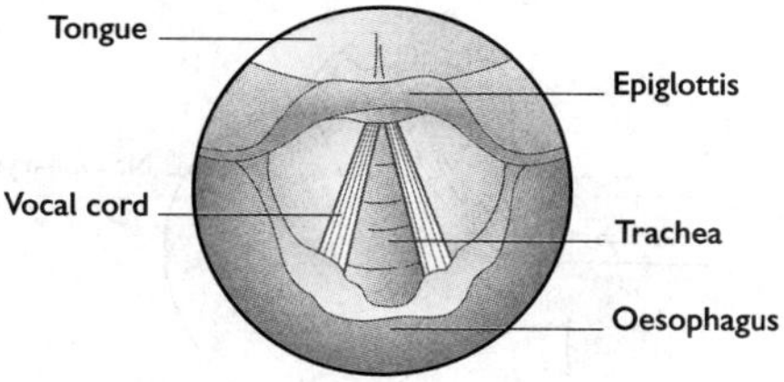

(B) Structures which should be visible at laryngoscopy.

Laryngeal mask airway (LMA)

Contraindications, consent, equipment and positioning as for intubation. Sizes: women 3 or 4, men 4 or 5.

Procedure as for intubation. Check equipment and check that cuff on LMA works and there is no leak; apply a small amount of lubrication to the top of the LMA around the cuff. Once the patient is adequately pre-oxygenated and sedated, remove mask, tilt head backwards (avoid if C-spine injury) and open mouth. Standing at the patient's head take the LMA in your right hand holding it like a pen with the black line of the LMA shaft facing you. Slide the LMA along the roof of the mouth firmly and smoothly. Keep advancing until the mask of the LMA disappears from view and it reaches a natural stop. Inflate the cuff with the required volume of air (documented on the LMA itself). Attach the CO_2 monitor and re-inflating bag to the LMA and gently squeeze. Once satisfied with the position of the LMA, secure it in place with tape and continue to ventilate, giving sedatives/hypnotics as required.

Confirmation the chest should rise and the CO_2 monitor should detect CO_2 as the chest falls (expiration). Auscultate in both axilla to listen for breath sounds. If unsure, remove, re-oxygenate with a bag and mask and attempt once more.

Complications failure to ventilate the patient revert to bag and mask ventilation ±Guedel/nasopharyngeal airway and reattempt once more. If still unsuccessful revert to bag and mask ventilation ±Guedel/naso-pharyngeal airway until expert help arrives.

Safety never undertake this procedure on your own. If in doubt, bag and mask ventilate a patient until expert help arrives. You will never be criticized for supporting an obtunded patient's breathing with bag and mask ventilation alone, but you will be if you unsuccessfully undertake a procedure you are unfamiliar with and untrained to perform.

Hints and tips speak to a friendly anaesthetist and ask to go to theatre to watch and help at inserting an LMA and other airway skills. Consult Chapter 6 of the *Advanced Life Support Providers' Manual* (5th edition 2006).

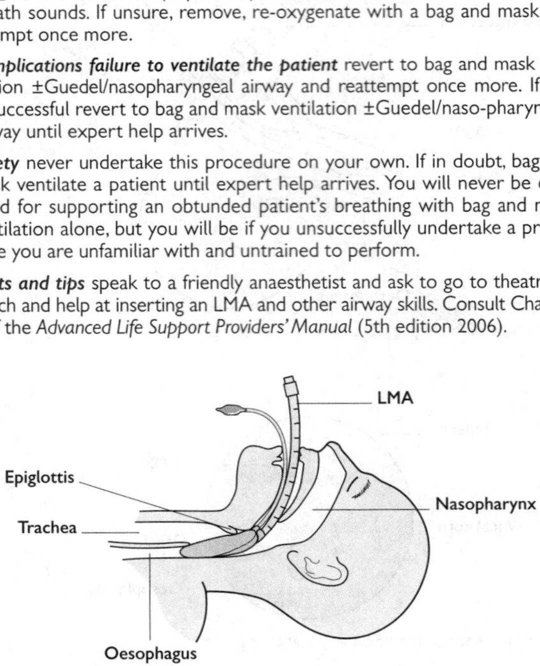

Position of an LMA once inserted.

Urethral catheterisation

Indications monitor urine output, urinary retention, incapacitation (eg ↓ GCS), incontinence, urological investigations

Contraindications ***absolute*** patient refusal; ***relative*** suspected urethral injury, urethral strictures/fistulas, active UTI

Consent verbal; explain why a catheter is required

Site via urethra into bladder

Equipment catheter pack (kidney dish, bowl, cotton balls, sterile towel and gloves), Foley catheter (10–16F), antiseptic solution, gauze, 10ml 1% lidocaine/lubricant gel in pre-filled syringe, 10ml saline-filled syringe, catheter bag

Checks no latex allergy/UTIs, correct sex catheter

Patient position lying on back, genitalia exposed (legs apart in women)

Procedure wash hands and wear sterile gloves. Prepare the equipment, using aseptic technique. Ask an assistant to pour antiseptic solution into the sterile bowl.

Male create a hole in the centre of the towel and drape it over the patient with the penis through the hole. Hold the penis with gauze in your non-dominant hand. Retract the foreskin and clean the penis with antiseptic. Hold the penis upright and instil 10ml lidocaine gel into the meatus. Occlude the penile tip to help push the gel along the urethra. Allow 2min for the anaesthetic to take effect, lubricate the tip of the catheter with lubricant. Put the kidney bowl between the patient's thighs and place the draining end of the catheter in it. Using your clean hand insert the catheter tip into the urethra and advance. Continue to advance the catheter to the hilt once urine starts draining to make sure the catheter balloon is within the bladder. Inflate the balloon with 10ml saline via the side port. Stop if there is pain or discomfort. Disconnect the syringe and pull back the catheter until you feel resistance. Attach a draining tube and bag to the free end of the catheter. Clean and redress the patient. Always replace the foreskin.

Female nurses usually perform female catheterisation. Drape the sterile towel between the patient's thighs. Separate labial folds with your non-dominant hand and clean with antiseptic solution. The urethra is between the vagina and clitoris. Continue as for a male patient.

Confirmation urine drains freely, no pain on inflating balloon

Complications pain, infection, local trauma, haematuria, strictures (long-term), retention on removing catheter

Safety never force the catheter or fill the balloon under force

Alternatives suprapubic catheter – seek senior advice (see p589)

Hints and tips

- Double glove on your dominant hand and remove the top glove once you have finished cleaning the genitalia so that you remain sterile when handling the catheter
- Avoid touching the lubricant gel with the hand holding the catheter as this makes the catheter slippery and difficult to grip and insert
- Try not to touch the catheter; it usually comes in a plastic cover which can be shuffled down or torn away as you insert it into the urethra
- If you feel resistance at the prostatic urethra hold the penis vertically and try to advance the catheter
- The urethra is 4–7cm in women so urine should be seen after 8cm; the male urethra is much longer (20cm) so the catheter must be inserted further
- If no urine appears check the catheter is in the correct place and advanced far enough; flush the catheter with saline to make sure it is not blocked with lubricant gel – if you still do not get urine, **do not** inflate the balloon, remove the catheter and seek senior advice
- Urine samples can be taken from a catheter (CSU)

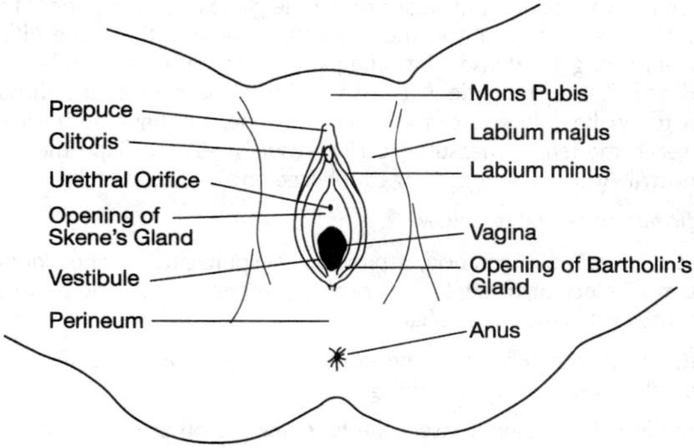

Anatomy of the female genitalia for catheterisation.

Nasogastric tubes (NG tubes)

Indications stomach emptying eg bowel obstruction (wide-bore or Ryle's tube), nutrition (fine bore)

Contraindications absolute basal skull fracture, facial trauma, patient refusal

Consent verbal; explain why a NG tube is required and warn the patient about initial discomfort (which does improve)

Site inserted into the stomach via a nostril

Equipment non-sterile gloves, NG tube, lubricant jelly, glass of water, adhesive tape, drainage bag and bowl (or spigot)

Checks make sure patient is alert, with no history of head injury. Use an appropriate sized tube. Gauge the length of tube to insert by measuring the distance from the nostril to angle of the jaw and from angle of the jaw to the xiphisternum.

Patient position sit the patient upright with head against a pillow

Procedure wash hands and wear non-sterile gloves. Ask the patient to take a sip of water and hold it in their mouth. Cover the tip of the NG tube with lubricant gel and insert into the patient's nostril. Aim the tube directly backwards. Once the patient feels the tube at the back of the throat ask them to swallow so you can advance the tube. Continue advancing until you reach the length measured earlier (usually ~40cm). Tape the tube to the nostril. Attach a drainage bag to the free end of the NG tube.

Confirmation see table below

Complications pain/irritation, aspiration, oesophagitis, tracheal/duodenal intubation, electrolyte depletion, local tissue necrosis, gastric perforation, tube may curl in mouth or pharynx

Safety check the tube is in the correct position with a CXR, essential before the tube is used for feeding

Alternatives if you cannot insert the tube, try the other nostril or consider passing it orally (only if patient unconscious); see next page for other options

Hints and tips use a chilled NG tube as these are less flexible.

Methods of confirming NG tube placement	
Chest X-ray	Essential before a fine-bore feeding tube is used and recommended for a wide-bore tube. Check tip of NG is visible below diaphragm and not in bronchial tree (check local policy if F1s are allowed to check NG position – may need to be senior).
NG aspiration	Aspirate fluid and test pH (stomach fluid usually acidic, pH <4). This does not confirm the NG tube is in the stomach.
Air injection	Listen for air over the stomach as 20–50ml of air is injected. This does not confirm the NG tube is in the stomach.

Replacing a suprapubic catheter

Indications long-term catheter due for change (every 8–10wk) or problem with catheter (blocked, leaking, UTI)

Contraindications absolute patient refusal; ***relative*** suprapubic stoma only recently created (<3d), bleeding disorder/anticoagulant therapy

Consent verbal (p69)

Site suprapubic catheter site, usually in the midline about 10cm below the belly button

Equipment sterile dressing pack, sterile gloves, new long-term catheter (usually 16F) and appropriate syringe with water for inflating balloon, sterile lubricating anaesthetic gel, cleaning solution, new drainage bag, 20ml syringe, disposable gloves and waste bag

Patient position lying supine, exposing suprapubic catheter site

Procedure wearing gloves empty current catheter bag. Deflate existing balloon with 20ml syringe, emptying syringe if there is more than 20ml in the balloon. Gently but firmly remove the old catheter and put in a waste bag. Clean hands, put on sterile gloves, prepare sterile trolley with dressing pack and remove perforated end of new catheter. Place sterile drape over insertion site, making a hole in the drape if necessary first. Clean insertion site, then apply some anaesthetic gel over the site and a small amount into the site; wait for 2 minutes for anaesthetic to work. Take the catheter in its plastic cover and pass the tip into catheter site, avoiding touching the rubber directly. Gently feed catheter in all the way. Connect to new drainage bag. Wait for urine to flow out of the catheter before inflating the balloon; volume of water to inflate balloon is stipulated on catheter and its packaging. Withdraw catheter to ensure balloon is working and catheter cannot fall out. Document in patient's records the date and the sizes and types of catheter taken out and then put in.

Confirmation urine flowing freely

Complications bleeding at catheter site or blood-stained urine after new catheter sited (common and if minor not a concern), patient discomfort, catheter site closes up after removal of old catheter (uncommon with mature catheter sites, but can occur with freshly formed stomas (<3d)

Safety only undertake catheter changes on mature, established stomas as newly created ones (<3d) may close immediately after removing catheter

Hints and tips if in doubt, speak to a urology nurse or the urology specialist. Sometimes the old balloon won't deflate, or the old catheter won't pull out – there are numerous reasons for this; speak to your senior or the urology nurse specialist/urology StR on-call.

Replacing a PEG feeding line

This is usually performed by a gastroenterologist or an endoscopist.

If the PEG has just fallen out it is possible to apply lubrication and insert a large urinary catheter into the hole to prevent the hole closing up. This may prevent the need for an operation.

Ascitic tap

Indications diagnosis from ascitic fluid

Contraindications ***absolute*** patient refusal; ***relative*** abnormal coagulation, local infection

Consent verbal; explain why a tap is required

Site left/right iliac fossa, horizontal to the umbilicus, but lateral to the mid-inguinal point (see diagram opposite). Avoid the suprapubic area with the bladder and inferior epigastric arteries.

Equipment sterile gloves, antiseptic solution in a bowl, 10ml 1% lidocaine, swabs, green (21G) needle, 20ml syringe, sterile adhesive dressing

Checks INR, seek advice if abnormal, empty bladder

Patient position lying flat on their bed, tilt bed slightly to one side

Procedure percuss the abdomen to assess the location and extent of the ascites. Wash hands and wear sterile gloves. Using aseptic technique clean the target area. Infiltrate around the area with 1% lidocaine initially into subcutaneous, then deeper layers towards the peritoneum. Allow 2min, then insert a green needle with a 20ml syringe vertically into the skin. Advance whilst aspirating until fluid flashback is seen (usually straw-coloured; may be bloodstained). Obtain 20ml fluid, then remove the needle and apply a sterile adhesive dressing.

- *Send fluid for* FBC, bacteriology (M,C+S, ±ZN stain/TB culture), biochemistry (protein, glucose, LDH, amylase), cytology

Confirmation fluid aspirated from abdominal cavity

Complications pain, bleeding (local or perforated viscus), perforated bowel/bladder, infection (skin or peritonitis), fluid leakage from wound

Safety do not have repeated attempts, if unsuccessful contact a senior and consider performing under ultrasound guidance

Alternatives therapeutic paracentesis (see box opposite)

Hints and tips avoid sites close to old surgical scars to avoid going through adhesions; in obese patients use a bigger needle. Afterwards lie the patient with the puncture site upwards to minimise fluid leakage.

Diagnosis of ascites

	Transudate ascites	**Exudate ascites**
Total protein	<30g/l	>30g/l
Aetiology	• Cirrhosis • Nephrotic syndrome • CCF	• Infection (>250 white cells/mm^3) • Pancreatic cause • Malignancy • Budd–Chiari syndrome

Therapeutic paracentesis

Ascites may need to be drained for symptomatic relief, to reduce infection risk and prevent respiratory compromise. Drainage should take place over <6h to reduce the risk of infection. Up to 6l can be drained in this time so long as 100ml salt-poor albumin IV is given for every 1.5l ascitic fluid drained to prevent hypotension. The patient's FBC, U+E, LFT and INR should be checked after the procedure.

A Seldinger paracentesis set is used. The procedure is similar to an ascitic tap except that a guide-wire is inserted through the needle followed by the drain over the guide-wire. The drain must be removed within 6h.

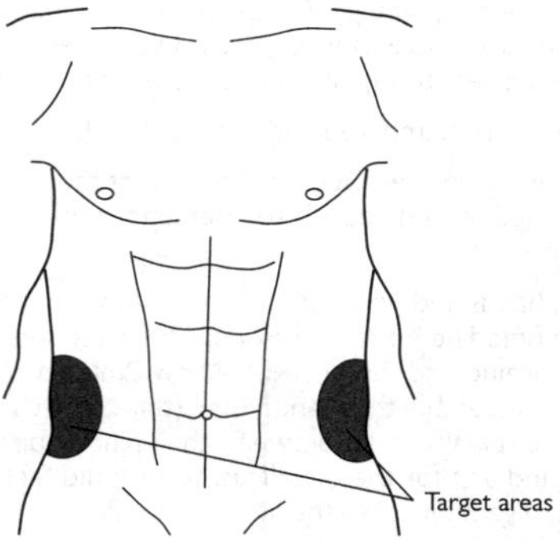

Target areas for ascitic tap at the level of the umbilicus, 3–4cm lateral to the mid-inguinal line.

Lumbar puncture (LP)

Indications suspected meningitis, encephalitis, subarachnoid haemorrhage, investigation of other neurological conditions

Contraindications ***absolute*** patient refusal, ↑intracranial pressure (see p300, check CT), infection at the site, cardiorespiratory compromise (treat first, including antibiotics); ***relative*** bleeding diathesis/anticoagulation, spinal deformity

Consent verbal; explain why the lumbar puncture is required

Site draw a line between the iliac crests and feel for a gap in the spine where the line crosses it, this is L3/L4. Ask the patient if this feels like the middle of their back. The cord ends at L1/L2, so never do LPs above the L2/L3 interspace; mark the spaces using arrows away from the spine.

Equipment 2ml syringe, orange (25G) needle, 1% lidocaine, antiseptic, gauze, lumbar puncture pack, sterile gloves, 3 specimen pots labelled 1/2/3 (or 4 pots if you suspect SAH), fluoride oxalate blood tube (p557)

Checks check pots are numbered and the assistant knows this

Patient position lying on their side on the edge of the bed with their back exposed, legs curled up and neck flexed (fetal position). Their body should be 90° to the floor.

Procedure wash hands and wear sterile gloves, gown and mask. Clean area thoroughly with Betadine® or chlorhexidine. Infiltrate subcutaneously with 2–3ml of 1% lidocaine and 25G needle. Allow 2min to take effect during which you should assemble the manometer (thin tube, check the numbers match up). Insert spinal needle between the spinous processes with the bevel facing up and aim for the umbilicus. You should feel resistance from the supraspinous ligaments then the ligamentum flavum and dura followed by a lack of resistance as you enter the subarachnoid space. Withdraw the stylet and look for clear fluid (do not panic if you see blood, this is probably a spinal vessel – withdraw and use a lower space), if there is no CSF pull back 2–3cm and realign. If the patient feels pain shooting down their leg you are hitting a nerve root so withdraw, then next time head more towards the midline. Once CSF is seen attach the manometer and measure pressure (7–20cmH_2O is normal). Use the three-way tap to drain the manometer fluid into the three specimen pots (10 drops in each) and the fluoride tube (six drops). Withdraw the entire needle and cover the wound with a sterile plaster. Take a blood sample in a fluoride oxalate (p557) tube and send for glucose levels. Advise the patient to lie flat for 1h and ask the nurses to check neurological obs and BP.

Confirmation CSF fluid seen

Complications headache post-procedure (worse sitting up, occurs within 24h and lasts 3–4d, p301), infection, trauma to nerve roots

Safety never do this procedure for the first time on your own

Alternatives can be performed under X-ray guidance though this is rare; there is no equivalent, consider asking a senior to help

Hints and tips position is everything; explain exactly what you want the patient to do, make sure their back is straight and their legs are tightly curled up. If you are having difficulty finding the midline, ask the patient if it feels to the left, right or middle. Make sure the needle is horizontal.

CSF samples send sample 2 and the fluoride tube for biochemistry (protein, glucose, pH), samples 1 and 3 to microbiology for M,C+S (consider requesting viral culture/PCR) and the fourth in a brown envelope (away from light) to biochemistry for xanthochromia if SAH suspected.

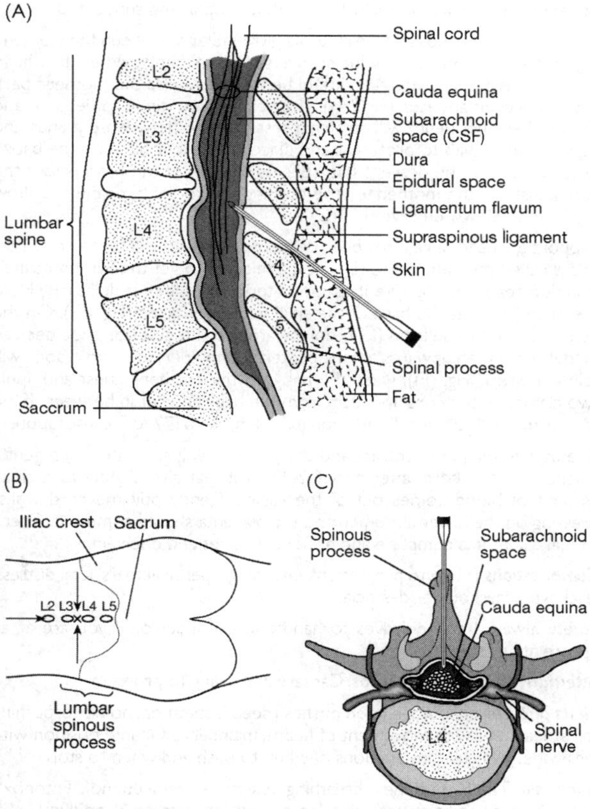

(A) Anatomy of a lumbar puncture. (B) Position and surface anatomy for a lumbar puncture. (C) Cross-section of the spine during a lumbar puncture.

Normal vaginal delivery

The first stage of labour often takes many hours. Monitor maternal HR, BP, temp, contractions and fetal HR every 15min. Second stage begins once the cervix is fully dilated – see below.

Consent verbal; explain that you will help her deliver her baby

Equipment sterile gloves, cord clamp x 2, cord scissors, swabs, Syntometrine® injection (ergometrine 0.5mg and oxytocin 5units given IM into the thigh as the baby's anterior shoulder is delivered), neonatal resuscitaire, name tags for baby

Patient position usually on her back with legs open and supported

Procedure wash hands and wear sterile gloves. Stand between the women's legs slightly to one side with sterile swabs to hand. When the head becomes visible (crowning) it should be facing towards the mother's back with its occiput anterior (Fig. (A)). The head will continue to descend and the mother's perineum will stretch; press the skin between the anus and vagina with a swab to protect it and place your other hand on the baby's head to control the descent (Fig. (B)). As the top of the head passes the vagina instruct the mother to stop pushing and to pant; meanwhile allow the head to slowly emerge (Fig. (C)).

Support the head once it has been delivered; the head will turn to one side, this is called restitution (Fig. (D)). Ask a midwife to get the Syntometrine® injection ready and to give it as the anterior shoulder is delivered. Hold the head firmly at the base of the skull with two hands (Fig. (E)). On the next contraction pull the head downwards so the anterior shoulder can be delivered then upwards for the posterior shoulder; the whole body will follow quickly (Fig. (F)). Place the baby on the mother's chest and apply two clamps to the cord 15–30cm from the baby and cut in between. If the baby is not well crash-call the neonatal team; see p172 for resuscitation.

The uterus will now contract and the placenta will separate. Keep gentle traction on the cord; after about 2–5min it will give slightly as a small amount of blood comes out of the vagina. Gently pull the cord whilst pressing on the lower abdomen and the placenta should come out. Check to make sure it is complete and has two arteries and one vein.

Complications failure to progress, haemorrhage, perineal tears, fetal distress, fetal hypoxia, shoulder dystocia

Safety always have midwives to hand and call a senior if you are at all unsure at any stage

Alternatives ventouse, forceps, Caesarean if failing to progress

Hints and tips encourage good pushes (deep inspiration, no noise, pushing for at least 20s with movement of head), maintain a suitable position with legs wide, give clear instructions of when to push and when to stop

Analgesia TENS machines, breathing exercises, paracetamol, Entonox® (nitrous oxide and air), pethidine (early–mid 1st stage only), epidural

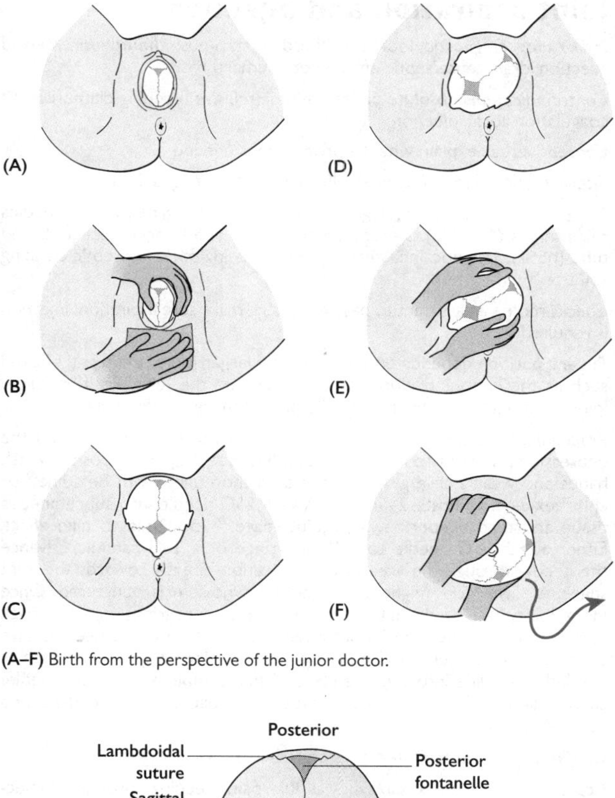

(A–F) Birth from the perspective of the junior doctor.

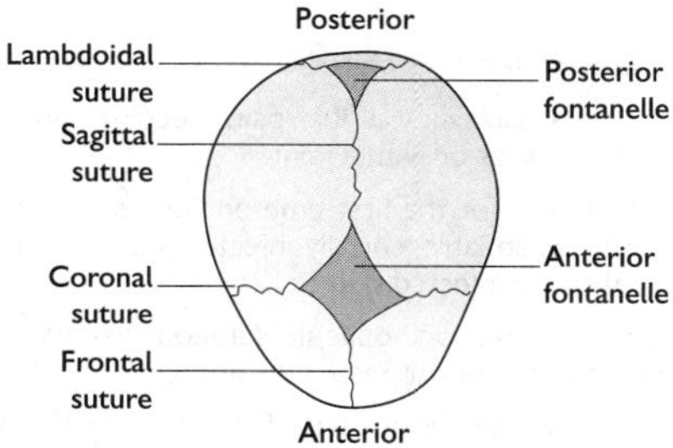

(B) Palpable anatomy of the fetal skull.

Joint aspiration and injection

Indications ***diagnostic*** look for blood/crystals/pus; ***therapeutic*** steroid injection, drain tense/septic effusion or haemarthrosis

Contraindications ***absolute*** patient refusal; ***relative*** bleeding diathesis/anti-coagulation, local infection

Consent verbal; explain why the procedure is needed

Site any synovial joint (eg wrist, elbow, shoulder, knee, ankle)

Equipment 2, 10, 20ml syringes, orange (25G) and green (21G) needles ±IV cannula (16–18G), 3 specimen containers and fluoride oxalate blood tube (p557), 1% lidocaine, sterile gloves, dressing pack, antiseptic cleaning solution

Checks recruit an assistant to pass you things, make sure aspiration/ injection is required

Patient position depends on joint; easier if larger joints are slightly flexed such as the knee and elbow as this opens up the joint. Position larger joints over a few pillows to make the patient more comfortable.

Procedure for aspirating knee identify lateral border of patella and the depression posterior to it over the joint line (see diagram opposite). Wash hands and wear sterile gloves. Clean area thoroughly with Betadine® or chlorhexidine. Infiltrate 2–5ml of LA with 25G needle into subcutaneous tissue and then deeper towards joint space. Allow 2min to take effect. Either attach 21G needle to a 10ml syringe or a 16G cannula; advance the needle through the area of LA infiltration directly towards the joint space. A slight 'pop' might be felt as the synovium is punctured. Once in the joint space fluid will be easily drawn into the syringe, or a flashback in the cannula will be seen; if using a cannula then remove the needle, leave the plastic component in place, and attach a syringe. Aspirate as much as needed and divide into specimen pots. Once complete withdraw needle/ cannula and apply plaster to skin. Medial approaches are also described (*OHAM7* p946).

Confirmation fluid aspirated, tension relieved

Complications failure to tap synovial fluid, pain, bleeding, subsequent infection of subcutaneous tissues or within joint

Safety never perform this for the first time on your own; always perform aspiration aseptically, as an iatrogenically infected joint is disastrous; avoid advancing needle through infected skin

Alternatives seek help from orthopaedic surgeon/rheumatologist; some radiologists perform this under ultrasound guidance

Hints and tips thick viscous effusions are difficult to draw up through small needles, so use a larger needle or cannula. Always speak to the relevant laboratory beforehand and enquire what volume and in which container they need their sample.

Joint injection

Steroid injections are used for a number of inflammatory disorders, but should be performed by an expert. If there is doubt whether a joint is infected or not, then steroids must not be injected into that joint (*OHCS7* p708).

Synovial fluid in health and disease

Aspiration of synovial fluid is used primarily to look for infectious or crystal (gout and pseudogout) arthropathies.

	Appearance	Viscosity	WBC/ml	NØ
Normal	Clear, colourless	High	<200	<25%
Non-inflammatory[1]	Clear, straw	High	<5000	<25%
Haemorrhagic[2]	Bloody, xanthochromic	Variable	<10,000	<50%
Acute inflammatory[3]	Turbid, yellow	Reduced		
• Acute gout			~14,000	~80%
• Rheumatic fever			~18,000	~50%
• Rheumatoid arthritis			~16,000	~65%
Septic	Turbid, yellow	Reduced		
• TB			~24,000	~70%
• Gonorrhoeal			~14,000	~60%
• Septic (other)[4]			~65,000	~95%

[1] eg degenerative joint disease, trauma.

[2] eg tumour, haemophilia, trauma.

[3] Includes eg Reiter's, pseudogout, SLE etc.

[4] Includes staphs, streps, Lyme, and pseudomonas (eg post-op).

For inflammatory causes of arthritis: Synovial fluid WBC >2000/ml is 84% sensitive (84% specific); synovial fluid neutrophil count >75% is 75% sensitive (92% specific) NB: not all labs are equally skilful.

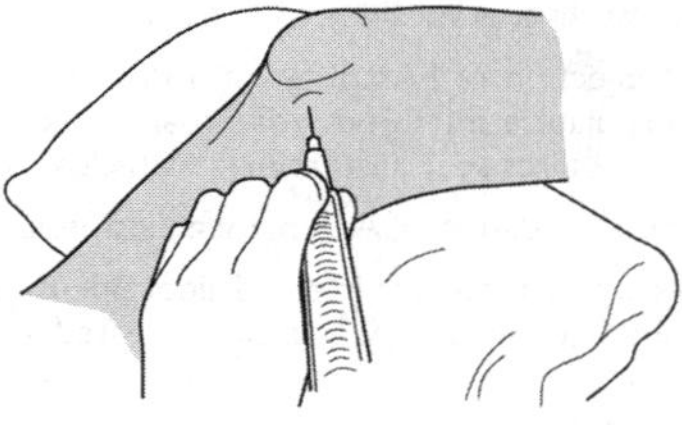

Aspirating a knee joint; rest the flexed knee on a pillow.

Local anaesthetic (LA)

Local anaesthetics (LAs) should not be used without knowledge of their side-effects, toxic doses and properties. A basic understanding about this drug class is essential as it will improve the patient's outcome.

Indications suturing, wound cleaning, FB removal, cannulation, cardiac arrhythmias, minor and major surgery (cataracts/hip replacement); topical preparations for cannulation, catheterisation, corneal anaesthesia

Types of block a ***field block*** is infiltration of LA into the tissue around a wound; this numbs small cutaneous nerves. In a ***peripheral nerve block*** a specific nerve is anaesthetised (eg digital, median) with subsequent dermatomal anaesthesia. A ***spinal anaesthetic*** blocks motor and sensory nerves below the level at which it is injected (often L3/L4). For full descriptions see *OHCS7* p634.

Which LA to use most wards will stock lidocaine (formerly lignocaine); 1% lidocaine solutions are usually sufficient. Other LAs are more likely to be used in the operating theatre or the ED. Different LAs vary in their speed of onset and duration of action. The table opposite shows the basic properties of commonly used LAs.

LAs with adrenaline (epinephrine) the vasoconstricting action of adrenaline prevents the LA from being rapidly redistributed by the circulation, prolonging its action at the injection site and allowing a larger dose to be administered. It is especially useful for scalp and facial anaesthesia. LAs with adrenaline must **never** be used near end arteries, (fingers, toes, penis, nose, ears) as this may lead to ischaemia/gangrene.

LA toxicity this usually occurs when serum concentrations peak (usually 45–60min after use). The symptoms and signs of toxicity are shown opposite. The *toxic dose* of LAs represents the maximum dose that should be injected into the tissues.

Management of LA toxicity if suspected, stop any further injection or infusion of LA, check ABC and give 15l/min O_2; midazolam 1–4mg/STAT IV increases the convulsion threshold and may prevent seizures; consider:
- ***Intubation*** if conscious level falls or seizures are resistant to conventional therapy (p284)
- ***CPR*** if there are signs of cardiovascular collapse (p208)

Allergy to LAs this is rare and much more likely with the ester group of LAs (cocaine, tetracaine (formerly amethocaine)) than the amide group of LAs (lidocaine, bupivacaine, prilocaine); treat as for anaphylaxis (p206)

Bier's block an IV injection of LAs distal to a double-cuffed tourniquet, often used to manipulate a fractured wrist in an awake patient (*OHCS7* p742). IV use of LA requires specialist training with close supervision.

Alternatives Entonox®, sedation ±LA, general anaesthesia ±LA

Hints and tips LAs sting as they are injected; lidocaine is less painful if it is diluted, warmed and injected slowly. LAs are 'activated' by alkaline conditions and so are much less effective when injected into inflamed/infected tissues which have a lower pH.

Commonly used local anaesthetics and their properties

Local anaesthetic	Onset	Duration	Toxic dose
Bupivacaine (Marcain®)	Medium	Long	2mg/kg
Levobupivicaine (Chirocaine®)	Medium	Long	2mg/kg (data lacking)
Lidocaine	Fast	Medium	3mg/kg
Lidocaine (with adrenaline)	Fast	Medium	7mg/kg
Prilocaine (Citanest®)	Fast	Medium	6mg/kg
Ropivacaine (Naropin®)	Medium	Long	3–4mg/kg

Calculating LA concentrations

Multiply the percentage solution by 10 to give the concentration in mg/ml

% solution	mg/ml
0.25%	2.5mg/ml
0.5%	5mg/ml
0.75%	7.5mg/ml

% solution	mg/ml
1%	10mg/ml
2%	20mg/ml
4%	40mg/ml

Maximum doses of lidocaine without adrenaline /kg

Volume in brackets represents ml of 1% lidocaine solution

Weight (kg)	Maximum dose
50	150mg (15ml)
60	180mg (18ml)
70	210mg (21ml)

Weight (kg)	Maximum dose
80	240mg (24ml)
90	270mg (27ml)
100	300mg (30ml)

Symptoms and signs of systemic local anaesthetic toxicity

Mild toxicity	• Tingling around the mouth • Metallic taste • Tinnitus • Visual disturbance • Slurred speech
Moderate toxicity	• Altered consciousness • Convulsions • Coma
Potentially fatal toxicity	• Respiratory arrest • Cardiac arrhythmias • Cardiovascular collapse

Suturing

Indications the two main indications for skin suturing are:
- Wound closure
- Keeping drains and lines in place

Contraindications absolute patient refusal, foreign body in wound, wound infection, old wound (>12h except on face), bite

Consent verbal (in the ED), written (elective surgery), common law (emergency surgery)

Site appropriate to wound/drain/line site

Checks tetanus status (p357), no infection or foreign bodies, no neurovascular deficit requiring referral, no damage to the underlying structures (eg tendons); if in doubt ask for senior opinion

Patient position patient lying in a comfortable position which exposes the wound site

Equipment sterile drape, sterile gloves, sterile water, 10ml syringe, green (21G) needle, orange (25G) needle, local anaesthetic (LA), appropriate suture material, suture pack (toothed forceps, needle-holder, scissors, gauze), assistant to hold the local anaesthetic

Anaesthetic prepare the sterile pack on the trolley with sterile gloves open and antiseptic solution in the receiver. Wash hands and put on sterile gloves. Draw up LA using a green needle and a 10ml syringe. Change to an orange needle for infiltration. Clean the skin with antiseptic solution and use the sterile drape to cover the area except for the wound. Warn the patient and insert the LA needle (it is less painful to go through the walls of the wound than through the skin). Draw back to check you are not in a blood vessel then infiltrate superficially. Allow 2–5min for the LA to work. Use this time to prepare your suture material and hold it with the needle facing upwards in the needle-holder. Before starting to suture, ensure the skin is numb.

Suturing starting at the middle of the wound, pick up the skin edge with the toothed forceps and pass the needle perpendicularly through the skin 5mm from the wound edge and into the wound just under the dermis. Grasp the needle point with the needle holder and pull it through gently. Hold the other skin edge with toothed forceps and again pass the needle through the skin, this time through the dermis first, up to the surface about 5mm from the wound edge. Pull most of the suture through then grasp both ends of the suture, tighten and oppose the skin edge so the edges are slightly everted but without tension. Hold the free end of the suture with the needle-holding forceps and make 3 knots around the forceps (anticlockwise, clockwise, anticlockwise). Make sure you 'lock' each knot by pulling the knot initially in the direction of the wound and then perpendicular to it. Cut the ends of the knot about 1cm long. The knots should lie to the side of the wound not on top of it. Repeat the procedure with sutures 5–10mm apart, depending on the area being sutured. When you have finished, clean the wound, apply a dry dressing and tell them when the sutures will need to be removed (see opposite).

Confirmation stitches apposing wound edges but not under tension

Complications infection, poor healing, hypertrophic/keloid scarring

Safety avoid touching the needle by using the needle-holder; when you do not need the needle keep it back to front in the needle-holder, with the point covered by the needle holder

Alternatives steristrips and glue (p356); staples have a lower infection rate, but can cause prominent hypertrophic scarring and require staple removers to take them out (may need to attend ward)

Hints and tips

- Make sure you and the patient are in comfortable position with good lighting before you start
- Use toothed forceps on skin as blunt forceps crush the tissue
- Local anaesthetic can be dangerous, see p598; adrenaline helps haemostasis, but should not be used on extremities
- Avoid nylon sutures for drains as this is often uncomfortable
- Consult a senior if the edges need a lot of tension to meet; you may need to use deep or subcutaneous sutures
- See p356 for treatment of wounds
- Get senior help early; if the sutures do not look right the patient will have the scar for life and it is often simpler to start again
- Operations are judged by the scars; take time to make them look good

Suture size and suggested dates for removal of sutures

Location	**Absorbable?**	**Suture size**	**ROS at day**
Face and neck	No	6/0	3–4
Lips/mouth/tongue	Yes	6/0 vicryl	N/A
Chest/abdomen	No	3/0	7–10
Limbs	No	4/0	5–7

Types of suture material

Non-absorbable sutures	**Absorbable sutures**
Nylon (ethylon)	Vicryl
Prolene	PDS
Silk	Monocryl

Wound care advice for patients

- Keep the wound area clean and dry for at least 48h
- Seek medical help if the wound looks infected, ie redness, swelling, tenderness
- Avoid heavy lifting for at least 6wk (except for scalp or face wounds)
- Drive when you can perform an emergency stop and check the view over your shoulder (see p646)

Chapter 12

Interpreting results

Full blood count (FBC)

There are three main components: red cells (haemoglobin or Hb), white cells (leucocytes or WCC) and platelets (plts). Remember these components represent the three cell lines from bone marrow.

Main FBC abnormalities

Anaemia	↓Hb	p332
Acute blood loss	FBC initially normal	p212
Infection/inflammation	↑WCC, ↑plts	p392
Haematological malignancies	↑↑WCC	p336
Bone marrow disorders	Persistent change in ≥1 cell line	p336

Hb – red bloods cells (♂ 13–18g/dl: ♀ 11.5–16g/dl)

- ↓*Hb* Anaemia, classified according to MCV, see p333 for causes, investigations and management
- ↑*Hb* Dehydration (p317), secondary polycythaemia eg heart/lung disease, polycythaemia vera (p336). Consider prophylactic LMWH (p346–7) due to the increased thrombosis risk

Reticulocytes (50–100 x 10^9/l or 0.5–2.5%) these are immature red cells released from bone marrow in response to haemolysis or blood loss (response detectable after a few hours, not acutely). They are also raised secondary to inflammation and infection.

WCC – white blood cells (4–11 x 10^9/l)

Causes of abnormal WCC

Cell		Causes
Neutrophils (2.0–7.5 x 10^9/l)	↑	Bacterial infection, inflammation, acute illness, myeloid leukaemia, steroids
	↓	Viral infection, sepsis, drugs (chemotherapy, steroids, carbimazole), splenomegaly, bone marrow failure, ↓B_{12} or folate, autoimmune disease
Lymphocytes (1.3–3.5 x 10^9/l)	↑	Viral infection, inflammation, lymphocytic leukaemia
	↓	Steroids, chemotherapy, HIV, autoimmune disease, bone marrow failure
Eosinophils (0.04–0.44 x 10^9/l)	↑	Parasitic/fungal infection, asthma, atopy, lymphoma
	↓	Rarely pathological

Plts – platelets (150–400 x 10^9/l)

Causes of abnormal plts

↑	Inflammation, infection, acute illness, recovery from splenectomy, essential thrombocytosis, polycythaemia [rubra] vera
↓	Heparin (in 5%), idiopathic thrombopenic pupura (ITP), chronic alcoholism, bone marrow failure, DIC, viral infections, splenomegaly, HELLP

Clotting

Clotting is often measured before procedures and operations if there is suspicion of an abnormality (eg jaundice). It is also measured to allow correct dosing of warfarin and heparin. See p345 for clotting defects.

Causes of abnormal clotting

Test		Causes
INR(0.8–1.2)	↑	Warfarin, liver disease, DIC, sepsis, deficiency of factors II, V, VII or X, heparin
	↓	Rarely pathological
APTTr(0.8–1.2)	↑	Heparin, haemophilia A+B, von Willebrand disease, DIC, sepsis, deficiency of factors II, V, VII, IX, X, XI or XII, liver disease, warfarin
	↓	Rarely pathological
INR and APTTr	↑	DIC, sepsis, liver disease, warfarin, heparin

Cardiac markers

The types of cardiac markers measured differ between hospitals, however most will measure creatine kinase (CK) and a troponin (either I or T). These tests are used to diagnose myocardial infarction and acute coronary syndromes, especially to distinguish from stable angina.

Causes of abnormal cardiac markers

Test		Causes
CK(25–195u/l)	↑	MI, rhabdomyolysis (muscle breakdown – check renal function), exercise, recent surgery, hypothyroidism
	↓	Rarely pathological
Troponin	↑	MI (only raised after 6–12h), small rise may be seen with CRF, PE, septicaemia
CK and troponin	↑	MI

Inflammatory response

Acute or chronic inflammation can affect a wide range of blood results, including:

- ↑ ESR
- ↑ CRP
- ↑ Ferritin
- ↑ Plts
- ↑ WCC
- ↓ Albumin

A very high ESR (>100mm/h) should raise suspicions of giant-cell arteritis (p389), polymyalgia rheumatica (p411) or myeloma (p336).

Urea and electrolytes (U+E)

These are measured to assess renal function and the concentration of the two main electrolytes in the blood.

Main urea and electrolyte abnormalities

Dehydration	↑urea, ±↑Cr	p317
Acute renal failure	↑K^+, ↑↑urea, ↑Cr	p316
Chronic renal failure	↑urea, ↑↑Cr, ↓Hb	p321
Upper GI bleed	↑↑urea, others normal	p245
Addison's disease	↓Na^+, ↑K^+, ↑urea, ↑Cr	p421

Urea and creatinine

Urea and creatinine (Cr) are metabolic waste products excreted by the kidney. An increase in either measure suggests a degree of renal dysfunction. If both urea and creatinine are raised the patient has renal failure. Check previous U+E results to distinguish between chronic and acute renal failure. Acute renal failure is an emergency, see p316.

Causes of abnormal urea and creatinine

Test		Causes
Urea (2.5–6.7mmol/l)	↑	Dehydration, excess protein intake eg upper GI bleed, acute illness, pre-renal failure
	↓	Rarely pathological, can be caused by a lack of protein eg alcoholism, anorexia, liver failure, malnutrition
Creatinine (Cr) (70–150μmol/l)	↑	Renal failure, may be acute, chronic or acute on chronic; muscle injury
	↓	Rarely pathological
Urea and creatinine	↑	Renal failure, check K^+ and ECG

Sodium and potassium

Numerous diseases can affect electrolyte levels, these are discussed in the section on electrolyte imbalance. Small changes in K^+ can induce fatal arrhythmias in the heart so abnormal K^+ levels should be treated as an emergency (p326).

Abnormal sodium and potassium

Electrolyte		Causes
Na^+ – Sodium (135–145mmol/l)	↑	See p328
	↓	See p328
K^+ – Potassium (3.5–5.3mmol/l)	↑	Urgent ECG, inform senior, see p327
	↓	Urgent ECG, inform senior, see p327

Liver function tests (LFT) and amylase

These are measured to detect jaundice, liver disease, biliary disease and pancreatitis. Liver dysfunction may affect clotting, particularly INR.

Main liver function abnormalities

Pre-hepatic jaundice	↑bilirubin (unconjugated), ↓Hb, ↑reticulocytes, ↓haptoglobin	p268
Hepatic jaundice	↑bilirubin (mixed), ↑↑ALT/AST, ↑γGT	p268
Cholestatic jaundice	↑bilirubin (conjugated), ↑↑ALP, ↑γGT	p268
Hepatocellular damage	↑↑AST/ALT, ↑γGT, ↑ALP	p265
Liver failure	↑bilirubin, ↑INR, ↓albumin	p264
Alcoholism	↑γGT, ↑MCV, ↓plts	p116
Pancreatitis	↑↑amylase, ↓Ca^{2+}, ↑glucose, ↑↑CRP	p241
HELLP (pregnant)	↑AST/ALT, ↑γGT, ↓Hb, ↓plts	p438

Liver function tests

See p263 for the investigation and management of liver disease.

Causes of abnormal liver function tests

Test		Causes
ALT (or AST) (3–35u/l)	↑	Liver disease/damage, biliary disease, alcohol, muscle damage, MI, pancreatitis
	↓	Rarely pathological, consider ↓vitamin B6
ALP(40–120u/l)	↑	Biliary disease/damage, liver disease, alcohol, bone disease (especially Paget's), pregnancy
	↓	Rarely pathological
γGT(10–55u/l)	↑	Biliary or liver disease, alcohol
	↓	Rarely pathological
Bilirubin (3–17μmol/l)	↑	Jaundice (p268 – haemolysis, liver disease, obstruction), Gilbert's syndrome
	↓	Rarely pathological
Albumin (35–50g/l)	↑	Dehydration
	↓	Inflammation, cirrhosis, malnutrition, pregnancy

Amylase

Causes of abnormal amylase

Test		Cause
Amylase (0–120u/dl)	↑	Acute or chronic pancreatitis, abdominal disease (eg perforation), burns, anorexia, salivary adenitis, renal disease
	↑↑↑	Acute pancreatitis (eg 3x upper limit of normal)

Calcium and phosphate

Calcium and phosphate are electrolytes predominantly stored in bones. Blood levels are affected by many diseases including parathyroid and bone abnormalities.

Main calcium and phosphate abnormalities

Bone metastases	↑Ca^{2+}, ↑ALP	p330
Hypoparathyroidism	↓Ca^{2+}, ↑PO_4^{3-}, ↓PTH	p331
Hyperparathyroidism	↑Ca^{2+}, ↓PO_4^{3-}, ↑ALP, ↑PTH	p330
Myeloma	↑Ca^{2+}, ↑urea, ↑Cr, ↓Hb, ↑ESR	p330
Paget's	↑↑ALP, ↔Ca^{2+}, ↔PO_4^{3-}	p330

Causes of abnormal calcium and phosphate

Test		Causes
Ca^{2+} – Calcium (2.12–2.65mmol/l)	↑	Primary/tertiary hyperparathyroidism, malignancy (myeloma, bone metastases, PTH-related peptide secreting tumours), excess vitamin D supplements, sarcoidosis
	↓	Vitamin D deficiency (Asians, Africans, chronic renal failure), hypoparathyroid, acute pancreatitis, alkalosis, magnesium deficiency
PO_4^{3-} – Phosphate (0.8–1.25mmol/l)	↑	Chronic renal failure, ↓PTH, myeloma, excess vitamin D, rhabdomyolysis, cell lysis (eg post-chemo), acidosis
	↓	Malabsorption/malnutrition, alcohol, ↑PTH, burns, alkalosis, post-DKA treatment

Effects of parathyroid hormone disease on blood tests

Disease	Ca^{2+}	PO_4^{3-}	PTH
Primary hyperparathyroidism	↑	↓	↑
Secondary hyperparathyroidism	↓	↓	↑
Tertiary hyperparathyroidism	↑	↓	↑
Hypoparathyroidism	↓	↑	↓

Endocrine tests

Cortisol

Short Synacthen® test

- Take blood for cortisol ideally at 9am. Occasionally ACTH is also tested; it needs to be transported on ice. Call biochemistry to check which bottle to use.
- Give 250μg Synacthen® IM/IV
- Take blood for cortisol 30min later
- A baseline or 30min cortisol level above 550nmol/l is normal and excludes primary adrenal insufficiency
- If 30min cortisol <550nmol/l and ↓ACTH → ACTH deficiency
- If 30min cortisol <550nmol/l and ↑ACTH → Addison's disease

Glucose

Interpretation of oral glucose tolerance test

Fasting glucose	Glucose after 2h	Diagnosis
Any	≥11.1mmol/l	Diabetes
≥7mmol/l	Any	Diabetes
<7mmol/l	7.8–11.0mmol/l	Impaired glucose tolerance (IGT)
6.1–6.9mmol/l	≤7.7mmol/l	Impaired fasting glucose (IFG)
<6.1mmol/l	≤7.7mmol/l	Normal

Thyroid function

	T_4	T_3	TSH
Hyperthyroidism	↑	↑	undetectable
T_3 hyperthyroidism	normal	↑	undetectable
Subclinical hyperthyroidism	normal	normal	↓
1° hypothyroidism (thyroid disease)	↓	↓	↑↑
2° hypothyroidism (pituitary disease)	↓	↓	↓ or normal
Subclinical hypothyroidism	normal	normal	↑

Electrocardiogram (ECG)

Examine all ECGs in a systematic manner to avoid missing the basics.

Check patient details, date and time of ECG, speed of paper (25mm/s)

Rate at 25mm/s each large square represents 0.2s and each small square 0.04s. To calculate rate divide 300 by the number of large squares between one R wave and the next R wave (see Table below).

Large squares	Heart rate (bpm)	Large squares	Heart rate (bpm)
1	300	2 3/5	115
1 3/5	188	2 4/5	107
2	150	3	100
2 1/5	136	4	75
2 2/5	125	5	60

Rhythm Sinus rhythm each QRS has a P wave before it. ***Atrial fibrillation*** no P wave and the QRS complexes are irregularly irregular. ***Atrial flutter*** the baseline is described as saw-tooth and the QRS are often regularly spaced. ***Ventricular rhythm*** QRS is wide (>0.12s or >3 small squares) and has no association with P waves. ***Nodal rhythm*** P wave may be absent or part of the QRS complex, but rhythm is regular. ***Regularly irregular*** rhythms suggest a degree of heart block (p197).

Axis this is surprisingly easy. Look at lead I and count the number of small squares that make up the height of the R wave. Next count the number of small squares that make up the Q or S wave. Work out the difference between the R and Q/S wave (ie R wave squares – Q/S wave squares). Do the same for lead aVF.

Draw a large cross (below) and plot the numbers for lead I and aVF. The line between where they meet and the middle is the cardiac axis. An example is shown where lead I has a 10 square R wave and 7 square S wave (10 – 7 = 3) and lead aVF has an 8 square R wave and 1 square S wave (8 – 1 = 7). The normal axis is from –30° to +90° (below).

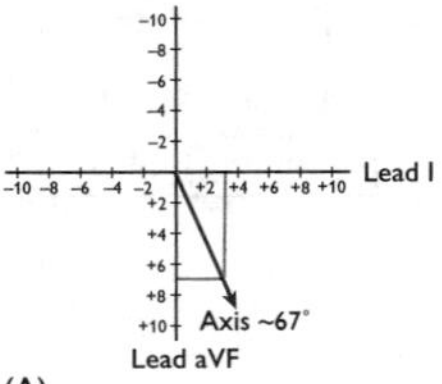

(A)

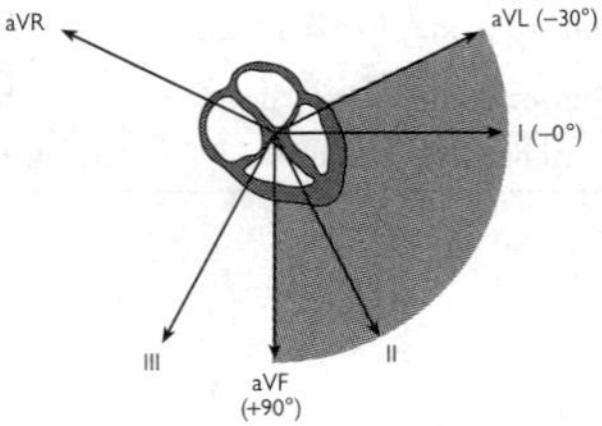

The table below shows a quick way of working out the rough position of the axis by comparing the size of the R wave to the size of the Q wave.

		Lead I	
		R > Q/S	R < Q/S
Lead aVF	R > Q/S	0 to 90°	90 to 180°
	R < Q/S	0 to –90°	–90 to 180°

P wave absent in AF (p188), atrial flutter (p188) and heart block (p197). Bifid P wave suggests left atrial hypertrophy. Peaked P waves are seen in right atrial hypertrophy (eg pulmonary hypertension) and transiently in ↓K^+.

PR interval normally 0.12–0.2s (3–5 small squares). Longer in heart block (p197) and shorter in WPW (p189).

QRS complex normally <0.12s (<3 small squares). Wider QRS implies ventricular rhythm (eg 3rd degree heart block) or bundle branch block (causes below). Paced rhythms may also have wide QRS complexes.

Hypertrophy left (*LVH*) sum of S wave in V3 and R wave in aVL >28mm (men) or >20mm (women)[1]; right (*RVH*) R>Q or S wave in V1, deep S wave in V6, T wave inversion in V2, ± V3, ± V4, right axis deviation.

ST segment usually level with baseline; elevation >1mm (causes below, infarction p180); depression >0.5mm suggests ischaemia (p181–2).

T wave inversion (pointing down) in leads I, II or V4–V6 suggests ischaemia. Often peaked in ↑K^+ and acute MI, flattened in ↓K^+.

Other components of the ECG

- ***QT interval*** is often calculated by modern ECG machines, though can be worked out manually (p190)
- ***U wave*** (positive in most leads) follows the T wave and precedes the P wave; if present it implies ↓K^+ though can be a normal finding
- ***δ wave*** a slurred upstroke to the QRS complex found in conduction defects eg Wolff–Parkinson–White p189
- ***J wave*** an upwards wave seen immediately after the QRS complex and before the T wave in hypothermia

Hints and tips being able to read an ECG systematically is much more important than a spot ECG diagnosis. The common ECG abnormalities which should not be missed are: AF, MI or ischaemia, LBBB/RBBB, 3rd degree heart block and ventricular tachycardia.

Electrocardiograph

Normal ECG

PR interval	0.12–0.20s
QRS interval	<0.12s
QT interval	0.33–0.43s

PR and QT intervals vary with heart rate

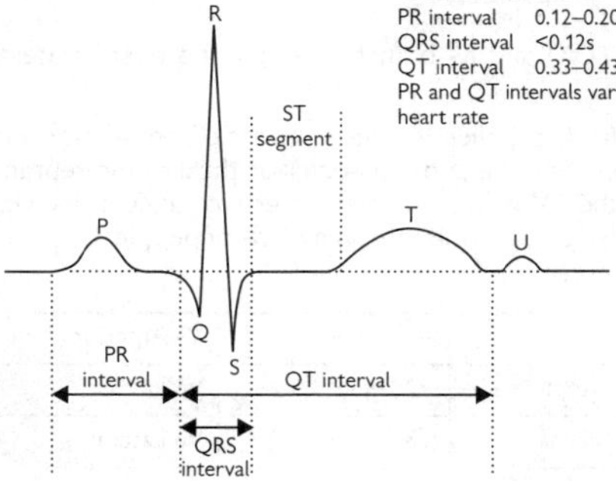

1 Cornell Criteria

Causes of . . .	
ST elevation	STEMI, pericarditis, ventricular aneurysm, LBBB, hypothermia, coronary artery spasm (Prinzmetal's angina), early repolarisation (early takeoff)
LBBB	Acute MI, ischemic heart disease, hypertensive heart disease, cardiomyopathy, aortic valve disease
RBBB	Normal, heart failure, PE, pulmonary hypertension
Left axis deviation	Left ventricular hypertrophy, inferior MI, left anterior hemiblock, hyperkalaemia
Right axis deviation	Right ventricular hypertrophy, chronic lung disease, normal in children, left posterior hemiblock

Coronary artery territories and the ECG

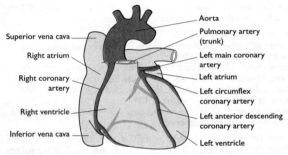

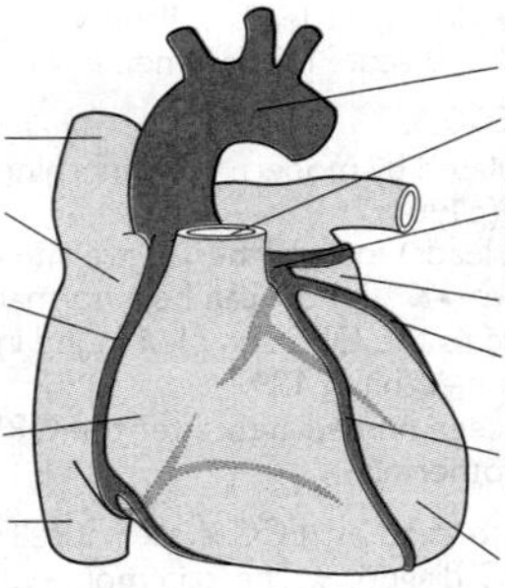

Simplified structure of the heart and its coronary blood supply.

Left anterior descending artery (LAD) and its many branches supply the anterior and anteriolateral walls of the left ventricle, and the anterior two-thirds of the septum

Left circumflex artery (LCX) and its branches supply the posterolateral wall of the left ventricle

Right coronary artery (RCA) supplies the right ventricle, the inferior and posterior walls of the left ventricle and the posterior third of the septum; the RCA also gives off the AV nodal coronary artery in ~85% of individuals, with the LCX supplying this in the remaining 15% of people.

I Lateral	aVR	V1 Septal	V4 Anterior
II Inferior	aVL Lateral	V2 Septal	V5 Lateral
III Inferior	aVF Inferior	V3 Anterior	V6 Lateral

Territories of the heart on the ECG.

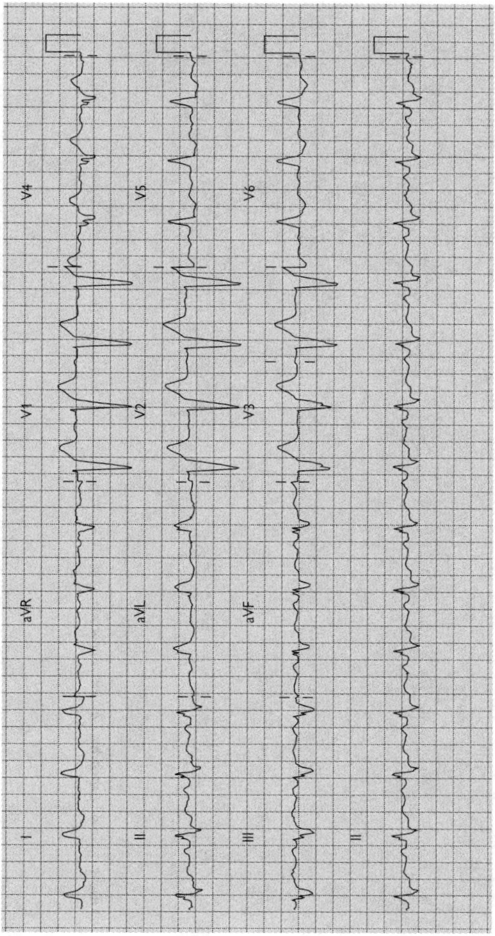

(A) **Left bundle branch block:** Note W pattern in V1 and M pattern in V5/V6, also no Q wave in V5/V6 and inverted T wave in I and aVL. Remember 'William Marrow'.

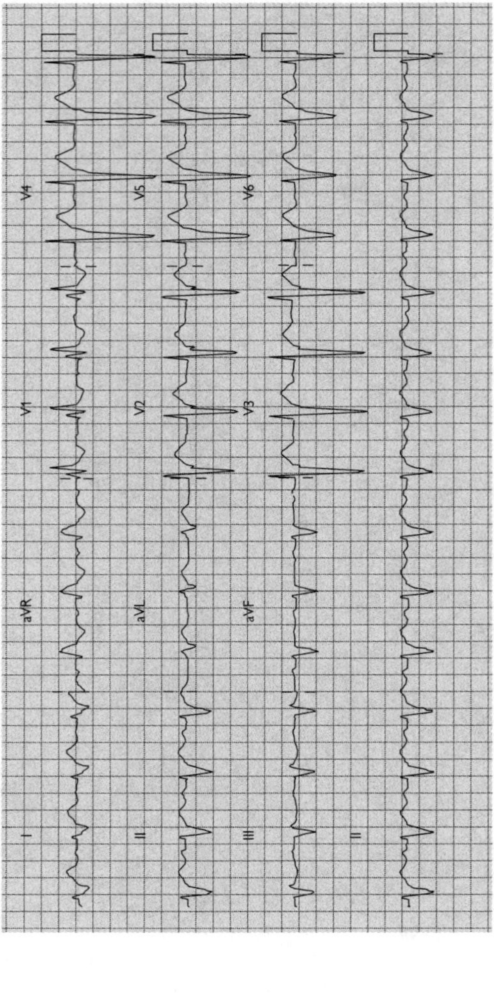

(B) Right bundle branch block: Note M pattern (RSR) in V1, W pattern in V5/V6 and inverted T wave in V1. Remember 'William Marrow'.

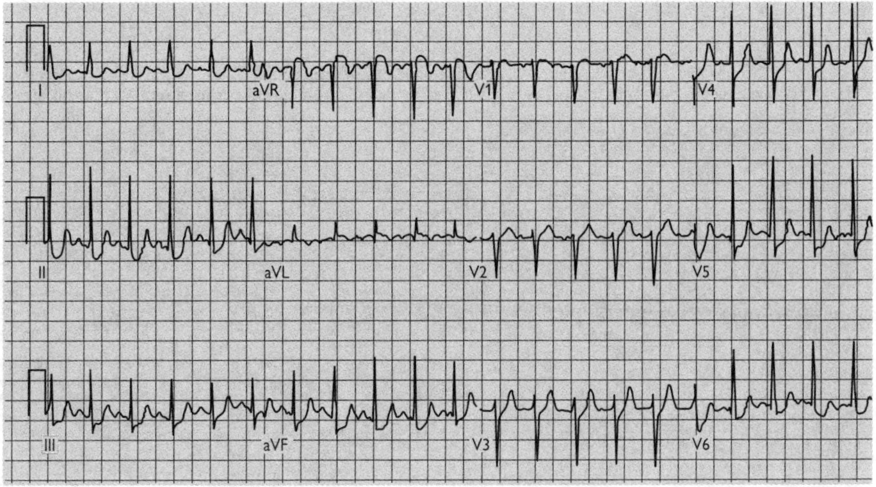

(C) **Acute inferolateral ischaemia:** Note ST depression in leads I, II, II aVF and V3 to V6, also T wave inversion in AVR (normal variant) and aVL.

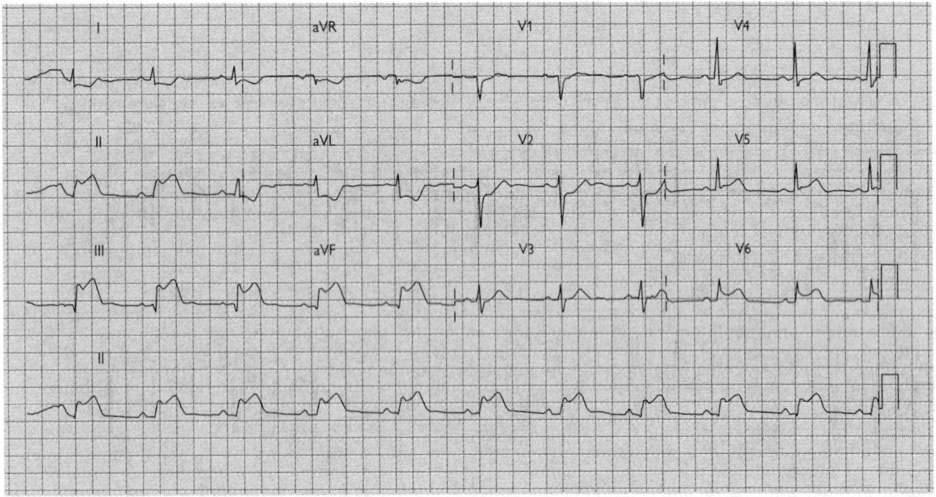

(D) **Acute inferolateral myocardial infarction**: Note ST elevation in leads II, III and aVF (inferior leads) and also in V5 and V6 (lateral leads). The ST depression in I and aVL are reciprocal changes and often seen with large infarcts.

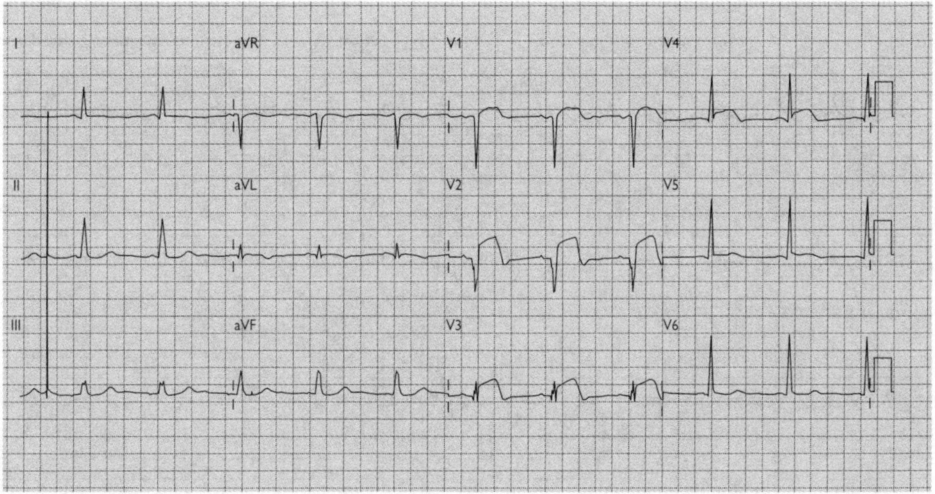

(E) **Acute anterior myocardial infarction**: Note the ST segment elevation in leads V1 to V4 and slightly in V5 and the evolving Q wave.

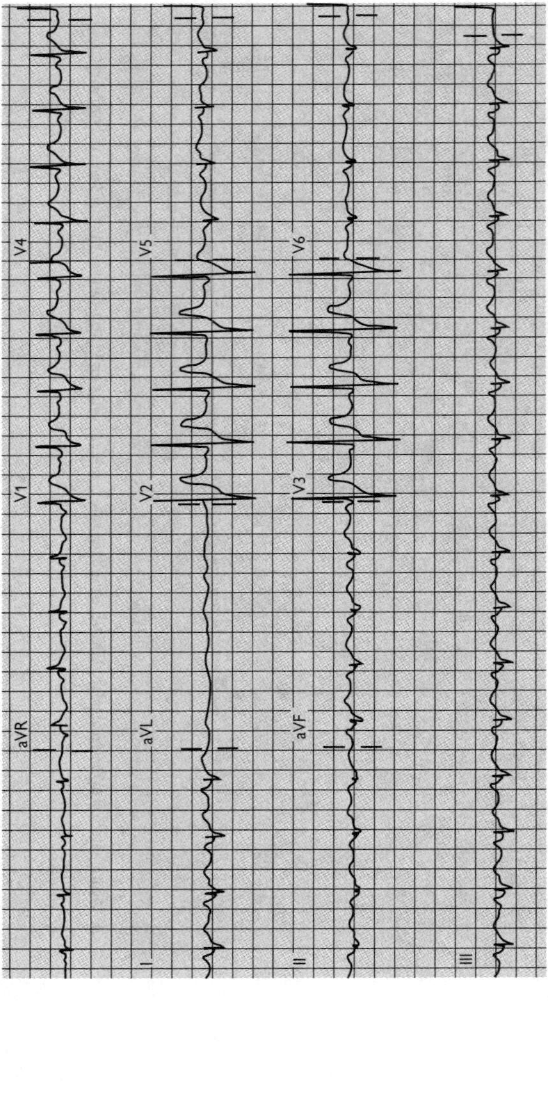

(F) **Acute posterolateral infarct:** Note dominant R wave and ST depression in V1/V2 and ST elevation in V5/V6.

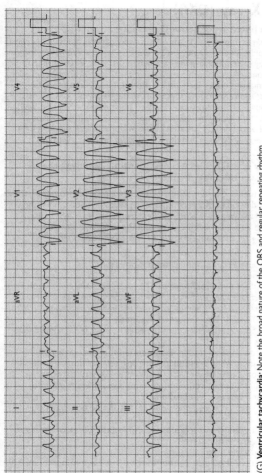

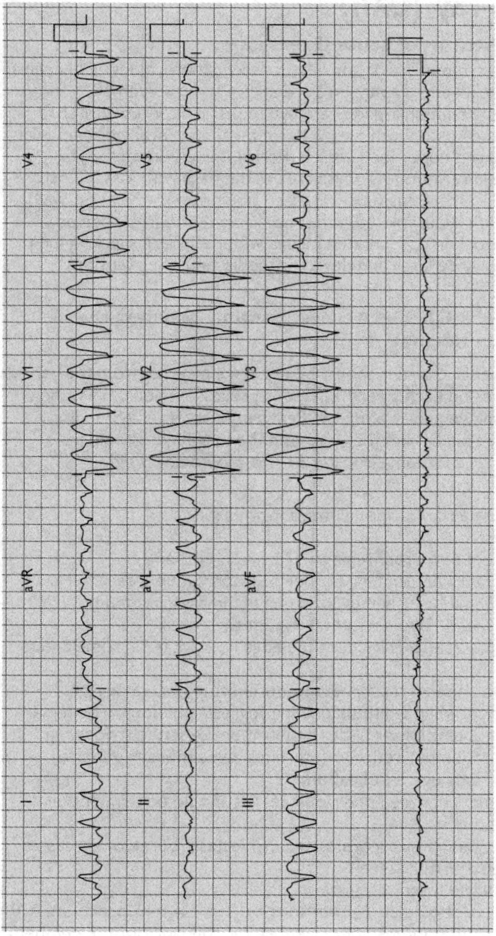

(G) **Ventricular tachycardia:** Note the broad nature of the QRS and regular repeating rhythm.

Chest X-ray (CXR)

The main patterns of acute disease are:

- ***Pneumonia*** asymmetrical shadowing (consolidation), blunting of angles, blurring of heart and diaphragm borders, air bronchograms
- ***Pulmonary oedema*** enlarged heart, symmetrical hazy/reticular shadowing, blunted costophrenic angles or pleural effusions, indistinct hilar vessels, enlarged upper lobe vessels, Kerley B lines, distinct septa
- ***Pleural effusion*** featureless white area at the base with loss of costophrenic angle ±meniscus (upper surface sloping up to the chest wall)
- ***Asthma/COPD*** hyperinflated, flattened diaphragm, barrel chested
- ***Pneumothorax*** line of separated pleura with peripheries lacking lung markings – may be large and deviating mediastinum (eg tension)

Adequacy of a CXR – interpret cautiously unless the following are normal

- ***Rotation*** medial clavicles should be the same distance from the vertebral bodies on each side; the spinous processes should be in the middle of the vertebral bodies • ***Penetration*** intervertebral discs should be visible behind the heart and the lung fields should have markings • ***Inspiration*** ≥7 posterior ribs should be visible

Develop a routine so you spot all the abnormalities:

- ***Lung outline***
  - *blunting/loss* of costophrenic and cardiophrenic angles
  - *indistinct heart border*, lung border or diaphragm edges
  - *pneumothorax* best seen by inverting the image or rotating by 90°
  - *Kerley B lines* 1–2cm horizontal lines at the edges
  - *pleural plaques/thickening* does the edge look whiter in some areas?
- ***Lung fields***
  - *colour* too dark suggests pneumothorax, emphysema or high penetration, while white shadowing suggests pulmonary oedema, pneumonia, effusion or under-penetration. Describe shadowing as nodular (lumpy), reticular (fine lines eg pulmonary oedema) or alveolar (fluffy eg consolidation).
  - *vascular markings* the upper lobe vessels should be thinner than lower lobe ones
  - *cavities* ie dark circles, consider bronchiectasis, bullae or abscesses (may have a air/fluid level)
  - *localised white lesions* eg carcinoma
- ***Lung size*** there should be 7 posterior ribs (see diagram opposite), ≥10 hyperinflated, ≤6 poor inspiratory effort; for anterior ribs the numbers are two lower, ie ≥7, 6, ≤4
- ***Diaphragm***
  - is there a pneumoperitoneum (perforated bowel), thin black line under the diaphragm
  - is the right side slightly higher than the left? If not consider excess chest or abdomen pressure
  - are the domes convex? Flat suggests hyperexpansion

- ***Mediastinum***
  - this should be <8cm wide at the aortic arch, wider suggests swelling eg aortic dissection or lymphadenopathy
  - the heart should be <50% the width of the chest on a PA (non-portable) film, larger suggests cardiomegaly
  - is there collapse or consolidation behind the heart?
- ***Trachea*** should be central and uncompressed
- ***Hila*** these should have a concave shape with distinct vessels
- ***Bones*** look at the spine, clavicles, scapulae, shoulder and ribs. Look for fractures, osteolytic and osteosclerotic lesions. Is the spine straight?
- ***Soft tissues*** surgical emphysema (pneumothorax), breast lesions

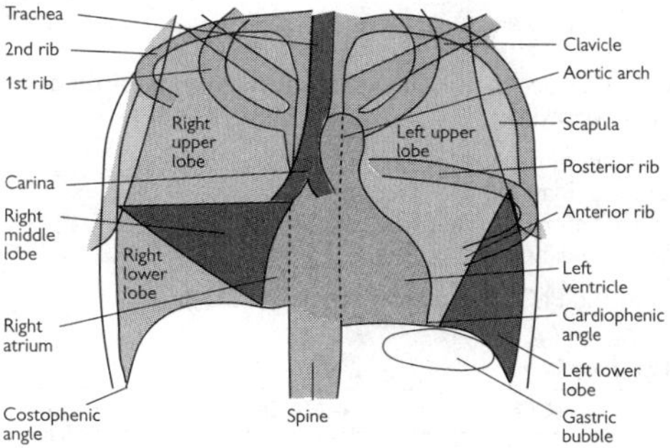

Major features on an AP CXR.

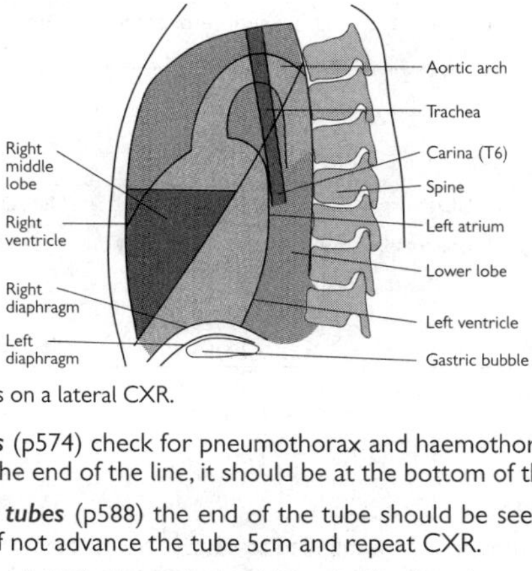

Major features on a lateral CXR.

Central lines (p574) check for pneumothorax and haemothorax; note the position of the end of the line, it should be at the bottom of the SVC.

Feeding NG tubes (p588) the end of the tube should be seen below the diaphragm; if not advance the tube 5cm and repeat CXR.

Chest drains (p580) the end should be inside the chest wall without touching the opposing wall, ideally angled downwards for effusions and up for pneumothoraces; note the size of pneumothorax or effusion.

Arterial blood gases (ABG)

Arterial blood gas (ABG) analysis calculates PaO_2, $PaCO_2$ and HCO_3^- in a heparinised specimen (can also be undertaken on venous or capillary blood or on fluid aspirated from the chest or abdomen), as well as the pH, O_2 saturation, base excess, anion gap and on some machines concentrations of Na^+, K^+, Ca^{2+}, Cl^- and lactate. For advice on how to perform an ABG see p562.

Normal ranges (patient breathing room air)

pH	7.35–7.45	HCO_3^-	22–28mmol/l
PaO_2	10.5–13.5kPa	Base excess (BE)	−2 to +2
$PaCO_2$	4.5–6.0kPa	O_2 saturation	95–100%

NB Note that a normal pO_2 in a patient on a high inspired concentration of O_2 is very worrying.

First look at the pH:
- pH <7.35 = acidaemia
- pH 7.35 to 7.45 = normal pH
- pH >7.45 = alkalaemia

Next look at the $PaCO_2$ and bicarbonate (HCO_3^-):

Types of acidaemia

	↓HCO_3^-	↔HCO_3^-	↑HCO_3^-
↓$PaCO_2$	Metabolic acidosis	x	x
↔$PaCO_2$	Mixed acidosis	x	x
↑$PaCO_2$	Mixed acidosis	Acute respiratory acidosis	Chronic respiratory acidosis

Types of alkalaemia

	↓HCO_3^-	↔HCO_3^-	↑HCO_3^-
↓$PaCO_2$	Chronic respiratory alkalosis	Acute respiratory alkalosis	Mixed alkalosis
↔$PaCO_2$	x	x	Mixed alkalosis
↑$PaCO_2$	x	x	Metabolic alkalosis

x – incompatible

Base excess

This is the amount of 'base' needed to restore pH to the normal range
- Base excess >+2, patient has excess base present (ie alkalosis)
- Base excess <−2, patient has insufficient base present (ie acidosis)

Causes of acid–base disturbance

	Acidosis	Alkalosis
Metabolic	Shock DKA Renal/liver failure Drug overdose (eg TCA) Renal tubular acidosis Lactate (p215) Refer to 'anion gap' below	Vomiting Diarrhoea Hypokalaemia
Respiratory	Severe asthma/COPD Severe pneumonia Severe pulmonary oedema Myasthenia gravis Drugs (eg sedatives, opiates) Chest trauma/scoliosis Obesity	Hypoxaemia Cranial lesions (eg stroke) Anxiety/hyperventilation

If all else fails calculate the anion gap or speak to a biochemist

If the differentials for a metabolic acidosis are still unclear then calculate the anion gap which should answer any remaining problems (see below); alternatively ask a senior or speak directly to the clinical biochemist in the laboratory

The anion gap

This is calculated by $([Na^+] + [K^+]) - ([Cl^-] + [HCO_3^-])$

Normal value is 10–18mmol/l

It helps to distinguish the different causes of a metabolic acidosis:

- ***Raised anion gap***
  - lactic acidosis (p215 shock, sepsis/infection)
  - urate (renal failure)
  - ketones (DKA, alcohol, starvation)
  - drugs/toxins (salicylates, biguanides, ethylene glycol, methanol)
- ***Normal anion gap***
  - renal tubular acidosis
  - diarrhoea
  - drugs (acetazolamide)
  - Addison's disease
  - pancreatic fistula
  - ammonium chloride ingestion

Respiratory function tests

Peak expiratory flow rate (PEFR)

Indications used for the diagnosis, monitoring (eg daily diary/obs) and severity assessment of obstructive lung disease (asthma and COPD).

Method reset the tab and fit a clean mouthpiece. Ask the patient to stand up and hold it in their hand (not covering the scale), breathe in deeply and blow as hard and fast as they can (with encouragement), they do not need to exhale maximally. Use the best reading of three attempts.

PEFR[1]	>80%	80–50%	55–33%	<33%
Asthma severity	Normal	Mild–moderate	Severe	Life-threatening

[1]Compared with best or predicted (see chart on opposite page)

Spirometry

Indication diagnosis and monitoring of respiratory disease.

Before testing leave out morning inhalers or nebulisers (unless severely ill) to allow reversibility assessment.

Method usually performed by trained technicians in a respiratory function laboratory. The patient must inhale as deeply as they can then exhale as fast and as long as they can manage. This is difficult enough without COPD. The following measurements are made:

- **FEV_1** forced expiratory volume in 1s, the volume exhaled in the first second after deep inspiration and forced expiration, similar to PEFR
- **FVC** forced vital capacity, the total volume exhaled from deep inspiration to maximal exhalation

Beyond spirometry respiratory function laboratories can also measure:

- **RV** residual volume, the volume of gas remaining in the lungs after a maximum expiration
- **TLC** total lung capacity is the combination of FVC and RV

	Obstructive	Normal	Restrictive
FEV_1	↓↓	Predicted	↓
FVC	↓	Predicted	↓↓
FEV_1/FVC	<75%	75–80%	>80%
RV	↑	Predicted	↓
TLC	↑	Predicted	↓

Obstructive asthma, COPD, emphysema.

Restrictive interstitial lung disease, sarcoid, connective tissue disorders, neuromuscular disease (including myasthenia gravis and Guillain–Barré).

Other spirometry measurements

Reversibility asthma (a reversible obstruction) is diagnosed if there is ≥250ml and ≥15% improvement in PEFR or FEV_1 with bronchodilators. Asthma can coexist with COPD (non-reversible obstruction).

Gas transfer also called *transfer factor*, is measured using carbon monoxide. It is reduced in emphysema, acute asthma, anaemia and interstitial lung disease and increased with chronic asthma, left heart failure, polycythaemia and exercise.

Flow volume loops graphical representations of the results with volume on the x-axis and flow rate on the Y-axis. Exhalation is above the line and inhalation below the line. There are four main patterns:

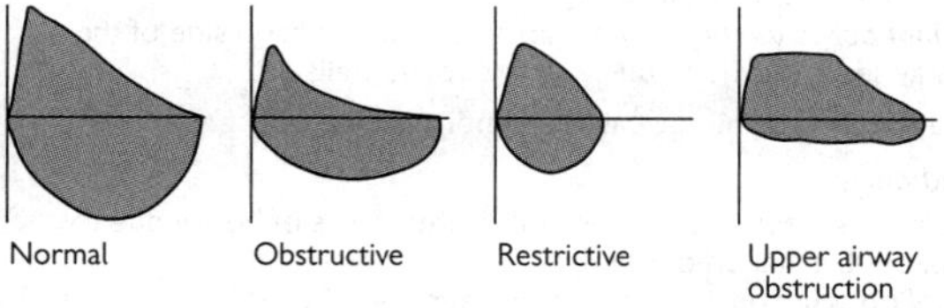

Upper airway obstruction lesion occluding the bronchi, trachea or larynx associated with stridor, see p230.

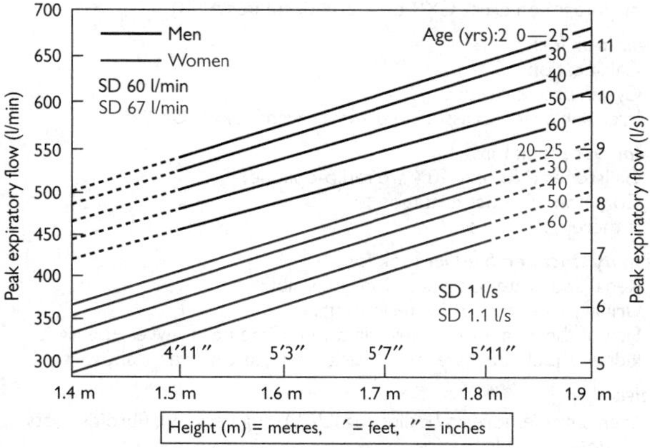

Normal peak expiratory flow values.

Abdomen X-ray (AXR)

The main patterns of acute disease are:

- ***Bowel perforation*** free gas seen on lateral decubitus abdominal film or erect CXR underneath the diaphragm
- ***Dilated loops*** of small bowel >2.5cm or large bowel >6cm (see table opposite)
- ***Sigmoid volvulus*** grossly dilated loop of bowel ('coffee bean' shaped)
- ***Constipation*** faecal loading in the large bowel, often starting from the rectum
- ***Gallstones/renal stones*** calcifications in the RUQ or along the urinary tract; 10% of gallstones and 90% of renal stones are visible on AXR
- ***Chronic pancreatitis*** calcified specks in the epigastric/pancreatic area
- ***Chronic renal failure*** small kidneys
- ***Abdominal aortic aneurysm*** wide aorta on the left hand side of the spine; may see a calcified outline of the aortic walls

Develop a routine so you spot all the abnormalities:

Bowel pathology

- *Bowel gas* (best seen in a supine film) dilated loops of bowel due to mechanical obstruction or paralytic ileus
- *Fluid level* obstruction, ileus, gastroenteritis
- *Stomach* dilated in pyloric stenosis; look for linitis plastica ('leather bottle stomach') in advanced stomach cancer
- *Gas outside the lumen* bowel perforation (look for air under the diaphragm on erect CXR or lateral decubitus AXR)

Liver look for:

- Calcification
- Cysts/abscess cavities
- Irregular opacities associated with malignancy (1° or 2°)

Biliary tree look for:

- Gallstones (NB only 10% are radio-opaque)
- Common bile duct dilatation
- Is there a stent *in situ*?

Urinary tract and bladder look for:

- Renal and ureteric stones (90% are visible)
- Urinary catheters or ureteric stents
- Size of the kidneys, obvious dilatation of the pelvicalyces; the right kidney should be lower than the left one, as the liver is above it

Pelvis

- *Uterus/ovaries* foreign bodies (eg IUCD, ring pessary), fibroids, cysts
- *Prostate* size, calcification

Bones

- *Lytic lesions (dark)* think bronchial/breast/renal carcinoma, myeloma
- *Sclerotic lesions* think prostate/breast carcinoma, Paget's disease
- *Fusion of the vertebrae/sacroiliac joints, curving of the spine* degenerative disease, scoliosis, ankylosing spondylosis

Other soft tissues

- *Psoas muscle* if absent, think of ascites, haematoma or retroperitoneal mass

Hints and tips

- AXRs are daunting to interpret initially, so it's important to keep in mind what you are trying to confirm/exclude on it
- Stand back and approach things in a systematic manner
- Take the findings on AXR together with the clinical picture and discuss what management is necessary with the rest of your team

Large bowel vs. small bowel obstruction

	Small intestine	**Large intestine**
Number of loops	Lots	Few
Distribution of loops	Central	Peripheral
Diameter of loops	>2.5cm	>6cm
Haustrae[1]	No	Yes
Valvulae conniventes[2]	Yes	No
Faeces present	No	Yes

[1] Haustrae folds which do not completely cross the bowel lumen wall.

[2] Valvulae conniventes folds which do completely cross the bowel lumen wall.

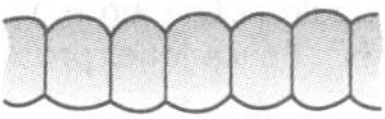

Small bowel with valvulae conniventes

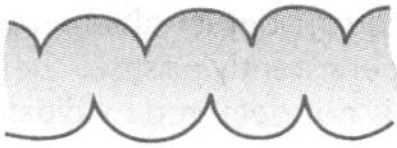

Large bowel with haustrae

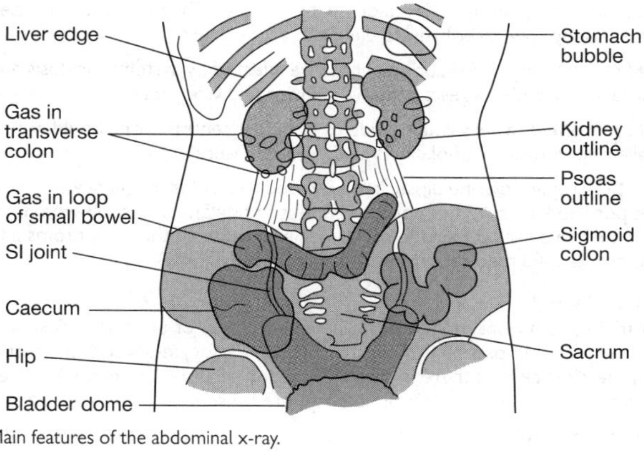

Main features of the abdominal x-ray.

Urine tests

Urine samples should be 'mid-stream' (MSU) to limit contamination, alternatively they can be taken from a catheter (CSU).

Dipstick

UTIs can be asymptomatic and urinary symptoms (dysuria, frequency, urgency) can be present without a UTI. This table gives the chance of a positive urine culture from dipstick readings. Dipsticks are not sensitive:

	Leucs +ve	**Leucs –ve**
Nitrites +ve	>95%	90%
Nitrites –ve	70%	<20%

Nitrites are produced by Gram-negative bacteria (eg *E. coli*) and suggest urinary tract infection (UTI).

Leucocytes (white cells) are raised from inflammation of the kidneys and urinary tract, most commonly UTIs, but also stones, trauma, neoplasia, infection of related structures (eg prostate, appendix) and renal disease.

Blood dipsticks detect haemoglobin and may distinguish this from blood cells. Send the urine for microscopy if either are seen. A positive dipstick with no red cells on microscopy suggests myoglobinuria or haemoglobinuria. See p314 for the causes of haematuria.

Protein dipsticks detect albumin which should not be present in urine. If protein is persistently positive then see p315. Bence-Jones protein (seen in myeloma) is not detected by dipsticks.

Glucose should not be present in urine but is common with ↑age; its presence suggests, but cannot diagnose or exclude, DM (see p276).

Ketones are raised in DKA (along with glucose). They can also be raised after fasting, low carbohydrate diets and acute illness.

pH normal range 4.5–8; urine pH can be affected by systemic acidosis and alkalosis. Acid ph suggests systemic acidosis and vice versa.

Specific gravity a very rough guide to urine concentration; it should not be relied upon (urine osmolality is a superior measure).

β-hCG a separate urine dipstick can be used to test for pregnancy; it should be positive within 12d of conception. It is important to test all women of reproductive age to exclude pregnancy as a cause of their symptoms and before harmful medications or investigations (eg X-ray).

Microscopy

A mid-stream urine (MSU) or catheter specimen of urine (CSU) should be sent for microscopy if there are nitrites, leucocytes, blood or protein on the dipstick or if there is clinical suspicion of a UTI. In children a clean catch, catheter urine or suprapubic aspirate is used.

White cells >10/mm^3 is abnormal; same causes as leucocytes on dipstick.

Bacteria may be seen on simple microscopy and this is highly suggestive of a UTI; Gram staining may help identify the pathogen. The sample needs to be cultured for complete identification.

Red cells >2/mm^3 is abnormal; see p314 for management of haematuria.

Casts hyaline and fine granular casts are not significant; dense granular, red-cell and epithelial casts suggest renal disease; white-cell casts are found with pyelonephritis.

Culture and sensitivity

Samples sent for microscopy are routinely cultured over 48h. The culture is said to be positive if >100,000 colony forming units/ml are present. The sample is recultured in different mediums to determine the bacteria present and their sensitivity to antibiotics. A mixed culture (more than one organism present) suggests a contaminated sample. Urine culture is not 100% sensitive or specific – it can often be wrong and require repeating.

Biochemistry

Sodium concentration is a useful test in acute renal failure. A low urine sodium (<20mmol/l) suggests hypoperfusion, eg hypovolaemia, while a raised concentration (>40mmol/l) suggests acute tubular necrosis. It is also used in the assessment of hyponatraemia (p328).

Urine osmolality is a measure of the concentration of the urine; the normal range is 500–800mosmol/kg. It is used in the investigation of renal disease and diagnosis of diabetes insipidus (p322). In acute renal failure it can help distinguish between prerenal failure (>500mosmol/kg) and acute tubular necrosis (<350mosmol/kg).

24h urine protein total protein and microalbumin can be measured, total protein is the more common test; microalbumin is used to detect developing renal failure in diabetics and a value of >30mg/24h is abnormal. Urine creatinine should also be measured to determine GFR.

24h Protein	Significance
<150mg	Normal
150mg–3g	Proteinuria, probably renal if >2g (p315)
>3g	Nephrotic syndrome (p315)

Creatinine clearance the excretion of creatinine per minute can be calculated from a 24h urine collection and this gives an estimation of the glomerular filtration rate (GFR), p321.

Catecholamines/VMA if a phaeochromocytoma is suspected a 24h urine sample is analysed for free catecholamines (eg adrenaline) or their metabolites (eg vanillylmandelic acid, VMA).

Toxicology urine can be screened for a wide range of recreational and medical drugs. Dipsticks give results in <10min while lab-based tests can often take several days.

CSF

Microscopy

Red cells (0 per mm^3) these are raised from a bloody tap (more in the first bottle than the third) or from a subarachnoid haemorrhage (same in first and third bottles), however the two can only be distinguished reliably by measuring for xanthochromia (subarachnoid only). High levels of blood cells will disrupt the measurement of WBC and protein. The following calculations may help:

- True CSF WBC = CSF WBC – (bld WBC x CSF RBC ÷ bld RBC)
- True CSF protein = CSF protein – (RBC ÷ 100)

White cells (<4 per mm^3) raised levels in infection or 48h post-subarachnoid, levels tend to be higher in bacterial meningitis. The main type of white cell suggests the infectious agent:

- *Neutrophils/polymorphs* (normal 0 per mm^3) bacterial infection
- *Lymphocytes/mononuclear* (normal <4 per mm^3) viral infection or TB

Bacteria a Gram stain may show bacteria in the sample; this is always pathological; talk to a microbiologist about treatment.

Biochemistry

Protein normally <0.4g/l; levels >1.0g/l are usually only seen in bacterial or TB meningitis. Less dramatic rises can occur in all types of meningitis and also multiple sclerosis or Guillain–Barré.

Glucose (>2.2mmol/l or >70% plasma) reduced in meningitis, especially bacterial meningitis.

Xanthochromia is a yellowing of the CSF caused by the breakdown of blood; it is present 4–12h following a subarachnoid haemorrhage

	Normal	Bacterial	TB	Viral
Appearance	Clear	Cloudy	Clear	Clear
White cells	<4 x 10^9/l	5–2000 x 10^9/l	5–500 x 10^9/l	5–1000 x 10^9/l
Type of cell	None	Neutrophils	Lymphocytes	Lymphocytes
Glucose	>70% plasma	Very low	<50% plasma	>70% plasma
Protein	<0.4g/l	>1g/l	>1g/l	0.5–0.9g/l

Culture

Bacteria it can take several days for bacteria to grow but the majority are positive within 48h. It may take a further 24–48h to identify the type of bacteria and its sensitivity to antibiotics. Liaise with a microbiologist.

TB culture can take weeks because it is a slow growing bacteria. It may be possible to detect TB sooner using PCR. Talk to the laboratory technicians and microbiologists.

Autoantibodies and associated diseases

Autoantibody	Disease (% frequency where known)
Acetylcholine receptor	Myasthenia gravis (80%)
Antinuclear (ANA)	SLE (95%), RA (32%), JIA (76%), chronic active hepatitis (75%), Sjögren's syndrome (70%), systemic sclerosis (64%), normal 'controls' (0–2%)
Anticardiolipin	Primary antiphospholipid syndrome
Anticentromere	CREST variant systemic sclerosis
Anti-Ro	Sjögren's syndrome, subacute cutaneous lupus, SLE (30%), systemic sclerosis (60%), interstitial pneumonitis
Anti-La	Sjögren's syndrome (65%), SLE (15%)
C-ANCA	Wegener's granulomatosis (90%), MPA (11%), Churg–Strauss syndrome
P-ANCA	Churg–Strauss syndrome (60%)
dsDNA	SLE (60%)
ssDNA	SLE (70%), autoimmune rheumatic disease, inflammation
ENA	Includes: Anti-Ro, Anti-La, Anti-Jo-1, RNP, Scl-70, Anti-Sm
Gastric parietal cell	Autoimmune gastritis, pernicious anaemia
Glycolipid	Multi-focal motor neuropathy, Guillain-Barré syndrome, Miller–Fisher syndrome
Glomerular basement membrane	Goodpasture's syndrome
IgA-endomysial	Coeliac disease
Anti-Jo-1	Myositis
Mitochondrial (AMA)	Primary biliary cirrhosis (>95%)
Rheumatoid factor	RA (50–90%), SLE (15–35%), systemic sclerosis (20–30%), juvenile RA (7–10%), polymyositis (5–10%), infection (0–50%)
RNP	SLE and MCTD
Anti-Scl-70	Systemic sclerosis
Anti-Sm	SLE
Smooth muscle (SMA)	Chronic active hepatitis (40–90%), primary biliary cirrhosis (30–70%), idiopathic cirrhosis (25–30%), viral infections (80%), 'controls' (3–12%), autoimmune sclerosing cholangitis
Thyroid peroxidase	Hashimoto's thyroiditis (>80%), Graves' disease (50%)
Thyrotropin receptor	Graves' disease (50–80%)

Skeletal radiographs

Identification check the radiograph for the name of the patient and when the image was taken; check if the image is of the left or right side.

Bones for each bone follow the edge of the cortex around the whole circumference, looking for steps or cracks; does the bone look normal, or clearly very bowed or angulated around a fracture. Check the consistency of the bone matrix itself; is it uniformly pale and very opaque (osteopenic) or dense and very mineralised (sclerotic); are there cysts (lytic lesions) or patches of more dense bone (sclerotic lesions or callus)?

Joints always check the joint above and below the bone in question, eg elbow and wrist when looking at the radius or ulnar. Does the joint look normal, are the bones involved in the articulation in their normal position, is the distance between these bones increased or decreased? Re-check for breaks in the cortex of the bones within the joint (intra-articular fractures).

Soft tissue signs soft-tissue **oedema** is often subtly seen on some radiographs, suggesting there is overlying swelling; this is especially seen around peripheral bones/joints (wrists, hands, ankles, feet etc). Very occasionally **gas** can be seen on radiographs, and appears black; this can arise from gas-forming bacterial (classically *Clostridium* species), but also from open wounds. **Bleeding** and oedema adjacent to some joints gives rise to specific features; one of the best examples of these is the anterior fat pad sign of the elbow. Small amounts of intra-articular haemorrhage force a normally hidden fat pad to appear on the lateral elbow radiograph, anterior to the distal humerus. The presence of this sign strongly suggests there is a peri-articular fracture. The posterior fat pad is often seen even in the absence of trauma/injury.

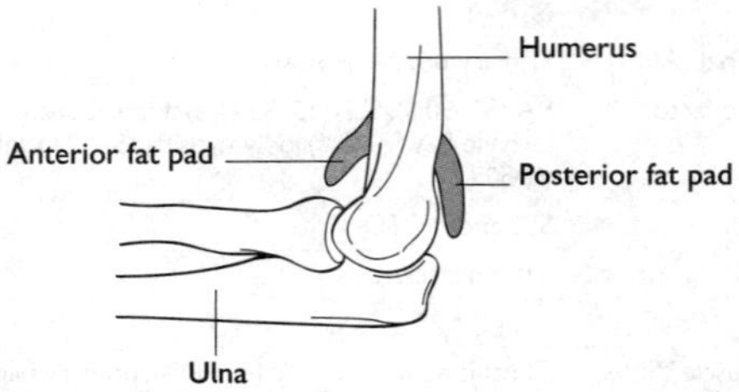

The anterior and posterior fat pads on a lateral elbow x-ray.

If all else fails sometimes it is difficult to see a radiological cause of the patient's complaint. Always ask a senior to review the radiograph or show it to a senior radiographer or the radiologist who is 'hot reporting'.

PACS **P**icture **A**rchiving and **C**ommunication **S**ystem is an electronic system which most hospitals are now using to store their radiology images on. Viewing the images is undertaken on-screen and various manipulations of the image can be performed by the user such as inverting, rotating, magnifying and altering the contrast – this makes finding fractures much easier.

Describing fractures	
Side	Right or left, dominant or not
Bone	Clavicle, radius, tibia etc
Location	Proximal, midshaft, distal
Type	Simple (2 bits), comminuted (≥3 bits), oblique, spiral
Shape	Displaced, angulated, impacted, rotated
Joint surface	Intra-articular fracture or not, dislocation
Complications	Compound (open fracture, p353), neurovascular involvement

Fractures in children children's bones are still growing and generally softer and more malleable than adult bones. The greenstick fracture is a fracture of the shaft of a long bone, but like a green twig, snapping it often only breaks just one cortex rather than both (the classical definition of a fracture is a break to both cortices). Greenstick fractures are most common in the forearm. Fractures at the growing ends of bones usually take on one of five forms (see Salter Harris classification below) and must be managed carefully to ensure the bone continues to develop/grow normally.

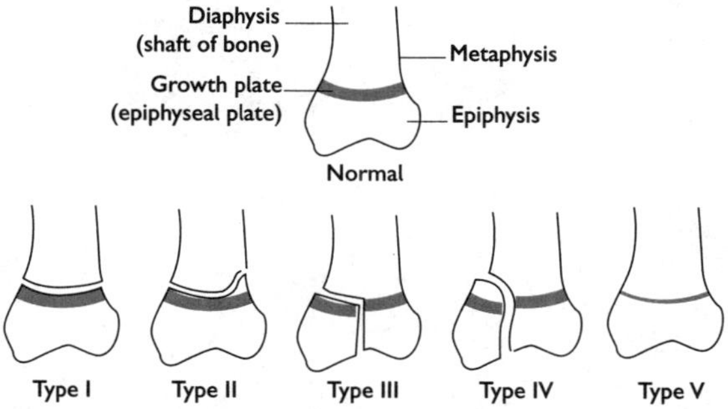

Salter Harris classification of growth palate fractures.

Pathological fractures are fractures at a site where the bone is weakened, usually where there is a cyst, metastatic lesion or inherited defect.

For specific bones/joints			
Hip	p355	Elbow	p502
Knee	p355	Wrist	p354
Ankle	p355	Hand	p354
Foot	p550	Back	p505
Shoulder	p501	C-spine	p360

Salter-Harris classification of growth plate fractures

Chapter 13
Appendices

Useful numbers and websites

Medical organisations

General Medical Council (GMC)
- 08453 578001 www.gmc-uk.org
- Registration issues 08453 573456

Postgraduate Medical Education and Training Board (PMETB)
- 020 7160 6100 www.pmetb.org.uk

British Medical Association (BMA)
- 020 7387 4499 www.bma.org.uk

Medical Defence Union (MDU)
- 0800 716 376 www.the-mdu.com
- 24h help 0800 716 646

Medical Protection Society (MPS)
- 08457 187 187 www.medicalprotection.org
- 24h help 0845 605 4000

Medical Doctors' and Dentists' Defence Union of Scotland (MDDUS)
- 0141 221 5858 www.mddus.com
- 24h help 0141 221 5858

Counselling lines

BMA Counselling Service
- 08459 200169

Doctors' Support Network (mental illness)
- 0870 321 0642 www.dsn.org.uk

Sick Doctor's Trust (alcohol and drug addiction)
- 0870 444 5163 www.sick-doctors-trust.co.uk

Financial organisations

Wesleyan Medical Sickness
- 0800 092 1990 www.wesleyan.co.uk

BMA Services
- 0800 358 0014 www.bmas.co.uk

Other

Gay and Lesbian Association of Doctors and Dentists (GLADD)
- 0870 765 5606 www.gladd.org.uk

Medical Research Council (MRC)
- 020 7636 5422 www.mrc.ac.uk

Medical Women's Federation
- 020 7387 7765 www.medicalwomensfederation.co.uk

Médecins Sans Frontières (MSF)
- 020 7404 6600 www.msf.org

Voluntary Services Overseas
- 020 8780 7500 www.vso.org.uk

Wellcome Trust
- 020 7611 8888 www.wellcome.ac.uk

(Royal) College of

Anaesthetists	020 7092 6000	www.rcoa.ac.uk
Emergency Medicine	020 7404 1999	www.emergencymed.org.uk
General Practitioners	020 7581 3232	www.rcgp.org.uk
Obstetricians and Gynaecologists	020 7772 6200	www.rcog.org.uk
Ophthalmologists	020 7935 0702	www.rcophth.ac.uk
Paediatrics and Child Health	020 7092 6000	www.rcpch.ac.uk
Pathologists	020 7451 6700	www.rcpath.org
Physicians	020 7935 1174	www.rcplondon.ac.uk
Physicians of Edinburgh	0131 225 7324	www.rcpe.ac.uk
Physicians of Ireland	018639 700	www.rcpi.ie
Physicians and Surgeons of Glasgow	0141 221 6072	www.rcpsg.ac.uk
Psychiatrists	020 7235 2351	www.rcpsych.ac.uk
Radiologists	020 7636 4432	www.rcr.ac.uk
Surgeons of Edinburgh	0131 527 1600	www.rcsed.ac.uk
Surgeons of England	020 7405 3474	www.rcseng.ac.uk
Surgeons of Ireland	00 3531 402 2100	www.rcsi.ie

A selection of medical websites

For doctors

www.emedicine.com
www.gpnotebook.co.uk
www.bmjpg.com (BMJ publishing)
www.library.nhs.uk (NHS library)
www.bnf.org

For patients

www.netdoctor.co.uk
www.patient.co.uk
www.macmillan.org.uk (cancer)
www.medlineplus.gov (USA based)
health.allrefer.com (USA based)

A selection of locum agencies

NHS Professionals	0845 606 0345	www.nhsprofessionals.nhs.uk
JCJ	0800 590 979	www.jcj.co.uk
Pulse	0800 980 3315	www.pulsestaffing.co.uk
Medacs	0800 037 5050	www.medacs.com
Nationwide Locum Service[1]	0845 650 7018	www.nlsandumrweb.co.uk

[1] Specifically for overseas doctors

Height conversion

Metres (m) to inches (inch), multiply by 39.37 (12 inches to the foot)
Inches to meters, multiply by 0.0254

m	inch	feet	inch
1.36	53.5	4	5.5
1.37	54	4	6
1.38	54.5	4	6.5
1.40	55	4	7
1.41	55.5	4	7.5
1.42	56	4	8
1.43	56.5	4	8.5
1.45	57	4	9
1.46	57.5	4	9.5
1.47	58	4	10
1.48	58.5	4	10.5
1.50	59	4	11
1.51	59.5	4	11.5
1.52	60	5	0
1.54	60.5	5	0.5
1.55	61	5	1
1.56	61.5	5	1.5
1.57	62	5	2
1.59	62.5	5	2.5
1.60	63	5	3
1.61	63.5	5	3.5
1.62	64	5	4
1.64	64.5	5	4.5
1.65	65	5	5
1.66	65.5	5	5.5

m	inch	feet	inch
1.67	66	5	6
1.69	66.5	5	6.5
1.70	67	5	7
1.71	67.5	5	7.5
1.73	68	5	8
1.74	68.5	5	8.5
1.75	69	5	9
1.76	69.5	5	9.5
1.78	70	5	10
1.79	70.5	5	10.5
1.80	71	5	11
1.81	71.5	5	11.5
1.83	72	6	0
1.84	72.5	6	0.5
1.85	73	6	1
1.87	73.5	6	1.5
1.88	74	6	2
1.89	74.5	6	2.5
1.90	75	6	3
1.92	75.5	6	3.5
1.93	76	6	4
1.94	76.5	6	4.5
1.95	77	6	5
1.97	77.5	6	5.5
1.98	78	6	6

Temperature

Degrees Fahrenheit (°F) to degrees celsius (centigrade °C)

$$°C = (°F - 32) \times 0.56$$

Degrees celsius (centigrade °C) to Degrees Fahrenheit (°F)

$$°F = (C \times 1.8) + 32$$

Pressure

Millimetres of mercury (mmHg) to kilopascals (kPa)

$$kPa = mmHg \times 0.113$$

Kilopascals (kPa) to millimetres of mercury (mmHg)

$$mmHg = kPa \times 7.519$$

Weight conversion

kg to pounds (lbs), multiply by 2.2046 (14lb to the stone; 16oz per lb)
Pounds to kg, multiply by 0.4536

kg	St	lbs	kg	St	lbs	kg	St	lbs
1	0	2.2	43	6	11	85	13	5
2	0	4.4	44	6	13	86	13	8
3	0	6.6	45	7	1	87	13	10
4	0	8.8	46	7	3	88	13	12
5	0	11	47	7	6	89	14	0
6	0	13	48	7	8	90	14	2
7	1	1	49	7	10	91	14	5
8	1	4	50	7	12	92	14	7
9	1	6	51	8	0	93	14	9
10	1	8	52	8	3	94	14	11
11	1	10	53	8	5	95	14	13
12	1	12	54	8	7	96	15	2
13	2	1	55	8	9	97	15	4
14	2	3	56	8	11	98	15	6
15	2	5	57	9	0	99	15	8
16	2	7	58	9	2	100	15	10
17	2	9	59	9	4	101	15	13
18	2	12	60	9	6	102	16	1
19	3	0	61	9	8	103	16	3
20	3	2	62	9	11	104	16	5
21	3	4	63	9	13	105	16	7
22	3	7	64	10	1	106	16	10
23	3	9	65	10	3	107	16	12
24	3	11	66	10	6	108	17	0
25	3	13	67	10	8	109	17	2
26	4	1	68	10	10	110	17	5
27	4	4	69	10	12	111	17	7
28	4	6	70	11	0	112	17	9
29	4	8	71	11	3	113	17	11
30	4	10	72	11	5	114	17	13
31	4	12	73	11	7	115	18	2
32	5	1	74	11	9	116	18	4
33	5	3	75	11	11	117	18	6
34	5	5	76	12	0	118	18	8
35	5	7	77	12	2	119	18	10
36	5	9	78	12	4	120	18	13
37	5	12	79	12	6	125	19	10
38	6	0	80	12	8	130	20	7
39	6	2	81	12	11	135	21	4
40	6	4	82	12	13	140	22	1
41	6	6	83	13	1	145	22	12
42	6	9	84	13	3	150	23	9

Body mass index (BMI)

BMI calculation

BMI = weight (kg)/height^2 (m^2)

eg: 77kg, 1.83m

77/(1.83 x 1.83) = 23 (normal)

BMI	Weight status
<18.5	Underweight
18.5–24.9	Normal
25.0–29.9	Overweight
>30	Obese
>40	Morbidly obese

Body mass index chart for adults

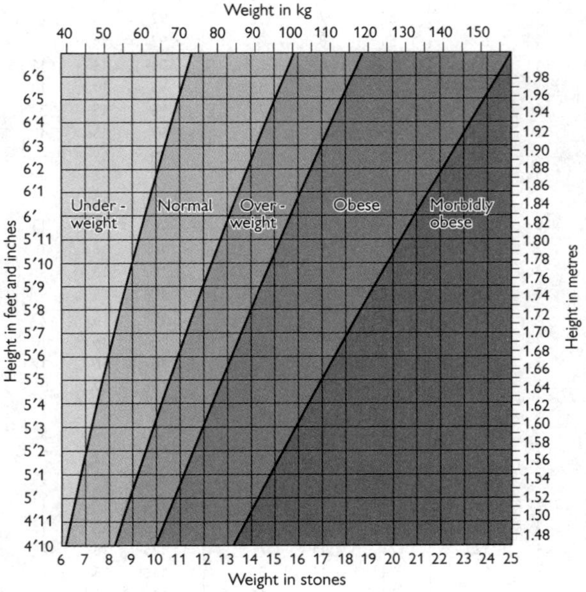

Plotting weight against height estimates BMI.

Boy's head circumference 23wk to 1yr

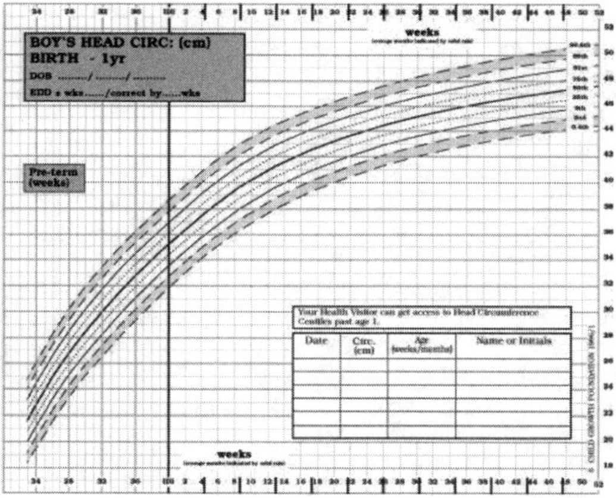

Girl's head circumference 23wk to 1yr

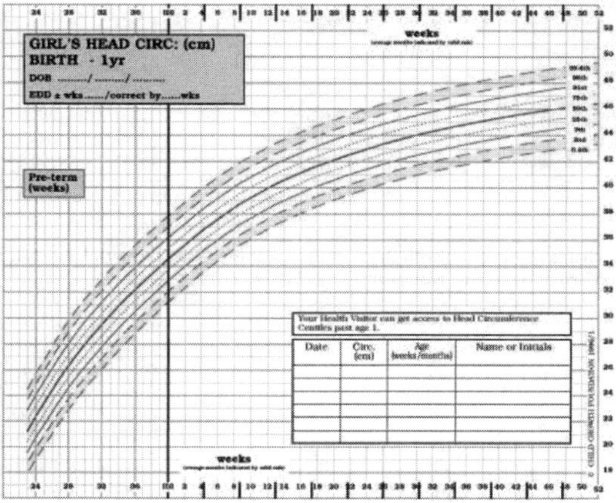

Growth charts reproduced with the permission of the Child Growth Foundation © further information from www.healthforallchildren.co.uk.

Boy's weight 23wk to 1yr

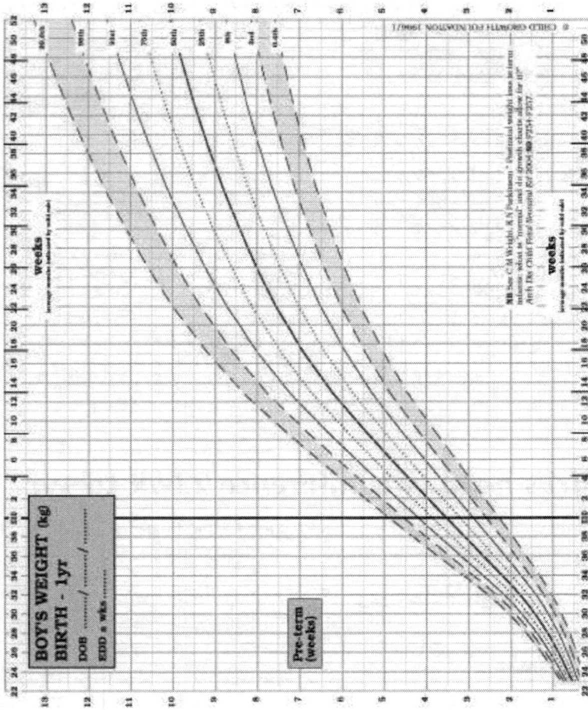

Growth charts reproduced with the permission of the Child Growth Foundation © further information from .www.healthforallchildren.co.uk.

Boy's weight 1yr to 5yr

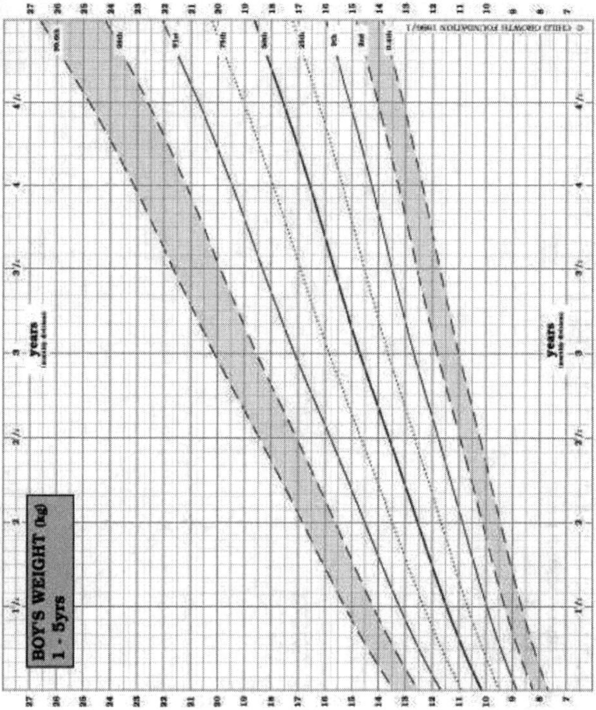

Growth charts reproduced with the permission of the Child Growth Foundation © further information from www. healthforallchildren.co.uk.

Girl's weight 23wk to 1yr

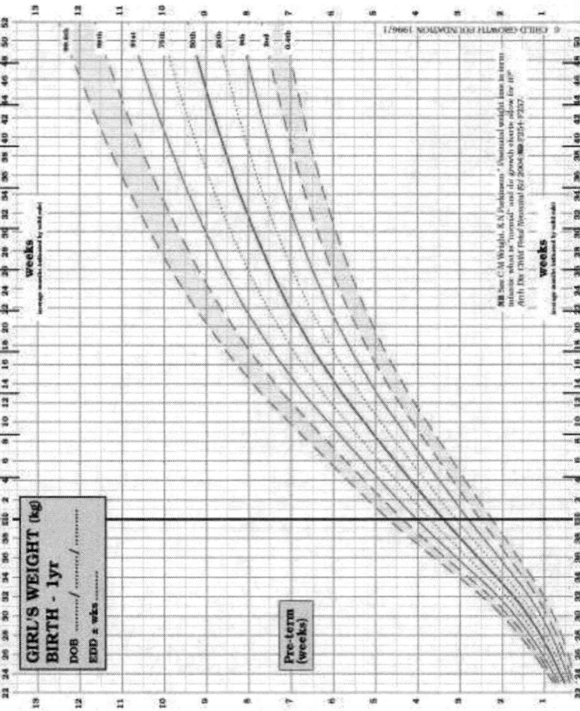

Growth charts reproduced with the permission of the Child Growth Foundation © further information from www. healthforallchildren.co.uk.

Girl's weight 1yr to 5yr

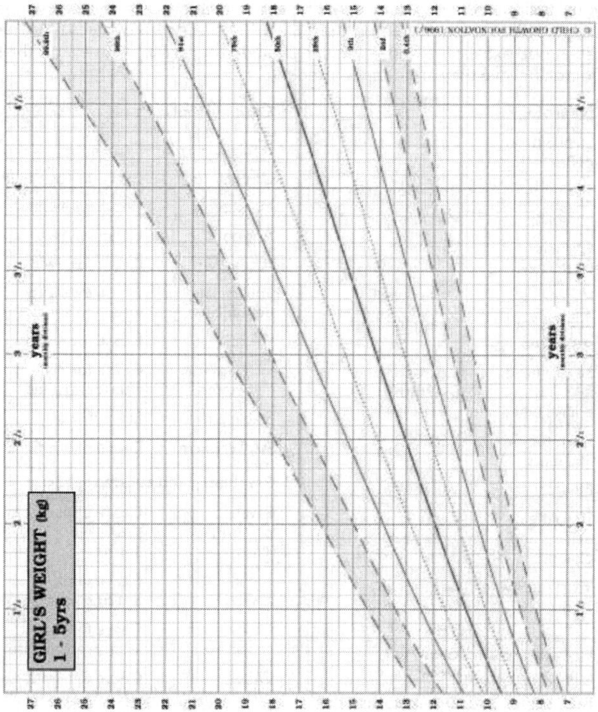

Growth charts reproduced with the permission of the Child Growth Foundation © further information from www. healthforallchildren.co.uk.

Driving regulations

The DVLA issues strict regulations about which medical conditions affect your ability to drive. A summary of this information is shown below, the full guidelines are available on the DVLA website (www.dvla.gov.uk). This list is not exhaustive and a patient should stop driving if they, or their doctor, believe they are incapacitated.

Neurology	
Stroke (mild deficit)	Cease for 1mth
TIA	Cease for 1mth
Disability	**Variable***
Chronic neurology	**Variable***
Meningitis	Drive if well
Seizure (or suspected)	**Cease for 1yr***
Severe head injury/intra-cranial bleed	**Cease for 6–12mth***
Brain tumours and mets	**Variable***
Neurosurgery	**Variable***
Visual field defects and diplopia	Cease driving (may be allowed if stable)
Visual acuity	Better than 6/12 corrected with both eyes
Unexplained syncope	**Cease for 6mth***
Recurrent severe vertigo	**Once attacks controlled***

Diabetes	
Diabetes on insulin or tablets	**Must be able to recognise hypo***
Diabetes on diet only	Drive if well
Recurrent hypoglycaemia	Cease until controlled

Cardiovascular	
Stable angina	Drive if well
Unstable angina	Cease until stabilised
MI/ACS	Cease for 4wk
Angioplasty	Cease for 1wk
Pacemaker	**Cease for 1wk***
Implantable defibrillator	**Cease 6wk after insertion/shock***
CABG	**Cease for 4wk***
Incapacitating arrhythmia	**Cease for 4wk after controlled***
Stable arrhythmia	Drive if well
AAA >6.5cm	**Cease driving***

Psychiatry and substance abuse	
Severe psychiatric illness	**Cease until stable for 3mth***
Alcohol abuse	**Cease until 6–12mth control***
Opioid, benzo + cocaine use	**Cease for 1yr after previous use***
Other recreational drugs	**Cease for 6mth after previous use***

Other	
COPD	Drive if well
Sleep apnoea + narcolepsy	**Cease until symptoms controlled***
Chronic renal failure	Drive if well
HIV	Drive if well

*Patient must notify the DVLA

If a patient refuses to notify the DVLA about a medical condition you have a duty to break confidentiality and inform the DVLA on their behalf.

Interesting cases

Note down any interesting or unusual cases which could be used for a teaching or a Grand Round case presentation.

Hospital number	
Details	

Hospital number	
Details	

Hospital number	
Details	

Hospital number	
Details	

Telephone numbers 1

Hospital:	Telephone:	
	Extension	Bleep
Consultants		
Consultant Secretary		
Registrar-level		
SHO-level		
F1		
Ward		
On-call 'registrar'		
On-call 'SHO'		
On-call F1		
Haematology		
Blood bank		
Clinical chemistry		
Microbiology		
Radiology		
ITU		
Porters		
Pharmacy		

Your firm's timetable 1

Time	Monday	Tuesday	Wednesday	Thursday	Friday

Telephone numbers 2

Hospital:	Telephone:	
	Extension	Bleep
Consultants		
Consultant Secretary		
Registrar-level		
SHO-level		
F1		
Ward		
On-call 'registrar'		
On-call 'SHO'		
On-call F1		
Haematology		
Blood bank		
Clinical chemistry		
Microbiology		
Radiology		
ITU		
Porters		
Pharmacy		

Your firm's timetable 2

Time	Monday	Tuesday	Wednesday	Thursday	Friday

Telephone numbers 3

Hospital:	Telephone:	
	Extension	Bleep
Consultants		
Consultant Secretary		
Registrar-level		
SHO-level		
F1		
Ward		
On-call 'registrar'		
On-call 'SHO'		
On-call F1		
Haematology		
Blood bank		
Clinical chemistry		
Microbiology		
Radiology		
ITU		
Porters		
Pharmacy		

Your firm's timetable 3

Time	Monday	Tuesday	Wednesday	Thursday	Friday

Index

Bold type indicates main references.

D

E

F

G

H

I

J

K

L

M

N

S

T

V

W